Business Basics for Dentists

Business Basics for Dentists

SECOND EDITION

James L. Harrison

University of Louisville
Louisville, KY, USA

David O. Willis

University of Louisville (Retired)
Louisville, KY, USA

Charles K. Thieman

Healthcare Practice Consultants, LLC
Louisville, KY, USA

WILEY Blackwell

Library of Congress Cataloging-in-Publication Data:
Names: Willis, David O., author. | Harrison, James L. (Dentist), author. | Thieman, Charles K., author.
Title: Business basics for dentists / James L. Harrison, David O. Willis, Charles K. Thieman.
Description: Second edition. | Hoboken, NJ : Wiley-Blackwell, 2024. | David O. Willis's name appear first in the previous edition.
Identifiers: LCCN 2023014965 (print) | LCCN 2023014966 (ebook) | ISBN 9781119892854 (paperback) | ISBN 9781119892861 (adobe pdf) | ISBN 9781119892878 (epub)
Subjects: MESH: Practice Management, Dental
Classification: LCC RK58 (print) | LCC RK58 (ebook) | NLM WU 77 | DDC 617.0068–dc23/eng/20230727
LC record available at https://lccn.loc.gov/2023014965
LC ebook record available at https://lccn.loc.gov/2023014966

Cover Design: Wiley
Cover Images: © Aja Koska/Getty Images; NESPIX/Shutterstock

Set in 9.5/12pt STIXTwoText by Straive, Pondicherry, India

SKY10055712_092023

Contents

SECTION 4 DENTAL OFFICE SUCCESS FACTORS

Preface

Surveys of new dental practitioners consistently rate practice management as the area where they were least prepared and found the most problems in practice. Dental schools do an excellent job of preparing graduates to handle dentistry's technical and patient treatment aspects. However, they do a less than excellent job preparing graduates to run a dental practice.

This problem comes from several sources. Most students do not enter dental school with a business background. They have taken scientific-based courses to prepare them for the rigorous dental curriculum and have not taken a business class in their predental curriculum. Many students have never had a dental-related job in the private sector. They depend on the professional mentoring of the faculty to prepare them for the world of dental practice.

Students are concerned with the immediate needs of learning dentistry, completing clinical requirements, and passing licensing exams – and that is where their efforts should go to their most immediate and pressing needs. They cannot run a successful dental practice until they graduate from dental school and earn a dental license.

National boards have tested students on fundamental scientific and clinical knowledge for years, not on how to operate a successful practice. Because many dental schools teach, in part, to prepare their students to pass these boards, curriculum time and faculty efforts are heavily weighted toward preparing students for this important milestone.

The economic environment of dental practice is changing rapidly, and educators have not kept up. In years past, if the new graduate knew dental techniques and treated their patients well, practice success was virtually assured. Today, new practitioners face a bewildering array of insurance plans, consumerism, corporate practices, large student debt payments, and regulatory requirements. In the face of this uncertain future, graduates want additional information to help them compete effectively in the new reality.

This book is primarily for dental students about to graduate, new graduates (in both private practice and other clinical settings), and recent graduates who have been out of school for five years or less. It is not written for well-established dentists who have practiced for 20 years, although they may find pearls to apply in their practices. Instead, the essential business information that new practitioners can apply in their practice situation to compete effectively is presented. It is not intended to be specific management advice for every management problem – readers should consult with accountants, management consultants, or mentors about specific problems – but if the issues can be understood, then the dentist will communicate more effectively with advisors and will understand and implement solutions and advice more effectively.

A dental practice is a small business that responds to business concepts and rules like any other small business. The only difference is that dentists sell dental services, not hardware, clothing, electronics, or automobiles. So it is essential to understand a business principle and then apply it to dental practices. In this way, a practitioner in New York City or Mayfield, Kentucky, can use the same business principle in different-looking practices.

The numbers given as examples or illustrations represent the United States as a whole. Some areas, especially large urban areas, have higher costs and fees than other small towns and rural areas. For example, typical wage rates for hygienists in large urban areas are currently $60 per hour; in many small to mid-sized towns, rates for hygienists are $35 per hour. Likewise, the fees charged are also generally higher in those urban areas. Therefore, the numbers shown may not represent a practice situation exactly, but the business concept behind the example is valid regardless of the practice area.

This book surveys the topics of operating a dental practice. As such, it is only an introduction to each of the topics. For example, although several pages are devoted to the methods of valuing a dental practice, experts have written entire manuals and even entire books on this subject alone. Other excellent texts, websites, and how-to manuals cover this book's topics. For example, the American Dental Association produces an excellent series of books that cover practice transitions, regulatory compliance, and many other management topics in a level of detail that cannot be put into one book. This book is only a starting place for studying management in the office.

This second edition has added more information about career planning. We have found that fewer graduates are directly entering private dental practice. As the practice world moves to more network practices, new graduates find more professional opportunities in those networks. Many use them as a stepping stone to an eventual private situation; others use them as a lifelong career option. Either way, the graduate still needs the information presented here to be a more effective employee.

We intend this book to be a text and a reference book. If the reader is a student, they may be required to read specific chapters to pass a test or course. A practitioner who has a problem with staff interactions in the office may pick up the book and read the chapter on how to motivate employees. Either way, the intention is to understand how business people think about problems and develop specific solutions to management problems. We hope that you find the information helpful in that regard.

JAMES L. HARRISON

DAVID O. WILLIS

CHARLES K. THIEMAN

Career Planning

Career development is becoming more critical for dental graduates in today's economic climate. Many students leave dental school with hundreds of thousands of dollars of student debt. Not only does the graduate need immediate income to make student loan payments, but the significant debt levels may also hinder their ability to secure loans at favorable rates. The increase in corporate and franchise practices provides immediate employment opportunities and increases competition in the local marketplace for start-up practices. Solo practitioners, who face increased competition as well, are often reluctant to take on an associate in the traditional role of owner and mentor. The complex dental insurance world makes practices less profitable than in the past, leading to further cash-flow problems for young practitioners.

Because of these economic constraints, graduates need to plan their career development. In the past, the simple answer was to "set up my practice." The plan may involve working in a corporate practice for several years to increase clinical and management skills or working in a public health setting to gain some student loan relief and build clinical skills. Most graduates still aim to practice ownership (solo or group), but now they must take an often-winding road to reach their goal. This section provides a way to plan a career in clinical dentistry. (In this book, we do not look at opportunities in industry or academia, only the various clinical practice opportunities.)

There are two general categories of income generation for new dentists. First, they can work for someone else (get a job). This option allows immediate income generation, but does not always provide long-term professional security. They can find employment with a private practicing owner-dentist as an associate dentist, with a Dental Management Service Organization (DMSO) as an employee dentist, or with the government through the public health or military systems. The second option is to own all or part of a practice. This option provides long-term security, but is often expensive and risky to establish. Here the graduate can buy an existing practice (buy-out), start a practice from scratch (cold start), or buy into an existing practice (buy-in) in a partnership arrangement. This section of the book examines each of these possibilities.

CONCERNS OF THE CAREER DEVELOPMENT PROCESS

The career planning process is concerned with three major concerns:

- **Establishing short- and long-term career goals**
  Everyone has a personal long-term career goal, and each of us takes a different path to reach those goals. Our short-term goals contribute to achieving our long-term career goals, and personal wants, needs, desires, and circumstances affect our career goals.

- **Understanding the difference between employment and ownership positions**
  Employment and practice ownership are two different concerns, and each has advantages and disadvantages that become decisive factors in career planning.

Business Basics for Dentists, Second Edition. James L. Harrison, David O. Willis, and Charles K. Thieman.
© 2024 John Wiley & Sons, Inc. Published 2024 by John Wiley & Sons, Inc.

- **Planning for career transitions**
  As professionals move through their careers, they must be sure that the transitions from one phase to the next are well planned. Otherwise, they may have made early decisions that either support or decrease the likelihood of making the next step in the plan a success.

OBJECTIVES OF THE CAREER DEVELOPMENT PROCESS

Given these three main concerns, we group the career development process's objectives into this section's major chapters. The issues that dentists should examine in their career planning process include the following:

- **Chapter 1: Career Planning**
  Everyone needs to examine their personal wants, needs, desires, and abilities when developing a comprehensive career plan. They also must make a realistic appraisal of opportunities and roadblocks that affect the process.

- **Chapter 2: Employment Opportunities**
  Many new graduates will enter directly into employment situations, whether in private practice (associateship), corporate, or government situations. To be successful, they must understand the nature of employment and the advantages of each type of employment position. They may use these situations as stepping stones to fulfillment of their long-term goal.

- **Chapter 3: Practice Ownership**
  An ownership position (either solo or in a group) has an entirely different purpose from an employment position. The owner is trying not only to make an income from the practice, but also to build personal wealth by increasing the value of the practice. These are generally "destination"-type opportunities, and most owners plan to be in their practice for their careers.

- **Chapter 4: Practice Transitions**
  Practice transitions involve changing employment or ownership positions, which may include starting a new practice, buying out an existing practice, or buying into an existing one. How a person goes about the process has important implications for financing and planning.

- **Chapter 5: Valuing Practices**
  If someone purchases all or part of a practice, they need to set a value so that they can borrow money to pay for the practice without placing a significant burden on the practice's cash flow. Therefore, the buyer needs to achieve a value that is consistent with business norms and will enable them to pay off the practice acquisition loan promptly.

- **Chapter 6: Securing Financing**
  When someone locates a practice to purchase and has a reasonable value associated with it, they need to find a lender who will lend them the money required for the purchase. Terms may differ for different lenders, and understanding these differences can help borrowers decide and negotiate an advantageous financing package.

Career Planning

CHAPTER 1

Don't confuse having a career with having a life.

Hillary Clinton

GOAL

This chapter aims to describe specific career planning decision points and processes.

LEARNING OBJECTIVES

After the completion of this chapter, the student will be able to:

- Describe the characteristics of dental practice as a career.

- Define professional options available to the new dental graduate.

- Describe career choice points that affect the career path.

- Describe personal and professional factors that affect the location decision.

KEY TERMS

career decision points   career path

Dentists have many professional options to use their skills and training. Some involve ownership, while others are employee situations. In this book, we only discuss practice-related options. The opportunities include:

- Employment
  - Private sector
    - Private associateship (non-owner)
    - Corporate employee (non-owner)
    - Industrial research
    - Corporate support
  - Public sector
    - Military/Veterans Affairs
    - Public health patient care settings
    - Dental education

- Ownership
  - Private solo practice (owner)
  - Private group practice (owner)

Business Basics for Dentists, Second Edition. James L. Harrison, David O. Willis, and Charles K. Thieman.
© 2024 John Wiley & Sons, Inc. Published 2024 by John Wiley & Sons, Inc.

CHARACTERISTICS OF DENTAL PRACTICES

Dental practices are unlike many other service businesses. Most dentists are still in individual practices, with few colleagues with whom to confer. They must personally deliver the service, which involves hard physical work. They cannot delegate most procedures and must be personally present for the procedures that they do delegate. This means there is little managerial leverage, so the dentist cannot play golf while the office operates. There is no managerial progress. Someone cannot work their way up the management line to become a regional manager or vice president. Most new graduates come to the workplace with high educational debt and must include that in their practice debt finance plan. Dentists' earnings typically peak at 45–50 years of age. After that, the physical nature of the work causes them to decrease the number of patient visits. Often dentists then look to add associates or plan to sell their practices. The question is whether to sell at the peak of the income-generating potential (and therefore at the highest price) or to "milk the cow" and take income from the practice as they continue to slow down.

COMMON MYTHS ABOUT DENTISTRY

There are several misconceptions about dentistry that will influence career choices.

DENTISTRY IS EASY MONEY

Many people outside the profession view dentistry as an easy way to make a lot of money. Although dentistry is still one of the more lucrative professions, those in the profession know it is not easy to make money. Dentistry is physically demanding work. Dentists often work long hours in contorted positions to make patients comfortable. Back and neck problems, repetitive motion injuries, and eye strain are common problems of seasoned dental practitioners. Dentistry is also emotionally demanding work. Many patients fear dental procedures or have unrealistic expectations about their desired outcomes. Staff members may have personal problems or interpersonal disagreements that affect the work environment.

A DENTIST MAKES MORE MONEY OWNING A PRACTICE

Dentists *might* make more money if they own their practice. Practice ownership requires knowledge, skills, and abilities that not all dentists have. Additionally,

owner–dentists need to spend time and emotional energy to operate the business side of effective practice. Not all dentists want to do this. Some are excellent clinicians but do not want the extra problems of ownership. They want to treat patients, not worry if the hygienist and assistant have interpersonal problems or fret about the changes in a local employer's dental insurance plan. These dentists are best off working for someone else, letting the owners worry about the management of the practice. They can make more money treating patients if they work with someone good at managing a practice or a network of practices. Someone who is excellent clinically, behaviorally, and managerially and loves all aspects of running a practice can make more money owning it.

BIGGER IS BETTER

Many dentists believe that a bigger practice is better. Personal wants, needs, and desires might lead someone to a smaller, more personal practice better suited to their temperament. A larger practice is not necessarily a more lucrative practice. Profits come from using the practice's resources to the maximum amount possible, regardless of size. A small practice can be as profitable as a large one. However, an extensive, well-run practice does have some advantages if the owner has the managerial expertise to make this larger and more complex business entity use all its resources effectively. A larger practice might show a higher profit if well run. A bigger practice may weather economic downturns more easily. When sold, larger, more profitable practices bring a higher price, although sometimes finding a buyer for these large practices is difficult.

STUDENT DEBT MAKES IT IMPOSSIBLE FOR A DENTIST TO BORROW MONEY TO BUY A PRACTICE

Dental graduates are carrying higher levels of student debt than before. Changes in the student loan programs have made it more difficult to consolidate these loans at low interest rates. Tax law changes have limited the amount of student loan interest graduates can deduct. Nevertheless, dentistry is still one of the higher-income professions. Banks and other lenders who make start-up and buy-out loans to dentists understand these problems. They will work with dentists to develop loan packages if the practice can support the cash flow needed to pay all expenses, including student loans. Not all practices will be profitable enough at a price that can support the cash flow required to make all the payments, however. This can result from the practice price being set too high, high overhead in practice, or the financial characteristics of the potential buyer. A graduate who does not have a high loan burden or who has a spouse who earns a significant income may show cash-flow needs that are much lower. This dentist may qualify to borrow for a practice purchase when someone else would not.

PUBLIC HEALTH IS FOR DENTISTS WHO CANNOT MAKE IT IN PRIVATE PRACTICE

It has become part of the professional culture that "good" dentistry is exquisitely done (expensive) reconstructive dentistry. True, dentists in the public care sector may not do much complex reconstructive dentistry because the organization's purpose is to provide more basic services to a larger clientele. This does not make dentistry or the dentist's application of their hard-earned skills of less quality or less critical. The public sector provides valuable services to a large segment of the population. Many dentists find satisfying and rewarding careers by devoting their skills to this style of practice.

A DENTIST DOES NOT HAVE TO TAKE INSURANCE PLANS IN PRACTICE

If a dentist is in a private ownership position, they make all the management decisions. Long-term, insurance-free practice is the goal of many practitioners. However, most do not get there. It takes a combination of location, clientele, management, clinical expertise, and time to develop a practice that does not participate in dental insurance plans. Someone may take plans in the short term with the aim to wean off them as they build a private clientele. As the economic environment and insurance industry change, more practices find the need to participate in insurance plans.

A DENTIST WILL BE IN THE SAME OFFICE THEIR ENTIRE CAREER

This used to be more accurate than it is today. In the past, the graduate would open or buy a practice and then build it over the years, and they would be in an ownership position immediately after graduation. New graduates today may work in several professional situations before arriving at their final practice setting. With the increasing number of employment opportunities, many dentists never reach an ownership situation, choosing to do clinical work in non-ownership positions for their entire careers. The old notion that private practice is the only good form of dentistry is dying out.

CAREER PATHS

Dentists now talk about career paths in which they have an ultimate, long-term goal but may take several steps to reach it. Short-term goals then support long-term goals. Each step in the short term should support the long-term intention. For example, the traditional path would be to finish dental school, go directly into a pediatric dentistry residency, and then open a practice. A new graduate who has high student debt may take a different career path. In this path, someone may graduate and join a public health practice that offers loan forgiveness. They can build speed and confidence while working with young patients in the clinical setting. They then attend residency and join a group pedodontic practice. Career paths are different for everyone depending on their circumstance. Graduates with an immediate family member who has a career in dentistry or other healthcare profession are at an advantage. They generally have a deeper understanding of a healthcare career and often have a built-in entry into a practice situation. Graduates with a history of working in private industry or government use that knowledge to their advantage.

Each person makes career path decisions based on their situation at the time of the decision. Specific decision points direct and influence decisions. These include the following.

THE DESIRE FOR INCOME

If someone desires a high income (as opposed to an adequate income), then a long-term plan should include a private practice ownership option. Specialist dentists' incomes are higher than generalists'. Short-term options might include associateships or military practice to build skills and knowledge while someone pays down debt and accumulates assets. If a high income does not drive a person's professional needs, other desires can be driving forces.

DEBT LOAD

If a dentist has a small or no student debt at graduation, then they are in the fortunate position of being able to take on debt for a practice purchase or personal needs. Heavy student debt may limit practice options to those showing excellent cash flow. Short term, a graduate might need to practice in an associateship or corporate practice for several years to pay down debt, or find a public health practice that includes loan payment or forgiveness.

THE DESIRE TO BE THE BOSS

Most dental students claim to want to "be their own boss," but when they face the reality of the debt load, managing the business, and the extra time necessary, many decide that the trade-offs are not worth it. Part of the old culture of the profession was that the ultimate form of professional effort was a private individual practice, and that notion has changed. Currently, many corporate and public practices use the entirety of someone's professional skill, care, and expertise without practice ownership. If someone is fiercely independent and wants to make or break it on their skills, then private practice is the place.

THE DESIRE TO LIVE IN DIFFERENT LOCATIONS

Some people enjoy the idea of moving and living in different places. Others know where they want to settle and live the rest of their lives. If someone fits into the first group, then practice ownership is a problem. Practice ownership is a long-term commitment, and it takes many years to fully recover the investment (time and financial) that someone makes when establishing a practice. They may not find a willing buyer for a practice when they want to sell it or have licensing problems in a new location. Network practices, the military, and public health practices are all more conducive to moving to different areas and experiencing different cultures.

THE DESIRE FOR PERSONAL OR FAMILY TIME

Some people love dentistry and would do it 24 hours a day if they could. Others enjoy time away from the office for personal or family activities. Some like to take time every week, while others prefer to take periodic time off for travel or other similar activities. Where a person falls on this continuum is also essential in helping to decide career points. It is not easy to take much time off in an individual ownership position and maintain a high income. Patients want work done, staff members want to get paid, and income stops when the dentist is not there. They can set their hours and take time during the week, but taking many extended blocks is more of a problem. It is easier to take time in a group practice where others can cover for a dentist and share costs. The easiest way to take blocks of time is to work in an employment situation with guaranteed time off (such as military or public health). Often, people in this situation will work more hours during the week but will have the flexibility of blocks of vacation time.

OTHER DECISION POINTS

There are many other career decision points. If someone enjoys doing research, they obviously will be in a situation in industry or academia where they can do this activity, and where someone wants to live influences the path as

well. If a dentist wants to live in a specific rural area, the only option may be private ownership. Some people prefer working in an organization with many other people; some prefer working alone.

LOCATION DECISIONS

Regardless of the specific career option, the dentist's first decision is where they want to live. Several factors contribute to this decision.

PROFESSIONAL FACTORS

The single most important professional factor is the dentist-to-population ratio. This ratio describes the number of dentists to treat a given population in the area. It is an indicator of the potential viability of a dental practice. It is usually expressed as a ratio such as "1 : 2300," which says that there is one dentist for every 2300 people in the service area. There may be a need to modify the ratio because it is a general number. The dentist should check that the ratio represents the area in which they are interested. (The numbers may be for the entire county or part of an urban area.) Moreover, the ratio includes both specialists and generalists. If the dentist is a generalist, they probably want to take the specialists in the area out of the equation. The ratio also includes a simple count of all licensed dentists. This includes retired, part-time, and non-practicing dentists. If the dentist can, they should play with the numbers to arrive at the number of full-time equivalent (FTE) generalists per population. (Someone who practices half-time represents 0.5 FTE dentists.)

Healthy ratios are generally between 1 : 1800 and 1 : 2500. The military has traditionally believed that one dentist can treat 800 soldiers (but the military has 100% utilization). Higher-income areas tolerate lower ratios as people buy more dental services. Rural areas traditionally have a lower utilization rate than urban areas. A ratio of 1 : 2500 or 1 : 3000 may be required in these areas to suggest enough patients. The dentist can get these ratios from the American Dental Association (ADA), which has several publications that summarize economic factors for dentists across the country. In smaller communities, the graduate can get a phone book and talk to people in the area. The dentist can probably develop an accurate ratio with information from the local chamber of commerce.

The number and type of other dentists in the area are deciding factors. The potential practitioner should feel comfortable with the professional community they will work within, the local dental society, and civic organizations. They should also be sure there are adequate specialists for referral and consider staff availability. A new practitioner may need to train staff, or there may be training programs nearby.

PERSONAL FACTORS

Personal desires are probably the most important practice location decision. The dentist should decide where they want to live and move there. If they are not personally satisfied, then even excellent professional opportunities will not compensate for their lack of personal fulfillment. The dental practitioner should also consider their aspirations, career, and life plans. They should decide their preferred lifestyle. Each person has preferences for climate, culture, and recreational opportunities. Some want a rural lifestyle where hunting, fishing, and hiking opportunities abound. Others would not live anywhere that does not have an entire arts community and excellent country clubs. Everyone must reconcile their preferred practice pattern with their preferred personal style. They may want a crown and bridge–style practice but prefer a remote rural location. The two might not be compatible. Therefore, everyone must be realistic in their assessments.

The next most significant factor in dentists' general location decisions is spouse and family desires. Where someone wants to go is only part of the lifestyle decision, and if they are married the spouse is generally involved in the decision process. A professional or working spouse needs personal growth opportunities as much as the dentist does.

ECONOMIC FACTORS

Once someone has decided on one or several general areas to live in, they should then look at the area's economy. As a service provider, a dentist depends on other businesses to provide employment so that people have money and insurance to afford dental care.

The dentist should examine the economic base of the area. They should find out the sources of income for people in the area. Primary industries, such as mining, farming, and manufacturing, bring money into the local economy. (Each primary industrial dollar circulates eight times in a local economy before dissipating.) From there, the money flows to the secondary industries that support the primary industries, such as construction and retail stores. Tertiary industries, such as dentistry, provide services to the employees of other industries. The dentist should look for broad-based primary industries in the selected location. Several industries in a town provide a strong economy. The dentist should be prepared for a boom-and-bust economy if the area has a single primary

industry (such as one large manufacturing plant or a mining-based economy). Everyone has money when the mines (or other primary industries) are busy. If the mines shut down, miners do not buy shoes or build houses, and construction workers and sales people do not go to the dentist. In contrast, a well-diversified primary industrial base can absorb an individual sector shutdown without leading to a general economic collapse.

Several indicators help to gauge the economic health of a community. Most patients consider dental care a deferrable expense rather than a medical necessity. As such, it is highly dependent on disposable income. (Disposable, or discretionary, income is what is left over after people have paid for necessities, such as food, housing, and clothing.) Higher disposable incomes generally mean a better dental economic location. Economic growth in an area means that people's incomes are growing and more people are moving into the area. These people will need a dentist. High-growth areas are also good locations. Some areas have a high turnover rate (people move frequently), while others are more stable. It is easier to establish a practice in an area with a high turnover than to break into a stable area where most people already have a dental provider. However, in the high turnover area, the practitioner will need to continually grow the practice as patients they previously attracted leave through the revolving door.

There are many places to find this information. A call to the local chamber of commerce is an excellent place to start. The chamber's job is to encourage commerce in the area. They already have much information about the potential town. Census data is helpful for comparisons. The problem with census data is that it is usually old by the time a person can get to it. Many states have state data banks that the dentist can call to find the information needed. Additionally, much of this information is readily available on the Internet.

PROFESSIONAL HISTORY

The dentist's professional history may limit their options or allow a particular option to be realistic.

DEBT LOAD

A person's debt load (especially student debt) influences whether an option is acceptable. Bankers have regulators and overseeing committees they must satisfy. If the dentist has so much debt that they are at risk of not being able to make the regular payments on some of their loans, the bank may not loan additional money for a practice.

PRODUCTION HISTORY

The practitioner must show that they can handle the volume of a practice that leads to adequate profit and cash flow. If someone is looking at a practice that needs to generate $900 000 annually to meet projections, the practitioner must show that they can do that much dentistry. Suppose they had previously been an associate generating $800 000 annually or in an Advanced Education in General Dentistry (AEGD) or military practice where they generated significant production. In that case, a lender could infer that they could reasonably handle the practice, but not so with a new graduate who was busy treating two patients daily.

PRACTICE CHARACTERISTICS

The characteristics of the practice the dentist is considering establishing or purchasing influence the viability of the option. If a practice has a large contingent of discounted insurance plan patients, the dentist will have to produce even higher amounts of dentistry to see adequate cash flow through the practice. Lower levels of discounted insurance participation lead to higher margins, but less dentistry is being done. In these practice opportunities, the dentist must have a marketing plan to generate the private-pay patients required for profitability.

CASH-FLOW PROJECTIONS

These factors all come together in the cash-flow projection. Suppose the practitioner can show through a realistic cash-flow projection that they can service the practice debt, generate an income to live on (including personal debt payments), and pay taxes. In that case, the practice option is viable, and if not, then it is not a viable option at this point.

CAREER PLANNING PATHWAYS

Given these decision factors, we provide the career pathway flowchart in Figure 1.1 as a helpful way to think about career paths. We discuss each option in more detail in later chapters of this section.

The first and most crucial task for any dental student is to finish dental school. Until a person does this, no other career decision has any meaning. That is not to say that they should wait until graduation to begin making these plans. Some dental students cannot see that there is a life after dental school with no fixed curriculum, where everyone makes the same choices. For these reasons, we discuss making decisions after graduation, but not waiting until after graduation to make the decisions.

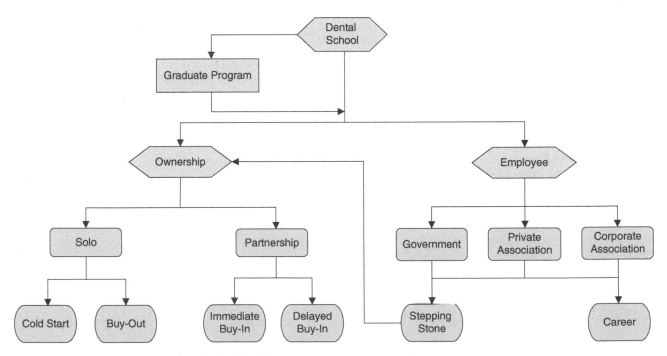

FIGURE 1.1   Career pathway flowchart for dental graduates.

GRADUATE TRAINING

The initial decision point after graduation is whether to pursue graduate training or move directly to a practice option. Graduate training may take the form of additional general training or specialty training. Regardless, this only delays the career decision for several years.

Advanced Training in General Dentistry

There are two options for general dentistry training after dental school: AEGD and general practice residencies (GPRs). AEGD programs focus primarily on dental treatment. They generally occur in a dental school environment and are the halfway point between dental students and practicing dentists. If someone feels they need time to become a more competent technical dentist before going into practice, an AEGD may benefit them. AEGDs usually do not require participants to be on call, and the dentist will not get the same level of medical/hospital experience as they might in a GPR. GPR programs are frequently held in medical facilities. These programs concentrate on dentistry as it relates to whole-body medicine. As such, participating dentists are included in medical rotations, sometimes functioning almost as overflow physicians at some time in the program. Like being a physician, most require participants to have on-call shifts. Because GPRs do not focus exclusively on dentistry, participants gain a wide variety of exposure and experiences. These experiences are beneficial for those considering oral surgery and emergency care specialties.

Specialty Training

A dental specialty is an area of dentistry that the ADA has formally recognized through its National Commission on Recognition of Dental Specialties. Currently, there are 12 dental specialties recognized by the National Commission. This commission sets standards for recognition and policy guidelines for its Boards and Organizations. They all require the completion of an advanced education program. These are:

- Dental Public Health
- Endodontics
- Oral and Maxillofacial Pathology
- Oral and Maxillofacial Radiology
- Oral and Maxillofacial Surgery
- Orthodontics and Dentofacial Orthopedics
- Pediatric Dentistry
- Periodontics
- Prosthodontics
- Dental Anesthesiology
- Oral Medicine
- Orofacial Pain

The graduate needs to research the specialty they are considering. Dental specialties have associations where professionals can meet, network, and discuss their work. If someone is interested in a dental specialty, there are few better places to look than the corresponding professional association. They should spend time shadowing and talking to mentors about the specialty to ensure it fits their desires and interests. This can also give insight into the daily life of a specialist. Internships/externships are usually done in an academic or hospital setting. This offers insight into a typical day in residency and often goes more in depth into the different treatments and procedures.

Graduates should consider the economic effect the delay will have on starting their careers. Most specialty programs do not pay residents, and most practitioners must pay tuition to attend. (Hospital-based residencies, such as a GPR or oral and maxillofacial surgery, generally pay a modest stipend.) So, income will be lost for two to four years while the graduate completes the program. However, this may be offset by the higher income levels many specialty practitioners earn.

EMPLOYEE OR OWNER POSITION

The next central decision point is whether to become an immediate owner of a practice or to work as an employee, long or short term. This may be a decision that is made for the graduate. As already described, there may not be a purchase opportunity, or the graduate may not be in a financial or experience position to own a practice. Many graduates use employment (government, private, or corporate) as a stepping stone, building clinical and managerial skills while paying down debt and building financial assets. After several years, they may be in a better financial position and purchase a whole or part interest in a practice. Others may use the employment situation as a career option. When someone is in an ownership position, they may loop back to an employee situation by selling their practice, often to a corporate entity, and working for that corporation.

Employment Opportunities

CHAPTER 2

A *man's got to know his limitations*.

Harry Callahan, *Magnum Force*

GOAL

The goal of this chapter is to describe common issues in employment situations for dentists.

LEARNING OBJECTIVES

At the completion of this chapter, the student will be able to:

- Describe standard methods of compensation for dentists.

- Describe standard associate-owner arrangements in dentistry.

- Differentiate between an employee and an independent contractor.

- Describe the advantages and disadvantages of working as an associate in private practice.

- Describe the advantages and disadvantages of working for a corporate practice.

KEY TERMS

arbitration
associateship
associateship contract
BSA (business service agreement)
buy or sell provision
career benefits
claims-made policy
commission
DGP (dental group practice)
direct pay
dispute resolution
DMSO (dental management service organization)

draw against future earnings
employee benefits
employee dentist
employee insurances
employee status
employment contract
government employment
incidents of ownership
independent contractor
mediation
military
non-competition agreement
non-disclosure agreement

non-solicitation provision
paid time off
percentage of collections
percentage of production
public health
restrictive covenant
salary
tail coverage
termination for cause
total compensation
variable commission
wage

Business Basics for Dentists, Second Edition. James L. Harrison, David O. Willis, and Charles K. Thieman.
© 2024 John Wiley & Sons, Inc. Published 2024 by John Wiley & Sons, Inc.

Many new dental graduates take employment positions initially out of dental school. This may be to hone clinical skills, pay down debt or build assets, improve practice management knowledge, or because they do not want the involvement of practice ownership. Regardless of the reason, the critical point about employment is that the dentist is there to make money for the employer, whether a private practitioner, network practice, or governmental organization. If the dentist does not make money for the employer, they will not be there long. The dentist should understand that employee positions are not about them but about the organization. The dentist is valuable so long as they contribute to what the organization does.

GOVERNMENT EMPLOYMENT

MILITARY

One option for employment is to become a dentist in the Armed Forces. The US Army, Navy, and Air Force all recruit dentists to serve as commissioned officers in their Dental Corps. Both active duty and reserve components recruit dentists with a US dental degree and a license to practice dentistry. Students may also be eligible for special programs covering tuition and providing a monthly wage while in dental school. Graduates will serve in the military as dentists for a set time, depending on the program.

Dental Corps members are responsible for the dental health of military personnel and their family members. Many dentists are stationed stateside in the medical clinics of military bases, and others are assigned tours of duty at US military bases worldwide. Responsibilities may include the emergency medical treatment of service members in deployed places near combat or participating in humanitarian missions in the United States and overseas.

As a military member, a dentist will be eligible for all the benefits and privileges that any other service member enjoys (Box 2.1). Military dentists work at modern dental facilities, use modern technology, spend quality time with patients, and maintain a flexible schedule. Additional bonuses and retention incentives are available to dentists.

The Health Professions Scholarship Program (HPSP) is a program that a dental student can apply for that will pay for three years at an American Dental Association–accredited program (DMD/DDS). This scholarship covers tuition, books, equipment, supplies, and a monthly stipend (income). Since the military pays for schooling, it requires a minimum four-year commitment to military service upon graduation.

| BOX 2.1 | CURRENT EMPLOYEE BENEFITS OF MILITARY DENTISTS |

- Medical, dental, and life insurance
- Substantial retirement plans
- Housing allowances
- 30 days paid vacation each year
- Signing bonus
- Health professions loan repayment
- Special pay incentives
- Advanced training opportunities
- Dental officer retention bonus

The military reserve Dental Corps employs dentists in the armed services. Some reservists are former active-duty service members, and others have only served in the reserve Corps. There are several scholarship and loan forgiveness programs for Corps participants. Reservists can maintain active employment in the civilian world, using the reserves as part-time employment. The reserve dentist should remember that they can be called to active duty at any time and with very short notice. This might be a problem, especially for a dentist who owns a solo private practice.

PUBLIC HEALTH

The uniformed dental officers of the United States Public Health Service Commissioned Corps serve in the Indian Health Service, the United States Coast Guard, the Federal Bureau of Prisons, and the National Health Service Corps. The Commissioned Corps is governed by the Surgeon General and falls under the Department of Health and Human Services rather than the Department of Defense. Even though the Commissioned Corps is not an armed service, officers may be called to assist in public health response to man-made and natural disasters. Officers enjoy the same benefits as their military counterparts.

The Health Resources and Service Administration (HRSA) operates Federally Qualified Health Centers in many areas of the United States. These are community-based healthcare providers that offer primary care services in underserved areas, both urban and rural. Examples of Federally Qualified Health Centers include Community

Health Centers, Migrant Health Centers, Health Care for the Homeless, and Health Centers for Residents of Public Housing. There are strict guidelines they must follow to qualify as a health center. Many include dentistry in their services and have loan repayment and scholarship programs for participants through the National Health Service Corps (NHSC).

Some state and local governments provide dental services for their citizens. They often target these programs at specific high-need groups, such as homeless populations or underserved geographic areas. There is tremendous variation in the expectations and compensation in these programs. Some of these employment opportunities for dentists are full-time, while others rely on part-time area practitioners. Some offer full benefit packages; others use independent contact dentists. Many new practitioners use these opportunities to supplement their income as they build a practice.

PRIVATE PRACTICE/ASSOCIATE ARRANGEMENTS

An associateship occurs when one dentist (generally a junior dentist) works for another dentist (generally the senior dentist) who owns the practice. The essential characteristic of this arrangement is that the practitioners are not equal. One controls the workplace or the work of the other. The owner–dentist may take any form of business (proprietorship, partnership, LLC, or corporation). The non-owner dentist may have one of two types of status. They may be an employee of the practice or have an independent practice within the owner–dentist's practice (independent contractor arrangement).

Many associateships are part-time. The owner–dentist knows they have more patients than they can see, but they do not have enough patients to keep two dentists fully busy. In these cases, the new dentist often works in a second associateship or salaried position when they are not at the primary office. They must ensure they do not violate restrictive covenants or other agreements in the primary office.

There are several common scenarios of owner–dentists seeking associates. Regardless of the specific scenario, the best associateships are where the owner can provide an adequate patient pool to keep the employee busy.

- **The owner–dentist has many "extra" patients and office capacity (space and staff)**
  This scenario is the best for both parties. The owner–dentist can refer new patients to the associate. The office has unused capacity, so the associate adds few additional costs.

- **The owner–dentist has one or more unused operatory for the associate**
  The key to this scenario succeeding is an adequate patient base for the owner to share with the new associate. That means the owner–dentist must be as busy as they want, with excess patient flow.

- **The owner–dentist is not busy and wants the associate to help share costs**
  This common situation leads to many problems, often resulting in the two practitioners competing against each other for the patient base. If the owner–dentist is not busy, they need to increase their patient base through marketing or other methods rather than trying to decrease costs through engaging an associate.

- **The associate can use the office when the owner is not there**
  This scenario works for the new dentist to build a patient base, and it works well if the new dentist wants to continue to work the "off" hours (evenings and weekends). Once the new dentist establishes a patient base, then they look for a new office (or establish an office) to work more reasonable hours. The owner–dentist often provides space and materials, and the associate generally provides staff.

- **The owner has a second office for the new dentist to work in**
  The owner may have established or purchased an office in a nearby location or town. They want someone to work the practice, often with potential buy-in opportunities. There is not much mentoring in these situations; each dentist (owner and employee) is busy working in their respective offices. These are usually good opportunities to do a large volume of dentistry under the management tutelage of a senior dentist.

- **The owner provides primary care or managed care patients for the associate**
  In some associateships, the owner–dentist gives the associate all the excess discounted insurance patients or assigns the associate to do all the primary care, with the owner doing the advanced (and costly) complex restorative care. The only way these scenarios work is if the owner pays a salary to the associate. If the associate's compensation is based on production or collections, they may find insufficient profit in these situations to adequately fund the associate's lifestyle.

OWNERSHIP

A true associateship arrangement involves a senior owner–dentist and an employee dentist. This can take one of two forms.

Employer/Employee

One form of associateship is the pure employer–employee relationship, in which the associate is a professional employee of the practice (proprietorship, partnership, LLC, or corporate). As an employee, the associate participates in office benefit plans like other employees. The practice withholds income taxes and matches Social Security taxes the same as other employees. The owner is in clear control of the situation. A restrictive covenant (covenant not to compete) is common in employee situations. (Note: the effectiveness of these restrictive covenants varies by state.)

Independent Contractor

The second type of relationship is called an "independent contractor." In this arrangement, the associate dentist contracts independently for the owner–dentist. Several advantages exist for the owner–dentist in this arrangement. Because the associate is independently employed, they are a proprietorship and file their own Schedule C. The owner does not pay matching Federal Income Contributions Act (FICA) tax and pays no unemployment tax on the associate. The owner does not withhold income taxes. Instead, the associate estimates and files quarterly like any other proprietorship. The associate does not participate in any office retirement plan or benefit plans offered to other employees. The downside for the owner–dentist is that a restrictive covenant is virtually non-enforceable in an independent contractor arrangement. By definition, if the associate is *independent,* they can work for any dentist (or for themselves) where and when they see fit. If the associate leaves the practice, they are ethically and legally obligated to inform patients so that the patients can receive continued care. Otherwise, this may put the associate in the position of being forced to abandon the patient. (The owner can have a non-solicitation clause for employees and patients not under the care of the associate.)

Many owner–dentists want to have the best of both situations. They want to avoid the tax consequences of the additional employee, but they also want the advantage of a restrictive covenant; they need to choose one or the other. The Internal Revenue Service (IRS) has several guidelines for determining whether a relationship is

BOX 2.2	CHARACTERISTICS OF AN INDEPENDENT CONTRACTOR

- Worker personally delivers the service
- There is a continued (ongoing) relationship
- Worker must work on employer's premises
- Worker uses employer's equipment or materials
- Owner controls employees (hiring, firing, and paying)
- Worker cannot work at other locations
- Worker cannot suffer a loss

an employee–employer or independent contractor relationship. Box 2.2 shows that most dental associateships are employer–employee relationships, and the only true independent contractor relationships are space- and time-sharing arrangements.

COSTS

Most associateship arrangements result in increased costs for the owner. The owner must hire additional clinical assisting staff for the employee practitioner. The number of front office staff often needs to expand significantly if they offset hours so that the junior dentist is in the office for hours when the owner is not. Office space may even need to increase. The new dentist is usually not as productive as the owner–dentist, leading to decreased relative revenues. Often the owner–dentist spends time with the new dentist that they formerly spent seeing patients, decreasing income further. For all these reasons, associateships typically lead to decreased income for the owner–dentist for the first year. By the second year, however, the younger dentist's production should increase and cash flow should improve enough that the owner–dentist can see some profit from the arrangement.

The practice typically pays costs for the associate with a couple of exceptions. (This varies by geographic area.) Before applying the percentage, the owner generally deducts the lab bill and extraordinary costs (such as implant parts) from the production (or collection) amount. This results in sharing these costs on a percentage equal to the percentage income split. (Box 2.3 gives an example of lab bill allocation.) Direct professional costs (such as malpractice insurance and continuing education expenses) are paid by either owner or associate, and the owner usually pays other costs (supplies, staff, etc.).

BOX 2.3	EXAMPLE ASSOCIATESHIP FINANCIAL ARRANGEMENT

	Associate pays (1)		Owner pays (2)		Split, off the top (3)	
	Associate	Owner	Associate	Owner	Associate	Owner
Fee		$1000		$1000		$1000
Lab (3)						$200
						$800
Split	$350	$650	$350	$650	$280	$520
Overhead costs		$300		$300		$300
Lab (1, 2)	$200			$200		
Net	$150	$350	$350	$150	$280	$220

Assumptions: $1000 procedure, $200 lab bill, 65/35 split, and $300 overhead costs.
There are three scenarios:

1. Associate pays the lab bill after the split.
2. Owner pays the lab bill after the split.
3. The lab bill is subtracted from the gross ("off the top") before the split.

ADVANTAGES

There are many advantages to associateships for both the owner and junior dentist. The associateship can act as a trial period before a partnership or buy-in. This gives both sides a chance to decide if they are compatible enough to establish a long-term professional relationship. The junior dentist invests a minimum amount of money. These people often have high educational debt loads and probably cannot borrow enough money for a practice purchase or start-up. If they require expansion, the owner–dentist has the financial resources to afford it. There should be few ego conflicts since there is a delineated hierarchy. Associateships should be excellent learning opportunities. The senior dentist can learn new techniques and materials from the new graduate. The associate learns practice management, patient interaction skills, and clinical efficiency in practice. Due to economies of scale, the now larger practice may afford equipment and personnel that would not be profitable or feasible in a smaller practice. If the associateship leads to buy-in or buy-out, the owner sells, and the associate buys the practice at the peak of its income-generating potential.

DISADVANTAGES

Associateships have no incidents of ownership for the associate. It is a job, pure and simple, not a co-ownership arrangement. Associates often believe they have "helped build the practice," increasing its value through their efforts. They believe the owner should give them some consideration in compensation or a buy-in valuation. On the other side, owners contend that they have paid a good wage for the associate's work. The associate has no more claim on the increased value of the practice than does a hygienist or assistant. This conundrum has led to more than one associate buy-in offer failing to complete. The answer lies in communication and openness from the beginning.

Associateships face many of the same difficulties as other group practices. With more than one dentist in the office, staff can become disoriented, unsure who to go to for what problem. There are more management problems for the owner because the practice is now larger. These occur in accounting, staffing, and scheduling issues. Often owners see a drop in income for the first year of an associateship. This is due to increased expenses, the extra time required to help the associate (fewer patients seen), and a possible decrease in the patient pool as they share the patient pool with the associate.

Most associateships (80–90%) end without forming a partnership. When they end, many associates find that a restrictive covenant they signed as part of the employment agreement excludes them from a particular area. An associate should be sure that if they cannot live by the restrictive covenant, they do not sign it. (This may mean that they do not begin the associateship.) This problem is especially acute in associateships that have lasted for several years.

When there is no real buy-in, the restrictive covenant forces the associate to uproot from the area, though they have established ties in the community and want to stay.

WORKING FOR CORPORATE NETWORK PRACTICES

Rather than have one practice with 50 dental practitioners, networks of practices may have 50 locations, each with one practitioner. In these, the owners attempt to gain the savings of large groups but retain the intimate nature of the individual practice. There are two common forms of organization. One is a dental group practice (DGP), where non-dentists own the practices. The other is a dental management service organization (DMSO), in which the parent company owns most of the practice's assets and provides support services under a strict contract. State laws regarding ownership of professional practices play a large part in which form is common in each state.

Corporate networks claim to be more efficient than individual practitioners. Much of this comes from their size, which allows them to negotiate volume discounts that the small, individual practitioner cannot. The networks negotiate lower costs (volume discounts) for dental supplies and office products. They often establish a corporate laboratory or negotiate volume discounts with existing dental labs. Their knowledgeable background ensures they negotiate favorable leases and find better locations for new practices. They develop competitive staff compensation packages that are market driven but not too generous. The parent company can also negotiate higher reimbursement from third-party carriers (insurers). If they control a large share of the dental marketplace, they may threaten to leave the insurer's network of providers if they do not increase reimbursements for their practices.

OWNERSHIP

A common form of ownership is a DGP in which the parent organization owns the individual practices directly. Here, the dentist is an employee of the parent corporation. The parent corporation (DGP) compensates the individual dentist for the dentistry that they do. Supply and demand determine the pay scale. The DGP pays what it must pay to get enough skilled dental providers. Often the parent will provide significant employee benefits as part of the total compensation package. Some DGPs allow more senior dentists to buy an ownership interest in the parent through employee stock ownership programs (ESOPs) or other forms of ownership involvement. They often offer these through a retirement plan or bonus options. Some DGPs

have a co-ownership arrangement with the individual practitioner. The parent organization may own a controlling portion (say 51%) of the practice and the practitioner may own the remainder. When the practitioner leaves or retires, there is a ready buyer for the practice.

A DMSO is an arrangement common in states requiring dentists to own dental practices. Here, the parent company owns most of the tangible assets of the practice (e.g. dental equipment and the building). Depending on state law, the dentist continues to own the intangible assets. The DMSO then has a contract (business service agreement, BSA) with the dentist or professional corporation to provide management and other services for the dental practice. These services often include purchasing or leasing office space and equipment, scheduling, billing patients, filing insurance claims, hiring employees, marketing the practice, and managing bank accounts for the practice. The Professional Corporation (PC) owns the patient records and provides all professionally licensed services (i.e. patient care as defined in the practice of dentistry in each individual state). The PCs often must be owned by a licensed dentist or a dentist licensed in that state. The contracts often have strict buy-out and restrictive covenants that make it difficult and expensive for the dentist to leave the practice and compete directly with the former DMSO. These arrangements vary by state depending on the individual state's laws.

The ownership structures can get quite complex, and several investors can own the DMSO. The investors can be internal, usually founding owners. They might be investors from the outside – generally from private equity groups. The investor with the greatest percentage of equity or stock ownership owns the majority control of the DMSO. The minority investors have input into the company's operation, but the controlling interest determines the final say/control. Most private equity investments in DSOs are majority ownership, although some DSOs are funded by private equity investment taking a minority position. Many evolving DMSOs are founder owned. However, growth and the need for capital to fund it lead to outside investment and the help of a private equity relationship.

COMPENSATION

Dentists often earn a percentage of production or collections in corporate network arrangements. If production is the basis of compensation, then net production (production minus adjustments) is often used, especially in areas where a large portion of the dental market includes managed care (reduced payment) plans. Supply and demand in the area determine the specific percentage. The parent company often offers employee benefits (such as health insurance, paid vacation, or retirement plan contributions) that add to the total compensation value – a typical percentage of compensation runs at 25–35%, with employee benefits added to this. Because there is no ownership interest for the provider, the difference between this and the office profit ratio (typically 40%) is income to the parent company. The parent company deducts corporate costs (administrative, training, etc.) from this to calculate corporate profit. The cost of doing the dentistry (i.e. hiring dental practitioners) is a cost of doing business for the parent company. It is income for the individual practitioner. Some companies offer bonus plans based on set production amounts that give the associate dentist a more significant percentage compensation on these production or collection amounts. Other companies offer bonus plans that allow practitioners to split a percentage of the profits after all expenses are paid, including provider pay and parent company fees. In multiple practitioner practices, the percentage is based on the percentage of production that each practitioner brings into the practice.

OWNERSHIP OPPORTUNITIES

Many DMSOs allow dentists to own stock at the DMSO level. This encourages a partner through the growth and value of the DMSO. The ownership levels and stock distribution vary from one organization to the next. However, the goals of these structures are similar – to enhance ownership/partnership engagement, better align interests with the dentist and with the growth of the business beyond their practice, and enhance retention of the dentist in the organization long term.

Advantages

There are advantages over practice ownership to both new and experienced practitioners for working in a corporate network. The practitioner does not invest, nor is there a long-term commitment to the practice location. The arrangement can be a good learning experience if the parent company values clinical and management training for practitioners. The practitioner has an immediate "paycheck" without worrying about debt repayment or cash flow. A practitioner might make a higher income than in a privately owned practice because the parent company uses its management systems and expertise to manage the practice. The dentist spends time seeing patients, which helps to generate additional income. There is less of an emotional and time commitment for the practitioner. If the hygienist quits, the parent company will find temporary coverage and hire a replacement. The dentist's free time is for personal use, without worrying about the practice's

business. Dentists can often move within the network's practices without losing income or benefits.

Disadvantages

There are also disadvantages (when compared to practice ownership) to working in a corporate network. First, it is a job; the owning parent company is the boss. Many dentists enter the profession to enjoy self-reliant independence, which does not occur in this practice form. Often the practitioner will work more hours and work the less-desirable weekend or evening off-hours than in an established private practice. If a dentist wants to leave the network, a restrictive covenant may severely limit their practice opportunities. The dentist has no ownership interest, therefore no equity build-up. The dentist has no practice (asset) to sell at retirement or leaving. A corporate opportunity may not be available where and when the practitioner wants. Suppose the dentist is managerially, clinically, and behaviorally competent. In that case, they can make a higher income in an ownership situation because they gain the value of ownership (both profit and equity build-up). Finally, the parent company may fail or be bought by another management company with a different philosophy.

METHODS OF EMPLOYEE COMPENSATION

Total compensation includes more than the base pay, although that is the most obvious and essential point most people use as a determinant. However, when an employee calculates their total compensation, they need to think of how they are better off financially and personally from the employment. They may prefer a lower base pay if it is paired with needed employee benefits. Here, we look at all the forms of compensation that an employee might encounter.

DIRECT PAY

There are many direct pay formulas, each with advantages and disadvantages for the employer and employee. Most involve some variation of a salary or per diem (daily rate), a wage (hourly rate), or a commission (percentage of collections or production). Each has advantages and disadvantages, but any system should provide profit and incentives for both sides (Box 2.4). These formulas only discuss direct monetary compensation, and employee benefit plans may significantly increase total compensation.

Direct pay is the cash (check, direct deposit) the employee receives for doing the work for which they are hired. Government taxes and requirements reduce direct pay. For example, the federal government requires that employers withhold an estimate of what they will pay at

- Allow reasonable profit for the owner.
- Allow reasonable compensation for the employee.
- Provide incentives for the employee to produce.
- Provide incentives for the employee to collect.
- Provide incentives for both to be efficient.
- Be fair to both.

year-end in federal income taxes from their employee's regular paychecks. (This required amount is based on IRS tables.) The employer must also withhold a certain amount from employees for Social Security and Medicare taxes. The employer must send this withheld money to the government (with the employee's name attached). At the end of the year, the employee determines the amount of tax owed and then compares this to the amount withheld along the way. If too much was withheld, they get a refund. If too little is withheld, they owe an additional tax payment. Many state and local governments have similar withholding systems that employers must follow. Owners also reduce pay based on the benefits package that they offer. For example, the employer may have a retirement plan in which it matches an amount that it withhold from an employee's pay. Alternatively, it may partially fund a medical insurance plan. (Generally, the amounts an employer withholds for these benefit plans are not taxable income for the employee.)

Several types of direct payments are common in dentistry. They include the following.

Salary

A salary is a negotiated amount that the employer pays, regardless of how much work the employee does. The salary may be based on a weekly or daily (per diem) amount. Salaries are manageable from a bookkeeping sense. Salaries provide a known budgeting amount for both the owner and the employee. This provides substantial financial security for the employee. There is no problem allocating or dividing accounts receivable in case of a break-up because all the accounts are the owner's. The owner does not pay the employee based on the accounts. However, salaries provide no incentive for the employee to produce or collect. Employees soon realize that their remuneration will be the same if they see 2 or 20 patients daily. The owner takes a risk that the employee–dentist may cost more than they produce, leading to a financial loss for the employer. This loss may be from employee abilities, inadequate patient base, excessive insurance plan adjustments, or unrealistic expectations of the parties involved.

Wage

A wage is like a salary; it is based on the number of hours the employee works. This limits, to a degree, the loss that an employer might suffer if there are inadequate patients; then, the employer can limit the employee's hours (and therefore compensation). This transfers some financial risk from the employer to the employee.

Percentage of Production

Many employers base compensation on a percentage of production. This may be gross production (the total dollar value of the dentistry done) or net production (the value of the dentistry less any required insurance plan adjustments). Most practices use net production as the basis for compensation.

This method has the advantage of quick cash flow (and therefore more security) for the employee. It induces the employee to produce because this directly ties compensation to the amount of dentistry they do. Because the employee has no control over the credit and collection policies of the office, this method adds fairness in that they are not held accountable for collection failures. Some owners who base compensation on this method lower the percentage paid to consider the uncollectible amounts or charge back to the associate when they write off the bad account. There is no problem with accounts receivable if there is a breakup because the employee–dentist has already been compensated for production.

Percentage of Collections

Another standard compensation method involves paying the employee a percentage of the amounts collected from what the employee produced. Many established private dentists like this method because it resembles the problems of collection and cash flow faced by the established practitioner. This method also provides an obvious incentive for the associate to produce and collect. In this situation the owner is less likely to lose. However, this method involves more complex bookkeeping. The office must specifically allocate the work done by each provider to that employee and track the associated collections. The employee has a problem with delayed compensation. This means that the money may come into the office several months after the production. It is challenging to develop a family budget, especially for a new practitioner. A significant problem is the disposition of accounts receivable in case of break-up. Suppose the employee is paid based on collections. In that case, they must access the patient financial records to verify that the owner has made appropriate compensation payments after the employee leaves the practice. The owner may not be as diligent as the employee would like in making collection arrangements. A common solution is for the owner to pay the employee 80% of that employee's accounts receivable. The owner then collects the accounts.

A common point of negotiation (for both production and collection-based compensation) is whether to credit the employee with production attributed to the dental hygienist they "cover." Employers claim that they are paying the salary and other costs of the hygienist, and the employee seeing these patients generates additional work that leads to compensation. Employees claim that they are using their clinical skills, knowledge, expertise, and abilities to do the exam and review the hygienist's work. A common resolution is to credit only the exam (and often radiograph) portion of the visit to the employee's production.

Combination Methods

There are many combinations or variations of these methods. Some have a base salary with a bonus for production. Many offices use a variable commission, paying a higher commission percentage for monthly production amounts. This provides incentives for the associate to produce at higher levels. Because the employer has already paid fixed costs, these higher production levels are also more profitable for them.

Some employers offer new dentists an initial salary to develop personal cash flow and then switch to a commission basis when the employee has developed a sufficient patient base and clinical skills. Other employers help new practitioners to weather initial cash-flow problems by offering a draw against future earnings. The owner pays the employee a percentage of production or collections in this arrangement. The employer pays an initial fixed monthly amount, like a salary, regardless of the employee's earned compensation. Once the employee's commission is above the "salary" amount, the employee pays back the difference by continuing to take the same draw until they make up the difference. (Box 2.5 gives an example of this arrangement.)

EMPLOYEE BENEFITS

Benefits are additional value besides money that the employer offers to the employee as a condition of employment. These may be as various insurances (medical, disability, life, malpractice), paid time off (holidays, vacation, personal or sick days), additional compensation (bonus plans), or financial inducements (retirement plan contributions or dependent care allowances). Benefits are valuable for the employee dentist from a financial perspective because the total value of the benefit comes to them free of income or Social Security taxes. Benefits cost the owner the cost of the benefit, although the owner offsets part of the cost through the tax deductibility of the benefit. (Chapter 27 discusses benefits in more detail.)

Common Benefits

The possible list of fringe benefits is endless. Most employers offer employees a set package of benefits to compete with other employers in the area. There are significant accounting and tax compliance issues with benefit plans, so most employers do not change them frequently. If the dentist is an employee, they are generally eligible for those employee benefits. These benefits fall into three general categories:

- **Employee insurances** are the most common group of benefits and are also the costliest group. Depending on the size of the employing organization, it may be required to offer some of these to employees.

- **Career benefits** include those that directly affect the dental professional. The employer may pay for (or reimburse) costs associated with continuing dental education. Often, the employer will give specific courses or topics to attend. They may reimburse other professional costs, such as licensure renewal fees or malpractice insurance premiums.

- **Paid time off** is an essential benefit for many employees, which may come as holidays, vacation days, or sick

---

BOX 2.5	EXAMPLE – DRAW AGAINST FUTURE EARNINGS

Month	Employee production	Employee commission	Employee compensation	Monthly shortage/overage	Total shortage/overage
1	$5 000	$1 650	$5 000	−$3 350	−$3 350
2	$10 000	$3 333	$5 000	−$1 667	−$5 017
3	$15 000	$5 000	$5 000	$0	−$5 017
4	$20 000	$6 600	$5 000	$1 600	−$3 417
5	$25 000	$8 250	$5 000	$3 250	−$167
6	$30 000	$10 000	$9 833	$0	$0

Assumptions: The employee earns 33% of production as a commission. The employer will pay the employee a monthly salary of $5000 as a draw against future earnings.

days. Many employers combine vacation and sick leave into a "personal leave" for either purpose. Employees who are producers (like dentists) must understand that their time off is very costly for employers. Not only does the practice miss the employee dentist's production, but they must pay support staff and services and deal with scheduling problems when the employee dentist is out of the office. This also debunks the notion that some employees believe they should be allowed as much time off "without pay" as they want.

Funding Benefit Plans

There are two ways to fund benefit plans: the owner can either pay the entire benefit amount or share the cost with the employee. The more the employer pays, the richer the benefit becomes for the employee. Whenever a dentist evaluates an employment situation, they should remember to include the value of the benefits offered in the total compensation. Remember, the benefits to the employee must come from somewhere, and they generally come from a lower income for the owner, dentist, or corporation.

TOTAL COMPENSATION

Total compensation then includes more than the base pay. When an employee calculates their total compensation, they need to think of how they are better off financially and personally from the employment. One person may value paid time off more than self-reliance, and another may value the relationship between hard work and the outcome of higher pay.

Box 2.6 shows how these forms of additional compensation add to the total compensation package.

BOX 2.6	DENTIST TOTAL COMPENSATION: SALARIED EMPLOYEE VS. COMMISSIONED EMPLOYEE VS. INDEPENDENT CONTRACTOR				

	Employee salary	Employee commission	Independent contractor		Assumptions
Base pay					
Production	$500 000	$500 000	$500 000	500 000	Doctor production
Base pay	$125 000	$125 000	$125 000	25%	Base pay as % of production
FICA match (7.65%)	$9 563	$9 563	$0	7.65%	FICA match
Employee fringe benefits					
Medical insurance	$4 800	$4 800	$0		Office pays medical insurance @ $400/mo
Life insurance	$1 200	$1 200	$0		Office pays group life insurance @ $100/mo
Long-term disability insurance	$4 800	$4 800	$0		Office pays group long-term disability insurance @ $400/mo
Retirement plan	$3 750	$3 750	$0		Office matches 3% retirement contribution
Career benefits					
Annual dental license	$300	$300	$0		Office pays the annual dental license
Malpractice insurance	$900	$900	$0		Office pays the annual dental malpractice insurance premium
CE tuition	$1 000	$1 000	$0		Office pays $1000/yr for CE course
CE travel	$1 000	$1 000	$0		Office pays $1000/yr for CE travel
Paid time off					
Holidays	$0	($11 538)	($11 538)		Assumes 6 non-working holidays/yr
Vacation days	$0	($28 846)	($28 846)		Assumes 3 weeks (15 days) vacation/yr
Sick days	$0	($9 615)	($9 615)		Assumes 5 sick days/yr
				260	Working days/yr (52 wks × 5 days)
Total compensation	$152 313	$102 313	$75 000	$1 923	Production/day (Production/working days)

CE, continuing education; FICA, Federal Insurance Contributions Act.

It also shows how the various types of relationships affect employee compensation. This example assumes a rich benefits package. All three dentists produce the same amount of dentistry and are compensated at the same rate (25%). The office provides fringe benefits for employee dentists but not for independent contractors. The commission-based dentists do not receive any compensation for days out of the office. That production is lost as compensation, and they would have to produce more in the remaining days to compensate for the lost production. While this chart does not represent any specific practice opportunity, it illustrates the value and cost of employee benefits to the employee and owner of various employment relationships.

EMPLOYMENT CONTRACTS

Regardless of the employment situation, the parent organization will probably ask the dentist to sign an employment contract. (In a private practice associateship, they are called *associateship contracts*.) The employee should also want a contract to spell out expectations for both sides. While these contracts define the employer's expectations of the employee, they also define what the employee dentist can expect from the employer. Good contracts are written ones. While a verbal contract is legal in many situations, if a dispute arises it can be challenging to define what the two sides agreed upon.

Every contract is negotiable until the parties sign it. If an employee dentist has questions or qualms about the wording or intent of a contract section, they should resolve it with the employer before signing. If the employee dentist and the employer differ about a particular piece of the contract, then maybe the arrangement is not good. Both parties need to know this sooner rather than later. Individual private practices have more leeway in the contract negotiation process. Often the larger chains and networks have standard contacts with all their dentist providers. These can be "take it or leave it" negotiations.

Generally, the employee and owner discuss issues and resolve differences. Then the owner has an attorney draft the contract, including the points that they have resolved. The potential employee dentist should have an independent lawyer review the contract, looking out for their interests. (A lawyer represents the side that is paying them.) It is a few dollars well spent.

Employment contracts for dentists commonly cover several topics, including the following.

DURATION OF CONTRACT

Most contracts state a specific length of time during which the contract is effective, having a starting date and an expiration date. A new graduate should include a start date that allows leeway for licensing and credentialing. (If a new graduate does not obtain their license in time, this protects them from the contract becoming void because they did not start working on the effective date.) Some contracts have a trial period before the contract takes effect, including information about how the relationship will continue after the expired trial period. A renegotiable one-year contract is a common arrangement. Many contracts include a provision for an automatic extension or a date for a contract renewal discussion. For example, some contracts have an automatic renewal 90 days from expiration unless the employee gives notice of their intent to leave.

> **Example**
>
> This Agreement and the Employee's employment shall commence as of the effective date hereof and shall continue for a period of (____) year(s) or until terminated in accordance with provisions of Section ____ of Agreement ("Initial Term"). This agreement shall be automatically renewed for a successive one-year term upon the anniversary of such year and each year thereafter unless written notice of election not to renew is given by either party not less than _____ days prior to the expiration of the term then in effect, or unless this agreement has been otherwise terminated as hereinafter provided.

LEGAL CLASSIFICATION

Whether the employee dentist is an employee or an independent contractor has far-reaching implications for liability, financial matters, practice management, and taxpayer accountability. The key to this determination is the genuine nature of the relationship as represented in the agreement and practice, rather than what the practice calls the relationship. Historically, many associateships were called independent contractors, even though they should have been employer–employee relationships. The pay was often structured at a higher percentage of collections due to the additional taxes (employer portion of FICA) that the employee would have to pay as an independent contractor. A common current practice is for these relationships to be considered a true employee/ employer agreement.

It is the parties' intention that Dentist shall be an Independent contractor. As such, Dentist shall be accountable to company as to the results of Dentist's work only and not as to the manner or means by which such results were accomplished. This Agreement shall not be construed to create a partnership, joint venture, fiduciary relationship, principal-agent relationship, or employer-employee relationship between Dentist and Company, and neither party shall be liable for any obligation incurred by the other. Dentists shall not be entitled to participate in any of the benefits or other plans maintained by the company for its employees. Company shall not make any state or federal unemployment compensation payments on behalf of Dentist, and Dentist shall not be entitled to these benefits in connection with services performed under this Agreement. Dentist shall be responsible for and pay all taxes due in accordance with Federal, State, City, County, and other local tax laws, including applicable income taxes. The company will not withhold FICA from payments to the Dentist or make FICA payments on Dentist's behalf. The company will not withhold State or Federal income taxes from payments to dentists.

COMPENSATION

As discussed earlier, there are many forms that compensation can take. The contract should clearly describe how compensation will be determined and what reports will be provided to show that the pay is accurate. (Complicated pay or bonus programs can be challenging to understand and compute.) If an office has current or former associates, they are a good source of information in this area.

Pay is generally based on collections or production (adjusted collections, adjusted production). The adjustments are based on patient write-offs, insurance write-offs, and uncollectable accounts. One thing to note is that if the employee is paid on collections, there should be provisions in the contract that state how and for what time they will be paid for money received after they leave the office. If not, then much of their work over the last several weeks will not be paid.

Example

For each pay period, Employee shall receive an amount equal to thirty percent (30.0%) of their Net Collections for such pay period. For purposes of this Agreement, "Net Collections" means the sum of money Employer

actually collected during the pay period for services employee personally rendered, less credits and refunds paid and less cost of lab fees and implants. Net Collections shall not include any collections for services rendered by any individual other than Employee, including but not limited to hygienists, or any receipts collected after Employee's employment ends. In addition, Net Collections shall not include any receipts from designated health services as defined from time to time by the so-called Stark law.

Direct Pay

The contract should state clearly how the employee pay will be determined and how often the employer will pay the employee. Often contracts have examples of pay calculations.

Example

As compensation for all services rendered by the Dentist, Company will pay the Dentist an amount equal to the greater of:

I. Twenty-Five percent (25%) of the amount collected monthly by Company while Dentist is actively employed and which results from dental treatment performed by Dentist at the Office, less patient refunds for dental treatment performed by Dentist at the Office ("Earnings"); OR

II. a minimum base (annual gross salary) of One Hundred Twenty Thousand Dollars ($120 000) or a daily guaranteed rate ($450–$700) ("Minimum Salary"), payable in accordance with company's standard payroll schedule.

Some contracts will refer to a draw on future earnings or cumulative earnings and cumulative minimum salary, which means the amount of earnings and minimum salary, respectively, from the agreement's inception through the month of reconciliation.

Example

Earnings, Cumulative Earnings, and Cumulative Minimum Salary will be calculated and reconciled by the company monthly. If Cumulative Earnings do not exceed the Cumulative Minimum Salary, the Dentist will be paid the Minimum Salary for that month only. In each month in which the Cumulative Earnings exceed the Cumulative Minimum Salary, the Dentist will be paid the Minimum Salary plus the amount by which the Cumulative Earnings exceeds the Cumulative Minimum Salary, less the amount of any Cumulative Earnings previously paid to Dentist.

Employee Benefits

The contract should also list other forms of compensation in the form of benefits. Associates' benefits include continuing education, health insurance, malpractice insurance, retirement plan contribution, paid vacation, professional dues, paid sick time, life insurance, and disability insurance. Few employers offer this entire list of employee benefits, and some employers have cafeteria or cost-sharing benefit plans.

Examples

Employee Benefit Programs. Employer may, but shall not be obligated to, maintain one or more employee benefit programs from time to time. Employee acknowledges that their participation in any such employee benefit program is subject to the satisfaction of eligibility requirements. Plan documents shall control the terms of such programs.

Dental License and DEA Certificate Renewal. Employer shall pay directly or reimburse Employee for the cost of their [State] dental license renewal fee (excluding any late fees) and one-half of their DEA certificate renewal fee; provided, however, each amount paid or reimbursed by Employer shall be pro-rated over the term of the license or certificate (currently 24 months for the dental license and 36 months for the DEA certificate) and upon expiration or other termination of employment hereunder, Employee shall reimburse Employer an amount equal to the renewal fee paid or reimbursed by Employer multiplied by a fraction, the denominator of which is the term of the license measured in days, and the numerator of which is the term of the license measured in days minus the number of days Employee was employed by Employer after Employer paid the fee.

Continuing Education. Employer shall pay directly or reimburse Employee for up to $_____.00 per calendar year of expenses incurred to attend continuing education programs (including tuition/enrollment, reasonable food, travel, and lodging).

Amount of Time Off (Paid or Unpaid)

The contract should spell out how much paid time off (if any) the employer provides and how much unpaid time (if any) it allows. (Unpaid leave costs the practice lost production and employee expenses.)

Example

Time away from the practice for attending professional meetings, conventions, seminars, training and continuing education courses, vacation time and personal time shall be requested in advance and shall be taken at a time approved by Employer based upon seniority and workload, patient needs and other business considerations. Only one dentist may be away from the practice at the same time. Employee commits to working local school Spring Breaks. Employee shall be entitled to two calendar weeks of paid vacation time to be based upon the number of hours they normally work per week; all other time away from the practice shall be unpaid. Unused time may not be carried forward to the next calendar year.

FINANCIAL RESPONSIBILITIES

The contract should establish the employee dentist's financial responsibilities. The employee dentist may be required to pay for laboratory bills, the associate's malpractice insurance premiums, chairside assistants, equipment, supplies, or billing. In employer–employee relationships, the employer carries more of these expenses. In independent contractor relationships, the contractor carries more of them. It is common for some of these expenses to be split.

Example

Employee is responsible for all other costs and expenses, including but not limited to:

1. Employee's cell phone;
2. Employee's home internet;
3. Employee's continuing education costs more than $500 per year and professional meeting costs;
4. Employee's health insurance costs;
5. Employee's automobile expenses;
6. Employee's professional liability insurance expense; and
7. One-half of Employee's DEA certificate renewal fee.

CONTRACT DISSOLUTION

Equitable terms for termination should be determined at the onset of the relationship. The contract should state the days' notice required for termination by both parties. Generally, the employer will list for cause and without cause provisions. Termination for cause may include loss of dental or DEA license, a conviction for a felony, theft, or crimes of "moral turpitude." Ending a contract with cause may change the obligations of either side. Both parties should have equal notice periods. Often the employer will ask for more time due to the time it takes to find a replacement. Penalties for breaking the contract or leaving before the number of days' notice will also be listed as part of the contract. If there was originally a signing bonus or moving expenses, there might be requirements for returning all or a portion of this money outlined in the contract.

The contract should detail the settlement of practice-related expenses. Some contracts state that the employee dentist is responsible for the cost of any rework done or any patient refunds after they leave. Both provisions should have associated time limits. If an employee dentist is paid based on collections, the contract should detail how the practice will compensate the employee after they leave the practice. Often, for a period ranging from 30 to 120 days, the practice is responsible for collecting and paying the departing dentist. If the contract stipulates that the office does not pay the departing dentist after they leave, it should detail compensation for the employee's work in the last month.

What happens in the event of the death and disability of either owner or employee is stated in most contracts. In some situations, the contract defines the division of patient records and office staff.

Most agreements require the departing employee dentist to purchase two years of malpractice tail coverage. Many employers will purchase a claims-made policy because it is less costly. Tail coverage (extended reporting) shields the associate from all claims arising from professional services provided while the claims-made policy was in place but reported after the policy ended. Generally, employment contracts will require two years of tail coverage.

Example

Terminating Events. Employment hereunder shall terminate when:

A. Employee dies;

B. Either party gives the other party at least sixty (60) days advance written notice of termination;

C. Employer, at its option, elects to terminate employment, with or without advance written notice, for any of the following reasons:

  1. Employee's unexcused failure for seven or more consecutive days to render active, full-time service hereunder. For purposes of this Section, scheduled time off, sickness, and disability shall be considered excused absences;

  2. Employee's conviction or indictment of a felony involving moral turpitude;

  3. Employee's abusive use of alcohol, drugs, or other substance;

  4. Employee's theft or embezzlement of any form from Employer or harassment of any employee of Employer;

  5. Employee's [State] dental license or controlled substance registration certificate is revoked or restricted;

  6. Employee breaches this Agreement and fails to cure the breach within 30 days of a written demand from Employer to cure such breach; or

  7. Employee's disability. Employee shall be deemed to be disabled if

     a. a physician selected by Employer determines that Employee is unable to perform the clinical and administrative duties hereunder on a full-time basis as a result of one or more physical or mental disabilities (resulting from an illness, disease, accident, or otherwise), or

     b. employee misses the equivalent of 20 full work days, consecutive or otherwise, as the result of one or more physical or mental disabilities (resulting from an illness, disease, accident, or otherwise). Employer's option to terminate Employee's employment shall be in addition to all other rights and remedies of Employer, at law or in equity.

CONTRACT MODIFICATION AND DISPUTE RESOLUTION

The contract should state how to resolve a significant disagreement over contract provisions. Mediation and arbitration are both types of alternative dispute resolution (ADR), which means they are alternatives to litigation. Court battles are costly and may take years to resolve. Mediation and arbitration are similar in that they bring parties in conflict together outside the courtroom to resolve a dispute, but each has its own method. Mediation is intended to lead to a voluntary agreement, although either side can still go to court for a resolution. With arbitration, the arbitrator's decision generally is final and binding on both parties. When agreeing to mandatory arbitration, the parties should be aware that they are waiving their right to have a court (or a jury) resolve any dispute that may arise.

Mediation Example

In the event of any dispute, claim, question, or disagreement arising from or relating to this Agreement, the Parties hereto shall use their best efforts to settle the dispute, claim, question, or disagreement. To this effect, they shall consult and negotiate with each other in good faith and, recognizing their mutual interests, attempt to reach a just and equitable solution satisfactory to both parties. If they do not reach such solution within a period of 60 days the parties will conduct two mediation meetings and if they do not reach such solution within a period of 60 days, then, upon notice by either party to the other, all disputes, claims, questions, or differences shall be finally settled by arbitration.

Arbitration Example

The validity, interpretation, construction and performance of this Agreement shall be governed by the laws of the (Specific State). Any action with respect to this Agreement shall be submitted to binding arbitration before one arbitrator, who shall be selected by the American Arbitration Association. Any arbitration hereunder shall be administered by the American Arbitration Association under its rules governing commercial disputes. The arbitration shall be conducted in (County and State). The administrative fees and expenses shall be paid by the party who initiates the arbitration. Each party shall be responsible for the party's own attorneys' fees and other costs. However, the arbitrator may award reasonable fees and administrative costs to the prevailing party. The award of the arbitrator shall be final and enforceable in the courts of the (Specific State) and/or in Federal District Court.

BUY OR SELL PROVISIONS

The contract can also include a future buy-out or buy-in to a practice, partnership, or professional corporation. The terms of the agreement can specify the price of the sale or buy-in, and if it does not state an amount, then a method should be set for how and when an evaluation would be done. The contract can also include financing arrangements for any future buy-out or buy-in to a partnership or professional corporation. A right of first refusal allows the parties to set forth future intentions in case of death or disability.

Example

If Dr. A, the practice's dentist owner, becomes disabled or dies during the term of this agreement, Doctor B, the associate, will be given the first right to purchase the practice at its fair market value, which will be determined independently by the average of three external appraisers.

RESTRICTIVE COVENANTS

Many employer–employee agreements include restrictions. A restrictive agreement can take the form of non-competition, non-solicitation, or non-disclosure. These agreements vary tremendously from state to state in their enforceability. They generally include penalties for the departing dentist if they break these provisions. These covenants are enforceable in many (but not all) states if they serve a useful purpose and are reasonable in scope, geography, and time. (There is no universal standard for "valid" or "reasonable" in these decisions.) In states that allow them, most courts will uphold the enforcement of reasonable restrictive covenants that protect valid business interests but do not violate "public policy." Public policy is what the court perceives as the common good. It is influenced by the availability of dentists in the area, the disruption of the doctor–patient relationship, and the patient's right to choose their dentist. However, the cost and effort of litigating these issues are high. If the employee believes that they cannot live by the provisions of the restrictions in the future, then they should not sign the contract.

A **restrictive covenant** (often called a **non-competition agreement**) prohibits an associate, almost always an employee, from practicing dentistry within a particular geographic area for a set length of time, after leaving the employer. On termination of the associateship, the covenant is meant to prohibit the associate from opening a competing office nearby and transferring patients away from the owner–dentist. It is based on the idea that an owner–dentist has a valid business interest (the patients/clients of the business) that should be protected. This protects the employer for the effort, time, and money they have put into building their practice.

A **non-solicitation** provision, enforceable in many areas of the United States, typically declares that the departing dentist will not solicit any patients or employees of the current practice. Only a few states allow limits on accepting businesses or hiring new workers. Instead, these provisions may bar the former employee from contacting former customers or coworkers or asking them to come as patients or employees. Often these are limited to patients treated by the associate or employees who have worked directly with the employee.

A **non-disclosure agreement** forbids an employee (or former employee) from exposing sensitive trade secrets and other proprietary business information while on the job, afterward, or both. These may include patient lists, referral lists, and office policy or procedure manuals.

Example

Noncompetition.

A. *Covenants*. While Employee is employed by Employer and for a period of twenty-four (24) months after my employment hereunder ends ("Restricted Period") for any reason, with or without cause, Employee will not (except when acting on behalf of Employer), directly or indirectly, on their own account or on behalf of, through, or in conjunction with any other person (including without limitation, their spouse or as a principal, agent, consultant, officer, director, manager, employee, shareholder, partner, or member) through any means, including but not limited to the use of social media:

1. Practice dentistry or own, manage, operate, join, have an interest in, control or participate in the ownership, management, operation or control of, be employed by, assist in, act as a consultant to, provide capital or financing to, be directly or indirectly connected with, rent property to, or have any direct or indirect financial interest in, any dental office that is within five (5) miles of the Location ("Protected Territory");

2. Send any announcements to or solicit in any fashion any of the patients of Employer or advertise in the Protected Territory for the purpose of soliciting patients residing or working in the Protected Territory;

3. Encourage any patient of Employer to switch to another dental office or encourage any patient to discontinue or reduce the services acquired from Employer; or

4. Hire or attempt to hire, or go into business with, any individual who is employed by Employer.

B. *Additional Covenant*. Prior to termination of employment, without the actual knowledge of Employer, Employee will not discuss with any patient of Employer their intention to terminate employment with Employer or their plans following termination of employment unless they enter a business or activity other than dentistry when such employment ceases.

C. *Permitted Exception*. Notwithstanding *Section 5.4A*, Employee may passively own for investment purposes only not more than 3% of any publicly-owned company that engages in dentistry in the Protected Territory.

D. *Waiver of Right to Protest*. Employee agrees the duration, geographical limitations and description of the prohibited conduct described in this Agreement are reasonable and they have received valuable consideration for the covenants contained herein. They expressly waive the right to protest the reasonableness of the duration, limitations, and prohibited conduct specified in this Agreement.

E. *Extension of Restricted Period*. Should Employee violate this *Section 5.4*, then the Restricted Period shall be extended for a period of time equal to the period during which said violation or violations occurred. If Employer seeks injunctive relief from said violation in court, the running of the Restricted Period shall be suspended during the pendency of said proceeding, including all appeals by Employee alleged to be in breach of this Agreement. This suspension shall cease upon entry of a final judgment in the matter.

PREPARING FOR EMPLOYMENT

Preparing for employment starts with understanding and setting short-term and long-term goals. Sitting down and writing out on paper what the graduate is looking for in employment is critical in directing the search. These goals should be specific in what the graduate is looking for and how it will help them meet their long-term goals. Reaching long-term goals might take several job opportunities to find the correct position.

SEARCHING FOR EMPLOYMENT OPPORTUNITIES

Dentists looking for employment following graduation can approach their job search in one of two ways: reactive or proactive. Reactive job search tactics entail looking for job opportunities and applying for those that appeal. As a result, when a dentist sends their résumé to recruiters or answers a job board advertisement, they are at the mercy of others.

In a proactive job search, a dentist chooses the companies and jobs they want to apply for. This way, rather than hoping for an excellent job to come their way through recruiters and job boards, they earn the position that they chose and worked for. The applicant should have a solid résumé and LinkedIn profile before starting a job hunt, as companies may use these as a screening method. The following are some proactive job search strategies:

- Identify key contacts and networking opportunities.

- Research the companies and offices.

- Leverage networks.

- Reach out to hiring managers.

NETWORKING

Networking is identifying and interacting with others to exchange information and develop professional or social contacts. Identify who the contact network is; some examples might include family and friends, job contacts, social networks, activities and involvement, faculty, students, alums, and staff, to name a few. An email can be sent to ask a question, and extending an invitation to meet for coffee or virtually is a great way to start the process. Joining professional associations and attending their events is very helpful in meeting dentists in a particular area.

RESUMES AND CURRICULA VITAE

Depending upon the job opportunity, a dentist may need to prepare a resume or a curriculum vitae (CV) or "course of life."

A CV is a detailed compilation of academic credentials, job history, and accomplishments. It is generally presented in chronological order, beginning with education and training. Since the CV includes all research publications, presentations, and coursework, it is generally longer than a résumé. It is used in academic or research settings, for which a chronology of academic or research growth is essential. This may be used in applying for an academic position, grant, fellowship, or advanced education program (residency).

A résumé is generally shorter and more focused on the job at hand. It summarizes someone's education, skills, and work history. It allows the applicant to present important achievements for a particular job or job setting. It is standard for private-sector jobs, where past performance is more important than academic training.

When preparing a résumé, the applicant must realize that many companies today use applicant tracking software (ATS). Since 2008, almost all Fortune 500 companies have used ATS. Every corporate job posting receives an average of 250 résumés. From those, the company will choose four to six candidates to interview and select one of those for the position. Most ATS uses keyword searches to select résumés. Therefore, applicants should use the job posting language to describe their skills and experience. The ATS also screens for spelling and grammar. The applicant should make sure to proofread, and have others proofread, the résumé before sending it out.

Résumés should contain the following four categories: contact information, education, skills, and work experience. This information can be presented in chronological or functional order, or a combination of the two.

- A **chronological** format is the most common résumé type and is preferred by recruiters. This résumé lists the most recent position first.

- A **functional** résumé focuses on skills and experience. Instead of the work history section at the top of the résumé, the functional format might have a professional experience or accomplishments section that lists various skills developed over the years. This type of résumé is helpful for people who are new to the workforce, have limited work experience, or have gaps in their employment. By highlighting skills rather than work history, the applicant can emphasize how they are qualified for the job.

- A **combination** format is a mix of chronological and functional résumés. It highlights relevant skills while providing chronological work history. The work history is not the focus and typically does not take up much space on the résumé. This type of résumé helps the applicant highlight what makes them the best fit for the job while giving the employer the information they want.

A non-traditional résumé has a unique format that includes photos, graphics, illustrations, graphs, and other visuals. It might be an online résumé or a physical résumé with infographics. On a social networking platform, it may be a video or a CV. The purpose of this type of résumé is to stand out from others who are applying for the same job. While such résumés are unique, the applicant must remember that the goal of a résumé is to secure an interview. If the applicant provides a picture or a video on the résumé, the employer might judge them, for good or bad, before they can meet them.

One challenge new graduates often face when developing a résumé is their lack of work experience in dentistry. The graduate should highlight their experiences in training (school) in specific clinical rotations and the experiences they have had while working in those clinics. Another way to highlight the desire to learn and grow is to take formal continuing education courses. A category can be added to the résumé that highlights the courses taken above and beyond the education of the dental school curriculum. Listing skills related to new dentistry technologies, such as digital technologies and lasers, are essential to highlight. Finally, any externships, volunteer clinics, or leadership must be noted. Following are some examples.

- **Continuing Education**
  - Advanced Adhesive Dentistry & Dental Materials by Dr. Jose Smith & Dr. James Smith
  - Caries Management by Risk Assessment (CAMBRA) by Dr. Hank Firestone
  - How to Improve Patient Engagement by Rebecca Jones
  - Treatment Planning Guidelines for Esthetics by Dr. Leon Harrison, University of Louisville and Seattle-Jefferson County Dental Society and Foundation

- **Skills**
  - Optical Scanner – trained in the use of Sirona Primescan
  - Trained in Anatomage (Invivo 6) – digital treatment planning for surgically guided implant surgery
  - Used 3D printing (EnvisionTEC) to fabricate models and occlusal splints

- **Volunteer Clinics**
  - GKAS (Give Kids a Smile) participant 202X, 202Y
  - Church mission to Haiti to treat indigent populations July 202X
  - Local Dental Society Community Outreach Program June 202X

INTERVIEWING TECHNIQUES

One thing that every job search in every career has in common is that no one knows what is best for the applicant but themselves. One person's ideal situation may not be everyone else's. Dentistry can be stressful even when it provides the best challenges and opportunities for growth. The applicant decides what kind of environment or opportunity will advance their career. One of the essential things an applicant can do before an interview is to sit down and write out what they are looking for in a position. Mentorship, income, new technology, or continuing education opportunities might be on their list. Some people make a list and rank the items from most important to least important. Others divide the list into "must have" and "nice to have" items. This process helps focus on what the applicant is looking for in a practice or other opportunity.

Before the interview, the applicant needs to research the practice and its personnel. They should examine its website to learn about the staff and the practice and review how long staff members have worked there. The website should show the type of dental practice the applicant would be joining.

The applicant should "look the part" and dress appropriately. If the applicant is a new graduate, showing up in scrubs does not set the proper tone for a new dentist. Clothes should be at least business casual. More formal business attire is appropriate if the practice is traditional and formal. If the practice has a more relaxed and informal "vibe," more relaxed clothes and personal appearance are appropriate. The applicant should remember that this is not a time to make a personal statement about dress and appearance; it is a time to fit into the conventional way the practice operates.

THE INTERVIEW ITSELF

Interviewing for a job position is like dating. There may be a series of interviews as the applicant and potential employer get to know each other better and probe more deeply to find out if the applicant is a good match for the position. The first interview is a chance to get to know each other, and it is an opportunity for the applicant to understand the practice's vision and philosophy on patient care. It is also a chance for the practice owner to assess the applicant's interpersonal skills and see if their personality would be a good "fit" for the practice. The applicant should be less worried about the details and more concerned about finding a situation to help them reach their long-term goals. A second or third interview allows both sides to reaffirm their initial impressions and probe further into any area of concern.

Applicants often find it helpful to do a mock interview with a friend, classmate, or significant other acting the part of the interviewer. The "interviewer" can assess both verbal and non-verbal responses from the "interviewee," offering constructive feedback. Making a video recording (on a phone) can be very useful in showing the interviewee how they will appear in the session.

The following are common questions that begin an interview:

- What can you tell me about yourself?
- What are your greatest strengths?
- What would you consider your weaknesses?
- What are your unique qualities?
- Why are you applying for this position?
- What is your desired salary?

These are common questions about experience and background:

- Can you explain your educational background?
- Where did you attend dental school? Can you describe your program?
- Will you tell me about a time when you overcame a difficult situation at work?
- What did you like best about your previous position?
- Have you considered opening your own practice?
- What have you done to continue your professional development in current dental techniques and procedures?
- Do you have any dental specializations (pediatric, sedation)?
- What is the most important thing you have learned in your years of experience?

And here are some common questions that probe experience more deeply:

- How can you determine if a patient needs a dental x-ray?
- What types of local anesthesia would you use to complete a filling?
- Have you ever had to help a patient who was uncomfortable with a dental procedure?
- Can you describe your bedside manner with patients?
- How would you explain a dental health problem to a patient? For example, how would you explain to a patient that they need a cavity filled?

- Can you describe your most challenging procedure? What was the outcome?
- How long would it take you to perform an extraction?
- What was your average production rate in your previous position? How effective was the practice at seeing patients in a timely way?

The interview is also a time for the applicant to learn about the dental practice. This comes in several forms. One is asking the interviewer direct questions. The applicant can also assess the atmosphere of the office. Furthermore, they can ask for specific "numbers" or reports about the practice.

The following are questions that an applicant might ask a future dental employer:

- Why is the owner hiring?
- What are your expectations of a new associate?
- Does the practice plan to recruit new patients?
- How do new patients come into the practice?
- Which patients would I see? How would that affect my bottom line?
- Has the practice had a previous associate? What went well? What did not go so well?
- Can you show me a case you have been working on?
- What systems do you have in the office (i.e. new patient, financial arrangements, recall program, cancelations/no-show policy)?

If the initial interview goes well, both sides may want to probe for additional information. Often practitioners are reluctant to give detailed practice information to anyone, and they want to be sure that the applicant is sincere and may be a good fit for the position. At that point, the applicant might ask for additional reports from the practice that pertain to their employment opportunity. (For example, how much income the practitioner makes is not material to the agreement, but the number of recall patients that flow through the practice monthly is essential for the applicant to know.)

Some reports an applicant might request from the practice are the following:

- Current year/previous year production/collection report per doctor.
- Total practice write-offs.
- Production report by procedure code and category.
- Total hygiene production.

- Number of new patients per month.

- A copy of the schedule for the past two weeks (this will give a good idea regarding how full the schedule is and which procedures are being done).

- Total number of active patients.

- Re-care (recall) percentage.

Some common red flags to look for when interviewing a practice are these:

- The practice does not want to provide any practice numbers or reports.

- There are not enough new patients and no plan for the associate to gain patients.

- The office has many insurance write-offs or a low collection percentage.

- There are not enough chairs for the new associate. A minimum of two chairs per doctor should be available.

NEGOTIATING THE CONTRACT

Depending on the employer, a job applicant may have considerable room to negotiate provisions in a contract or very little room. Most large DMSOs have standard contracts and give little room to negotiate. Theirs is often a "take it or leave it" approach to negotiation. They are often concerned that if they concede a point for one practitioner, others will want the same or more provisions changed. Smaller and more individual practices generally have more negotiating room.

Both employer and potential employee should enter the negotiation in good faith. The intention is to reach an agreement that both sides think is fair. The employer will present a preliminary agreement on the contract's provisions. At this point, the applicant goes to the list of items they were looking for in a position (from the interview step). If there are "must have" items not in the preliminary agreement, they present them to the employer. Then the applicant works down the list to the less essential items. The art of negotiating is to find a compromise position that both sides can accept. For example, the employer and applicant are $20 000 per year apart in income, and neither side wants to give in. A solution may be to develop a bonus plan that allows the new practitioner to meet their income needs while keeping the employer from a potential ongoing financial loss. Alternatively, one side may accept one provision if the other accepts changes to a different one. However, each side must have a bottom-line number for each negotiating point. If they do not satisfy that point, they will walk away from the negotiations.

Practice Ownership

My son is now an "entrepreneur." That's what you're called when you don't have a job.

Ted Turner

GOAL

This chapter aims to describe common issues in practice ownership for dentists.

LEARNING OBJECTIVES

At the completion of this chapter, the student will be able to:

- Describe the characteristics of dental practice ownership.

- Differentiate between the two ways to make money in dentistry.

- Describe the advantages and disadvantages of individual practice.

- Describe the advantages and disadvantages of individual group practice.

- Describe the advantages and disadvantages of true group practice.

- Describe the advantages and disadvantages of franchise practice ownership.

KEY TERMS

compensation
compensation for doing dentistry
compensation for ownership interest
corporation
dividends
franchises as ownership
incidents of ownership

individual group practice
individual practice
methods of production cost allocation
ownership compensation
pass-through entities
payment for production
proprietorship

relative value units
salary
salary with commission
single-owner LLC
solo group practice
true group practice

Business Basics for Dentists, Second Edition. James L. Harrison, David O. Willis, and Charles K. Thieman.
© 2024 John Wiley & Sons, Inc. Published 2024 by John Wiley & Sons, Inc.

Owning a dental practice is the dream of most dental school graduates. However, that ownership comes with both costs and advantages. A dentist will spend additional time managing the business of the practice. Most dentists get into the profession because they want to treat patients, not realizing the time and emotional energy they must devote to running a successful business. However, the upside of ownership is the pride, happiness, and financial return that come from running a successful practice.

In the past, the only type of practice ownership was the independent individual practitioner in a cottage industry business. Now there are large and small groups, franchises, and network practices that open many more possibilities to new graduates than were available previously.

CHARACTERISTICS OF PRACTICE OWNERSHIP

Doing dental services does not require owning a dental practice. Likewise, dentists can own a dental practice and not personally do any dental services by hiring another dentist to do them instead. If dentists separate, in their minds, owning a practice from doing dentistry, they can better understand the characteristics of practice ownership.

INCIDENTS OF OWNERSHIP

Business owners have certain rights in the business that non-owners, such as employees, do not. These incidents or rights of ownership result from someone putting their capital (money) at risk in the business (Box 3.1). Because they have taken on the risk associated with ownership that workers have not, then owners have the benefits that

BOX 3.1	INCIDENTS OF BUSINESS OWNERSHIP

- Ability to make a profit from the business.
- Decision-making authority (may be delegated).
- Increased responsibility and liability.
- Can pledge assets (for a loan).
- Gain in the value of the business.

result, whereas workers do not. Dentists can profit (or incur a loss) from business activities, whether they do dentistry or not. This is the basis of network practice entities. Dentists may choose (through a profit-sharing plan) to share those profits with workers, but it is unnecessary. If the business shows a loss, workers will not accept paying for a loss; they will go elsewhere to work or not work at all. The person who owns the business can decide how it will operate and whom they will hire to do the various functions. They have the responsibility for ensuring that the business is operated effectively. They also have liability if the business (or someone working there) injures someone or if the dentist directly injures someone through their negligence. Because they own the business's assets, they can pledge them as collateral for a loan or other purposes. If the business gains or loses value because of their management abilities, the dentist (as the owner) will enjoy the gain or suffer the loss in value. Workers do not share in this gain or loss. Associate dentists may not understand this difference clearly. They often feel that they have contributed to the growth in the value of a practice and should not, therefore, pay for that growth when they purchase (or buy into) the practice.

MAKING MONEY IN DENTISTRY

There are two ways to make money in dentistry. The first is to do dentistry, and the second is to have an ownership interest. People who own the practice and see patients make money both ways.

COMPENSATION FOR DOING DENTISTRY

Whether a dentist is a practice owner or an employee, they can earn money for dentistry. If they are a proprietor or a partner, they are an owner. They draw on the practice's assets (one of which is the office checking account), estimate their income tax liability, and prepay it quarterly to the Internal Revenue Service (IRS). Suppose they are an employee of an organization (such as a health center) or a practice corporation (even if they are the sole stockholder and provider). In that case, the corporation will pay them as an employee. The corporation will estimate its tax liability (based on IRS tables), withhold that amount, and send it to the government as prepaid taxes. The dentist receives the amount left after the corporation has paid estimated income taxes for them.

If someone practices in a corporate structure, they will earn pay for dentistry like any other employee. The corporation may pay them a commission (based on production or collections), salary, wage, or a combination method. If someone is a proprietor or a partner in a partnership, they pay themselves by drawing on the practice's assets. Some dentists take any money left over in the checking account at the end of the month as a draw. Others take a fixed amount (like a salary) for budgeting purposes and to ensure there is enough cash in the practice to pay regular bills. These people do not pay tax on how much money they take out of the practice (as a draw), but on how much profit the practice generates. Whether the person took any of it for personal expenses is irrelevant.

COMPENSATION FOR OWNERSHIP INTEREST

If a dentist is an owner, they may have a profit left in the business (practice) after paying all expenses (including paying dentists to do dentistry on patients). This is called *entrepreneurial profit*. If the dentist is an excellent manager, their entrepreneurial profit will be larger than if they are a mediocre or poor manager. They may distribute that profit to employees (as a bonus) or the practice owners as a reward for their investment in the practice. They may also combine these methods.

Business owners may distribute any profits to the owners of the business to compensate them for their ownership. If a practice is a corporation, the distribution is based on the number of shares owned. Dividends are from the corporation's profits. If the practice is a C corporation, the corporation must pay taxes on the profits first and then distribute them as dividends (where they are taxed again as personal income). To avoid this double taxation, C corporate practices usually pay out profit as bonuses, so this money is solely taxed once. Often these bonuses go only to the owner(s). S corporations (or "pass-through" entities) do not have this problem. They pass dividends through to the owners without paying taxes at the corporate level. Because these dividends are unearned income, the individual does not pay Social Security, Medicare, or self-employment taxes. Box 3.2 shows how a hypothetical practice might divide income and profit.

The owner may distribute any profit to any employee as a bonus, and the IRS considers this to be taxable income. They can distribute it by shares, based on production, or any other means the owners(s) choose. For example, someone may distribute profits only to certain dentists (owner or non-owner). It is entirely up to the owners what they do with the profits from the business.

INDIVIDUAL PRACTICE OWNERSHIP

An individual practice involves the most significant investment of someone's time and emotional energy and provides the greatest personal rewards when successful.

BOX 3.2	EXAMPLE OF PAYING FOR EQUITY (OWNERSHIP)

	Total	Owner #1	Owner #2	Associate
Production	1 800 000	700 000	600 000	500 000
Compensation for production (@ 25%)	450 000	175 000	150 000	125 000
Compensation for ownership	200 000	100 000	100 000	0
Total compensation	650 000	275 000	250 000	125 000

A group practice has three dentists, one associate (non-owner), and two owner dentists. Dentists are paid 25% of production, dividing any money left over (profit) equally between the owners. The practice produced $1.8 million last year. Total costs (not including payments for doing dentistry) were $1 150 000. The resulting compensation for the three dentists is shown in this chart.

Practice production	$1 800 000
Minus payments for production	−$450 000
Minus office costs	−$1 150 000
Equals business profit	$200 000

OWNERSHIP

One person owns an individual practice, which means the owner has complete control of and responsibility for the business. There are several forms that the business may take. From a management perspective, a business entity is not essential. (These forms are detailed in the chapter on business entities.) Briefly, the choices in the form of ownership for a solo practice are as follows.

Individual Proprietorship

In this form of ownership, there is only one owner regardless of how many employee dentists they may have hired. They take all profits to their personal taxes through Schedule C (Profit or Loss from a Business). The owner must apply for tax identification numbers through federal, state, and local taxing agencies. Individual states may have rules for registering the business.

Single-Owner LLC

As the name implies, this is a Limited Liability Company with a single owner. From a tax perspective, the IRS treats this practice as a sole proprietorship, and the owner–dentist gains some business liability protection in this form of business.

Corporation

A corporation is a business entity that is formed under state laws. States may call them an Association, Limited, Incorporated, or Company, depending upon the state. The ownership of a corporation is decided by who owns the corporation's stock. A solo dentist often owns all (100%) of the stock in their incorporated practice. Some states allow non-dentists to own stock in dental practice corporations, and others do not. The dentist is an employee of the corporation. They may also retain all management control by electing themselves as the President and Chief Executive Officer of the company. The IRS taxes corporations in several different ways.

COMPENSATION

The owner takes all profit from the business as compensation. This may be as compensation for dentistry or as business profit. The difference in the proprietorship or LLC practice is not meaningful because the owner is the business. In an individually owned corporate practice, the owner can characterize some profits from the business as dividends, which the IRS taxes differently than earned income.

ADVANTAGES

In the individual practice, the owner exercises complete control over the operational and strategic direction of the practice. It is their practice, and they can do what they want without compromising with other owners. If the practice increases in value, they enjoy the gain.

DISADVANTAGES

As an individual practitioner, the dentist has additional time commitments to manage the business, which typically amounts to several hours per week. Often, they may want another trusted practitioner to discuss clinical or management problems with. (Study clubs and mentors help to solve this problem.) They are responsible for the financial health of the practice. If they want to borrow money for a practice purchase or expansion, they have their credit rating and borrowing power to use.

The individual practitioner may find it more challenging to take time from the office for vacations or personal reasons. If they are not there seeing patients, their income decreases. Suppose they find a substitute for themselves when they are away. In that case, they pay the substitute most of what the owner would have taken as compensation for doing the dentistry, leaving only the entrepreneurial profit for the owner. Patients still want to be seen when the owner is gone, and employees still want to be paid. Without a large cash cushion, cash-flow problems can occur with time away from the office.

SOLO GROUP PRACTICES

This arrangement consists of independent practices physically located under one roof. Each dentist practices as a single practitioner (proprietorship or corporate). They may share ordinary overhead expenses, such as rent, business office, laboratory, or radiographic facilities. This form of practice is also called space-sharing, time-sharing, a cluster group, or a condominium arrangement. Individual autonomy is high. One dentist may own and rent the office space to another (time-share), or the participating dentists may jointly own the property (real estate partnership). The general purpose is to increase net income by reducing overhead and using facilities, equipment, and possibly staff more efficiently than the traditional individual practitioner. This occurs while maintaining the nature of a separate practice that many dentists cherish. For these reasons, this has become a popular method for established dentists to merge their existing practices.

The essential nature of an individual group is that the practices remain separate. Each practice has separate patient pools, (clinical) staff, billing, decision-making authority, and responsibility. This practice requires strict cost and income accounting because there is little sharing of authority or responsibility, only division of costs.

OWNERSHIP

There are many possible arrangements for individual group ownership based primarily on the control of the facilities:

- The facilities may be owned or rented by one dentist, who then sublets space to another during their off-hours (time-sharing).

- The facilities may be owned or leased by one dentist who rents space to another dentist during the same office hours (space-sharing).

- The facilities may be jointly owned or leased by two or more dentists who have separate treatment areas yet share the business office and reception areas and the costs associated with each (condo arrangement or real estate partnership).

Some or all practice participants may own the facilities as a management company, which provides, for a fixed or percentage fee, common management services such as scheduling, billing, and collections. They may jointly own the equipment through a leasing consortium of members who lease equipment to the practices. These umbrella organizations allow practitioners to enter or leave the group more easily. They also allow dentists who dislike management functions to concentrate on clinical patient care. They are usually formed as a pass-through entity so that expenses (e.g. depreciation) may pass through to the individuals.

COMPENSATION

Because each dentist operates a separate practice, compensation is based on collecting fees for individual services. Practices generally use separate accounting systems, so calculating compensation is straightforward. The individual dentist then pays the group's practice costs and any shared costs.

If standard business personnel and billing are used through a management company, the management group collects fees and allocates them to the individual practitioner. The group then deducts expenses, and the practitioner receives compensation directly from the management company. Suppose a percentage of the production compensation system is used instead of a collection-based system. In that case, the group either applies a standard collection ratio or charges back bad debts to the individual dentist's account. This prevents members of the individual group from sharing in the bad debt.

Owners of the management company receive a proportional share of any profits generated by the group based on the percentage equity interest of each partner.

COSTS

Efficiency in the individual group practice comes from sharing expenses for everyday concerns. These may include rent, utilities, supplies, waiting room, receptionist, business personnel, or other mutually agreed ordinary expenses. The more expenses shared, the more the savings. The individual dentist is responsible for any other costs associated with their practice, such as production (clinical) staff, associated lab bills, or professional education costs. The common costs are allocated among participants on several bases, including the following.

Fixed-Fee Basis

On a fixed-fee basis, the owner or owner organization rents the office and other agreed services for a fixed dollar monthly fee. This method is simple to administer and easily understood. However, this method charges the lower-producing members of the group more (i.e. a higher percentage) and typically benefits the higher producers.

Percentage of Production

In this method, the contract specifies the percentage of total monthly production that the renter pays for using the owner's office and supplies. Often dentists include a minimum or maximum dollar amount to protect parties from unexpected production levels.

Cost Ratios

Here, the individual's production is related to the entire group's production. The group assesses costs proportionally to everyone according to the production ratio. For example, if a dentist is responsible for 32% of the entire group's production, that dentist would be responsible for 32% of the costs for the month. This allocation assumes that supplies and other common expenses vary in concert with the production.

Combination Methods

Some dental groups combine the preceding methods. Fixed costs may be allocated on a straight percentage with the addition of variable costs based on production or a ratio of fixed costs.

ADVANTAGES

An individual group arrangement has several advantages over a "true" group practice or individual, freestanding practice. Because these practices are separate, there are fewer management disputes. The arrangement may be easy to administer because each practice maintains separate dental and financial records. Professional consultation and companionship are available, leading to improved emergency coverage shared between the patients. Patients may even perceive the group as a more modern practice. Finally, the common costs, such as rent or a business manager, may decrease, increasing the individual practitioner's net income.

DISADVANTAGES

An individual group arrangement also has several disadvantages. Competition among the practices may arise for patients and staff, particularly for new practitioners who participate in this type of group. The solution is a transparent allocation system for walk-in emergency or non-referral patients.

Because the public may perceive the practitioner as practicing with another dentist, their reputation may be either enhanced or tarnished by the acts of the other dentist. The courts may even hold someone to the liability requirements of a partnership if they offer themselves as a group practice. Disagreements over common areas and staff may develop. One dentist, for example, may feel that they should reprimand a receptionist for job deficiencies, but another does not. Similar problems may arise regarding the purchase of new equipment or costs associated with the redecoration of the reception room.

If one of the solo group members wants to sell their practice, there may be further problems. The existing practitioner may find it challenging to find someone who wants to come into a situation with other competing established practitioners. Patients may decide to leave the existing practitioner for the remaining one. The exiting dentist may not find someone the remaining practitioners want in the practice, but they may have no say.

The individual group generally does not benefit from the advantages of partnerships and true groups, such as shared treatment areas and clinical staff. Actual savings typically come at the expense of autonomy and independent decision-making ability. Individual groups do not increase efficiency unless the dentists share space or offset hours.

TRUE GROUP PRACTICES

True group practices are two or more dentists with a legal arrangement in which they share a common space, patient records, income, expenses and personnel in patient treatment, and business management of a standard dental practice. The true group may be either a partnership or a corporation, and a proprietorship is incompatible with a true group practice. The individual's autonomy and control are low, in deference to group control. True groups share expenses and compensate dentists based on a previously agreed formula. The essential nature of the true group is that the individual subordinates their managerial authority and decision-making to the group. Clinical decisions are affected to a lesser degree. True groups may consist of either one or multiple specialties.

The true group is a single practice entity, with the group controlling staff, patients, and expenses. (Many groups assign patients to doctors for continuity of care.) The critical point is that the group is the primary entity rather than the individual practitioner, as in the individual group. The practitioners share responsibilities, equipment, records, and often even patients. The group then compensates the dentists for doing dental or other practice-related services based on production, collections, or even hours worked. There may be different degrees of ownership – associate non-owner, management, equipment, or real estate umbrella partnerships – as in the individual group.

From the patients' perspective, true groups differ from traditional individual practices:

- Patients may identify more with the group than with the dentist. This eases or eliminates the direct monetary relationship between provider and patient in individual practice.

- Patients can usually use emergency and non-traditional hours more efficiently.

- There may be fewer choices regarding specialist referral, but the patient can get care in one office. If the group is multidisciplinary, the group's policies may dictate that practitioners conduct specialty referrals internally.

- The patient also perceives a greater continuity of care in case of death or disability of the practitioner, and can get comfort from a consultation that may occur within the group or complex care.

OWNERSHIP

True groups show many different forms of business organization. The practice, the management of the practice, the equipment, real estate, or the laboratory may each have distinct organizations that are a part of or separate from the practice. They may act as umbrella organizations or subcontractors for the practice itself. Each separate unit may be a profit center and charge the other units reasonable fees for the services provided.

The practice itself is either a corporation, LLC, or partnership. All the participating dentists are not necessarily owners of the practice, nor are they necessarily equal owners. They also may be simply employees compensated for doing dentistry but not sharing in the risks associated with ownership.

COMPENSATION

Compensation involves accounting for income from doing dentistry, specific costs associated with producing that dentistry, and specific costs for the individual dentist. Any money left over is entrepreneurial profit allocated among the owners, usually on a pro-rata ownership basis.

Compensation for Doing Dentistry

Total compensation for doing dentistry is a combination of income determination methods and a cost method.

Methods of Income Determination

There are several common methods of establishing income from dentistry.

Salary One method is to pay either a monthly salary or an hourly wage. This provides easy bookkeeping and gives income security, but lacks any production incentive. The group may lose money if an individual is not self-motivated or feels unjustly compensated. If, for example, all members receive the same salary but have significantly different production levels, the higher producers may become upset and feel inadequately compensated. Compensation by a salary encourages non-patient activities such as management duties, community activities, or part-time teaching in a university. Some groups structure a salary drawn against an average or minimum production level. This forces the participants to produce enough to at least "make their salary." For example, a dentist in the group may draw a salary of $10 000 per month. If the overhead averages 66.7%, they must produce $30 000 monthly to "make salary." If they only produced $20 000 one month, the salary would remain the same, but they would need to produce an additional $10 000 in a subsequent month to offset the underproduction.

Payment for Production Payment can be based on a percentage of production or collections. This is probably the most common method. Bookkeeping is more complex in this arrangement. However, computerized management systems simplify this activity. The non-owner practitioner has little incentive to spend time in non-production endeavors. If production is the income basis, then the practice uses a standard collection ratio (e.g. 96% of all charges collected) to estimate collections or charge bad debts back to the individual practitioner.

Salary with Commission Another common system is a salary base with a commission tied to production. Often a practice establishes a minimum for bonus compensation, which gives the participants the security of a fixed-base income but encourages and rewards production by the individual. This case presents an example of salary or commission compensation.

Relative Value Units A final variation is to set relative value units for each procedure. Relative value units assign values to procedures other than the traditional dollar amounts associated with individual services. These units may be based on the expected time required to complete a procedure, a dollar figure based on costs, specific practice incentives, or some combination. The practitioner is rewarded for this relatively established value. Relative value units encourage participants to do procedures that may be less profitable or more time-consuming, such as a simple alloy instead of a cast restoration. The practice then takes any efficiencies as profit. For example, a typical three-surface alloy may take 30 minutes of chair time and generate $150 of income. A casting for the same tooth may take 60 minutes of chair time but generate $1000 of revenue. A pure dollar relationship is 6.6 : 1 (1000 : 150), whereas the pure time ratio is 2 : 1 (60 : 30). A relative ratio may be arbitrarily set at two units for the alloy and seven units for the casting. Their relative value ratio is then 7 : 2. If the unit is defined as $50, then the dentist would be compensated $350 for the crown procedure (7 units × $50/unit) or $100 for the alloy procedure (2 units × $50/unit). This makes the casting somewhat less valuable for the provider (from a remuneration standpoint) and the alloy more valuable.

Methods of Production Cost Allocation

The primary methods for cost allocation involve deciding how two broad classes of expenses will be charged to each practitioner. These are the fixed office costs and variable costs of production. The importance is evident in a practice where the practitioners' production numbers are significantly different. If Dr. A has a large production relative to Dr. B, then Dr. A would prefer to divide costs equally; Dr. B would prefer to divide costs according to the production ratios because this would lead to a lower cost (and higher profit) for Dr. B.

There are standard methods of allocating costs.

Equal Shares Sharing expenses equally makes all costs fixed for the practitioners. The more costs they share equally, the more the higher-producing group members are helped financially.

Based on Production Sharing expenses based on a pro-rata share of production assumes that different practitioners use supplies and common services equally. Strict production-based cost accounting favors the lower-producing members of the group. Some procedures, for example periodontal therapy, use fewer lab charges and supplies than others, such as crown and bridge procedures. Practices often charge laboratory costs to the individual provider as a specific charge.

Individual Expense Accounting This method shares fixed expenses based on equal shares, with costs of production (variable expenses) based on production.

Specific Cost Allocation This method charges specific costs for a practitioner to that individual practitioner. These are costs that the individual might take as income, but instead decides to take as a business expense. Examples include retirement plan contributions, personal insurance benefits, automobile expenses, professional dues and publications, continuing professional education, and meeting expenses. Exceptions may include costs that all practitioners share equally. Examples might be dental association dues or standard malpractice insurance policy premiums.

Compensation for Ownership Position

Compensation based on the ownership position of the participants leads to incentives for owners to see the group succeed, incentives to control costs, and incentives to produce. Any money left over after paying for producing dentistry is business or entrepreneurial profit. They then split this based on the ownership interest of the practice.

The compensation formula must leave enough after paying for production to have meaningful compensation for ownership (Box 3.3). Usually, 10–15% is left for equity payment, and what associates in the area typically earn dictates the production compensation amount. (This would be the cost to the practice for hiring someone to produce the dentistry produced by the owner(s).)

ADVANTAGES

There are several advantages for dentists who practice in a true group:

- Professional consultation is readily available. In a true group, individuals succeed when the group succeeds. Concentrating on an area of clinical interest may be easier.

- The potential for higher individual incomes exists because groups share costs and greater efficiency develops with a larger practice.

| BOX 3.3 | EXAMPLE SPECIFIC COSTS ALLOCATION |

	Total	Owner #1	Owner #2	Associate
Collections	1 800 000	700 000	600 000	500 000
Gross production payment (@ 35%)	630 000	245 000	210 000	175 000
Specific charges	141 000	52 000	48 000	41 000
Net production payment	489 000	193 000	162 000	134 000
Office (shared) costs	1 061 000			
Business profit	250 000			
Divided by ownership		125 000	125 000	
Total compensation		318 000	287 000	134 000

A group practice has three dentists, one associate (non-owner), and two owner dentists. Dentists are paid 35% of production, less specific charges for their production (lab and implants), and personal expenses (auto, retirement plan, etc.). All common costs are paid by the practice, dividing any money left over (profit) equally between the owners. The practice produced $1.8 million last year. Shared costs were $1 061 000. The resulting compensation for the three dentists is shown in the chart.

- The practitioner has greater flexibility for personal time because other practitioners can share the patient load. However, group needs may temper individual autonomy in such time requests. An additional benefit of financial security exists for the practitioner in case of sickness, accident, or other disability. Other dentists are available to maintain the production of disabled practitioners.

- Many creative buy-ins, buy-outs, and retirement options are available to a group practice. There is a ready-made buyer in the group and generally a predetermined price. A group may be better able to offer financing for the purchase amount than an individual practitioner. No lag in patient treatment occurs if there is the death or disability of one practitioner. The quality of patient care may improve if active peer review and sharing of techniques and information occur. The quality of patient care may improve if active peer review and sharing of techniques and information occur.

DISADVANTAGES

Some disadvantages exist for the practitioner who is contemplating a group practice:

- There are different personalities to adapt to in the group.

- The individual generally loses some independent decision-making authority, and this loss increases with larger groups. Someone who seeks a high degree of autonomy should not consider a group arrangement.

- Depending on the circumstances, the dentist may lose the direct production–compensation relationship, which may be an advantage or a problem. If someone is interested in doing non-clinical duties (such as practice management, community work, or teaching), this can be an advantage for that person.

- The dentist–patient relationship may be lost in favor of a practice–patient relationship. This new relationship may be based on financial responsibility, treatment responsibility, or interpersonal relationships.

FRANCHISES AS OWNERSHIP

A franchise is a business arrangement in which the individual owns the business (practice). They contract with a parent organization for business guidance in an ongoing relationship. The owner must adopt the franchiser's methods and materials. This differs from a consulting relationship in that it offers advice for a short time. The owner is free to carry out the advice or not and can generally end the consulting contract whenever they wish.

OWNERSHIP

This allows the individual to retain ownership while tapping into the expertise of a proven organization. An individual owner (franchisee) must pay the parent organization (franchiser) both initiation ("front-end fees") and ongoing management fees for the use of the trademark, training, and advisory services. The parent then provides name recognition, management expertise, and a proven business formula for success.

There are no federal requirements for franchise information. Generally, states enforce laws and regulations on franchises in their state. The individual owner must enter these relationships cautiously and only with expert advisors.

COMPENSATION

Because the dentist owns the practice, the dentist's compensation is based on the practice's profit. The franchisee may pay significant fees to the parent company (franchiser) for the ongoing guidance and use of the trade name and procedures.

ADVANTAGES

The advantages of joining a franchise include the following:

- Name recognition of the parent organization. Everyone in the United States knows McDonald's corporate name, and the individual franchisee benefits from that kind of corporate image. Although not as prominent in dentistry, franchises can advertise on a regional level, increasing their presence in the dental consumer's mind. As patients move, they may seek out franchise dentists in their new locations.

- The franchiser has management expertise that the individual practitioner does not. (Dental schools train dentists to do dentistry, not run a business!) The franchiser brings management expertise, proven systems, and tested business methods to the individual franchise. The inexperienced individual franchisee would struggle for years to achieve this level of expertise.

- The franchiser offers training for staff and dentists, and this shares the knowledge of how to do business and patient procedures with the people doing them.

- The dentist keeps an ownership interest in the practice. Many dentists want to be practice owners for the autonomy and income that ownership offers.

DISADVANTAGES

Franchises have several disadvantages for dentists as well:

- The franchiser locks a dentist into a long-term relationship with the franchiser. Many dentists believe that once the practice is "up and running," they will cancel the franchise arrangement. That is not so. Most franchise contracts have significant costs associated with ending the relationship. After many years of practice, the ongoing franchise fee has become a sore point for many practitioners.

- If other franchises have problems, they may be guilty by association. For example, if another dentist in the franchise is guilty of drug charges, the public may associate "all of those dentists" in the franchise together.

- The parent franchiser company may fail, leaving the franchisee with significant legal and financial problems. The parent company may be sold to another who then changes the terms of contracts or does not offer the same level of services. Restrictive covenants may prohibit the franchisee from opening another practice nearby.

Practice Transitions

For many people a job is more than an income – it's an important part of who we are. So a career transition of any sort is one of the most unsettling experiences you can face in your life.

Paul Clitheroe

GOAL

This chapter will provide guidelines for a dentist when deciding on practice options. It also discusses factors that affect a practice's transfer.

LEARNING OBJECTIVES

At the completion of this chapter, the student will be able to:

- Differentiate between a buy-in, a buy-out, and a cold start.
- Describe the types of buy-in arrangements.
- Describe the types of dental practices that are typically for sale.
- Describe factors in locating a new dental practice.
- Describe various methods of financing the practice transfer option.
- Describe transfer considerations for each type of practice transfer option.

- Describe tax implications for each type of practice transfer option.
- Describe the typical process for each of the practice transfer options.
- Describe banks' typical process when evaluating a loan application.
- Describe the information that loan officers will require for loan processing.
- Define the more critical factors used in evaluating the economic state of a community.
- Describe the typical series of events in negotiating a practice transition.

KEY TERMS

bank financing
cold start
depreciation recapture

immediate buy-in
intrafamily transfers
sweat equity

walk-away sale

Business Basics for Dentists, Second Edition. James L. Harrison, David O. Willis, and Charles K. Thieman.
© 2024 John Wiley & Sons, Inc. Published 2024 by John Wiley & Sons, Inc.

Life transitions are a complicated, confusing, and exciting time for people. Most dentists now make several transitions in their professional careers, often moving from one employment situation to another. This chapter looks at the transitions involved in changing practice ownership: starting a practice, buying an entire practice, or buying into a practice and becoming a partner.

Selecting among these ownership transitions is, in part, a financial decision and, in part, a management decision. The buyer's quandary is, do they set up a practice or buy an existing practice? If they buy a practice, they buy an ongoing business with existing staff, location, patient base, and cash flow. If they set up a practice, they have complete control over the site and location, new equipment, and the facility they want. They must hire staff and generate patients, but both will be the ones they want. They will need to borrow additionally for working capital, but they are not paying for the patient base. From a purely financial perspective, it is possible to develop a spreadsheet that purports to show the outcome of the buy or start-up decision. It is based on the assumptions that the spreadsheet creator uses, however, and it can show either outcome as superior. Generally, purchasing a practice in a more competitive dental marketplace comes out ahead financially because of the built-in patient base and the resulting immediate cash flow. This is especially true for more experienced practitioners. In a less competitive area where someone can be busy from the first day, they do not need the additional cost of buying a patient base. It becomes less expensive to establish a practice.

STARTING A DENTAL PRACTICE (DE NOVO)

Starting a practice is also called a *De Novo* because the person starts from the beginning.

RELATIVE ADVANTAGES AND DISADVANTAGES

There is no single transition path that is appropriate for all practitioners. Starting a practice poses issues that some may see as advantages and others as disadvantages.

Advantages

The advantages of a de novo relate to the fact that a dentist can make the dental practice exactly what they want it to be. It is their practice, including business systems, practice philosophy, and managed care participation. The location, the design of the office, and the staff will all be what the dentist wants, not what a previous owner wanted. New offices and equipment need less maintenance and repair. New practices may be less expensive because the buyer is not paying for "goodwill." If the area chosen is in high need of dentists, the newcomer does not need to buy goodwill. If someone can be relatively busy from the beginning and grow at an acceptable rate, they do not need to pay someone else for a patient pool.

The dentist controls the regional and specific site location of the practice. They may want to buy into a practice in a particular area, but if no dentists are interested they obviously cannot buy in. That is not the case with a practice set-up. Similarly, the office design and equipment selection will fit their criteria, not what exists in the facility.

Dentists can grow professionally with the patient pool when they start a practice. Initially, their clinical speed will not be as high as it will be later. (Clinical speed comes from decision-making, not just hand skills.) So clinical speed increases as the patient pool and practice "busyness" increase.

Disadvantages

On the downside, starting an office from scratch can be more expensive because the dentist generally buys new equipment and supplies. Establishing a new practice takes six months from the idea to the first patient visit. If the dentist is not working or in school during this time, they have lost a half-year's income, adding to the expense. New offices take much time, effort, and many headaches to develop.

A new practice does not have a patient base. Depending on the area, it may be easy or difficult to market and build a patient base. Because of this, new dental practices generally have cash-flow problems. New practitioners must borrow additional working capital (often about three months' expenses) to weather this problem. Insurance plan participation currently drives dental marketing in many areas. These plans result in lower income from plan-fee requirements, leading to lower cash flow and lower profit in new practices in these areas. Because of this, bankers are warier about financing a practice that does not have a demonstrated cash flow.

LOCATING THE PRACTICE

The first problem a dentist faces in a de novo is finding a location for a new practice. These are two different problems. The first is finding a general region, and the second is finding a specific site.

Regional Location

Many new dentists had already decided when they entered a dental school where they planned to practice. They are from a specific town or area and have always wanted to return to that area to practice. Their decision is easy – the decision is tougher for the buyer with no pre-established region to move into. The latter must examine their desires and then do a lot of homework to find an area that meets their needs.

Site Location

Once someone selects a region or general area to practice in, the next decision involves picking a specific site for the practice. Marketing gurus say that there are only three factors to consider in developing a successful business: location, location, and location. Although this is an oversimplification, it points to the importance of specific site selection in practice development.

There are many types of locations for dental offices, each with pros and cons (Box 4.1). Freestanding buildings, either owned or leased, are becoming less common as commercial real estate gets more expensive. Medical office buildings are accessible to the public, have ample parking, and lend an air of professionalism. These landlords are used to the specific needs of professionals, which can be helpful. These sites are expensive, however. Many are condominium-type arrangements, in which someone purchases the office and then pays a fee to the condominium association for maintenance and repairs. Strip-type shopping centers have adequate parking and are generally on a significant road, giving high visibility. They are relatively expensive. The landlord is usually responsible for snow removal and other everyday maintenance items, although they generally charge the lessee

(dentist) a maintenance fee to cover these items. The lessee usually must purchase and maintain heating and air-conditioning units.

The practitioner should check the types of businesses the property owner caters to. A dentist probably does not want a pawnbroker, tattoo parlor, or head shop opening next to their office. Large shopping malls are the highest-cost location. Set-up costs are high because most retail space is not set up for plumbing, electrical, and other dental office improvements. Malls often charge high rent and sometimes a percentage of gross sales. The practitioner should try to negotiate this out of the lease. Like in strip malls, the practitioner is usually responsible for utility upkeep. General office buildings may be the least expensive alternative. Location and parking may or may not be optimal. The advantages of these sites are on a case-by-case basis.

Visibility The dental office should be easily seen by as many people as possible. The dentist should try to find a busy street or major thoroughfare to place the office in. They want to be seen often enough that they lie in the back of people's minds. When people decide to look for a dentist, the dentist that they have passed by frequently is one of the first names that pop up. People must know where the practitioner is.

The practitioner needs to invest in a good sign. This sign ought to "cut through the clutter" of the other signs that compete for people's attention. That is not to say that sign must be the biggest, but it must be as large as the others. That also does not mean they need a flashing neon sign unless the office is on the strip in Las Vegas. Signage is even more important if the office is in a retail center or an office building. In these cases, the sign is the dentist's drive-by visibility.

BOX 4.1	TYPES OF LOCATIONS FOR DENTAL OFFICES	
	Set-up cost	Lease cost
Location strip mall	Medium	High
Major mall	High	Very high
Medical office building	High	High
Individual office building	Very high	High
Leased building	Medium	Low

Accessibility   The dental office must be easy to get to. The practitioner should imagine how a receptionist would tell people how to find the office. They ought to be able to describe the location in 15 words or fewer. "Right across from the hospital in the Doctor's Park Office Building, Suite 221" is accessible for most people to find. "Take Main Street south to the third light; right on Oak for two blocks, then down the alley on the left for 200 feet" is not easy. The dentist must ensure adequate parking and an accessible entrance and exit from the street. (Modern dental patients expect adequate parking.) If they are practicing in an urban area, they should consider the location of public transportation. The practitioner should also be sure that there are no physical barriers to entry (e.g. steps without a disabled-accessible ramp). In a new office, the practitioner must meet building codes regarding disabled accessibility. The architect or designer will know the codes.

Zoning   Before signing for any property, the practice owner must be sure that the zoning will allow a dental office on the site. The practitioner must take care, particularly in residential areas, that they have permission before committing any money. Zoning changes do not always go as expected. Legal fees can mount quickly if a citizen's action group or another developer wants to challenge a zoning request.

DEVELOPING THE FACILITY

Once the practitioner decides on a location, they must develop the facility where they will practice.

Lease versus Buy

Most dentists today lease space for their offices. Many who do own are owners in a condominium arrangement. Many owners believe that owning their building insulates them from the problems of having a landlord. That is true, but it brings with it the problems of ownership. When the plumbing breaks down, the practitioner is responsible for fixing it. Changing tax laws may reduce or increase the value of ownership.

If a dentist is going to lease, they must know that most commercial property is priced on a square-foot-per-year basis, such that "$13 a foot" for a 1000 square-foot office is $13 000 yearly or $1083 per month. Depending on the state of commercial real estate in the area, the practitioner can negotiate specific clauses into the lease. They want the property owner to pay as many ancillary costs as they can negotiate. These include general maintenance, plumbing, heating and air conditioning, snow removal (if

appropriate), and cleaning of the common areas. Leasehold improvements (improvements that the practice owner makes to the landlord's property) are expensive for a dental office. This is primarily because of the extensive plumbing needs. (Each operatory requires hot and cold water, waste, air, vacuum, nitrous, oxygen, and electrical outlets.) Many dentists have negotiated a given amount (e.g. $10 000) for leasehold improvements. Others have gotten months of free rent while the owner–dentist makes the improvements. When a dentist negotiates any of these items, they should be sure that they write these items into the lease. The landlord may be noble and true. However, if the landlord sells to another party, there is no record of verbal agreements. Many landlords want a professional office in their space. Dentists are excellent, high-class, long-term tenants. So, the practice owner does have some bargaining leverage.

Designing the Office   The owner–dentist should get a book on dental office design and visit as many offices as possible, asking other practitioners for suggestions for improving their space. The office owner is going to have to live in the space for many years to come, so they need to make it a place with which they are comfortable. The office owner may consult an interior decorator or designer to assist with color and wallpaper selection.

If the practitioner builds a freestanding building (shell) from scratch, they will probably use an architect or construction engineer familiar with dental office construction needs. Most full-service equipment dealers have one or more staff members familiar with dental office design. Most will work with the practitioner and complete the design for free (or at a nominal cost), with the understanding that the dentist is going to buy the equipment from that dealer. These dealers may also help them find space. They know the building codes related to dental offices and the requirements for inspection and certification for a particular state. They may even have several general contractors they have used who are familiar with dental practice construction.

The office owner must let the designer know what they want in an office design. The designer will probably bring a couple of preliminary designs for review. The practitioner needs to study the designs to find the features of each that they do and do not like. They should then take suggestions back to the designer and continue doing this until they are happy with the design. Once construction begins, changes become *very* expensive. The office owner will probably want a general contractor if they are making substantial changes to an existing office space. Again, the equipment dealer can help them find one.

General Design Decisions

There are unique design criteria for operatories and x-ray areas. The dentist must decide if they want open operatories or closed rooms. Either one works, depending on the office owner's style. Pass-through x-ray heads save costs if they can be designed to reach chairs in both operatories. They often cannot, however. The type of equipment being bought may determine, in part, the design of the operatories and support areas. Traffic patterns should be convenient for patients, staff, and the dentist. The office owner must place high-traffic areas near the front, making patient traffic patterns as short as possible. This also relieves congestion in hallways. The hygienist probably will see more patients a day than the dentist. Therefore, the hygienist's operatory should be nearer to the patient reception area.

The dental office must have a centrally located sterilization area. Employees will need a large counter space for breaking down trays and cassettes; a deep double sink to wash instruments; another for packaging and autoclaving; and more for preparing and storing sterile trays and cassettes. A dental office will need a minimum of 10–12 ft of counter space for efficient instrument sterilization. If the office has cabinets below and above the counter, there must be enough space for office sterilization procedures. Many people use the lab for this space. Separate areas, however, are a better idea.

Some areas are low-use areas, which need to be away from high-traffic areas. Staff lounge areas and mechanical rooms are often noisy and smelly; those should be away from patient treatment and traffic areas. Private offices are luxuries and should also be out of the traffic flow. There need to be public restrooms if the office is in a stand-alone building or is freestanding. These restrooms need to be near the patient waiting room but under the control of the staff. (It is amazing what kids try to flush down the toilet.)

Most designs do not have a large enough business office area. Dental business offices need significant counter space for electronic gadgets, such as a computer, printer, fax, copier, answering machine, and maybe an old-fashioned typewriter. The more storage, the better. As paper patient chart numbers increase, so do storage requirements. (Electronic charts do not have this problem.) Front-office personnel should not make collection or other private patient calls within hearing of patients in the reception room or treatment areas. The office should have a separate room, near the business office but closed off with a door, for making these telephone contacts. There should be a counter, at elbow height near but out of the patient flow, for patients to write checks or sign charge slips. It must also include a pen.

The reception area ought to be just that. Patients should be received, not made to wait there. If the dentist and patients are both on time, there is minimal waiting. Rural practices and practices that see many children will often have family members waiting for the patient to receive treatment. In these cases, a larger waiting room is helpful. The lab is a seldom-used area and should be in a peripheral, low-use section. The same goes for the private office. If a dentist sits at a desk, they are not seeing patients or generating any money. The office should be a low-priority, low-use area as well. Many dentists like a consultation area for patient treatment plan presentation and financial arrangements. If the office owner wants one, it should be a separate room near the patient traffic flow area.

Ordering Equipment and Supplies If a dentist purchases new operatory equipment, they must be sure to order it several months before they need it. Most of the equipment will be in stock, but some critical pieces (like a compressor) may be back-ordered (not in stock). The equipment supplier will help the office owner by providing lists of instruments and materials. The owner will also need to order business office equipment and supplies, including accounting packages, patient records, and office stationery.

STAFFING THE OFFICE

The practitioner must begin to staff the office at least six weeks before opening. This assumes that it will take them three weeks to find the right people, two weeks before those people can come to work, and a week of training and preparation. Practitioners can use friends and family for mock patient visits and phone calls to prepare for the first day of patients.

The dentist should try to find an experienced front-office person at the beginning of practice. An experienced person can help to set up the office systems and be aware of forms and procedures that the dentist does not know. Eventually that person may leave, but by then the office will function smoothly, and the office owner will be much more knowledgeable about how they want to operate.

FINANCING THE OFFICE

Most banks and finance companies will qualify a dentist for a line of credit. The office owner then taps into this line whenever a bill comes due. The practitioner needs to be sure to establish a line of credit for working capital as well. As a rule, they need to plan on three months' expenses as needed for working capital.

If the practitioner is going to own their building, they will probably need to arrange finance. Banks are generally willing to lend 80–90% of the cost of appraised real estate, and the office owner will need to come up with the remainder as a down payment. If they are also buying a practice or equipping an office, they may be entering into more debt than the banks will allow.

BUYING AN EXISTING PRACTICING (BUY-OUT)

Another option for a dentist to enter practice is to buy an existing practice.

Most dentists hire a consultant to help with a practice's valuation, purchase, and transfer. Someone may do this once or twice in their lifetime, and a transition consultant does it many times yearly. Usually, the seller will hire a broker to value, advertise, and sell the practice. Most brokers charge a percentage of the sale price to the seller as a commission. (Some charge a flat fee.) Some brokers claim to work for both sides in a transfer. It is not easy to represent both sides when one side is paying the broker, and the other is not. The buyer should have a different advisor work with them. Although an added expense, it is worth it (financially and emotionally) to have someone who is looking out for the buyer's interests in the process.

REASONS TO BUY AN EXISTING PRACTICE

For some reasons it makes sense to buy an existing practice rather than starting a practice from scratch. Some of these reasons relate to a dentist's particular style. A decision that makes good sense for one dentist may not fit the personality, style, or goals of another. Other reasons are financial, and a particular purchase deal might make better financial sense than starting a practice. A dental graduate should explore both areas before making an informed purchase decision.

All these discussions assume that the buyer can maintain the practice's production at the current level. A new practitioner looking at a large, established practice may not have the skills and professional maturity to handle a large practice. It would be foolish to pay top dollar for a productive practice when the production would decrease dramatically the first day they took over. So, purchasing a practice is a more significant advantage for an experienced clinician who can maintain high production levels.

Advantages of Buying a Practice

From a financial perspective, purchasing a practice may allow the buyer to make more money than a cold start. This occurs more in areas where patient competition is higher because the dentist has a built-in patient pool. The buyer will have a full book of patients from the first day, and they will have more cash flow because of those immediate patient visits. When starting a practice from scratch, a dentist may lose time when the office is not open because of construction delays or equipment delivery schedules. A dentist generally buys new equipment for a new office. Although this equipment needs fewer repairs, it costs more for the initial outlay. If the practitioner purchases the accounts receivable of an existing practice, they will not need as much working capital or start-up cash. A buying dentist probably will not need to recruit staff for the office immediately. Hopefully, existing staff will remain when the new dentist takes over.

From a personal perspective, purchasing a practice may decrease stress. The buyer knows that the practice can succeed. They do not have to worry about construction problems and delays. There is an immediate cash flow. The buyer has the reputation of the departing dentist to rely on. Often, the new dentist may gain the departing dentist's expertise by using a long-term consulting agreement. When someone purchases a practice, they buy the ongoing business systems: the accounting, inventory, and patient billing systems do not have to be set up.

Disadvantages of Buying a Practice

All the advantages come with a price; the financial price is called *goodwill* or the value of the ongoing business concern. (Chapter 5 discusses goodwill in more detail.) The buyer is paying the departing owner extra money, above the cost of the readily apparent assets of the practice, with the expectation that the practice's profit will flow to the new dentist. If the new dentist pays too much for the practice, then the payments will eat up any increase in the long-term money generated over a cold start. Similarly, if someone does not get a good transfer of patients (at least 90%), the practice price may be too high. From a financial perspective, buying a practice gives the new dentist higher costs than starting a practice from scratch, but an immediate cash flow to help cover those costs. The practice's value (cost) is a critical factor in the decision. If the area needs dentists and the new dentist can be busy when they open the door, it generally makes financial sense to start rather than buy out a practice.

As a dentist ages, the patient pool typically ages with them as children grow up and move away. If someone is buying the practice of an older dentist, then they may need to do significant marketing to gain a younger patient pool. Some older dentists have not updated their equipment in many years. If a dentist buys such a practice, they need to include the cost of significant facility and equipment updates in their estimate of what the practice will cost them.

From a personal perspective, the buyer buys the outgoing dentist's reputation, good or bad. It takes many years to change a community's perception of a dental practice, even if the practitioner has changed. Suppose the previous dentist's style was to fix holes in people's teeth. In that case, it will take a considerable amount of time for a new dentist to change the character of the practice to one of comprehensive periodontal and restorative services. If the new dentist is completely changing the character of the practice, why buy it? The immediate cash-flow advantages may not be worth the extra effort.

TYPES OF PRACTICES FOR SALE

Dentists who sell their practice typically fall into one of six groups. Understanding these groups is essential so the buyer can negotiate more effectively for the practice.

Retiring Dentists

Retiring dentists make up the first group. These older dentists are usually more concerned with finding the right person to care for their beloved patient pool than getting an excellent price. Depending on their practice style, they may have a large portion of the patient pool that needs advanced periodontal and restorative needs. The new owner–dentist must continue carefully with these patients to introduce them to modern dentistry's advantages without insulting the former dentist as providing out-of-date dentistry.

Young Dentists Changing Career Paths

Many dentists who have been in practice for several years decide to change their career paths. This often involves specialty training or moving to military or public health career options. Depending on the history and price of these practices, they can be an excellent opportunity. The buyer should be careful if the practice has shown good growth and profitability, because these young practices can show good gross income, but because of managed care and other write-offs have poor profitability.

Dentists with Personal Problems

Often, dentists who have significant personal problems may be selling their practices. This may involve a nasty divorce, depression over the death of a loved one, personal bankruptcy, or other personal problems. The buyer should approach these practices with caution. The potential buyer might be buying a host of issues, such as the dentist's reputation in the community, unpaid tax liens, future divorce court problems, or competition from the former dentist after they have resolved their problems.

Dentists with Health Problems

The potential buyer may occasionally find a practice available from a dentist with a disabling health problem. This may be the result of an accident or disease. The negotiations for many of these practices can be complex. The owner does not want to leave the practice; their medical condition is forcing them out. Here, the buyer needs to be careful not to pay too much through sympathy for the other dentist's condition. However, the buyer also does not want to offend the seller by being insensitive to their needs. If the seller has accepted their condition, the buyer can generally find a reasonably priced, valuable practice.

Death of a Dentist

If the owner–dentist dies unexpectedly, the most critical issue for all concerned is time. The longer the practice remains closed, the more patients will find another provider. After about three months of inactivity, there is very little goodwill value left in the practice of a dead dentist, and a buyer will pay for the equipment and other hard assets at that point. If the buyer is fortunate enough to buy and practice in the office soon after the other dentist's demise, they will get a fair value and save the estate a significant amount of money. Although it sounds cold, contacting the estate soon after the dentist's death helps preserve the practice's value for the estate. It can get complicated, but it is absolutely in the survivors' best interest to sell the practice as quickly as possible.

Entrepreneur Dentists

Some dentists think highly of their business and clinical skills, and they believe that no one can establish a practice like they can. They then establish practices with the notion of selling them to young dentists. Although these may be acceptable practices, they are often overvalued. Nevertheless, the selling dentist is quite a business person and can sound quite convincing in discussions with potential buyers.

TYPES OF BUY-OUTS

Buy-outs fall into three general classes.

Walk-Away Sale

In this sale, the (previous) owner walks away from the practice when the buyer purchases it. In this scenario, the buyer owns the practice upon closing the purchase deal. The next day, the buyer is in the practice, and the previous owner is not. The buyer and seller need arrangements to handle accounts receivable, patient questions, and staff concerns.

This is not to say that this type of transition is always a complete surprise. Often negotiations are private, with an announcement when the parties sign and complete the deal. Two interested groups are the staff and the patients. Staff members want to know that they will still have a job under similar terms and conditions as they did previously. The buyer should hold a staff meeting with the outgoing dentist to assure staff members that this is the case. Patients may have a long-trusted relationship with the previous practitioner. The owner needs to write a letter to patients of record, informing them of their intention and urging patients to remain in the practice to see the new dentist for their dental care.

Transition

In this buy-out, the (previous) owner works for a short time to help in the transition. This may be from a few weeks to six months. This transition helps comfort the new dentist by knowing they have someone to ask questions and help with clinical or management problems. Sometimes, the new dentist pays the outgoing dentist a consulting fee (as part of the purchase price). Generally, the new dentist finds that they do not need the outgoing dentist as much as they thought. Instead, the outgoing dentist begins to be a burden. Staff are not sure whom to report or complain to, patients often still want to see the outgoing dentist, and some departing dentists give unwanted opinions about changes the new dentist wants to make.

Trading Roles

In this buy-out, the (previous) owner works long term as an associate in the practice for the new owner. The problems are like with a transition, in that staff and patients may show allegiance to the former owner. This buy-out works best if the new owner has done an extended associateship in the practice before the buy-out. In this way, patients and staff members become familiar with both dentists.

WHAT A DENTIST IS BUYING

When someone purchases a dental practice, they are paying in the hope that the profit the practice has shown in the past will come to them. The buyer buys dental equipment, charts, goodwill, and other assets because they believe they can use them to make money. They do not buy them because they have intrinsic value or are collectors' items. The assets are only instrumental to what the buyer is purchasing, which is the demonstrated profit of the ongoing concern of the practice as a business entity.

The buyer hopes that the profits of the practice will transfer to them. To help this, the new dentist wants to make a few changes to the office until the patients have transferred their allegiance to them. (Generally, this is one or two recall cycles.) The more alike the new dentist and the departing dentist are, the more likely it is that patients will transfer and remain. Patients select a practice for their reasons, not the dentist's reasons. The patient pool that the departing dentist has built over the years selected that dentist for their reasons; the buyer should try to cater to them.

FINANCING THE PURCHASE

Many buying dentists become too concerned with the simple price of the practice. Instead of asking "How much is the practice?" they ought to ask "How much will I make when I buy the practice?" The method of financing the practice sale dramatically affects the financial outcome of the practice transfer. Chapter 6 discusses these options.

TRANSFER CONSIDERATIONS

There are several unique issues to consider in transferring practices from one owner to another. A brief discussion of several of these issues follows.

Buying a Practice and Real Estate

Some practices are in freestanding office buildings. If a dentist buys this practice, they need assurances that it can stay in the same exact location to transfer income-generating potential. The departing owner may want to sell the building to the buyer, or the owner may want to continue to own the building but offer a long-term lease. The owner may retain and lease the building to add to retirement or investment income. The new owner must ensure that a long-term lease is included in the practice purchase. An advantage for the buyer is a right of first refusal to purchase the building if the owner decides to sell it.

If the owner insists on selling the building with the practice, the buyer faces additional financial problems. Valuing the building is relatively easy: a reputable real estate appraiser can appraise the real estate. Securing financing for real estate may be more difficult. Many buyers are financially stretched to purchase the practice, have little collateral to pledge, and are concurrently borrowing to buy homes, cars, and other personal items. Buying a piece of real estate may increase the new dentist's debt level beyond what a banker believes is prudent. Understandably, the banker might not finance the loan.

On the other hand, real estate is tangible. Bankers may be willing to finance a higher percentage of the value of real property than intangible property such as goodwill. (Bankers often require 20% of the property value as a down payment, financing the remaining 80%.) The dentist should perform careful cash-flow and pro-forma income analyses here. If the numbers look right, the buyer might work with the bank for the real estate loan and use owner financing for the practice purchase (or vice versa). If the buyer purchases the real estate, they must allocate the price to land and building. Buildings are depreciable, and the land is not depreciable. The buyer wants to allocate as much as reasonable to the building.

Price and Other Considerations

The price that someone negotiates ought to be based on the actual value of the practice. Whether or not they can afford the price may be determined by other considerations thrown into the equation. For example, the whole deal may be contingent on the owner financing half the practice. Part of the price may be paid in consulting fees that the buyer pays to the seller. These fees come out of practice profits over time and so do not come into the stated price for the practice. They do affect the extended price of the practice, however. The owner may agree to stay for a certain length of time to aid in the transfer by introducing patients to the new owner, and even by doing some work on those patients for a reduced (or no) fee to the buyer. All these side deals can help justify the price or make the buyout work; they should not be overlooked. Nevertheless, the buyer must also not allow them to sell a bad deal. If the practice is overpriced, the potential buyer must not purchase the practice.

Intrafamily Transfers

The IRS looks closely at Intrafamily transfers. It realizes that many small business owners might want to transfer a business to their children or relatives at less than its actual value to avoid taxes. The IRS rule in these cases is "substance over form." This rule means that the reality of the transfer governs how it is taxed, not merely what the dentist says the form is. If the transfer is a gift, then the value of the practice is included in the Uniform Gift and Estate Tax. The transfer is then taxed as a gift. This frequently happens when someone sells their practice to a child for much less than the actual value and reports the transaction

as tax law requires. It is difficult for the IRS to track a dentist who closes the doors to the practice and then their child establishes a practice the next day in the exact location under a new name.

Accounts Receivable

The issue of purchasing accounts receivable is often contentious in practice purchases. The seller believes the accounts receivable should carry a higher value than the buyer. The buyer would like immediate cash flow without getting an additional line of credit for working capital, but only if the price is right. Buyers have the additional trouble of educating patients about an accounts receivable purchase. Many patients want to pay the departed dentist, not the new one, and others do not want to pay either one. The buyer cannot aggressively pursue these accounts without risking offending the patient pool, which they have just paid a considerable amount of money for as goodwill.

It is generally easiest to keep the accounts receivable out of the purchase price of a dental practice. (The buyer will usually need to borrow working capital.) The previous owner can collect the accounts as aggressively as they wish, and the new owner is relatively immune from patients' anger in this situation. The other standard method of handling these accounts is for the buyer to use typical collection methods to collect the accounts for the seller. (The buyer generally uses the seller's name for one year.) The seller then deducts a nominal amount, such as 10%, for collecting the accounts and then sends the remainder (90%) to the seller. After six months, the buyer may turn over any uncollected accounts to a collection agent.

Minimizing Change

As a rule, new practitioners should make as few initial changes as possible in practice. They should not rush in to paint the walls or hang new wallpaper. They have paid for the patients, and the buyer wants them to think that nothing has changed until the patients become accustomed to the new practitioner. If changes are required for safety reasons (e.g. the previous owner did not take good health histories), the new dentist must do what they need to be safe. However, if a picture is not straight on the wall, the new dentist should let it remain crooked for a year. After the patients have bonded with them, the buyer can make cosmetic and structural changes. The new dentist should also try to keep staff for the initial period because many patients are as close to the staff members as the dentist.

Length of Overlap

Many new dentists want a long period when the seller remains in the office. The belief is that this period of overlapping clinical time helps transfer patients. It only helps a small amount. (If they have taken care of the other factors, the patient transfer will occur.) What often happens is that the buyer, because of insecurity in their management and patient relations abilities, wants the seller to stay on as a crutch. However, the seller will get in the way after the first month. Patients will want to continue to see the seller if they think there is a choice. Staff will take problems (real or perceived) to the former owner. By the second month, the seller will be a problem. The buyer will want the former dentist out of the office by the third month. The buyer needs to use a good letter of introduction and other methods to encourage an immediate transfer and quickly get the seller out of the practice.

Patient Records

Sellers need access to records if a former patient sues them. Otherwise, the buyer generally buys the records. That means the buyer has bought exclusive business rights to the information in the records. The medical information in the record belongs to the patient. Suppose the patient requests that the dentist send their records to another dentist. In that case, the new dentist has an ethical obligation to send that information (written and radiographic) so that the patient's health is not compromised. The dentist does not send originals, only copies. (Many states allow the dentist to charge a nominal amount for copying records.) The dentist may not refuse to send a copy of the record because a patient still owes money (that is a separate issue) or because they do not like the other dentist. A dentist may (in most states) require the patient's signature to release medical information.

Buying Out an Incorporated Practice

Most dental practice business purchases are asset purchases. When someone buys the stock of an existing corporation, they take over the corporation and everything that comes with it. This includes assets and liabilities, leases, accounts, and unknown liabilities (such as employee claims against the previous business). When someone purchases an asset, they acquire only the assets and any liabilities the contract identifies. For these reasons, the buying dentist will purchase the assets, leaving the corporate shell with the previous owner. Buyers should be sure to list any assets or liabilities they want in the purchase agreement. For example, the previous owner (corporation) may have a lease on equipment that the buyer may or may not want to continue.

TYPICAL ORDER OF BUSINESS

Practice purchases follow similar patterns. The details of the individual practice purchase are different in each one, but the two parties must resolve many common issues for the purchase to work. The first thing to decide is if the seller wants to sell the practice. Often practitioners feel pressure from family or peers to retire or sell for other reasons. The owner, however, really does not want to sell. It may sound like a good idea initially, but as they draw closer to making the deal, the seller begins to get cold feet and back out of the sale. Other times, a retiring dentist may visit their accountant and find out that the deal they are negotiating does not leave enough money, after taxes, to fund the retirement as envisioned by the owner. Regardless of the reason, many sellers decide to back out of the sale late in the process. The buyer must try to be sure that this dentist wants to sell.

In all negotiations, the buyer must remember to produce at the seller's level, or higher, for the numbers to make sense. Otherwise, the profitability of the practice goes down. The buyer is buying the income generation of the practice. For example, assume a seller is producing $600 000 per year. The buyer buys the practice, but they can only do $400 000 of production. The buyer has suddenly turned that practice that makes $600 000 into a practice that produces $400 000 overnight. Would the buyer have bought the practice for the same amount if it produced $400 000? Probably not. The buyer must also keep the overhead at the seller's level. Otherwise, profits go down. If the owner's spouse worked in the office for free, profits would go down when the new owner hires someone to replace the previous owner's spouse. (Unless the spouse agrees to work free over the long term for the new dentist, which is an unlikely scenario!) The buyer will also have increased costs from equipment and supply changeover and from making a large mortgage payment to the bank.

Locating a Practice

The most difficult step may be finding a practice for sale in the area where the dentist wants to buy. In some areas, there may be only a few dentists. None of them may want to sell. Metropolitan areas offer more dentists wanting to sell at any given time but more new dentists looking to buy. The prospective buyer may not find a practice where they want when they want to buy it. Often the selling dentist does not want anyone else (like patients or other dentists) to know that they are selling their practice. They will generally use a practice broker or local accountant to develop confidential leads. If buyers have not expressed an interest in that broker, they may miss the opportunity. (Even if the buyer has, the broker may select someone else as the "chosen one" for this practice.) Equipment dealers and supply representatives often know who is looking to sell a practice. Many new dentists have found practices when working for temporary agencies. The best way to find a practice is to network with other dentists; a dentist should let other dentists know they are looking in an area. A potential buyer needs to be diligent and attend the local dental society meeting, join a study club, or become a member of the local professional community. A practice broker can help the potential buyer find and develop possible practices. The potential buyer ought to talk to everyone they can and let their intentions be known.

Investigating the Practice

When the dentist finds a potential practice to buy, they need to thoroughly investigate the practice to confirm the accuracy of the seller's information and ensure there are no hidden problems. This process is called "due diligence." Most dentists use an accountant, management consultant, or another professional familiar with transitions to help with the analysis. Initially, the buyer will meet the selling dentist and examine the office. They should ask questions about the organization and operations of the practice. The buyer needs to look at the schedule book and determine the number of patients available for transfer. During the initial visits, the owner probably will not give the buyer access to detailed financial records because the owner wants the buyer to be serious about the practice before showing tax returns and other crucial financial information. The selling dentist will decide if the buyer is the person that they want to take over the practice. Part of their assessment is an appraisal of the buyer's financial condition. The owner will want to know if the buyer has money or collateral to arrange finance or if they will need to offer owner financing.

Some selling dentists have brochures describing their practice. Others have a few numbers jotted down on the back of a napkin. Regardless, when someone is seriously discussing buying the practice, the seller must provide some essential things. One is a recent equipment appraisal done by a reputable supply house. Secondly, the seller will need to provide the last three years' tax returns for the office. (The buyer will need this for their financial analysis and for the banks to make theirs.) The notion is that anyone can put numbers on a piece of paper. What they report to the IRS is usually the most accurate information. Some practices, mainly if the seller owns multiple practices grouped on their tax return, will have an accountant's report that breaks this practice's numbers out from the others. Some selling dentists will require that a buyer signs a non-disclosure form. This says that the buyer agrees not to share this information with anyone except their professional advisors. This is reasonable because it often contains sensitive personal financial and tax information. Other dentists ask the buyer to sign a form of a restrictive covenant that says if the seller shows their financial information, they agree not to set up a competing practice in the same area. The buyer must avoid such arrangements if the seller is interested in staying in the area. They are often promoted by dentists who think much more of their practices than they should.

The buyer may want to have help in negotiations. Often the selling dentist will have professional help in developing a practice value and identifying potential leads. These people may claim to be able to represent both sides, and that is difficult for anyone to do. The seller usually pays the broker anywhere from 5% to 10% of the purchase price as a sales commission. The buyer should see where the broker's loyalties lie. The buyer needs to consult an accountant or management consultant to ensure that someone looks after their interests. (The buyer will pay this person a reasonable amount for their time, effort, and knowledge.)

Making an Offer

The owner–dentist needs to state (in writing) the price that they are asking for the practice. (Often, they ask the buyer to propose a price. The seller needs to make the first offer.) The buyer can then accept or reject the offer or make a counteroffer. A counteroffer says, "No, I do not accept your offer, but I would buy the practice at this price and for these terms." Any offer or counteroffer needs to be in writing. At this point, the buyer begins negotiations. They probably do not want to make a low counteroffer, but they also do not want to make one that the owner instantly accepts. The buyer negotiates what they believe is the fair value of the practice. They cannot worry if the seller is going to lose money; that is the seller's problem. The buyer does not want to bail the owner out because they made bad business decisions in the past. On the other hand, the buyer does not want to foul a deal that does make sense by insulting the seller with a lowball offer.

Most offers contain contingencies. These are qualifiers that the buyer or the owner must meet before the deal can proceed. Some common contingencies in offers include:

- The buyer must gain acceptable (to the seller) financing from a bank.

- The buyer must gain a dental license for the state of practice.

- The equipment must be in good working order at the time of transfer.

- The owner will agree to a restrictive covenant of X miles and Y years.

- The owner will write a letter (acceptable to the buyer) to all the practice's current patients, informing them of the transfer and urging them to continue patronage.

When the buyer has negotiated an acceptable deal for both sides, they send a letter of acceptance. (The buyer can consummate the deal with a handshake, but many people have been disappointed by final contracts or sales because of what one side "thought" was in the offer.) This letter spells out the buyer's offer and conditions. At this point, some sellers want the buyer to put down some "earnest money" to show that they are serious; others do not because they figure that the buyer has come this far, so they must be serious.

Securing Financing

The buyer should not wait until this point to talk to a banker. As soon as they find a desirable practice, they ought to begin discussions with a banker to determine what the banker needs to make a loan. (Many dentists begin talking with a banker before they find a practice.) Bankers can also act as advisors and ensure that a buyer does not make too many mistakes. The buyer should talk with colleagues to find out which banks are making loans to professionals and should talk with more than one bank. Different banks have different strategies regarding the types of clients they are trying to gain: one bank may not be seeking professional clients, whereas another may. Chapter 6 describes the typical types of loans that a dentist can find for practice purchases and the type of information that a banker will want to have.

Making the Transfer

Once the details have been ironed out, the transfer itself is almost anticlimactic. The buyer will get together with the seller, often at the banker's office, sign a few papers, and the buyer is a practice owner! However, the buyer's job is not over. (They should have done the following tasks before the closing date.) The buyer needs to find an accountant who they are comfortable with and who has other dentists as clients. The seller must transfer the lease for the office from them to the buyer. The buyer needs to contact the various utilities (water, gas and electric, telephone, etc.) to be sure that the account will be in the buyer's name. The buyer will need to pay any utility deposits as well. (Often, sellers include the deposit cost in the practice purchase price. The buyer pays the seller, and the seller calls the utility and transfers the deposit to the buyer's name.) They must call insurance agents (workers' compensation, business liability, malpractice, and office overhead) to ensure their coverage is in effect. The buyer must secure a federal tax identification number if they do not have one. They need to check if they need a state or local tax number or account. The buyer should find out if they can convert any reserve in the seller's unemployment account into their name. They must call their software vendor to change the name in the office computer system and the support contract if there is one. The buyer needs to open an office checking account at a local Federal Reserve bank and get an office checkbook. They should call the disability insurance agent to ensure they are covered for the new expected income level. Finally, the buyer needs to take their spouse or significant other out to dinner, celebrate the accomplishment, and contemplate the future.

BUYING INTO AN EXISTING PRACTICE (BUY-IN)

Buying into a dental practice is similar to buying out a practice, and the buyer should select a location and specific practice in the same way. The practice is valued similarly, and the issues of transferring ownership are comparable. However, there are a couple of significant differences that change the game dramatically:

- The buyer is buying only part of the income-generating potential of the practice. When they purchase a practice outright, the buyer buys all the income generation of the practice. When buying into a practice, the buyer must ensure adequate patients for the new number of practitioners.

- The dentists are forming or joining a group practice. Group practices have problems and advantages that differ from individual practitioners. (See Chapter 3.) When someone puts money on the table for a buy-in, they make a decision that is difficult to undo, and the buyer must be sure that it is the correct one.

Advantages of Buying into a Practice

When someone buys into a practice, they know that the dentist's owner believes in it. Otherwise, they would not plan to stay. Like buying an entire practice, the buyer has the advantage of an ongoing business with continuing cash flow, staff, patients, and equipment. If the price is right, then the buyer ought to make more money, in the long run, than when establishing a practice from scratch. New practitioners have the advantage of an experienced practitioner on the premises for clinical and management advice. The buyer also has all the advantages that a group practice shows.

Disadvantages of Buying into a Practice

The most significant disadvantage of buying into a practice relates to the group that results. If someone does not want a group practice situation or is unsure about future partners as coprofessionals, then they should not get involved in this type of relationship. Another problem happens if the original dentist wants to retire or leave and wants to sell their portion of the practice. However, the new dentist may be busy enough that they do not want to buy the other half of the practice. This leaves the older dentist to find someone else to buy their half. It can be a problem finding someone, especially someone the new dentist is compatible with. This means that once dentists establish a group practice, they will probably be involved in a group for the rest of their careers.

The second major problem occurs if the buyer ends the professional relationship. Who will buy the buyer's part interest in a dental practice? They will probably discount the value of their portion of the practice to compensate for the new owner's uncertainty about moving into an established practice. If the buyer tries to split the group up, the contract will probably have significant restrictions and covenants for future practice.

As these two examples show, when dentists plan a group practice, one of the first tasks is to decide the process and procedures if the group dissolves.

TYPES OF BUY-INS

There are several types of buy-in arrangements.

Immediate Buy-In

An immediate buy-in is rare. Because a buy-in implies some form of group arrangement, most dentists want to ensure they are compatible with the rest of the group. They often use an associateship to test the compatibility of personalities, practice styles, and philosophies. The times that immediate buy-ins occur are generally either family members buying into a family practice or former (or present) employees who have completed dental school.

Associateship Leading to Buy-In

The most common scenario is an associateship that leads to buy-in. Many practitioners establish associateships with this intent. However, both dentists need to understand that the associateship is not a guarantee of a buy-in. It is a trial period to see if the practitioners are compatible and if the practice can sustain two practitioners. The associateship trial period makes sense because a decision to buy in is tricky to change.

Trading Roles

The most challenging type of buy-in occurs when the new dentist buys into a practice (or buys out the entire practice) and the former owner then works for the new owner. This usually occurs after an associateship. The original owner–dentist often wants to begin slowing down in anticipation of retirement, but they also want to keep professionally active. The most significant problems come from staff disorientation. The staff members have a history of dedication to their former employer. Changing those allegiances can be difficult, especially when the new owner makes significant personnel changes.

WHAT A DENTIST IS BUYING

Like an outright practice purchase, the dentist is buying the ability to make money from the practice. That takes two forms: producing dentistry and ownership in the practice. The owner has an investment in equipment, intangible assets, and financial assets, and they expect and deserve a reasonable return on those assets. This is the pure "profit" that the practice generates.

When there is one owner–dentist, they have 100% of the decision-making authority. When there are two equal partners, each has 50% decision-making authority. It is possible to reach an impasse on essential decisions if the two disagree. (In a publicly traded company, the owner can quickly sell their share in the market; not so with closely held companies.) If there are three or more owners, one owner can lose decision-making authority if the other owners "gang up" against the lone disagreeing owner. Ownership interest is worth less when there are many dentists because one owner's decision-making authority is diluted. Typically, practices decrease about one-third in value in these cases. The problem with this scenario is that the other owners can now force someone out at a discounted price, leaving them with a more valuable practice than they paid for. This becomes a complex and potentially expensive proposition. So, a practitioner needs to work with an experienced transition consultant and lawyer when buying or selling partial interests in practices.

FINANCING THE PURCHASE

Financing a partial practice purchase differs from a total buy-out, because the existing owners will remain and ensure that the practice remains profitable. There are two options commonly available for financing buy-ins.

Bank Financing

Banks are usually willing to finance a significant part of a buy-in if the buyer can meet several conditions. Bankers are more comfortable lending money when a buyer can show a strong cash flow. If the dentist has been an associate in the practice, they can generally show a production level and cash flow that satisfy the banker's risk aversion. Bankers also know that many groups do not last and want to see a well-crafted partnership agreement.

Sweat Equity

Generally, the dentist only needs a portion as a down payment for this option, and they will pay the rest over time through their practice profits. This is the more common form of buying into ongoing practices.

BUYING INTO A CORPORATE PRACTICE

When dentists buy into a corporate practice, they buy stock as the ownership indicator. The corporation owns the assets, and so the corporation claims the depreciation and other deductions. The stock that someone purchases is a capital asset. It is neither depreciable nor deductible. Instead, they pay a capital gain or loss on the stock when they sell it. (This may be 30 years from the date of buy-in.) For example, if someone buys half a $500 000 practice, they will pay $250 000. If the entire purchase amount is for stock, the buyer has $250 000 committed that they can neither claim as a deduction nor as depreciation. If that same purchase were a proprietorship, the buyer would have most of the cost they could have claimed as a depreciation deduction, decreasing taxes significantly. To avoid this tax implication, most corporate buy-ins have complex buy-in agreements that make the arrangement fairer between the buyer and seller. Often an interest rate is assigned in the buy-in package (e.g. prime plus one percentage point), and the buy-in payments are determined by incorporating interest rate computations or amortization.

When someone buys stock in the corporation, buying it from individual stockholders is generally better rather than from the corporation itself. This gives some immediate cash to the seller(s) as a return on their investment. Buying from individuals is cheaper as well. Assume that someone wishes to buy half an existing corporate practice from a single owner whose stock value is $50 000. If they buy stock from the existing stockholder, they pay $25 000 for half of the owner's stock, the remainder financed through decreased income. If the buyer instead buys an equal share

from the corporation, they must buy $50 000 of stock from the corporation to have an equal portion of the stock. However, if the table turns and the stockholder leaves (because of death, retirement, etc.), the corporate practice is ongoing. The corporation generally makes the stock repurchase. This allows the ownership ratio to remain the same, with the purchase being accomplished with pretax money from the corporation, as opposed to spending personal funds to buy the stock of the departing member.

TRANSFER CONSIDERATIONS

Merging an Associate into a Mature Practice or Partnership

This arrangement implies that an associate working for another dentist (without ownership privileges) is now offered partial ownership of the practice. The associate generally does not have the same level of financial resources, and as a result this process is different from merging mature practices. The concept of taking a junior partner is a dynamic process that often stretches over several years. It begins with realizing the mutual need, usually through an associateship or trial period arrangement. A partial buy-in of the new partner culminates in a partnership.

There are many advantages to this process of partnership evolution. The parties generally make no future financial commitments in the trial period. There are minimal financial investments, yet mutual financial benefits. Because there is a junior–senior relationship, there may be fewer ego conflicts and an opportunity for a positive mentoring relationship. If problems arise, they are usually about personnel issues and patient disposition in case of a break-up. In addition, the junior partner may find that their income goes down when the buy-in begins. This is the result of a new monthly practice purchase payment.

Owners and associates must remember that an associateship is not a guarantee of future ownership and an associateship is an employment situation. At best, associateships only express the intent of the parties to form a partnership. Associateships are trial periods to see if the practitioners are compatible enough to form a group and if the practice can sustain the practitioners. The owner–dentist looks at several factors regarding the associate when considering a partnership:

- **Did the associate earn their salary?**
  Unless a partnership is for non-financial reasons (such as a merger with a relative), the associate must prove that they produce sufficient income. When the buy-in

begins, the associate will pay the lender a significant amount of their production to pay off the purchase. The associate must ensure their potential income is high enough during the buy-in period to maintain an acceptable personal living standard.

- **Are the two people compatible personally?**
One of the most common reasons partnerships break up is over personality conflicts that escalate into significant business disagreements. All dentists must be sure that there is both behavioral and philosophical compatibility before making a long-term commitment.

- **Is there a sufficient patient base for two productive practitioners?**
Usually, an associate does not reach full productive potential for several years. Often established practitioners know that they have more patients than they need but do not know if they have enough for two practitioners. In these cases, the practice patient base must increase to allow adequate patient flow for both practitioners.

- **Did the associateship meet its patient treatment objectives?**
Part of the initial reason for an associateship may have been to retain referrals within the practice, to add new techniques to the service mix, or to serve a new population base. Did this happen as expected, or will a partnership need to develop a new and different set of objectives?

- **Has it been enjoyable and professionally rewarding?**
Some people thrive on camaraderie and interaction in sharing space with another practitioner; others consider it bothersome. The practitioner should make an honest appraisal of the professional nature of the partnership.

STEPS IN FORMING A GROUP PRACTICE

Merging a junior partner involves the same problems as forming a group of established practitioners. There are several steps that the owner–dentist should take:

- **Determine the form of the new group**
Decide whether the group will be a partnership or corporation, individual group, or true group.

- **Have the practice valued**
Until both parties know how much money they will need, deciding whether the buy-in is feasible is impossible. Dentists who are unsure how to proceed with a valuation need to secure sound professional counsel.

- **Decide all the issues that are important in a group practice**
These issues include which advisors to use, how to divide income, allocation of costs, any ancillary agreements, required physical changes in the facility, necessary staff changes, disposition of present and future accounts receivable, and what happens on the dissolution of the practice.

- **Write a partnership agreement**
Consult with an attorney to develop a document that details the issues.

- **Determine the percentage to sell**
If all dentists are equal partners, the new dentist will buy a proportional share. If the existing practitioners(s) wish to retain control, they will sell less than a proportional share. The partnership and its attending aspects (i.e. when the parties sign the papers) control when the transition begins, not when someone makes the last payment. The senior dentist should immediately expect to share authority.

- **Determine the amount of down payment required, if there is owner financing**
If the owner is financing part of the sale, the buying dentist must make a down payment. The owner may require between 10% and 25% of the purchase price as a down payment. If the buyer borrows the down payment from a bank, the bank may require a first mortgage on that part of the practice, subordinating the seller's debt in case of default.

- **Determine interest, terms, and length of payback of the note if there is seller financing**
If the seller is financing the sale, they usually give the buyer an interest rate like the bank. This will often provide the seller with an acceptable rate of return while compensating for the risk. The owner should also decide if there will be a prepayment clause and if the loan will be assignable to another party. The parties must decide what happens if either party wants to end the relationship before the buyer completes the note. Accumulated cash and interest may be repaid, or penalties may be levied. Terms will not alter the value of the practice, but they may make it easier for the buyer to finance the purchase.

- **Have all documents drafted**

  An attorney should draft all the necessary legal papers. In a partnership buy-in, the list of legal documents would include the following:

  ○ A bill of sale that transfers a share of the titles of assets that will be sold.

  ○ A sale contract (contract of purchase) that stipulates the terms of the sale of the assets, and must include any covenants, restrictions, hold harmless clauses, and an allocation of the assets bought.

  ○ A promissory note (of security interest) that is the buyer's promise to pay for the assets and that offers security or collateral if they default on payments.

  ○ A partnership agreement that specifies the rights and responsibilities of the members in the new partnership.

- In a corporate buy-in, the papers required include the following:

  ○ A buy–sell agreement (or stock purchase agreement) that defines how shares in the corporation are bought or sold.

  ○ An employment agreement that specifies the new dentist's job with the corporation, including income determination formulas, work schedules, benefits, and other duties and rights that come with the job.

DENTAL SERVICE ORGANIZATION BUY-IN

An associate pursuing a career path with a dental service organization (DSO) and with the long-term objective of becoming a practice owner should inquire about the present ownership choices in the parent company and local practice(s) and how exactly one becomes an owner. DSOs differ significantly in ownership choices and organizational structure, though they have some common traits and interests. (Some DSOs might not provide any possibilities for practice ownership.) Some DSOs merely hire dentists as staff members without giving them a chance to hold any stock in the parent company or any part of the local practice. Dentists choose their career paths for various reasons and should look at the benefits of each option.

DSO ownership plans can be grouped into three basic options: ownership of stock in the larger DSO company, ownership of the clinical side of one or more local dental practices, and ownership of the business side of one or more local dental practices.

- **Option 1: Corporate equity ownership in the bigger DSO**

  The associate dentist can hold company shares in the larger, often privately held DSO, but not ownership in the local office or practices where the dentist now practices. (The term "privately held" designates stock not offered for sale to the general public.) Corporate shares of stock may be included in the remuneration packages for dentists of a DSO with this sort of ownership, particularly as part of a retirement portfolio benefit.

- **Option 2: Stock ownership in the local practice (clinical side)**

  Most states have laws requiring dentists to legally own all of the clinical portions of their businesses. In these circumstances, the newly hired associate dentist could pair up with an experienced dentist or dentists and have ownership of the clinical side of the practice. The corporate entity would still own all the hard assets and the business side of the dental practice.

- **Option 3: Ownership of the local practice's business side.**

  The associate may also own a share of the company that runs the dental office, which is a less typical type of DSO ownership. As the company primarily holds assets, this form enables the associate to participate in the asset base of the business entity. It allows for establishing an equity stake in the local business entity. The associate has an asset that may be passed to another dentist and contributes to the business entity's rise in value.

It is likely that mixtures of ownership options 1 and 2, and even all three levels, will emerge for competitive reasons as more and more DSOs create new models. These newer business structures would provide a larger range of ownership positions that would align with dentists' conventional ownership possibilities.

A dentist who is pursuing a career path with a DSO and long-term practice owners should consider the following:

- Which current ownership choices are available for the local practice(s) and the parent corporation?

- How does an employee transition to ownership?

- How will the ownership position's (stock's) worth be determined? There are several ways to value a dental business, and an associate should, at the very least, be aware of the fundamental procedures and how ownership finance will be set up. As with any business choice, the associate should obtain the independent advice of an attorney and a financial advisor with knowledge of purchasing dental practices.

- How will the stock or ownership interest be sold if the dentist decides to leave the company?

- What happens to the dentist's ownership interest if the company sells to or is bought out by another company?

Valuing Practices

CHAPTER 5

Price is what you pay. Value is what you get.

Warren Buffett

GOAL

This chapter will provide guidelines for the dentist to use when evaluating a practice for purchase and discuss factors that affect the practice's price.

LEARNING OBJECTIVES

At the completion of this chapter, the student will be able to:

- Describe the basic approaches to practice valuations:
  - Summation of assets
  - Capitalization of income
  - Cash flow feasibility
  - Comparable sales.

- Discuss the advantages and disadvantages of the various asset valuation methods.

- Describe factors that contribute to the valuation of a practice's "goodwill."

- Describe two common methods for valuing accounts receivable in practice transfers.

- Discuss the tax implications of practice assets for the buyer and seller.

- Describe the method of valuing corporate practices.

- Describe the three classes of assets purchased in practice sales.

KEY TERMS

book value
corporate ownership
fair market value
goodwill

intangible assets
minority interest discounts
practice price
practice value

replacement value
value and price

Business Basics for Dentists, Second Edition. James L. Harrison, David O. Willis, and Charles K. Thieman.
© 2024 John Wiley & Sons, Inc. Published 2024 by John Wiley & Sons, Inc.

Existing dental practices have value for dentists who want to begin a practice. They can avoid start-up problems and gain a continuing business with patients and cash flow. The problem is deciding how much they will pay to buy an ongoing practice compared to other professional options. In this sense, the actual price is irrelevant. "How much does the practice cost?" is the wrong question. The right question is "How much will I make while I pay off the practice loan compared to other options?" A dentist can live comfortably while paying off a practice loan if a practice is fairly valued.

WHY VALUE A PRACTICE?

There are several common reasons dentists might want (or need) to set a value for a dental practice. Unfortunately, the most common is to figure out the value of shared assets in a divorce settlement. As a rule, all assets gained in a marriage are common assets, and spouses must divide the value in a divorce. (Some states consider them to be personal assets.) The dental practice is often an essential and contentious marital asset to divide. A dentist may also want a value attached for buying (or selling) the entire practice or buying into a practice as an owning partner. The third common reason for valuing a practice is for general financial and estate planning purposes. If, for example, someone wants to know how much retirement income to expect from the sale of a practice, they need an accurate estimate of its value.

A dentist will probably use someone who is an expert in practice valuation to help in setting a price and in the practice transition. They will do this once or twice in a career, and the experts do it many times a year. They know how to set reasonable values, find buyers, and set up financing plans and tax compliance. Dentists should concentrate on their area of expertise, clinical dentistry, and hire a consultant to help with other business areas.

GENERAL RULES OF PRACTICE VALUATION

There are several general rules to remember when valuing practices.

VALUE DOES NOT EQUAL PRICE

The value of the practice is an estimate of its financial worth. The value depends on the formulas used to determine that value. The price for the practice is determined by how badly the seller wants to sell and how badly the buyer wants to buy that practice. If a practice is in an isolated rural area, few people may be willing to move to and live there. The seller in this case would be much more willing to sell the practice for less than the financially determined value.

THE BUYER IS BUYING THE INCOME-PRODUCING CAPACITY OF THE PRACTICE

The buyer does not buy dental chairs, handpieces, x-ray processors, or patient charts. What they buy is the proven ability of the practice to make money. All the assets are incidental to (though supportive of) that purpose. A practice that makes no profit has zero value. A buyer might purchase the physical assets (equipment), but there is no value placed on the ongoing concern of the practice. A sizable gross production with corresponding significant expenses may lead to no profit or a loss, where the owner is essentially working for free. Gross production, then, is not a good determinant of the value of a practice. As shown on tax returns, net income is a much more helpful determining factor. A common pitfall is a departing dentist claiming that the practice is much more profitable because they have consistently taken a certain amount of cash per year out of it in unreported cash. The seller claims the price should be much higher than the numbers warrant. The purchaser cannot verify these illegal activities, so they must disregard them in the valuation estimate.

THE PRACTICE VALUE IS THE "FAIR MARKET VALUE"

The Internal Revenue Service (IRS) definition of the fair market value (FMV) of any transaction is the "price that property would sell for on the open market. It is the price that would be agreed on between a willing buyer and a willing seller, with neither being required to act, nor having reasonable knowledge of the relevant facts" (IRS Publication 561). Essentially, this says that the value is whatever the seller can get for it in an honest transaction on the open market. The price paid becomes the value. The FMV is related to the motivation of both the buyer and the seller.

A DENTIST DOES NOT BUY THE PRACTICE'S "POTENTIAL"

A buyer purchases the expectation that the present or historical profits will be transferred to them. Future profits are uncertain and depend primarily on the buyer's ability to improve the practice. Many purchasers end up overpaying for a practice based on the misguided belief that they should pay for the practice's potential. If a new dentist doubles the profit in a practice, they should reap the rewards of that increase, not the departing dentist. So, a purchaser only buys the proven profits from the practice.

METHODS OF VALUING ASSETS

Several methods help determine the value of the various components of a practice. Each has strengths and weaknesses.

- The fairest method is the FMV. The FMV is an estimate of the willing buyer and willing seller method already described. Another way of viewing FMV is to think of an estimated price that someone would give at an auction, with interested, informed people participating. There are no "blue book" values. There are rules of thumb for determining FMV, some useful, some less so. Until the asset trades hands, neither the purchaser nor the seller knows its value.

- **Replacement value** is the cost of replacing the equipment with a new, similar asset. This method overstates the value because the asset sold is generally not new, and used assets need more repair and maintenance than new ones. A problem with this method is that there may not be a new similar asset from which to learn the value.

- Accountants often use the **book value** to calculate the value of assets. Book value is the purchase price reduced by any depreciation or amortization charges taken against the asset. For example, a dentist has a dental chair that they bought new for $20 000. After three years, the dentist has taken $13 000 in depreciation expenses. The value "on the books" (book value) is $7000 ($20 000 – $13 000). The problem with this method is that it is primarily determined by the depreciation method used. This is determined by the IRS estimate of a "useful lifetime," which may bear only passing similarity to the actual useful lifetime of the asset. Some methods speed up the depreciation deduction for tax purposes. To solve these problems, some accountants use an "economic depreciation" figure, which tries to account for actual useful lifetimes and depreciation methods. Although better than a straight book value method, it is still subjective, although accountants claim it is less so than appraisal methods. In the preceding example, the dental chair may have an actual useful lifetime (economic lifetime) of 15 years, although the owner depreciates it (for tax purposes) over 7 years. The "economic depreciation," based on a useful economic lifetime of 15 years, is $3/15 \times \$20 000$ or $4000. Based on this economic depreciation, the "adjusted book value"

of this asset is $16 000 ($20 000 – $4000). If the adjusted book values of all the office assets are added, an estimate of the value of the tangible practice assets can be derived. Similar calculations for financial assets, such as accounts receivable, can also be derived.

FOUR ASSET CLASSES

In valuing practices, a value may need to be placed on each of the four classes of assets (Box 5.1).

Physical (Tangible) Assets

These assets include in-place physical assets such as equipment (dental operatory and office), leasehold improvements, and furniture and fixtures. (This is usually a small part of the value of a practice.) Any methods can be used to value these assets, but the best is to have a reputable equipment dealer estimate the assets' FMV. All these assets should be free of liens, loans, or other encumbrances. That is to say, the seller must pay off any loans and clear any liens on all of the assets they sell.

Consumable supplies (inventories) can be valued by taking the purchase cost less useless supplies (considering shelf life). This is easy but time-consuming. Another estimate of the FMV of supplies is $8000 per dentist. This is also a small part of the purchase price, so the buyer should not worry about it (i.e. do not count matrix bands).

Placing a value on the leasehold improvements to the office is a disagreement in many practice purchases. Some advisors claim that leasehold improvements are separate tangible assets and should be valued by appraisal or

BOX 5.1	DENTAL PRACTICE ASSET CLASSES

Physical (tangible) assets
  In-place physical assets
  Leasehold improvements
  Furniture and fixtures
  Consumable supplies

Intangible assets
  Goodwill
  Restrictive covenants

Financial assets
  Cash on hand
  Security deposits
  Accounts receivable

Real estate
  Land
  Building

estimated through a useful lifetime of 20 (or 30) years. Most valuation experts claim that leasehold improvements are part of the ongoing concern value of a business and are, therefore, included in the value of the business's goodwill.

Intangible Assets

Intangible assets generally make up the most significant part of the total value of a dental practice. However, because they are intangible, they become challenging to value. These assets are called "Section 197 Assets" because that section of the IRS code defines them and how they are treated from a tax perspective. All Section 197 assets are depreciated over 15 years, regardless of the actual or expected useful lifetime. Box 5.2 details such assets.

Goodwill is the major intangible asset to be valued. It is an estimate of the expectation of future profits or transferability of the income generation of the practice. The more likely it is that the income will transfer to a new owner, the higher the value of the goodwill for the practice. This depends on the present owner of the practice, the new owner, the patient pool, and the other practitioners in the area. Other intangible assets, such as the use of the office telephone number, logos and letterhead, transfer of the office lease, and the right to patient records, are included in the value for "ongoing concern" as a subset of goodwill.

Goodwill is generally the most significant part of the value of a dental practice, often representing two-thirds to three-quarters of the total value. Many factors go into valuing goodwill for a dental practice, but the most important one is practice profitability. Often, a smaller-grossing practice with higher profitability will be more valuable than a higher-grossing practice with lower profitability. Some of the highest-producing practices may be the most difficult to sell because the prospective pool of buyers who can manage such a practice decreases as the size and value increase. The location of the practice may also affect the goodwill value. Areas that are more competitive paradoxically command a higher price for a similar practice. The buyer needs to buy the patient pool in a more competitive area, and the buyer does not need to buy the patient pool in a less competitive area. If it is relatively easy to generate, then there is no need to pay someone else for something that can be gotten for free.

Various restrictive covenants are separate intangible assets in a practice transfer. The most common is an agreement for the seller not to compete with the buyer (non-compete agreement). Any restriction must describe the particular area and duration. There may be restrictions on the solicitation of patients and staff ("non-solicitation" clauses) if the seller establishes a new practice outside the non-compete area. Conditions of redress (what happens if the covenant is broken) are also generally included. These are used in both buy-in and buy-out situations. Note that states differ tremendously in their application of these restrictions.

The high proportion of value assigned to intangible assets often leads to borrowing problems for prospective practice purchasers. Banks are under strict guidelines from regulatory bodies regarding the amount and percentage they can lend for unsecured and intangible assets. The bank may not be willing or able to lend the large amount required for a borrower to purchase a practice outright. Owner financing may be the only option to finance a large amount of goodwill.

Financial Assets

Financial assets are only valued if they change hands. Many practice transfers do not involve any financial assets. If the sale does not include accounts receivable, the buyer needs to borrow additional funds for working capital.

Cash on hand is valued dollar for dollar if it is transferred. Most practices have a petty cash fund for small purchases and a change fund to make changes for the few patients who pay in cash for their services.

Security deposits may transfer to the new owner, and utility companies (municipal water, gas, electric, telephone) may require a security deposit for the account. Rather than the seller getting reimbursed and the buyer paying a new deposit, these are often transferred to the buyer on a dollar-for-dollar basis. Other funds or accounts (e.g. unemployment reserve fund) may also be transferred.

The value of accounts receivable is often contentious. The problem is that the buyer must spend money to collect the account in postage, paper supplies, and staff

---

BOX 5.2	TYPES OF INTANGIBLE ASSETS

Goodwill
- Ongoing concern value
- Workforce in place
- Information base
- Know-how
- Customer-based intangibles
- Supplier based intangibles
- Franchise, trademark, or tradename

Restrictive covenants
- Non-competition agreement
- Non-solicitation agreement
- Non-disclosure agreement

salaries. The older the account, the less likely it is that the buyer will collect anything from it, so the accounts must be discounted from their face value to set a price. The question is by how much to discount them. One standard method is to use 80% of the value of all accounts 90 days old and less. Any debt over 90 days old is considered "bad" or uncollectible. More specifically, it will cost the buyer as much to collect these accounts as they will pay. The second method looks at the account's age and the office's historical collection effectiveness to set a multiple for each age category of the account. An office with an excellent history of collections (overall 98–99%) would be at the maximum multiple. An office at the other end of the scale (93%) would be at the low end of the multiple scales. (The two methods generally come out with similar values.)

Transfers often remove the accounts receivable from the purchase to solve the dispute over the value of the accounts. One common way is to require the seller to collect their accounts receivable using their own time, money, and resources, effectively removing the accounts receivable from the purchase. Other transfers have the buyer collect the accounts, allocating payments to the seller's or buyer's account for a given time (often 90 days). After that, the buyer turns all uncollected accounts to the seller for whatever continued action the seller desires. Generally, the buyer charges the seller a reasonable fee (e.g. 10%) as a cost of collections. The problem here is that the buyer is trying to gain the patronage of the patients and does not want to collect aggressively. So any aggressive collection efforts are made in the name of the selling dentist, not the current practice or buyer.

Real Estate

The final category of asset is real estate. Often the real estate is not part of the practice sale, and the seller cannot sell the real estate if the practice leases office space. (The seller may transfer a lease at favorable rates to the buyer.) The seller may not want to sell the real estate, preferring to retain the property and gain rental income from the buyer. The buyer should keep a lease with a favorable price and conditions for at least five years.

If the real estate is part of the practice sale, then a separate appraisal and loan are used for this asset class. Real estate is easy to appraise, and a loan for real estate is often easy to secure because it is a tangible asset.

METHODS OF PRACTICE VALUATION

Practice valuation is an inexact science at best. Depending upon the valuation's purpose, a different approach might be used. For example, dentists often must value a practice because of divorce proceedings. Some states require a specific valuation technique to ensure consistency. A banker may want to know that there is adequate cash flow for lending purposes. A comprehensive valuation uses several different methods to set values. Each method should begin to close in around a final value. There are four primary methods of valuation.

SUMMATION OF ASSETS METHOD

This method adds everything the practice owns (assets) and subtracts what it owes (liabilities) to set a value (Box 5.3). It answers the question: "What things of value does this practice have that I would want to buy?" As discussed earlier, tangible assets, such as equipment and supplies, are relatively easy to value. Most dental supply houses have people who are knowledgeable and capable of doing this. If real estate is to be sold, the buyer can get an appraisal. Banks and real estate appraisers do this routinely. Accounts receivable (if sold) can also be valued based on the practice's collection history. The problem then becomes how to set the value of the intangible assets. Several methods are frequently applied to estimate goodwill value. These include gross production and net income variations, often averaged over the past several years to account for practice growth or decline. A standard (and valuable method) is the weighted average of practice net income (adjusted for owner expenses) from the past three years. Any special accounting techniques (such as hiring family members or leasing from family partnerships) must be normalized. The value of leasehold improvements is generally included as a component in the estimate of goodwill, so it is not valued separately.

PROFIT CAPITALIZATION METHOD

This method is commonly used to value other types of businesses. It compares the dental practice (or other

BOX 5.3	SUMMATION OF ASSETS METHOD

Value of equipment and supplies
+ Goodwill
+ Financial assets
+ Real estate
− Liabilities

= Practice value

BOX 5.4	PROFIT CAPITALIZATION METHOD

$$\text{Value} = \frac{\text{Entrepreneurial profit}}{\text{Capitalization rate}}$$

Income
- Cost of services
- Overhead
- Depreciation
- Other expenses
= Profit before tax
- Taxes

= **Entrepreneurial profit**

Risk-free interest rate
+ Illiquidity premium
+ Risk-specific premium

= **Capitalization rate**

BOX 5.5	CASH-FLOW FEASIBILITY METHOD

Professional income (revenue)
- Normal business expenses
- Taxes
- Family budget expenses
- Retirement plan contribution

= Income available for debt service

business) to other investment opportunities (Box 5.4). It answers the question: "How much would a reasonable, non-dentist business person be willing to spend on this practice as an investment?" It does not ask how badly a dentist wants to practice in this office. However, if someone else were investing in this as a money-making venture, how much would they pay for it, expecting a reasonable return on investment? It assumes that the owner would hire a dentist (maybe themselves) to produce the dentistry (cost of services), pay the bills, pay taxes, and then have some profit. This "entrepreneurial profit" results from business acumen and savvy management techniques. That profit is then given a risk-adjusted investment value by dividing it by the cost of money, or the "capitalization rate." The actual computations take some understanding of financial principles, but the method is coming into more frequent use as business people enter the healthcare arena. This method is less useful in professional settings because the practice's success is tied closely to the individual practitioner's reputation and abilities. The reputation and abilities do not automatically transfer to the new owner as other branded products or services do.

COMPARABLE SALES METHOD

The comparable sales method is typically used to value houses and other real estate. If someone is viewing a three-bedroom house in a particular area of town, they look at the price the other comparable houses were sold for. Dentists can also find what other similar practices have sold for and say that this practice should sell for a similar amount. The problem with this method is to determine a "comparable" practice. Many practice brokers and consultants belong to trade organizations that compile all of the reported practice sales. This helps their members to determine comparable practices based on gross and net income, location, and many other factors. This method does not show if the cash flow supports the price (that takes another calculation), but it does say what price the practice would probably sell for on the open market. A broker or advisor has access to the practice sales data. Often this is used to value goodwill, with hard and financial assets valued separately.

CASH-FLOW FEASIBILITY METHOD

The cash-flow feasibility method gives an idea of the maximum someone could afford to pay for the practice or the maximum theoretical price (Box 5.5). It answers the question: "Can the practice meet normal business expenses, produce a regular income for the family budget, pay taxes, provide future financial security, and have enough left over to service the debt?" If the answer is "yes," then the practice is fairly valued. This method depends on the prevailing interest rates, the finance terms, and the specific family income needs. Many believe this is not a method of valuing a practice, but rather a way of reassuring the buyer about their choice. However, it does ensure that the practice value makes economic sense.

VALUING CORPORATE PRACTICES

The value of a practice is the same, regardless of the form of business. (That is to say, a practice has the same value, whether a corporation, a partnership, or a proprietorship.)

However, there are a couple of special issues to consider when transferring corporate practices.

Corporate practices have different tax reporting forms than proprietorships, which need to be adjusted to make them comparable. Generally, the doctor's income and employee benefits are included as corporate costs, reducing the apparent profit significantly. There may be dividend payouts or other accounting methods of distributing profits that should be reconciled.

The ownership interest of a corporation is its stock. In a perfect world, the value of the stock should be the practice's value. In the real world, the value of the stock of a dental corporation is difficult to determine. Some states require that dentists must own dental practice shares. Shares are not openly traded on the stock markets, so their value is difficult to set through regular supply-and-demand, open-market methods. Shares of stock are neither depreciable nor deductible for the buying dentist. Instead, a capital gain or loss on the shares is realized only when they are sold, possibly many years in the future. For these reasons, many corporate practice sales do not place the practice's total value into the stock. Instead, a nominal value is given to the stock, and the cost of the practice is made up to the seller through employment agreements or other methods of income transfer. This improves the tax advantages for the buying dentist. This is an area of great dispute with the IRS, so the buyer and seller must work closely with their advisors.

Suppose someone buys out or buys into an incorporated dental practice. The new owner shares in the assets and any corporate liabilities. For example, if a former employee sues for unjust dismissal, they sue the corporation, regardless of who the present owners are. If there are unpaid tax liabilities or penalties, similar consequences occur. Therefore, buying dentists need to protect themselves from assuming potential past liabilities. There are two ways of doing this. In a buy-out transfer, the buyer buys the practice's assets from the corporation, leaving the corporate shell with the previous owner(s). Any undiscovered liabilities are the responsibility of the original corporate owner. The previous owner can then dissolve the corporation when they choose, and the new owner can form a new business entity as they choose. The second method, more frequent with buy-ins, involves a side contract in which the selling dentist agrees to be responsible for any undiscovered liabilities. This method is not as clean as the first because the original owner can contest the details of the contract. Although this problem is not frequent, it can be significant when it happens.

| BOX 5.6 | PERCENTAGES OF REFERRAL BY SPECIALTY |

Specialty	Percentage
Endodontist	95%
Oral surgeon	90%
Prosthodontist	80%
Periodontist	75%
Orthodontist	35%
Pediatric dentist	20%

VALUING SPECIALTY PRACTICES

Specialty practices are valued in much the same way that general practices are valued. However, the referral basis of many specialty practices makes their valuation problematic for many buyers. The more a specialty practice depends on referrals, the lower its transferability of income generation is, and therefore the lower its value. That is to say, if an endodontist depends on referrals as the lifeblood of a practice, most referrals are generated because of that practitioner's relationship with referring dentists. The generalists may not continue to refer patients if a new endodontist buys the practice. A buy-in is less of a problem because the new co-owner should retain most of the referral base and income generation. The time the selling specialist remains with the practice to ensure a smooth transition becomes essential for the new specialist practitioner.

Different specialties have different percentages of referral and self-generated business (Box 5.6). Most pediatric dental practices generate the vast majority of their patients the same way generalists do, through direct contact with the public. A small percentage is referred from other practitioners. On the other hand, few people call an endodontist because they need a root canal.

TAX IMPLICATIONS OF PRACTICE SALES

Tax laws change frequently. Therefore, the tax implications of a practice purchase also change frequently, and the tax implications given here could change tomorrow. The buyer should have an accountant or tax attorney involved in any practice purchase. Box 5.7 gives a synopsis of the tax treatment of the various types of assets.

From the seller's perspective, there are two types of money received in a practice sale. One type is ordinary income and is subject to ordinary income tax. The second type of money is considered a capital gain. Capital gains

BOX 5.7	TAX TREATMENT OF THE VARIOUS TYPES OF ASSETS

Seller
Capital gain over basis
Depreciation recapture
Ordinary income

Buyer
Deductible
Depreciable over the useful lifetime (hard assets)
Amortizable over 15 years (Section 197 assets)

occur when a person buys a long-term asset (such as a dental chair) and then sells it for more than it is worth, thereby showing a gain on the capital investment. (There can also be a capital loss.) Capital gains are presently taxed at a lower rate than ordinary income. In addition, capital gains are not earned income and are not subject to self-employment tax (SETA) or Federal Insurance Contributions Act (FICA) taxes. Sellers then would prefer for the maximum amount of the sales price to be considered a capital gain.

One kink in this basic interpretation occurs when a seller has reported a substantial depreciation on an asset. For example, a dentist purchased a dental chair for $20 000 and has claimed, over time, $13 000 as depreciation on the chair, and he is now telling the IRS that the chair is worth $7000. If he sells that chair for $10 000, he has made a capital gain of $3000. Because the gain is a result of depreciation deduction, he must "recapture" that depreciation. The $3000 is therefore considered ordinary income for tax purposes. Ordinary income is the more highly taxed type of income for the seller. Some sellers may have depreciated all of their office equipment, meaning they must recapture all the value of the sold assets.

For the buyer, the money used to purchase a practice is two types of money (again, from a tax perspective). Some purchased assets, such as supplies, will be used up within one year and are an immediate deduction for tax purposes. When someone first purchases a practice, they have many deductions. Often this results in using the tax deduction against income taxed at a lower rate. Some assets are long-term (capital) assets. The buyer cannot deduct their cost immediately, but must spread the cost over the useful lifetime of the asset and take the tax deduction through depreciation. Hard, tangible assets have shorter useful lifetimes (three to seven years). According to the IRS, all intangible assets (such as goodwill or restrictive covenants) have 15-year useful lifetimes. Buyers are thus less concerned with the sale price allocation than the seller. However, they generally prefer to have the maximum amount allocated to tangible assets to take the more rapid depreciation deduction.

Usually, the buyer and seller will agree on the total price for the practice. After that, they will negotiate how they will allocate the assets for tax purposes. Depending on how they structure the deal, usually they will characterize soft assets as capital assets, and hard assets will be taxed as ordinary income. Sellers want to allocate more to goodwill because this is subject to lower capital gains tax rates. The IRS taxes hard assets as ordinary income for the seller. Buyers want the opposite. More money allocated to hard assets allows the buyer to speed up expenses and have shorter depreciation deductions (five to seven years). Goodwill amortization is spread over more than 15 years, slowing the deduction for the buyer. The objectives of the buyer and seller are then often at odds. Any negotiated amount must be "reasonable" and reported to the IRS. The buyer must file a form with the IRS when they purchase a business, such as a dental practice. This form describes the assets transferred and what price was given for each of them. In that way, the IRS can check to be sure that both the buyer and seller have correctly declared the value and type of assets sold.

Securing Financing

A banker is a person who is willing to make a loan if you present sufficient evidence to show that you don't need it.

Herbert V. Prochnow

GOAL

This chapter aims to explain the structure and use of various types of debt. It discusses specific types of loans and their use in personal and professional situations.

LEARNING OBJECTIVES

At the completion of the chapter, students will be able to:

- Define the common sources of loans for dentists.

- Discuss these types of debt instruments concerning the purposes, types, benefits, limitations, and uses for dental practitioners:
  - Bank note
  - Line of credit
  - Promissory note
  - Signature loan
  - Installment loan
  - Credit
  - Mortgage
  - Home equity loan.

- Define loan security and how it affects loans for dentists.

- Describe these types of interest rates:
  - APR
  - compound
  - fixed rate
  - prime
  - variable rate
  - simple.

- Discuss the tax implications of debt for practitioners.

- Describe how to control debt.

KEY TERMS

accounts payable	APR	bank note
after-tax interest rate	arm's-length transaction	banks
amortization	balloon payment	business plan

Business Basics for Dentists, Second Edition. James L. Harrison, David O. Willis, and Charles K. Thieman.
© 2024 John Wiley & Sons, Inc. Published 2024 by John Wiley & Sons, Inc.

collateral	lien	promissory note
compound interest	lien holder	secured loan
consumer debt	line of credit	signature loan
cosigner	loan security	simple interest
credit unions	marginal tax rate	Small Business Administration
down payment	mortgage	taxable interest rate
first lien position	non-taxable interest rate	term of a loan
fixed-rate interest	owner financing	unsecured loans
home equity loan	prime interest	variable-rate interest
installment loans	principal	working capital
interest	private banking	
interest-only payments	pro forma financial statement	

Debt can be a valuable financial tool, allowing a person to purchase goods or assets they could not otherwise afford. It can also be a significant drain on resources, especially if not managed properly. Usually, people use debt for large purchases (such as of a home or practice) when obtaining the item for cash would be difficult or impossible. The problem is, assuming debt means that a person must pay interest, add to the cost of the asset, and pay off the principal, reducing the funds available for other purchases or investment purposes.

Bankers and loan officers have several rules that they go by when qualifying a client for a loan (and, therefore, debt) (Box 6.1). Bankers do not simply make up these rules: the agencies that underwrite the loan require them. For example, the Federal National Mortgage Association (Fannie Mae) requires that the total monthly payment on all debt be no more than 36% of a family's gross monthly income. These debt payments include monthly housing costs, including taxes and interest, payments on installment credit, alimony, child support or maintenance payments, and any other payments on the non-income-producing property. Although some of these items (like taxes) are not debt, they are required periodic payments, so lenders treat them as if they were debt.

Most professionals incur debt at some point in their careers. Generally this is during the initial phases, when they buy practices, houses, and new automobiles. Often professionals enter the marketplace with a large amount of preexisting debt needed to finance their education. This student debt may be so large that it impairs their ability to secure additional personal or professional loans. Most bank loan officers understand professionals' significant potential earning power and work to develop them as clients.

As professionals move through their professional lifetimes, the need for debt usually declines as they pay off loans and accumulate assets. It is during the first several years that managing debt becomes crucial. Mistakes made early in a career can haunt a person financially for many years.

SOURCES OF LOANS

Banks are the best-known source of loans for professionals. However, there are many other potential sources of funds, and each has specific advantages and disadvantages.

BANKS

Banks are the most common source of funds for new practice loans. Bankers are in the business of lending money to people who they think will repay it. So, a dentist must convince the banker that they will repay the loan (Box 6.2).

There are two types of banks, national and local. (Actually, it is a continuum between these two ends.) National banks are larger and often have an entire division dedicated to working with professionals, called "private

BOX 6.1	ALLOWABLE DEBT LEVELS

Type of debt	Rule of thumb
Consumer debt	20% or less of gross monthly income
Housing costs	28% or less of gross monthly income
Total debt	36% or less of gross monthly income

| | BOX 6.2 | EXAMPLE BANK LOAN | | |

Year	Total payment	Principal	Interest	Remaining principal
1	77 228	42 971	34 256	357 500
2	77 228	47 002	30 225	310 497
3	77 228	51 412	25 816	259 086
4	77 228	56 234	20 993	202 851
5	77 228	61 510	15 718	141 342
6	77 228	67 784	9 443	68 179
7	77 228	74 062	3 637	0
	$540 593	$400 000	$140 593	0

Principal = $400 000

Term = 7 years

Rate = 9.0%

Dr. Jones buys a dental practice, securing an installment note for the amount shown. Her annual (estimated) payments are given. Loans are amortized monthly.

banking." The private banking section manages small businesses and other particular banking concerns. Large banks may have people within their private banking group who manage only professional (or even dental) practice loans. These people are knowledgeable about practice financing issues. The dentist may need to establish all professional (and often personal) bank accounts within the private banking section. However, it works well because the banker will know the dentist personally. On the other hand, local banks are variable in their understanding of dental office finance. Some small banks do not have private banking sections. Instead, the dentist may need to educate the banker about the specific problems faced by dental practices. (Bankers do not like to take risks they do not understand.) Many of these people are also knowledgeable and helpful to young professionals setting up their practice.

OWNER FINANCING

Many professional practices finance some portion of the cost through the previous owner. If a bank is unwilling to lend the entire amount, the owner may finance the remainder of the purchase price. The seller does this by allowing the buyer to pay part of the price over time to the owner rather than the lending institution. The seller will generally charge a comparable interest rate and require a promissory note detailing the loan terms.

Owner financing carries additional risk for the owner over simply getting the total purchase price as cash up front. If the buyer runs the practice into the ground, becomes disabled, dies, or is unable, for any reason, to pay off the loan, the owner may not receive the entire purchase price. Generally, the bank will require a first lien position on all tangible (hard) assets of the practice, which means it gets to sell the assets to satisfy its loan first. So, the previous owner may be left holding an empty bag. This may be the only way the owner can sell the practice for the price they want. If so, the buyer can expect to pay the owner a reasonable interest (comparable to a bank rate) for the portion they finance. The buyer may need to finance the down payment through a bank and arrange the rest of the purchase price as owner financing to make the buy-out work.

DENTAL SUPPLY COMPANY FINANCING

Most major national supply companies (e.g. Patterson, Sullivan-Schein) have arrangements with banks or finance companies that allow a dentist to borrow money to establish a professional practice. There is an obvious advantage for the supplier (the dentist buys equipment and supplies through them). The advantage for the dentist is that they may qualify for financing through these organizations when they may not qualify at the local bank. The downside is that the dentist often pays a higher interest rate than they would at the local bank. The finance company may also have significant prepayment penalties and other disadvantageous loan clauses. The dentist generally must buy their equipment through the supply company as well. Some only finance new practices, not buy-outs of existing practices. Others only offer to finance equipment purchases or upgrades. However, these companies know the dental marketplace, and if someone cannot gain financing through a bank, they may offer a method of financing the establishment of their practice.

FAMILY MEMBER FINANCING

Someone may be fortunate enough to have family members with sufficient assets to lend them for practice or personal needs. If this is the case, the dentist should structure the loan as an "arm's-length" transaction. This means that it is a bona fide business transaction, like someone else would negotiate at arm's length or without the benefit of family ties. The Internal Revenue Service (IRS) considers family loans partly as a gift if they are not negotiated at arm's length. This infers an actual interest rate and payback schedule.

A more common occurrence than an outright loan is when a family member guarantees the security of a loan by pledging assets or cosigning a loan for the young professional. Here, the family member has not provided the direct funds but has agreed to pay the loan cost if the borrower defaults and cannot pay.

MORTGAGE COMPANIES

Previously, the professional might have used a mortgage company primarily when purchasing a home, and they generally have not entered the commercial loan market. In the past several years, mortgage companies that cater to young professionals have emerged. They have found a niche in lending to professionals establishing their practices. Many of these clients have high student and other personal debts and do not qualify for traditional bank loans. They are still reasonable long-term lending risks because of their high expected incomes. Traditional banks may be unable to lend money to these people because of banking regulations. However, finance companies are not under the same guidelines. They may charge a higher interest rate and include prepayment penalties that make these loans less attractive compared to a traditional bank. Despite these shortcomings, many young professionals use them as a source of start-up financing.

SMALL BUSINESS ADMINISTRATION

The Small Business Administration (SBA) is an agency of the federal government whose charge is to help developing businesses secure start-up financing. It does not provide the loan proceeds but instead guarantees the loan through a local bank or lending agency. Usually, two or more banks must have turned a person down for a traditional business loan. That person may then contact an SBA officer who may help arrange for financing. The SBA often will only guarantee a loan for a start-up rather than a buy-out (because the latter is not a new business). It typically requires substantial down payments that young professionals cannot make. There is a considerable amount of paperwork involved in securing these loans. Some banks will not work with the SBA. Because the federal government backs the agency, the borrower is subject to the whims and attitudes of Congress and other governmental bodies. Availability and rules change constantly. Some young professionals have found success in this source of loans; others have not. While worth investigating, SBA loans are not a common source for new practitioners.

SWEAT EQUITY

Sweat equity occurs when someone works for another dentist, taking less pay but building up an equity or ownership position in the practice. The employee dentist shifts the decreased salary to the seller, who takes the amount given up as additional compensation. They value the practice and develop an imputed loan (with interest, term, principal, and possible down payment). These arrangements occur more frequently in buy-in situations. There are substantial risks for the owner–dentist in this arrangement. The purchasing dentist may decide during the buy-in that they do not like or want the practice. They may not be able to handle the load. Alternatively, the purchaser might decide they do not need to pay extra for this practice because they can quickly start their own. Because of these risks, these arrangements are tightly structured (from the seller's perspective), which leaves the buyer little room to change their mind. Box 6.3 gives an example of a sweat equity buy-in.

CREDIT UNIONS

Credit unions are like banks and savings and loans, except they serve a specific clientele (e.g. teachers, public employees, and dental association members). Their loans are usually for smaller personal purchases (automobiles, boats, etc.) rather than for business purposes. Credit unions often

BOX 6.3	SWEAT EQUITY			

	No buy-in		With buy-in	
	Owner	Associate	Owner	Associate
Collections	$600 000	$300 000	$600 000	$300 000
Payment for services	$200 000	$100 000	$200 000	$100 000
Equity buy-in			$70 121	–$70 121
Business profit	$100 000	0	$50 000	$50 000
Total compensation	$300 000	$100 000	$320 121	$79 879
Cost	$400 000			
Term	7 Years			
Interest payment/month	6%			
Payment/year	$5 843			
	$70 121			

This example assumes the associate will buy in for the given amount and will become an immediate equal owner. The providers receive 33% of production as compensation, and the business divides the profit equally among the owners. When the buy-in is complete, the equity payment ends.

offer better interest rates than traditional bank loans, but generally do not finance large business loans.

CREDIT CARDS

Every time a consumer purchases a credit card, they essentially borrow money from the issuing card's bank. Depending on the conditions associated with the card, there may be no interest accrued until the payment due date. Any balance left unpaid is subject to interest, often nearing 2% per month on the unpaid balance. (This is equivalent to approximately 24% per year.) Credit card debt is an expensive way to borrow money.

EFFECT OF CREDIT RATING

A person's credit history affects whether they qualify for a loan and the interest rate charged. Financial institutions generally use a person's credit score as the indicator of their credit rating. The credit score is based on their past use of credit and a history of paying it back on time. The higher their credit score, the better the credit risk a person is, and the lower the interest rate a banker will charge because they are surer that the person will repay the loan. Box 6.4 shows how a change in credit rating can make a massive difference in the interest rate and total payments over the lifetime of a loan. Before asking for a loan, a practitioner should check their credit rating and repair any problems in their credit history first.

BOX 6.4	CREDIT RATING IMPACTS		

Credit score	Interest rate	Monthly payment	Total loan cost
720+	5.0%	$1413	$118 725
675–699	6.5%	$1485	$124 735
620–674	8.0%	$1559	$130 924
	Principal = $100 000		
	Term = 7 Years		

This chart shows the effect of credit rating on a loan's interest rate. The interest rate then determines the monthly payment and total loan costs. The difference in the total loan cost on this $100 000 loan is $12 200 over the loan term. Larger loans will have a correspondingly more significant difference.

TYPES OF PROFESSIONAL DEBT

Debt incurred by professionals typically is in one of the following forms.

BANKNOTE

A banknote is the typical type of credit extended to professionals for business purposes. Banknotes are generally based on compound interest and amortized as with other compounded loans, and the practice's assets may partially or entirely secure them.

LINE OF CREDIT

Often, a borrower is unsure exactly how much money they need to borrow and when they will need it. Bankers solve this problem by establishing a line of credit. A line of credit allows a person to borrow up to a certain amount of money whenever they decide they need it. It is a prearranged loan that does not start until the borrower uses the money. For example, when someone starts a practice, they estimate their cash needs. Depending on the accuracy of the cash-flow projections, they might need cash to pay the bills at any time. Rather than borrowing a set amount (e.g. $20 000) and beginning interest payments on the entire balance immediately, the practice owner will generally establish a line of credit so that they will only borrow as much as they need when they need it. If they use $5000 the first month, they are only charged interest on $5000. The remaining $15 000 (of the initial $20 000) remains for the person to borrow when needed. The funds are in the bank, waiting, but the borrower is not charged interest unless they use it. Many practitioners have a standing line of credit at their bank as an additional source of quick cash beyond the emergency fund.

PROMISSORY NOTE

A promissory note is an agreement between two people, saying that one agrees or promises to pay a particular debt to the other. In the professions, promissory notes are seen in practice purchases in which the owner finances all or part of the purchase price. As a separate contract from the contract to purchase the practice, the seller will usually require the purchaser to sign a promissory note, which sets the terms for paying the principal and interest.

SIGNATURE LOAN

As mentioned, a signature loan is secured only by a signature and a promise to pay the entire loan. It is generally used for short-duration loans (one year or less) in which the borrower has an immediate cash need. Bankers will usually give signature loans to customers who have shown they have an excellent repayment history and only for limited amounts. Many practitioners have a standing line of credit that eliminates the need for signature loans.

ACCOUNTS PAYABLE

An amount that the dentist owes to someone else is an account payable. For example, if a practitioner orders dental supplies and the supplier sends a bill, the dentist has agreed to pay that debt. When they accept the merchandize, the dentist owes the vendor for the supplies. The dentist has an account payable until they pay the account in full. The vendor may charge interest or a service charge if the dentist does not pay it by the stipulated time. Charges that a practitioner makes on a professional credit card for meals, entertainment, or other professional expenses are a form of account payable.

TAX IMPLICATIONS OF DEBT

How the federal tax code views debt affects the cost of it and how to manage debt. The IRS views the interest on certain types of debt to be tax deductible. Notice that this is only the interest portion of the debt payment and solely for certain types of debt.

The types of interest presently considered tax deductible include home mortgages, second mortgages, business loans, business credit interest, some (limited) student loans, and particular investment interest expenses. Most personal debt interest is not tax deductible, including credit card interest, personal lines of credit, auto loan interest, and other personal loans. (Tax law is under the control of Congress, and these lists may change at any time.) Box 6.5 summarizes these categories.

The essential element of deductibility of interest is the resulting after-tax interest rate. By allowing deduction of the interest portion of the payment, the federal government, in essence, pays part of the interest. Assume that a person is in a 33% marginal tax bracket (that is, 33% of the next dollar earned will go to taxes). If that person has $1000 in interest payments that they deduct from their income before paying taxes, their taxable income decreases by $1000, and they pay tax on that lower income. That person saves $330 (33% of $1000). In other words, the $1000 interest only costs $670 ($1000 − $330). This decreases how much tax the person pays, affecting the actual after-tax rate.

Tax-deductible interest

Consumer

  Home mortgage

  Mortgage on second home (e.g. vacation)

  Home equity loan

  Certain student loans

Business

  Business debt interest

  Business credit interest

  Certain investment interest

Non-tax-deductible interest

Consumer

  Credit cards

  Auto loans

  Certain student loans

Business

  None – all business interest (that is a bona fide cost of doing business) is tax deductible, not taxable.

This chart shows which types of interest are tax deductible. This is the interest portion; it does not apply to the principal portion of a loan.

AFTER-TAX INTEREST RATES

Real interest rates, after tax consideration, then depend on the individual's nominal rate and marginal tax rate. This applies only to tax-deductible interest rates. Box 6.6 gives common combinations of interest rates and marginal tax rates. Assume, for example, that someone borrows money at 10% interest for a business (i.e. a tax-deductible purpose). If they are in the 15% marginal tax bracket, they save 15% of the 10% interest rate (1.5%) through tax deductibility. Their after-tax interest rate is 8.5%. This applies only to the interest portion of the loan payment, not the principal. The information in Box 6.6 makes comparing dissimilar loans or investments much easier.

NEGOTIATING WITH LENDERS

Bankers are in the business of lending money. However, they want to lend to people whom they believe will repay their loans as agreed. A banker will naturally ask many questions and gather much information to "qualify" a person for a loan (or to decide whether they are a good loan risk). The borrower should show the banker that they know what they are doing from a business perspective so that the banker will be more comfortable with giving them the loan. The borrower will probably need a formal practice valuation done by a reputable consultant, cash-flow projections, and sometimes a complete business plan. (Developing a business plan is covered Chapter 19.) The banker may have specific items they also want, such as the practice's tax returns and the seller's tax returns from the past three years. These are not simply hoops to jump through. The banker must take the loan application to the bank's loan committee to gain approval. A banker may not understand professional practices or a particular arrangement, but more than likely they do. The borrower should listen to the banker. If a banker does not believe the borrower can finance a practice at a given price and make it

| BOX 6.6 | REAL AFTER-TAX RATES |

Interest rate	Tax bracket				
	0%	15%	28%	33%	40%
8%	8%	6.8%	5.8%	5.4%	4.8%
9%	9	7.7	6.4	6.0	5.4
10%	10	8.5	7.2	6.7	6.0
11%	11	9.4	7.9	7.4	6.6
12%	12	10.2	8.6	8.0	7.2
13%	13	11.0	9.4	8.7	7.8
14%	14	11.9	10.1	9.4	8.4

"Tax bracket" is the marginal tax rate, and this is the percentage of tax paid on the next dollar earned. It consists of federal, state, and local income taxes.

work, the borrower should seriously reconsider the potential arrangement.

Most of the issues discussed in this chapter are negotiable. That is to say, the lender has some discretion in setting the rates, terms, and conditions of a loan. However, the banker must also gain approval from the bank's loan committee. This is a group of senior bank officers who act as a supervisory board, making the final decision on whether a loan is acceptable from the bank's point of view. Because the banker must represent the borrower in this meeting, the borrower should provide the bank with as much positive information as possible. The bank might ask the borrower to develop pro-forma financial statements or a complete business plan. Other times the loan application process may be a mere formality. Suppose someone is buying into the practice of a family member who is a longstanding, excellent customer of the bank (and will cosign the loan). In that case, the borrower may only need to complete a few forms to qualify for a loan.

CONDITIONS OF THE LOAN

A borrower might negotiate the specific conditions of the loan. Negotiating "interest only" for the first six months to a year is standard practice. This means that the borrower only needs to pay interest on the loan or even let the interest accumulate. This decreases payments in the first critical portion of the loan when start-up costs are high, and the cash flow may be at its lowest. If the purchaser does not buy accounts receivable, they will need to negotiate a line of credit for "working capital." The borrower might negotiate variable rates, longer-term, or even lower interest rates. Their bargaining position depends on their history with the bank and how much the bank wants to gain the borrower as a long-term customer. Suppose the borrower has presented a loan request to other banks or financial institutions. In that case, they might even have one bank match or exceed another bank's offer to gain the business.

The bank may not lend the borrower the total purchase price of a practice. Instead, the bank may require that the borrower pay part of the total purchase price as a down payment. (Common amounts are 10–25% of the purchase price.) This ensures that the person has a personal stake in the practice. Bankers assume that the borrower might work harder and be more serious about the practice if they have some money at stake. If the borrower does not have the money or assets for a down payment, they might convince the seller to lend the down payment in the form of a "second mortgage" or owner financing. The borrower

might also have a parent or other family member cosign a loan or pledge specific assets to secure the loan and qualify the borrower for the loan.

At larger banks, professionals usually deal with a bank employee in the private banking section. Private banking is the division of the bank that works with wealthy clients. (A starting dentist may not be wealthy yet, but the bank expects they will be.) Few professional practices file for bankruptcy, and few professionals default on loans. Private banking is much more personal than public banking. A dentist will have a specific loan officer assigned to their case, and they can work with the specific loan officer if cash-flow or tax problems develop in the practice. Some banks extend additional credit for purchasing a home or another consumer purchase through private banking. In return, the bank usually expects the dentist to maintain personal and professional accounts with that bank.

Different banks place different importance on loan factors, the factors that the bank might use to determine if it will lend money (Box 6.7). Many bankers value cash flow above all else. They want to be sure that the borrower will have enough cash flowing through the practice to pay the practice's bills, service the debt, pay taxes, and support a family (including student loan payments). If the practitioner can show the cash flow, the loan is good. Others require a down payment to ensure the borrower has some "skin in the game." Others may require a formal business plan (Box 6.8). Some will look at production history to be sure that the dentist can handle a practice of the size they want to purchase. Still, others place a high value on collateral and loan security. Bankers that understand dental practices realize the high student debt that many graduates carry. They will look at the cash flow (especially within a family budget) to ensure that the practice can also support this payment.

BOX 6.7   LOAN FACTORS

Can the borrower:

- Meet normal business expenses?
- Produce an income for the family?
- Service student loans?
- Service the practice debt?
- Pay taxes?
- Provide future financial security?

BOX 6.8	FORMS A BANKER MAY REQUIRE

Personal financial statements

Balance sheet	Required
Family income statement	Usually required
Last year's tax returns	If appropriate

Practice financial statements

Formal practice appraisal	Required if buy-in or buy-out
List of assets to be bought	Required
Pro-forma cash flow	Usually required
Pro-forma income statement	Occasionally required

Other practice information

Past tax statements (3 years)	Required if buy-out or buy-in
Partnership agreement	Required if buy-in
Lease	Usually required

If buying real estate

Real estate contract	Required

If doing a de novo start

Contractor's estimate for build-out	Usually required

If a cosigner is needed

Cosigner's personal financial statement	Required
Cosigner's credit report	Bank will do this

Other forms

Loan application	It depends on the bank
Business plan	Nice to have, often required
Credit report	Bank will do this

This chart summarizes many forms a bank will require before deciding whether to make a loan. Each bank has slightly different requirements. Some banks will require that their forms are used (e.g. for the balance sheet). Others may accept personally generated forms.

USE OF THE LOAN PROCEEDS

Bankers will look at the intended use of the loan proceeds when deciding the terms of the loan. If the dentist uses the proceeds for a practice purchase, they will generally secure the hard assets through a lien. A lien cannot secure the soft assets. Instead, the banker may ask for other security (such as a consigner). Similarly, working capital is not secured. Most practice loans include a line of credit for working capital wrapped into the overall loan package.

If the practitioner is borrowing money to purchase real estate along with the practice (e.g. an office condominium), the bank will usually make a separate loan for the real estate portion. It may require 10–20% of the value as a down payment. The bank generally extends this loan over a longer period (such as 20 years) to match the asset's lifetime and to lower the monthly payment. This is a secure loan because the bank files a lien on the real estate until the loan is paid in full.

Personal Financial Management

Money is central to our lives. It has the power to build up or tear down. It can grow and appreciate if properly managed or depreciate if mismanaged. Money can produce anxiety or joy – so can the lack of money. Money can lead to the gamut of human emotions, from happiness and jealousy to covetousness and rage. Money touches everyone in some way or another. It is used to buy power, control, and pleasure. It can easily be counted and becomes a surrogate for people's worth.

Money is also pervasive. There are entire broadcast networks devoted to money and investing. Daily publications and monthly magazines provide news about money and advise people on how to make it and keep more of it. Money dominates the news. Whether it is the collapse of a country's economy, wars over resources, riots and civil disturbance between those who have money and those who do not have any, money is the precipitating factor in many news stories. Money elects presidents, and financial scandal ruins promising politicians and other leaders.

Because money is so important, we need to plan for its use. We all need to do this, regardless of our professional situation. An employee in a government position will certainly have different financial needs and parameters than someone in a solo practice. The employer may provide specific insurance and other benefits solo practitioners must provide themselves. However, the planning process and the issues are the same.

Millions of dollars will pass through a dental office throughout a career. Dental employees depend on the dentist for their family's financial safety and security. Dentists will pay bills and taxes and still have a significant amount of money left for enjoyment. They then have to choose what to do with that money. It can be spent on themselves or their family, gambled away, saved for retirement, or given to churches or other worthwhile community organizations. Regardless, money needs to be managed to be spent wisely, saved, and invested appropriately. A plan to manage financial affairs is needed to accomplish these ends. This is called *financial planning*. Financial planning is developing and implementing coordinated plans to achieve personal and professional objectives. It is a long-term process that requires knowledge and work and may also require the expertise of professional money managers to help someone establish and reach their financial goals.

CONCERNS ABOUT THE FINANCIAL MANAGEMENT PROCESS

The financial planning process is concerned with three primary goals:

- **Balancing family spending**
  When someone earns money, they can either spend it or save it, and those are the only two options. They need an optimal mix given their family situation, goals, and ambitions.

- **Increasing net worth**
  As someone moves through their career, they should increase their net worth, and they accomplish this by increasing assets and decreasing liabilities.

Business Basics for Dentists, Second Edition. James L. Harrison, David O. Willis, and Charles K. Thieman.
© 2024 John Wiley & Sons, Inc. Published 2024 by John Wiley & Sons, Inc.

- **Planning for emergencies**

  Many dentists run into financial emergencies at some point in their lives. The issue is whether or not they have prepared for these emergencies. If allowances have been made, the emergencies will not be financially devastating.

OBJECTIVES OF THE PERSONAL FINANCIAL MANAGEMENT PROCESS

Given these three main concerns, the objectives of a financial plan are grouped according to familiar categories. However, these categories cannot be viewed in isolation because they overlap and feed into every other category. The issues that dentists should examine in their financial planning process include the following:

- **Chapter 7: Personal Money Management**

  As dentists move through their careers, they accumulate things of value, both physical (such as houses) and financial (such as investment portfolios). Paying the principal on loans yields a similar result because eliminating debt is equivalent to gaining a corresponding asset. These assets are then used for further investment, for family purposes, or to build an emergency fund for risk protection.

- **Chapter 8: Personal Insurance Needs**

  People face financial risks every day of their lives. These include the risk of premature death (before they have accumulated enough assets to care for their family's needs), the loss of income through a disabling condition, medical care expenses, and property and liability losses. People use insurance to protect themselves from these potential financial problems.

- **Chapter 9: Retirement Planning**

  No one provides business owners with retirement income except themselves. The government offers several tax incentives to encourage business owners to save for retirement. If a retirement plan can be integrated into office expenses, it can provide a comfortable income when business owners choose not to work.

- **Chapter 10: Personal Taxes**

  Taxes are a fact of life in the United States. However, personal and professional affairs can be planned to decrease tax burdens as much as possible within the laws and rules established by the taxing agencies.

- **Chapter 11: Estate Planning**

  As dentists accumulate wealth, they need to develop a plan for what happens to that wealth when (*not* if) they die. As small business owners, the practice may be one of the dentist's more significant assets, and proper succession planning helps protect the value of this critical asset. Additionally, people who have not accumulated a large amount of wealth need to be sure that their heirs are financially protected in case of premature death.

Personal Money Management

CHAPTER 7

Rule No. 1: Never lose money.
Rule No. 2: Never forget Rule No. 1.

Warren Buffet

GOAL

This chapter presents a description of the financial planning process. The relationship between practice development and personal needs will be stressed.

LEARNING OBJECTIVES

At the completion of this chapter, the student will be able to:

- Describe common issues of personal money management for professionals.

- Describe how personal lifestyle decisions affect the financial planning process.

- Describe how savings affect the financial planning process.

- Describe how to establish a personal credit rating.

- Describe how to manage personal credit cards.

- Describe the typical financial planning phases in a professional's life.

KEY TERMS

consolidation loan
credit card
credit rating (FICO score)
debit card

discretionary income
emergency fund
financial plan
identity theft

personal record management
safe deposit box

Many financial planning issues that young professional dentists face are the same as those for the general public. However, in other ways the issues for dental professionals are unique. They often start with high debt loads but balance that with high income levels. Dentists are frequently not employed by a company or organization that provides benefits such as medical insurance or a retirement plan. They are typically limited in how much income growth they can expect and must balance their income wants and needs with their desire for personal time. Because of these issues, new dentists must quickly learn how to manage money.

Business Basics for Dentists, Second Edition. James L. Harrison, David O. Willis, and Charles K. Thieman.
© 2024 John Wiley & Sons, Inc. Published 2024 by John Wiley & Sons, Inc.

PERSONAL MONEY MANAGEMENT

BECOME A GOOD MONEY MANAGER

Dentists need to become good money managers, in both their business and private lives. The first step is to learn all about money and how to use it. Becoming a good money manager does not just happen; it needs to be worked at, just like becoming a dentist. Dentists should study how to save, how to invest, and how to become wise consumers. They should subscribe to *Kiplinger's* or *Money* magazine. These are the two leading personal financial magazines, and they give valuable tips for saving, making, and investing money.

PERSONAL RECORDS

Dentists accumulate many vital personal financial records. Therefore, they should create a personal record management system, like the one developed for the office. Dentists should not let the paperwork pile up; they should work on records every month. They should get a safe deposit box at the bank, a fireproof safe at home, or a secure cloud storage vault for essential papers. These crucial papers include wills, insurance policies, names of advisors, and certificates of ownership, among others. Dentists should retain all tax records and related items for at least seven years and keep insurance policies as long as they are in effect.

GETTING PROFESSIONAL HELP

As professionals, dentists have skills and knowledge that members of the public do not have. Dentists not only work with patients to take care of their oral health, but also direct and intervene as professional expertise dictates. The same is true for managing financial affairs. A dentist may have a basic understanding of financial management, but there are times when the guidance of someone with expert knowledge in a specific area is needed. Dentists should become actively involved in their financial management and planning but use advisors' expertise when situations demand it.

Accountant

Most dentists go first to their accountants for advice about practice and personal finances. An accountant can be used to help with tax planning, setting up basic retirement plans, evaluating the numbers of the practice, and personal budgeting. Certified Public Accountants (CPAs) have different interests and expertise. Some work on any business or personal tax affairs. Some concentrate on professional practices (physicians, optometrists, or dentists). This latter group will often be in a better position to help with practice-specific questions (e.g. "Is it time to hire an additional hygienist?"). An easy way to find an accountant who serves mainly professional clients is to go to the local dental society meeting and ask several members whom they use. One or two names will probably come up repeatedly. Contact them, then interview them to see if they would be a "good fit" with your practice or personal needs and style.

Depending on the background and expertise of the accountant, additional help for investment planning, establishing estate plans, buying or selling or partnership opportunities, and a host of other advanced financial topics may be needed. Dentists often use a lawyer, financial planner, or management consultant.

Investment Advisor

The investment world is very diverse when it comes to advice on and executing (buying and selling) securities. There are full-service advisors, mutual fund companies, banks, and online Robo-investment advisors. The dentist must decide how much they want to be involved in regular investment decisions, what the level their current knowledge is, and how much time and effort they want to spend learning about the investment strategy and decision-making.

Insurance Agent

Dentists frequently have two insurance agents, one for their business insurance and another for their personal insurance. Some agents work only with one insurance company, and others are independent agents who shop around various insurance companies to find the best policy. Some insurers offer a package of products (e.g. various business insurances). Some include malpractice coverage, while others do not. Organized dentistry often endorses insurance plans for members. (This may be life, disability, or office insurance.) Agents are another source of contact with the insurance company. Dental practitioners should ask their colleagues for recommendations, then shop around for insurance coverage. An annual insurance review is prudent, as the need for different coverage changes as someone progresses through their career.

Management Consultant

The practicing dentist will use management consultants for two reasons – to address practice productivity problems and to help with practice transitions (buying, selling, or adding associates). As with other advisors, there will be a few advisors frequently mentioned by colleagues. Using someone with an excellent track record in helping other practitioners with particular issues is generally advantageous.

PERSONAL LIFESTYLE ISSUES

INCREASING LIFESTYLE AND INCOME

New dentists are typically like a kid in a candy store when they first start making money. They have been in college for 8–12 years, may be married, and have put off increasing personal spending and improving their lifestyle while in school. Suddenly, with new-found wealth, they buy too much (often on credit) and struggle for the next several years to pay higher bills with the growing take-home pay. The tendency is for lifestyle expenses to increase along with income. Every dollar they make is spent on a bigger house, a newer car, and various toys. It is easy for someone to listen to the tales of classmates and compare themselves to others, even though they may be in entirely different situations. Unfortunately, the solution is not a fun, warm process. Personal life expenses must be kept under control. It is easy to increase lifestyle to meet increasing income. Once accustomed to a particular lifestyle, it is difficult to cut back on spending, such as when starting a retirement savings plan. A solution is to develop and use a family budget. If income grows, the dentist can take half the increase and use it to fund spending or investment plans, using the other half to boost their lifestyle. This way, lifestyle increases (more slowly than without savings), and a savings or investment plan is painlessly funded. This approach does take discipline, however.

SPEND OR SAVE

When someone earns money, they can only spend or save it. As previously mentioned, after years of training most new dentists want to spend it immediately and enjoy it. Instead, they should get into the habit of saving. Dentists should start each budget period by saving at least 20% of their take-home pay, learning to live adequately on the remaining 80%. As their income increases, they should save as much of the increase as they spend. As Box 7.1 shows, saving even a dollar a day adds up to a sizable sum over time.

Separating Financial Needs from Wants

People want to buy physical goods, such as shoes and televisions, or intangible services, such as vacations or lawn-mowing services. Some of these are goods and services they need, and others they do not need but want. People need to have

BOX 7.1	SAVING (AND INVESTING) A DOLLAR A DAY			
	5%	8%	11%	14%
1 yr	$374	$380	$386	$392
5 yr	$2073	$2244	$2433	$2643
10 yr	$4736	$5592	$6651	$7966
20 yr	$12544	$18036	$26627	$40259
30 yr	$26416	$45728	$86628	$171179
40 yr	$46639	$107351	$266852	$701946

This shows how saving $1 a day adds up over time and the results for different interest rates and time periods.

reasonable housing, clothing, food, and insurance. They want a weekend getaway, a new designer purse, or a new fishing rod or shotgun. They should purchase these two types of goods and services differently. Everyone should buy their needs first. Only when they have satisfied their needs should they buy their wants. People can borrow to buy their needs if they must. However, they should never borrow for wants – they should only use savings or pay cash. This sounds easy. The problem is determining if a desire is a need or a want. Everyone needs housing, but do they need or want a larger house? People need recreation for their mental health and spiritual renewal, but do they need or want a week's vacation in Monaco? Often, people find that they can postpone or eliminate "wants" by making informed lifestyle decisions. This allows them to pay for "needs" or save for future "wants."

FAMILY PLANNING: THE COST OF A FAMILY

For many people, becoming a parent is their greatest adult challenge. These changing responsibilities, obligations, and commitments last a lifetime – once a parent, always a parent. No other life event causes people to become as thoughtful, careful, and focused on the future as having the moral, physical, and financial responsibility of raising children.

Children involve additional direct and indirect costs of increasing family size. Box 7.2 details some of these costs. No matter what people say ("Children are cheap. They hardly eat a thing!"), the simple fact is that having a family is expensive. For the dentist, these costs often come when the family budget is already thin because of the need to pay off student debt and initiate a dental practice. Family income gets squeezed even tighter if one parent quits work to care for children. Some estimates place the cost of

BOX 7.2	EXTRA COSTS FOR CHILDREN

- Babysitter or daycare expense
- Buying (and moving into) a larger home
- Remodeling or adding to an existing home
- Buying a larger or more reliable car
- Expanding insurance coverage
- Higher insurance premiums
- Moving to neighborhoods with better schools
- Sending children to private schools
- Paying for children's extracurricular activities
- Taking family vacations
- Paying increased medical bills
- Buying more or different food
- Buying more clothes and furniture
- Buying gifts for children

BOX 7.3	TARGET BUDGET AMOUNTS

Category	Percentage
Housing	30%
Food	20%
Debt payments	20–30%
Savings	5–10%
Miscellaneous or insurance	15%

raising a child to age 18 at nearly $500 000. This does not include the cost of college, professional, or graduate schooling. Having children is an expensive proposition indeed.

What should be done to prepare for children financially? The dentist should do the same type of financial planning as before children, have a budget, and stick to it. They should have an adequately funded emergency fund, more so now than before. They should expand savings and save for purchases, educational needs, and children's activities. The family should look closely at the impacts of having one or two working parents. One income means less money to spend and invest, but it also means one parent will be available to care for the children. Daycare is expensive! Family finances will be different (costs such as daycare and work expenses) and the family dynamic will be different. Everyone should balance the trade-off in finances with the non-material family life issues.

FAMILY BUDGET

Developing a family budget is the cornerstone of personal financial planning. A budget is a statement of how money has been spent in the past and estimates future income and expenses. As such, budgets become a target for day-to-day financial life. They also help identify spending patterns, coordinate savings, and improve living standards by

identifying areas of waste. Budgets are most often used when a family is having a financial problem. The family then helps set targets for spending and lets everyone know why spending is limited in one area or another.

Although each budget is unique for that person or family, some general targets for expenditure categories can be developed (Box 7.3). No more than 30% of take-home pay should be spent on housing costs, 20% on food (groceries and eating out), and 15% on other miscellaneous expenses. Debt payments (including student loan payments) should total no more than 30% of take-home (after-tax) pay. The budget should also detail paying 5–10% of take-home pay into savings (personal and retirement).

DEVELOPING THE BUDGET

Many families develop a budget only after they find a problem. "Where does the money go?" is a common starting point regarding budgeting and money management. Many websites, software apps, and financial self-help books can guide a family in developing a reasonable budget. Dave Ramsey and Suzi Orman are two famous personal financial planning personalities. Excellent apps that help with the budgeting (and financial planning) process include Quicken, Mint, EveryDollar, Tiller, and Fidelity Spire. All of these work on a common theme – we do not know where we spend our money until we write down where it goes, and only then can we develop a plan to improve our spending and saving habits.

Step 1: Write Down Income

Determine how much income flows to the family each month. Income is not just what is earned but all sources of money coming to the family budget. This may include grants, scholarships, family gifts, or other non-traditional sources. Often, money may come in a periodic large sum (such as a scholarship). Mast people break this down to a monthly amount for easy understanding.

Step 2: Write Down Expenses

The family should track their expenses for 30 days, placing each expense into a category (food, housing, car, etc.). This allows a better understanding of where they spend money each week and month. Start by listing all the family's expenses. Think about regular bills and irregular bills, and those bills that are paid bi-monthly or quarterly. Add these costs together with other costs, like food, gas, and entertainment. Every dollar spent should be accounted for. Software apps can quickly help families track large and small expenditures. Debit and credit card statements often help categorize expenses. This is an eye-opening experience as some families learn for the first time how much they are spending in each category.

Step 3: Look for Problem Areas

Subtract monthly expenses from income. Every dollar should be accounted for and placed in a category. Many families use a zero-based budget, which means they start at zero for each category (the base amount is zero), then justify all expenses in the category. Some expenses are necessary ("must-haves" such as food, shelter, clothing, and transportation) and some are optional (wants such as dining out or taking a vacation). If the family places all expenses in the "must-have" category, then additional sources of income or significant lifestyle changes are in order.

Step 4: Set Financial Goals

Effective money management starts with a goal and a step-by-step plan for saving and spending. Financial goals should be realistic, specific, have a timeframe, and imply an action to be taken. Each family should decide the financial goals that they are working toward. Some of these goals might be long term, like retirement planning; some might be short term, like saving for a car or a family vacation. The budget should not only include income and expenses, but also take into account the financial goals that the family has set.

Step 5: Monitor Progress

Even after someone starts a budget, they still need to stay on top of their expenses. Some people use spreadsheets or online tools to track their spending. Others follow Dave Ramsey, a popular radio host who teaches his clients to spend cash on food, gas, and entertainment items. He uses an envelope system to help people manage their day-to-day spending. Once the money in the envelope has been spent, they are done spending in that category.

SPECIAL CONSIDERATIONS

Many people work as independent contractors or are self-employed, which means they may have an irregular income. An irregular income comes in at different amounts, times, or both. When they make a budget, they need to base their income on their lowest-paid month from the previous year. They list their expenses and put an amount next to each item. They then can prioritize the expenses (must-haves or wants).

Once they have a bare-bones budget, they can plan for any additional income they bring in over the worst-case scenario. They might ask themselves: "If I had enough money for one more thing, what would it be?" They keep a prioritized list of what those items are. When they have additional money, they go to that list and use it as a guide to what they will use the rest of that money for. The list will change, and items will move up and down the list based on what is essential at a particular time.

HOW TO IMPROVE SPENDING HABITS

Whatever the present financial situation, there are only two things someone can do to improve it: earn more or spend less. Assuming they have maximized short-term earnings, there are several steps they can take to improve their spending habits. First (again), they must develop a budget. They should examine their spending patterns, looking for areas of wasteful spending or items that can easily be cut. They should write down their plan for financial improvement; it is too easy to devise a vague plan. Unless the plan is written down on paper, it does not mean anything. A person who wants to improve their spending should not use credit cards; many people get into severe financial trouble using credit cards. They should use checks or debit cards instead. Shopping trips should be separated from spending trips. Impulse buying leads to bad financial decisions. Expensive purchases should be compared on the internet or on a shopping-only (not purchasing) trip. No purchases should be made on the initial trip. When a decision has been made, the buyer should go on a buying trip to purchase the item; this way they will make a better buying decision. They should also quit smoking and other costly habits. Saving a dollar or all pocket change daily will quickly accumulate savings.

DEVELOPING PERSONAL SAVINGS

SAVING VERSUS INVESTING

Saving is holding on to money, stashing it away so it will not be lost. Gain is not expected. Investing is buying an asset (such as a stock or share of a mutual fund) that may increase in value over time. When someone invests, they hope for a gain but realize that a loss is possible. Both saving and investing are worthwhile goals in the right situation. If building an emergency fund or holding on to money for a short-term purpose, the safest bet is to ensure it is not lost. Money should be saved in a low-risk fund, such as a savings account or money market fund. If retirement is planned for 30 years hence, then the long-term gains hoped for by investing in a mutual fund are the better route. The value of the mutual fund may go down tomorrow, but it will hopefully (with wise fund choice) increase over the longer term. When someone invests, they take a calculated risk. This is not a pure gamble or game of chance. A saving method is more appropriate if they cannot afford to lose money.

EMERGENCY FUND

One of the most important financial tasks is establishing and saving an emergency fund. The emergency fund should consist of three to six months' take-home pay, depending on the amount and type of disability income insurance and other liquid assets available in emergency cases. The money should be put into a low-risk liquid investment such as a money market mutual fund or checking account. (Although this is not exciting, it is safe.) It is a form of savings used for emergency needs and not as a speculative investment. This fund might cover emergencies, including a car that dies, a short-term disability, or paying for medical treatment. It is not a vacation or Christmas savings plan. Other than emergency purchases, this fund allows the person to increase deductibles on all insurance policies, which saves substantial money in premiums. Establishing the emergency fund is one of the most critical *initial* financial planning jobs.

Get Adequate Insurance

Chapter 8 details the types of insurance a dentist might need. As a rule, dentists should not buy extended service contracts, a type of insurance. The dealer will try to sell an extended service contract when buying a television, refrigerator, automobile, or any other major purchase. These cover most repairs needed over the term of the contract. It is better to see if the item fails and then to pay to repair or replace it. The dentist should also never buy additional (credit or mortgage) insurance. These policies ensure that if one dies or becomes disabled, the policy will pay off a mortgage or car loan. These are expensive life insurance or disability policies. (Dealers sell them because they get a cut of the premium.) The dentist should have adequate life and disability insurance for their needs and then remember to refuse these additional insurances when buying a major

item. They should never buy insurance from someone who calls, because insurance policies should be investigated before buying. As a rule, consumers should shop around for insurance because it is a commodity item.

PERSONAL BANKING

BANKS

Many new graduates have never had the problem and luxury of managing significant amounts of personal money. Establishing a personal checking account and a professional (office) account is paramount. All checking accounts are not the same. Banks require different minimum amounts in an account, charge different service fees, pay different rates of interest, and may limit the number of checks that can be written. The dentist should shop for a bank that meets all their needs. Initially, they should find a checking account with low fees and minimum balances. They should look for accounts that pay more interest and charge lower fees as assets and savings grow. Many banks allow and encourage patrons to bank electronically, establishing monthly payments and transferring funds electronically to vendors. If the dentist is in private practice and borrowed money from a bank, that bank may require them to keep all accounts there. In this case, "private" banking services can also be used, which adds tremendous convenience to banking.

BANKING SERVICES

Banks provide many services besides checking accounts. Most offer e-banking, which improves convenience, and most banking can be done online. The banks loan money for small businesses or personal purchases and develop mortgages for large purchases. They offer credit cards for spending and often have accounts for credit card payments from patients. Many banks have unique small business divisions that offer payroll and other services to the small business owner. They have safe deposit boxes for critical personal and business records. They typically have investment advisors and retirement plan specialists to help people develop and nurture these accounts. One of the first professional relationships that a dentist should make is with a banker.

MANAGING CREDIT

CREDIT RATING

Establishing a credit rating is another crucial step in financial planning. The major credit bureaus keep credit ratings on all Americans using their Social Security numbers. This lets potential lenders quickly assess borrowers.

The lender can decide if someone is a reasonable lending risk by looking at how much they have borrowed before and if the loan was paid off promptly. The dentist should nurture their credit rating by paying off all debts and credit cards on time. A bad credit history will haunt a person for many years. It can lead to the denial of a practice, home, or other loan, of insurance or employment, or even of the right to cash a check or open a bank or credit card account.

The lending companies commonly report a credit rating using a Fair, Isaac, and Company (FICO) score, which was named for the company that developed the scoring system. (Some agencies use other, similar systems.) Scores range from 300 to 900, with most people in the 600–700 range. The higher the score someone has, the better their creditworthiness. A higher credit score means that it will be easier to get loans (and other forms of credit, such as credit cards), and the loans acquired will be at lower interest rates. Depending on the type of loan, lenders use the credit score, along with the entire credit report, differently. They place more (or less) emphasis on particular components of the score, depending on their product. If someone borrows $200 000 for a house, the lender will look at the person's score and history differently than if it was a loan for a $10 000 limit credit card.

Five major factors go into the calculation of a FICO score:

- **Past delinquencies**
  If someone has failed to make payments in the past, they are more likely to repeat the pattern.

- **How the credit has been used**
  If someone is close to the limit on a credit card (or worse, maxed out), they are at a greater risk.

- **The age of the credit file**
  Someone who has had credit for a long time has a track record and is therefore a better risk.

- **How often credit is asked for**
  Something may be awry financially if someone repeatedly asks for credit over a short time.

- **The mix of credit**
  With only one credit card, a person is riskier than someone with several forms of credit, such as a home mortgage and other loans.

All credit scores essentially begin at zero. Credit history is built up; it does not start at the top and is subtracted by poor credit choices. So, without borrowing money or having any credit (e.g. a credit card), a person does not have a credit history and is considered a poor

| BOX 7.4 | FREE CREDIT REPORTS |

Company	URL
Annual Credit Report	www.annualcreditreport.com
My Fico	www.myfico.com
Experian Inc.	www.experian.com
Equifax Inc.	www.equifax.com
Trans Union Corp.	www.transunion.com

credit risk in the eyes of the rating systems. With no credit history (i.e. someone who has never borrowed money), the banker will probably deny the application for a loan because the creditor does not know if the person is a reasonable credit risk.

Everyone should check their credit history and rating regularly (annually). One free credit report can be obtained from the major national credit bureaus. If a dentist plans to buy a house, borrow for a practice, or make another major purchase, they should check their history about three months in advance. If they find errors, this gives them enough time to change them. Box 7.4 gives the websites of the major credit houses: Experian, Equifax, and Trans Union. They and the other sites also have a wealth of information on managing credit and debt. Depending on the study cited, 1–50% of consumer credit reports contain errors. Some may be simple and inconsequential (such as a misspelling). Others may affect a credit rating for years to come. Fraudulent activity, such as identity theft, may even be discovered this way. Inaccuracies can be irksome to correct. The Fair Credit Reporting Act requires bureaus to respond promptly. However, the bureaus will not necessarily change someone's history just because they say so. (If they did, everyone would call and demand a clean credit history!) A person is essentially guilty until proven innocent. Proof and involving the creditor who sent in the inaccurate report are generally needed to clear an incorrect record and thereby increase the credit score.

DEBT MANAGEMENT

MANAGING CREDIT CARDS

Credit cards get more people into financial trouble than any other cause. Credit cards make it easy to buy things. When an item is purchased with a credit card, the issuing bank pays the merchant, essentially floating the credit card holder a loan for the amount of the item. The credit card-holder can then "borrow" up to the limit on the credit card. (Only the money in a particular account can be used with a debit card.) The credit card holder does not have to pay the bank for the item until the end of the month. That works well if the credit card balance is paid off at the end of each month. However, if it is not paid off, the bank charges the credit card holder interest, generally about 1.5%, on the unpaid balance. When compounded, that 1.5% per month equals nearly 20% per year. So, paying off a credit card balance is a wise idea. The problem is that it is easy to let the balances grow to overwhelming levels, and banks are too eager to let someone amass large credit card balances. The value of a credit card is being able to borrow money for purchases (up to the card limit) and the convenience of this form of payment. The apparent downside comes if balances are not paid off regularly or if someone borrows more than they can afford to pay off.

There are several common-sense solutions to the credit card problem other than using credit cards carefully and paying them off monthly. If someone has a credit card problem, use a debit card (instead of a credit card) because only the amount of money in the account can be spent. The bank will deny the merchant's authorization if there is insufficient money in the account to cover the purchase cost. This way, the person cannot overspend. Dentists should have one personal and one professional credit card. All professional purchases go on the professional card, and personal purchases go on the personal card. This keeps them more aware of the total credit card balance and prevents them from running up the total balance by having balances on several cards. (It is a good idea to have a "back-up" credit card with no annual fee. If a primary card is lost, stolen, or for any other reason becomes inactive, the back-up card can be used.)

If someone is using a credit card, they should shop for the best deal for their monetary circumstances. "Gold" cards have higher credit limits and more generous terms than regular cards. The catch is that someone must qualify with a good credit history and income. "Platinum" cards have even higher limits and requirements. Both cards have more advantages if someone is careful, but they offer more opportunity to bite off more than the person can chew financially if they are not careful. Some cards will rebate a percentage of the purchase (e.g. 2–3%) as a "cash-back" incentive or as points that can be used for travel or gift purchases. Many banks issue cards with the name of a sponsoring organization (such as an alumni association) on the card. A small amount of money goes to the sponsoring organization (instead of to the cardholder as a higher rebate). Dentists should avoid these cards; they are expensive. Most cards have an annual fee; this should be as low as possible. (Dentists should negotiate with a credit card issuer to eliminate the annual fee.) A low percentage interest charge is also ideal; however, there is usually a trade-off between the interest and the annual fee. Higher annual fees lead to lower interest rates. (The converse is true also.) If balances are paid off regularly, the lower annual fee is better. Interest rates should not affect this type of consumer. The lower interest rates are better if balances are not paid off in full. The cardholder should check when the payment due date is on a credit balance. Some cards require payment within 10 days. Others give the credit cardholder until the end of the month for payment.

While people use credit cards like cash, they are not just a transaction tool but can strongly affect their financial goals. Be sure to consider credit cards as part of the budget and debt management, and use them carefully and cautiously.

MANAGING STUDENT LOANS

Most new dental graduates carry a significant amount of student loan debt. This becomes a problem that affects every other area of personal financial planning. Unfortunately, there is no magic quick fix to student debt. The good news is that there are no significant delinquency or default problems with dental school graduates; they have a terrific track record for repayment. Dentists should practice good debt management habits and be persistent in paying off their loans. There are a few simple steps to get started. First, the dentist should know what they borrowed, who services the loan, and when it comes due. Secondly, they should identify and constantly review their repayment objectives. Thirdly, they must choose a repayment plan to help meet those objectives. These are the rules as of this writing (2023). New rules from the government or lenders could change them.

Step 1: Understand the Loan Portfolio

Understanding the loan portfolio is the first step in managing student loans. Most loan portfolios contain federal loans, campus-based loans, and private loans. Federal loans are referred to as direct unsubsidized and Direct PLUS (Grad PLUS) loans. Campus-based loans include Perkins, Health Professions Student Loan Program (HPSL), and Loans for Disadvantaged Students (LDS). These loans have different interest rates, capitalization, and grace and deferment periods. Private loans are not eligible for income-driven repayment (IDR) plans or public service loan forgiveness.

Interest Rates

Interest rates on direct unsubsidized and Direct PLUS (Grad PLUS) loans have fixed rates. Though these rates are fixed, the borrower may have different rates each year on their loans. Direct PLUS loans always have 1% higher interest rates than direct unsubsidized loans. Private loans will have variable or fixed interest rates, and their terms and conditions will vary according to the lender.

Capitalization and Compound Interest

Interest accrues on the principal balance of the loan. Interest does not accrue on outstanding interest while the borrower is enrolled as a full-time student or during repayment if they are enrolled in an income-driven repayment plan. Capitalization is the addition of unpaid interest to the loan's principal balance. After capitalization, interest will begin accruing on the new (and higher) principal balance. However, some events trigger the outstanding interest to be capitalized on direct loans. The eight events that trigger capitalization are:

- Default.
- The end of a forbearance period.
- The end of a deferment period.
- The end of a grace period.
- Failure to recertify income qualifications for an IDR plan.
- Loss of the "partial financial hardship" that qualified the borrower for an IDR plan.
- Loan consolidation.
- Changing from one repayment plan to another.

In the private sector, interest is capitalized daily or monthly, depending on the loan agreement. As already stated, when interest is capitalized, interest begins accruing on the new (and often higher) principal balance – a process referred to as compounding. It is essential to realize that borrowers utilizing IDR are not subjected to compounding interest.

Grace Periods

Typically, a student does not have to begin repaying their loans immediately after graduation. The period after graduation and before repayment begins is called a grace period. (Private lenders sometimes call grace periods "interim periods.") The standard length for the grace period is six months, but it can be extended for up to three years under certain circumstances. Each loan only qualifies for grace once. So, if someone graduates from a program and begins repayment but later decides to return to school, their loans will not reenter a grace period while they are in school or after their next graduation. For someone who enters repayment and returns to school, deferment may be an option; however, they should consider making qualifying payments in an IDR plan while a resident. Interest accrues during the grace periods for all unsubsidized loans. PLUS loans do not qualify for a grace period, and students are eligible for a six-month postenrollment deferment. Payments on these loans will begin simultaneously to the Direct Unsubsidized Loans. Graduates must read their loan agreement carefully and discuss the loan details with their lenders.

Step 2: Repayment Objectives

There are no wrong or right repayment objectives; this is a highly personal decision. These objectives might change and should be reviewed regularly. An aggressive strategy would reduce the impact of interest accrual and capitalization. There is no penalty for aggressive repayment of loans. Payments are applied to outstanding interest first before the principal, but should be confirmed with the loan servicer. Additional payments may be targeted on the most expensive loans. A cautious strategy might be utilized if someone needs to protect their income and maximize monthly cash flow. They might use a Public Service Loan Forgiveness program or repayment help in exchange for a service commitment.

Step 3: Choose a Repayment Plan

There are two primary choices for repaying a student loan: time-driven and income-driven repayments. Time-driven offers two options, a standard 10-year repayment or an extended 25-year repayment. (Larger loans might qualify for a 30-year repayment plan.) Income-driven plans base the loan repayment on the graduate's income.

Time-Driven Repayment

Time-driven repayment is not dependent on income. If a person does not select a payment option, they will be assigned a standard 10-year (120 level payments) plan. This standard payment can also apply to those borrowers who get into either IBR or PAYE (see later). At some point during these income-driven plans, if someone does not demonstrate partial financial hardship, their payment reverts to the original standard 10-year amount, which is a marker for the payments under an income plan (IBR, PAYE, and

REPAYE). As their income increases, borrowers will see their monthly payments under an income plan start to approach the standard 10-year amount. This standard plan is also suitable for someone with relatively low debt, a steady income moving into practice, or other resources to help with repayment, such as a spouse's income.

Another option for time-driven repayment is an extended 25-year (300 level payments) plan. To qualify for this option, the borrower must have more than $30 000 in student loans. With this plan, there is no penalty for aggressive repayment. This strategy might be helpful for someone with high debt who wants the same payment each month, who needs to show a lower debt-to-income ratio, or who can afford a higher payment but wants a lower required payment each month because of uncertain cash flow.

Income-Driven Repayment

IDR plans are designed for highly indebted borrowers who cannot afford repayment under other plans (most notably Standard 10 years). These plans are beneficial when the gap between federal debt and income is significant. The payments will change annually based on income and family size. These programs allow for a more manageable monthly payment and have the option of leading to loan forgiveness. The disadvantage is that the initial payments may not cover the interest, so the balance can grow in size. The debt remaining at the end of the term is forgiven but is considered taxable income. Debt forgiveness under these IDR plans is not dependent on the type of employment like other plans. PAYE forgiveness is forgiven after 20 years, while IBR and REPAYE forgiveness is after 25 years. The IDR has four options: Income-Contingent Repayment Plan (ICR), Income-Based Repayment Plan (IBR), Pay As You Earn (PAYE), and Revised Pay As You Earn (REPAYE). Most borrowers graduating now with income plans are likely using IBR, PAYE, or REPAYE.

While most graduates will select a payment plan and start actively repaying their student loans, some will need to postpone payments due to additional education or other life circumstances, such as short-term financial problems. Forbearance is when the monthly loan payments are temporarily suspended or reduced. The lender may grant the graduate a forbearance if they are willing but unable to make loan payments due to certain financial hardships (Box 7.5). During forbearance, principal payments are postponed, but interest continues to accrue. Unpaid interest that accrues during the forbearance is added to the principal balance (capitalized) of the loan(s), increasing the total amount someone owes.

BOX 7.5   LOAN FORBEARANCE

A forbearance may be granted for the following conditions:

- The graduate is unable to make scheduled loan payments for reasons including, but not limited to, financial hardship and illness.
- The graduate serves in a medical or dental internship or residency program and meets specific requirements.
- The total amount the graduate owes each month for all the direct loans is 20% or more of the total monthly gross income (for a maximum of three years).
- The graduate is serving in an approved AmeriCorps position.
- The graduate is performing a teaching service that would qualify for loan forgiveness under the Teacher Loan Forgiveness Program requirements.
- The graduate qualifies for partial repayment under the Student Loan Repayment Program, administered by the Department of Defense.
- The graduate is called to active duty in the US armed forces.

A deferment is a temporary postponement of payment on a loan that is allowed under certain conditions (Box 7.6) and during which interest generally does not accrue on Direct Subsidized Loans, the subsidized portion of Direct Consolidation Loans, Subsidized Federal Stafford loans, the subsidized portion of Federal Family Education Loan (FFEL) consolidation loans, and Federal Perkins loans. All other federal student loans that are deferred will continue to accrue interest. Any unpaid interest accrued during the deferment period may be added to the principal balance (capitalized) of the loan(s). The graduate should consider paying the interest that accrues during that period to avoid capitalization, whether choosing forbearance or deferment.

Student Loan Forgiveness

Some plans provide forgiveness of student loans. Public Service Loan Forgiveness (PSLF) is a program where the loans of borrowers who make 120 on-time payments on one of the IDR plans or standard repayment (10–30-year) loans would be paid off, while those employed by a 501(c)3 are eligible for tax-free forgiveness of their Direct or Direct Consolidation Loans (501(c)3 organizations are non-profit charitable organizations, such as churches and religious

BOX 7.6	LOAN DEFERMENT

The graduate may qualify for a deferment if they are:

- Enrolled at least half-time at an eligible postsecondary school.

- Enrolled in a full-time course of study in a graduate fellowship program.

- In an approved full-time rehabilitation program for individuals with disabilities.

- Unemployed or unable to find full-time employment (for a maximum of three years).

- Experiencing economic hardship (including serving in the Peace Corps) as defined by federal regulations (for a maximum of three years).

- Serving on active duty during a war or other military operation or national emergency and for an additional 180-day period following the demobilization date for a qualifying service.

- Performing qualifying National Guard duty during a war or other military operation or national emergency and for an additional 180-day period following the demobilization date for a qualifying service.

- A member of the National Guard or other reserve component of the US armed forces (current or retired) and are ordered to active duty under certain circumstances.

BOX 7.7	STUDENT LOAN FORGIVENESS

Service areas eligible for loan forgiveness:

- Emergency management.

- Military service.

- Public safety.

- Law enforcement.

- Public interest law services.

- Early childhood education.

- Public service for individuals with disabilities.

- Public service for the elderly.

- Public health.

- Public education.

- Public library services.

- Other school-based services.

organizations, educational and service organizations, and private foundations).

To qualify for PSLF, a borrower must work full-time as a W-2 employee, for 10 years, for a 501(c)3 organization that performs at least one of the services shown in Box 7.7. The borrower must be employed (as opposed to contracted) with the 501(c)3. If someone is classified as an independent contractor and receives a 1099-MISC tax form, their payments do not qualify for PSLF. Rules and regulations are constantly changing in these programs. Graduates can find updates on the website https://studentaid.gov.

Loan Consolidation

A Direct Consolidation Loan may make payments more reasonable by combining various federal student loans into one loan with one monthly payment. The graduate must apply for loan consolidation and select a repayment plan. Depending on the size of the student loans and how much they owe, they will have between 10 and 30 years to repay their Direct Consolidation Loan. Private education loans are not eligible for consolidation, but they may be considered when determining the maximum repayment period under specific repayment plans.

Loan consolidation can offer benefits to help manage education debt. Through consolidation, the graduate can achieve the following:

- Make lower monthly payments by increasing the repayment period.

- Make a single monthly loan payment on one bill to one lender.

- For loans other than Direct Loans (such as Perkins or FFEL loans), consolidation may give access to additional IDR plan options and PSLF.

The interest rate for Direct Consolidation Loans is fixed. This fixed rate is the weighted average of the interest rates on all of the loans consolidated, rounded up to the nearest 1/8 of 1%. There is no cap on the interest rate on a Direct Consolidation Loan. As with other types of student loans, anyone may prepay a Direct Consolidation Loan without penalty and change repayment plans if they find their current plan no longer meets their needs.

Although consolidation can help many graduates manage their monthly payments, there are some cases when a Direct Consolidation Loan may not work well. These are shown in Box 7.8.

| BOX 7.8 | LOAN CONSOLIDATION PROBLEMS |

Cases where consolidation does not work well:

- Any outstanding interest on the loans being consolidated will be capitalized immediately upon consolidation.

- Because Direct Consolidation Loans can have a repayment period of up to 30 years, the borrower may be increasing the total amount they pay in interest.

- If a graduate consolidates Perkins loans, they lose eligibility for cancelation benefits that are available only for Perkins loans, and they also lose eligibility for Perkins loan interest subsidy benefits.

- If a graduate consolidates existing Direct Loans or FFEL program loans, they lose any previously made qualifying payments toward PSLF or IDR forgiveness.

Bankruptcy

Someone can have federal student loans discharged in bankruptcy only if they file a separate action, known as an "adversary proceeding," requesting the bankruptcy court to find that repayment would impose undue hardship on them and their dependents. Bankruptcy courts do not utilize a single standard to decide whether ordering someone to repay their loans would cause undue hardship, but may consider the following factors:

- The debtor would be unable to sustain a modest quality of living if they were obliged to return the debt.

- There is reason to believe this hardship will last for the loan payback period.

- Before declaring bankruptcy, the debtor made good-faith efforts to repay the loan.

Bankruptcy courts can make several decisions based on someone's situation. As an example, the court might decide among the following:

- The debtor's loan may be dismissed entirely, meaning they will not have to pay anything back. All collection activities will end.

- The debtor's loan may be partially discharged, but they will still be responsible for paying back a portion.

- The debtor's loan may be required to be repaid but on alternative terms, such as a lower interest rate.

Death of the Borrower

Federal student loans will be discharged (ended) due to the death of the borrower or of the student on whose behalf a PLUS loan was taken out. If someone's parents have taken out a PLUS loan, it will be discharged if their parent dies or if they die.

PREVENTING DEBT PROBLEMS

With debt management, prevention is the best cure. Box 7.9 estimates the payments for various loans, knowledge of which is essential to ensure that payments fit the budget.

Keep a Reasonable Debt-to-Income Ratio

It sounds simple, but dentists should not borrow too much money and should keep an accurate eye on the budget. Most lenders set a limit of 35% of total pretax income for the total debt load, including home mortgages, automobile loans, credit cards, and other personal debt payments. A dentist may not qualify for certain types of loans if their debt payment-to-income ratio is too high.

Have a Specific Plan to Repay Debt before Borrowing

Dentists should work debt payments into their personal budget, ensuring they have the cash flow necessary to pay off the loan. If payments do not fit into the budget, something must be given up, either a present expense item or the anticipated purchase. Box 7.9 shows how to estimate the payment for a loan.

Avoid Impulse Buying: Plan and Save for Purchases

Many consumers get into debt problems from their credit cards. They look at a credit card bill at the end of a couple of months and realize that they have charged so many impulse purchases that they have reached their credit limit and now must aggressively pay down this expensive debt.

Pay Full Balances on Credit Cards Each Month

Credit card debt is one of the most expensive types of debt incurred. Most cards have a "grace period" built into payment schedules. The balance should be paid off in full each period so that interest payments on the accounts are not accumulated. The borrower borrows the bank's money for free if the balances are paid off. That is a good deal. Paying 24% interest per year is a bad deal. Make at least the minimum monthly payment on every card with a balance. Otherwise, the penalties add to the balances quickly. The

BOX 7.9	ESTIMATING LOAN PAYMENTS

Monthly payments on each $1000 borrowed

Years	4%	6%	8%	10%	12%	14%	16%	18%
1	$85.15	$86.07	$86.99	$87.92	$88.85	$89.79	$90.73	$91.68
5	$18.47	$19.33	$20.28	$21.25	$22.24	$23.27	$24.32	$25.39
7	$13.67	$14.61	$15.59	$16.60	$17.65	$18.74	$19.86	$21.02
9	$11.04	$12.01	$13.02	$14.08	$15.18	$16.33	$17.53	$18.76
10	$10.12	$11.10	$12.13	$13.22	$14.35	$15.53	$16.75	$18.02
12	$8.76	$9.76	$10.82	$11.95	$13.13	$14.37	$15.66	$16.99
15	$7.40	$8.44	$9.56	$10.75	$12.00	$13.32	$14.69	$16.10
30	$4.77	$6.00	$7.34	$8.78	$10.29	$11.85	$13.45	$15.07

Multiply the loan principal (in thousands of dollars) by the factor to determine the monthly payment amount.

Example 1: A new car is purchased for $30 000, and the entire amount is financed at 8% for five years. What is the monthly payment?
Payment = 20.28 × 30 = $608.40/mo.

Example 2: A dental practice is purchased for $200 000, and the entire amount is financed at 10% for seven years. What is the monthly payment?
Payment = 16.60 × 200 = $3320/mo.

borrower can direct more payment to one card if it is part of a strategy to pay off higher interest-rate cards first, which is generally a good idea.

GETTING OUT OF DEBT

If prevention has not worked and someone has too much debt, they should take several steps to reduce the debt load.

Understand There Are No Quick Fixes

Anyone can get into debt quickly, but it takes time to repay that debt. The first step is to begin *now*. The longer the person waits, the more interest accumulates. The person should admit to having a financial problem and begin working to solve the problem. If they are overwhelmed, they should seek professional financial help. A banker, accountant, or certified financial planner can help solve these financial problems.

Be Ready for Lifestyle Changes

Getting out of a large amount of debt will be painful. A significant amount of money will need to be paid to lenders for an extended time. Unless their income increases significantly, most people cannot maintain their lifestyle and pay off debt at the same time. Their lifestyle may need to be reduced. They should make a written plan because a plan is not confirmed until it is written on paper. The borrower should also take on no new debt. Credit card accounts should be closed, and a written accounting of all income and expenses should be maintained. A personal financial analysis should be done, and this information should be used to budget for spending. All extra income should be put toward paying off debt.

Work with Creditors

A debtor should not hide from creditors. Eventually, they will be found. Creditors want to be repaid and will work with the person to develop a payment plan that can be met. However, creditors must be kept informed. They may help by offering slower repayment plans or other methods that help the person get out of debt, which helps the creditor get paid the money owed.

Consolidate Debt When Necessary

Debt consolidation is when someone has several high-interest loans. Making these payments may be so challenging that the interest accumulates faster than it can be paid off. They are usually better off if they can borrow money at 10% to pay off an 18% credit card. (Origination fees and other consolidation loan requirements need to be researched.) In this way, the consumer can consolidate these expensive loans and, hopefully, pay off the debt more quickly. Note that this technique is primarily for people who are in debt trouble. Consolidation is not the simple panacea that some lenders make it out to be. The person now has one lender who may not be sympathetic to their problems.

Use Tax-Deductible Interest, If Possible

Sometimes, it is to someone's advantage to use home equity loans or business loans (working capital) to pay off debt. The interest rates (effective after-tax rates) should be compared to decide which is best.

Accelerate Debt Payments, If Possible

As a rule, the faster someone pays off debt, the less interest they will pay. Therefore, on the face of it, it is always a good thing to pay off debt as quickly as possible. However, there are several times when this rule of thumb may not be valid. Someone may need to stretch out a debt payment to have adequate cash flow for other budget expenses. Alternatively, they may have an incredibly low interest rate or generous terms on loans that make them attractive to keep.

A small additional payment makes a considerable difference to the total loan payout. Box 7.10 shows what happens to the number of payments when the amount paid each month is increased. Adding $50 per month to a 10-year loan will halve the number of payments made. (The principal paid remains the same but is paid more quickly and with less interest.) More significant savings are seen with more significant monthly additions. Most

BOX 7.10	MAKING LARGER LOAN PAYMENTS			
	Additional principal payment			
	+$50	+$100	+$200	+$500
Monthly payment	$1317	$1367	$1467	$1767
Term (years)	9.4	8.9	8.0	6.2

Assumptions:
    Principal = $100 000
    Interest rate = 9%
    Term = 10 years
    Normal payment = $1267/mo

Adding a few dollars to the principal in the monthly loan payment can significantly impact when the loan is paid off.

loans (especially mortgages) do not have prepayment penalties associated with paying off all or some of the principal early. If cash flow supports it, a person can get ahead financially by making an extra principal payment as often as possible.

Pay off Debt or Build Assets

Should someone use extra money to pay off debt, or should they save it? Paying off debt as quickly as possible has become fashionable. Being debt free should be a long-term financial goal. From a purely financial standpoint, a dentist should look at the after-tax return of the investment and the after-tax cost of the loan and then choose the one that gives a better return. If the interest rate is higher for the investment, they should invest rather than pay off the loan. If the after-tax interest rate of the loan is higher, they should pay off the loan. (See Chapter 16 for a discussion of this topic.) From a cash-flow perspective, cash may be needed for immediate necessities for the family or at the office. It is better to have an asset (the cash reserve) with a corresponding liability (the loan) than to have no cash and less of a loan. In the former case, the dentist may not need to go to a banker for an additional loan. In the latter case, when an additional loan is asked for the banker may balk, wondering why previously loaned money was not handled properly.

Once an emergency fund is built and an asset base established, then it becomes easier to put additional money into paying off debt. Again, comparing the expected return from investing with the savings from debt paydown is essential. A final factor is one's temperament. A dentist must be a disciplined enough investor to invest the money and not "blow it" on a purchase. Then the dentist must get the rate of investment return they anticipated. If the loan is paid off, the dentist should have a plan for the monthly payment that previously went to the loan payment. Finally, the dentist must invest that amount regularly, or it will be spent with nothing to show for it at the end of the pay-off period.

FINANCIAL PLANNING PHASES

There is a standard order of financial tasks for young professionals to consider (Box 7.11). These will be different for different life situations. A dentist who is single in a lucrative practice will have different constraints than a married dentist supporting a family in a start-up situation. Each person will enter the phases of financial planning more or less quickly and have different emphases within each phase than another person.

BOX 7.11	FINANCIAL PLANNING PHASES

Phase 1
Build the emergency fund
Buy appropriate insurance
Develop savings habit
Establish a family budget (spending patterns)

Phase 2
Increase emergency fund with income
Decrease insurance deductibles
Begin retirement savings
Begin children's college funds
Begin investment portfolio
Increase lifestyle (modestly)

Phase 3
Maximize retirement savings
Maximize personal savings and investment
Increase lifestyle
Buy toys

Phase 4
Maximize lifestyle
Donate wealth

PHASE 1: INCREASING DEBT

The first phase typically includes high debt levels because the graduate is making purchases (a practice or a home). The dentist should keep borrowing and spending under control. An initial task is that the dentist has adequate insurance. Part of personal insurance planning is to set the appropriate deductible for the circumstance. As the emergency fund is built, the dentist should increase deductibles and decrease the cost of personal insurance. They should build the practice or professional situation, growing earnings by making the practice profitable through increasing production and decreasing costs. The dentist should be sure that family spending patterns do not increase faster than income and saving increase. They should start funding an individual retirement account as soon as possible. This helps to build a savings habit or mentality, as opposed to a spending mentality. If a dentist moves from employee to practice owner, they face additional debt management problems, as detailed in Section 1 of this book.

PHASE 2: INCREASING INCOME

During the second phase, the practice begins to generate higher income. As income increases, the dentist needs to decide what to do with the additional money. Part of the increase (half) should be used to increase savings and begin investments. As income increases, so does the amount needed for the emergency fund. The dentist should fully fund this increased emergency fund and check that insurance benefits and deductible amounts are appropriate. They should start a practice retirement plan and save for their children's higher education expenses and personal investment portfolios. The dentist should estimate personal income taxes appropriately. As income increases, loan payments remain steady, and depreciation deductions decrease (generally around year 5). At this point, many dentists have not planned well for taxes and need to borrow cash to pay current taxes. Finally, once the savings habit has been developed, the rest of the increase should be used to improve the lifestyle.

PHASE 3: MAXIMUM CASH FLOW

During the third phase, the professional pays off the initial practice loan and the practice income is high. When that loan is paid off, the dentist should reallocate half the monthly payment to increase their retirement plan, use half of the remaining half to increase personal savings and investment, and the other quarter to increase lifestyle. Extra payments to retire debt to become debt free can now be made. At this point, the dentist can begin buying the toys (house on the lake, airplanes, etc.) they desire.

PHASE 4: MAXIMIZE LIFESTYLE

During the fourth phase, income is at its peak and expenses are at their lowest. The dentist has educated their children, paid off their house mortgages, developed their savings, and funded their retirement plans. At this point, working becomes a choice rather than a necessity. The practice and their personal life can be what someone wants them to be without worrying about money. Many people find that they have more time to devote to social and religious causes and discover additional activities to give their lives meaning.

Personal Insurance Needs

I detest life insurance agents; they always argue that I shall some day die, which is not so.

Stephen Leacock

GOAL

This chapter helps the student determine what personal insurance needs will be upon entering a professional situation. It suggests methods of obtaining the best buys in insurance.

LEARNING OBJECTIVES

At the completion of this chapter, the student will be able to:

- Discuss these types of insurance with respect to the purposes, types, benefits, limitations, risk management techniques, features, and tax consequences:
  - Medical (healthcare)
  - Disability
  - Life
  - Automobile
  - Homeowner's
  - Personal excess liability.

- Compare these types of life insurance:
  - Permanent (whole)
  - Universal
  - Endowment
  - Term.

KEY TERMS

actuaries
adjustor
any-occupation policies
automobile insurance
"back-to-work" clause
benefit
collision coverage
comprehensive coverage
cross-purchase agreements

deductibles
definition of disability
disability (income) insurance
elimination period
flexible-benefit plan
frequency of occurrence
guaranteed renewability
health maintenance organizations
  (HMOs)

homeowner's insurance
indemnify
inflation rider
insurance
insurer
liability
liability exclusions
life insurance
limitations of medical insurance

Business Basics for Dentists, Second Edition. James L. Harrison, David O. Willis, and Charles K. Thieman.
© 2024 John Wiley & Sons, Inc. Published 2024 by John Wiley & Sons, Inc.

medical insurance
non-cancellability
office overhead policy
ordinary life insurance
out-of-pocket expense
own-occupation policies
permanent life insurance
personal excess liability policy
point of service plan (POS)
policy

preferred provider organizations
(PPO)
premium
proven loss
pure life insurance
replacement cost provision
residual clause
riders
risk avoidance
risk management

risk reduction
risk retention
risk transfer
Social Security
term insurance
umbrella liability policies
uninsured motorists
universal life insurance
variable life insurance
whole-life insurance

The process of risk management involves identifying and managing a person's risk exposures to protect assets and income. People cannot live in a risk-free world, and there is always the possibility of loss. However, a person can protect their assets against significant, unexpected losses that could financially devastate themselves or others. Everyone needs to accept *some* risk. In analyzing risk, a person needs to separate those risks and determine which they can accept and which they need to manage through some type of insurance. This chapter discusses forms of personal insurance, and professional insurance is discussed in Chapter 28.

UNDERSTANDING INSURANCE

Insurance is one of the most-used risk management techniques. Insurance is available to cover almost any potential loss (Box 8.1), although here we are only looking at personal insurance. A person must decide if the loss is significant or common enough to insure against. (Someone may purchase flood insurance, but if they live on a mountaintop, why bother?) As a rule, if the loss can be self-sustained, it is cheaper, over time, not to buy the insurance and to self-insure and accept the loss. For example, a dentist probably should not buy dental insurance for their family because they can afford most dental costs incurred by family members. A dentist should probably buy medical and accident insurance because the potential loss would be significant. An automobile accident involving a week in hospital for one person can easily cost $100 000, not including liability if that person caused the accident.

Insurance is a commodity. That means the insurance is the same from one company to another (assuming comparable policies). Therefore, someone can shop for insurance based solely on price. Agents work for the insurer, not for the consumer. A person may pay extra for an extended insurance product, which means that they pay extra for convenience, familiarity with the agent, or broad forms of coverage. However, the insurance itself is the same. Insurance agents

are all different. The dentist should shop around for an insurance agent. Often, they will get better rates and better service if they have all types of coverage with one carrier, and may also get better rates if they stay with an insurer for several years without a claim.

Insurance aims to guard against an unexpected, significant financial loss. The basic theory of insurance is that many people pay a small amount (the premium) into a pool of funds. If any payers are unfortunate enough to suffer a significant loss, then part of the pool of funds covers that loss. For example, many people pay a small premium to an insurance company to cover if their home is damaged or destroyed by a disaster, such as a fire. Most people do not have any damage and therefore do not collect from their insurance company. However, if a fire damages a home,

| BOX 8.1 | **INSURANCE NEEDS FOR DENTISTS** |

Personal
Medical care expenses
Loss of income (disability)
Premature death (life)
Property and liability losses
Automobile
    Homeowner
    Excess liability (umbrella)

Professional
Professional liability (malpractice)
Business liability
Loss of use
Office overhead

Required business
Worker's compensation
Unemployment compensation
FICA (Social Security)

that home's owner will receive money from the pool (as a "payout") to cover the damages. However, insurance usually only reimburses for a *demonstrated* loss.

Insurance companies set premium rates based on several factors that influence their expected payout from the pool of premiums. The insurer needs to cover all expected losses and make a reasonable profit. The frequency of occurrence and the size of the typical award both influence the expected payout from the company. A person's history of claims, age, and other personal factors help determine the company's estimate of their particular risk as an insured party. Insurers use actuaries (like statistical accountants) to figure out risk tables and rates to charge their clients. For example, the chance of an 85-year-old man dying is much greater than that of a 5-year-old dying in a given year. The life insurance rates for the 85-year-old man will be higher than for the 5-year-old.

Insurers face the risk that more people will die, have a house fire, or have a car wreck in any given year than they anticipated. If that happens, they initially lose money, raise everyone's rates the following year, or cancel policies for the poorer risks. Most also carry insurance through Lloyd's of London or other insurance underwriters. They call this the secondary insurance market, which helps cover the insurers for significant losses, such as natural (hurricane) or human (terrorist) disasters. Insurers use other techniques to control how much risk they face. Copays, deductibles, payment limits, exclusions, and other riders all help control their potential losses.

Each person must decide when to use insurance. There are times when the law requires that they have insurance. (Workers' compensation and unemployment insurance are required insurance for employers. Most states require auto liability insurance.) Other than required times, a person should use insurance to help cover an unexpected, unpredictable loss that they would not be able to afford to pay out of pocket. The owner of a new $70 000 car often chooses to insure the car in case an accident causes such damage to the automobile that they cannot afford to have repaired. The owner of an old $1000 junk car may choose to carry no insurance on the vehicle. If they wreck the car, they lose the cost of the car. (Again, insuring liability, in case the owner of the junker caused the accident, is required by law in many states.) Other significant, unpredictable losses that can be insured against include damage to the home, hospitalization, loss of income because of a disability, liability as a professional (malpractice), or liability as a private individual (personal liability).

The person signs a contract (policy) with the insurance company. The contract states that the insurer (the company) will indemnify (make good a loss to) the policyholder in case of proven loss (as specified in the policy), given the restrictions written into the policy. Insurance companies usually sell policies through insurance agents. Agents may work for one company (a "captive" agent) or they may represent many companies (an "independent" agent), shopping around for the best rates for a given situation. A person's relationship with an insurance agent may be as close as that with an accountant, so they need to find a compatible agent. The buyer should be sure that the agent explains all the options of the policies and integrates the various types of coverage for the various insurances they purchase. The state where someone resides, not the federal government, regulates insurance companies and agents.

If a policyholder has a loss, the agent will be the initial contact with the company. The policyholder must understand that the agent does not decide whether the policyholder is reimbursed for a loss. The insurance company does that. The agent only acts as a go-between, often splitting their allegiance between the policyholder and the company. An adjuster is someone hired by the insurer to decide the amount of covered loss. After a car accident, the adjuster will determine how much it ought to cost to fix the car (and therefore the reimbursable loss). The agent will act as a best friend while someone is paying premiums. If that person files a claim, things change. The agents then play "good cop, bad cop" with the loss adjustors and the insurance company. Policyholders must remember that agents work for the insurer.

MEDICAL INSURANCE

Medical (healthcare) insurance originally reimbursed a person for high, unexpected medical costs, such as hospitalization. It has evolved into a mechanism to help pay for the costs of healthcare, large and small. The world of healthcare insurance is complex, and marketplace and governmental influences drive it. It is a constantly changing system, so here we only present the basics of health insurance.

Like other forms of insurance, health insurance is a contract that requires a health insurer or company to pay some or all of a consumer's healthcare costs in exchange for a premium. It pays different amounts for different types of care and who provides it. A person can generally shop for a healthcare insurance plan to find the one that best meets their needs. If, for example, they have a child with a developmental disability, they will need an entirely different plan from that for a healthy, single person with no dependents. If someone is employed, their employer may offer one insurance plan or a mix of plans from which to choose.

PAYING FOR HEALTHCARE

There are several ways in which insurers share the cost of healthcare with their plan participants. This encourages the consumers to become more knowledgeable and participate more in their healthcare decisions.

Premium

Medical insurance can be selected and paid for by the individual. If the dentist is employed, the employer often establishes a benefit plan that pays all or part of the insurance cost. The employee may be required to share in the cost through salary reduction. A general rule is that the more the purchaser (individual or employer) pays in premiums, the less the individual pays when seeing their healthcare provider. Premiums are paid each month. The government helps with premiums for low-income families.

Out-of-Pocket Costs

Out-of-pocket costs are consumers' costs for medical care that the insurer does not reimburse. Thus, consumers pay out-of-pocket costs and their monthly premiums, but the insurance contract has a limit on out-of-pocket costs. Once the consumer reaches that limit (an annual maximum amount determined in the contract), the insurance company pays all or a part of any further covered costs. Typical out-of-pocket expenses include the following:

- **Deductible**
  A deductible is the amount consumers owe for healthcare services before their health insurance plan begins to pay. (Premiums do not count toward the deductible.) For example, if a consumer's deductible is $1000, the plan will not pay anything until the consumer has paid $1000 for covered healthcare services. However, some healthcare services (often preventive services) are not subject to the deductible and may be covered by health insurance plans even if consumers have not met the deductible. Generally, the higher the deductible, the lower the premiums' cost. The insurance company will pay less because the insured pays more. The trade-off for a lower deductible is higher premium payments.

- **Copayment ("copay")**
  Copayments require the insured to pay a fixed part of the cost (e.g. $30) out of pocket, usually at the time of service. Often copayments are lower for preventive services. They are also lower for in-network providers than copayments for out-of-network providers. This encourages consumers to use the insurance company's network of providers. Copayments do not take the place of deductibles.

- **Coinsurance**
  Coinsurance is like a copayment. Here, the consumer pays a percentage (e.g. 20%) of the cost instead of a fixed amount. Coinsurance also does not replace deductible amounts; they are paid in addition.

Allowed Amount

An allowed amount is the maximum amount the insurer will pay for a covered procedure. (It is sometimes called an "eligible expense" or "negotiated rate.") If providers charge more than the allowed amount, consumers may have to pay the difference, especially if they see an out-of-network provider.

Balance Billing

Balance billing is when providers bill consumers for the difference between the provider's charge and the amount allowed by the health insurance plan. Say a provider charges $300 for a procedure and the insurance plan's "negotiated rate" is $200. The provider may bill the balance ($100) to the individual. However, if the provider has signed a contract with the insurer to be in their network of providers, they generally may not bill the balance. Out-of-network providers generally can. This is another incentive for the consumer to get care from a network provider.

TYPES OF HEALTH INSURANCE PLANS

Indemnity Plans

In the past, indemnity (traditional insurance) plans were the norm. In these plans, the patient went to the provider they chose, received care, and the insurance paid all or a portion of the bill. These indemnity plans – fee-for-service (FFS) plans – still exist, although they are becoming rare. Because the insurance company cannot enter into a contractual obligation with the providers, they cannot control the cost of care. So, these plans are often prohibitively expensive.

Flexible Spending Accounts and Healthcare Savings Accounts

Several types of accounts allow a person to deduct money from their pay (pretax) and then use that to pay for out-of-pocket medical expenses. Two common types are FSAs (Flexible Spending Accounts) and HSAs (Healthcare Savings Accounts). These are not actual health insurance plans, but savings plans that work together with a health insurance plan. A consumer uses money in the HSA or

FSA to help meet out-of-pocket expenses that the insurer does not pay. When a consumer uses an HSA or FSA to pay their qualified out-of-pocket medical expenses, they pay these on a pretax basis. The money someone contributes to an HSA or an FSA is not subject to federal income tax. However, there are strict rules on which expenses qualify. Companies establish FSAs as employee benefits. Individuals can use HSAs. Insurance companies, banks, or other financial institutions set up these accounts. An online search will find many companies to help a practitioner set one up. All these accounts have specific rules and are subject to the whims of Congress and the Internal Revenue Service (IRS). The practitioner needs to check with their advisor to get the right plan.

High Deductible Health Plan

A High Deductible Health Plan (HDHP) features higher deductibles than traditional insurance plans in exchange for lower monthly premiums. HDHPs are often combined with an HSA or an FSA to pay the higher deductible costs that the patient must pay. The patient pays the out-of-pocket expenses with tax-deductible contributions to the HSA or FSA. HDHPs are often called catastrophic health plans.

Managed Care Plans

Because of the high cost of medical insurance premiums, many individuals and employers buy managed healthcare contracts for their employees. These are generally not actual insurance products (which indemnify or agree to pay for a loss), but instead are forms of prepayment for care, which shift the risk of overutilization of health services from the insurer to the provider and the subscriber. Consumers with these private health insurance plans can generally choose between several types of care plans.

Managed care plans are networks of providers organized by the insurer to manage the patient's care. Health insurance companies contract with specific hospitals, doctors, pharmacies, and other healthcare providers to deliver medical services for agreed-upon rates. The plans that use these networks give consumers different levels of access to providers, with different premium price points, different consumer payment requirements, and different requirements for choosing providers.

- **Health Maintenance Organization**
  A Health Maintenance Organization (HMO) is a type of health insurance plan that usually requires the consumer to choose from a list of in-network doctors who work for or contract with the HMO. They generally have specific hospitals in their network as well. They require participants to be referred to a specialist by their primary care doctor. Typically, HMOs only pay for the care provided in their network (except for emergency care). HMOs generally charge only premiums. There are often no (or low) out-of-pocket expenses for the consumer. Premiums are typically lower in an HMO than in other plans because of the requirement to see a network provider.

- **Preferred Provider Organization**
  A Preferred Provider Organization (PPO) also creates a network of healthcare providers (doctors, hospitals, therapists). They have contracts with those providers that cover reimbursement and other care requirements. Consumers pay less if they use providers that belong to the plan's network (i.e. in-network providers). They can see out-of-network providers, but it will cost the patient more in out-of-pocket expenses. Patients do not need a referral to see a specialist. In exchange for greater access to providers, premiums are generally higher in a PPO than in an HMO.

- **Point of Service plan**
  Like a PPO, a Point of Service (POS) plan is a type of plan in which consumers pay less if they use doctors, hospitals, and other healthcare providers that belong to the plan's network. With this plan, consumers may go to out-of-network providers at a higher cost. Unlike PPO plans, POS plans require consumers to get a referral from their primary care doctor to see a specialist.

- **Exclusive Provider Organization**
  An Exclusive Provider Organization (EPO) is a managed care plan that covers services only if the patient uses doctors, specialists, or hospitals in the plan's network (except in an emergency). It generally does not cover services received outside the network; the patient must pay for these out-of-network services themselves.

Government Healthcare Plans

The US government provides insurance plans or direct care for a large segment of the population. Like private insurance, there may be small out-of-pocket expenses that consumers in these programs pay. Several of these programs are joint state–federal programs, so the funding, benefits, and terms vary from state to state. Depending on the dentist's history and present situation, they may qualify for one of these plans.

- **Medicaid**
  This is a joint (state-administered) health coverage program for low-income families and children,

pregnant women, some older adults, people with disabilities, and, in some states, other adults. The federal government provides a portion of the funding for Medicaid and sets guidelines for the program. States also have choices in how they design their programs, so Medicaid varies state by state and may have a different name in each state.

- **Children's Health Insurance Program**
  The Children's Health Insurance Program (CHIP) is a joint federal and state program that provides health coverage to uninsured low-income children. In some states, certain pregnant women are included.

- **Medicare**
  Medicare is a federal health coverage program primarily for people who are 65 or older. Some young people with disabilities or kidney failure also qualify. Medicare beneficiaries pay a premium or qualify for benefits coverage based on previous payment of payroll taxes.

- **TRICARE**
  TRICARE is the Department of Defense's healthcare program available to eligible members and their families of the seven US uniformed services: the Army, Navy, Air Force, Marine Corps, Coast Guard, Commissioned Corps of the US Public Health Service, and National Oceanic and Atmospheric Administration.

- **Veterans Administration health benefits**
  The Veterans Administration (VA) administers various benefits and services that provide financial and other assistance to service members, veterans, and their dependents and survivors. The VA provides medical coverage for eligible veterans who served in the US military.

PRESCRIPTION DRUG PLANS

Most health insurance plans include coverage for drugs and medicine prescribed by a physician. They use the term "formulary" or "drug list" to describe the list of prescription drugs that they cover. This formulary includes details about how much a consumer pays for each type of covered drug. Like other health insurance, there are various combinations of out-of-pocket expenses for the consumer.

Insurers group the covered drugs into tiers. (The plan may not cover all drugs.) Each of these tiers has a different consumer payment rate associated with it. This encourages patients to select lower-cost prescription (generic) drugs. For example:

- Tier 1 requires a $10 copayment.
- Tier 2 requires a $25 copayment.
- Tier 3 requires a $50 copayment.

The plan's formulary will list which drugs are in which tier.

GUIDELINES FOR CHOOSING A HEALTH INSURANCE PLAN

Choosing the right health insurance plan can be a complex decision. Here are a few recommendations, based on employee status:

- **Employee**
  The employer of an employee dentist will generally offer one or a limited number of related plans. These have different coverages and costs associated with them. The dentist should look at their past medical utilization to help determine future needs. Family plans will be more expensive (more people are covered) than individual plans. The dentist may opt for a higher-premium plan with lower out-of-pocket expenses if the employer pays part of the premium as an employee benefit, which decreases the cost. If the employer offers an FSA or similar plan, most people will take advantage of them to decrease out-of-pocket expenses.

- **Government plans**
  If the dentist qualifies for a government plan, this is usually the most cost-effective way to get coverage. Common qualifiers include low income and veteran status, and various state and national online portals help qualified people begin the decision process.

- **Self-employed**
  The self-employed dentist can buy insurance from a private company or an online government portal.

- **Practice owner dentist**
  Current law requires business owners with more than 50 employees to provide health insurance coverage. Smaller firms are not required but may opt to provide health insurance as a benefit to attract employees. There are several tax implications that the owner needs to discuss with their accountant. There are also rules about eligibility and payments. This is a complex process. The owner will probably need to contact a broker or a health insurance company directly to begin the process and ensure compliance. They may be able to include an FSA- or HSA-type account as well.

DISABILITY (INCOME) INSURANCE

The chance of someone becoming disabled at some point during their professional career is much greater than the chance of dying during that same time. According to the Social Security Administration, 25% of today's 20-year-olds can expect to be out of work for at least a year because of a disabling condition before they reach the average retirement age. Although death is undoubtedly a more critical event than disability, many professionals carry life insurance but do not include disability insurance as part of their financial risk management plan.

Flu can disable someone for several days; an actual disability is an inability to work for at least 30 days. Less than that is considered a simple illness. Disability insurance does not insure someone against becoming disabled and does not automatically pay if they become disabled. It does protect their loss of income if they are disabled. So, the more proper name for this type of insurance is disability *income* insurance. As with other insurable losses, a person generally needs to show the loss to collect the benefits. For example, a dentist must show that they lost $10 000 per month in income for the policy to replace it. If they only had $3000 per month of income, that is all the policy would replace, even if it had a $10 000-per-month face amount (limit). Disability insurance coverage, regardless of the source, usually only replaces about two-thirds to three-fourths of pretax income. (Usually, the benefits are tax free, so there is no need to include the cost of taxes in the benefit.) With multiple policies, disability income insurance will generally exclude or offset payments from other policies. A common "insurance with other insurers" clause reduces payments proportional to any other policies.

Disability can occur for many reasons. An automobile accident can leave someone unable to practice for the rest of their life. A skiing accident or a simple fall in the home can render them incapable for many months. Contagious diseases (e.g. hepatitis B, HIV) can leave someone incapable of practice. A heart attack can disable them for weeks or years. Modern medicine has changed many diseases, such as diabetes or cardiovascular problems, from deadly acute diseases to more chronic diseases. However, these lead to more disability claims. The most common long-term disabling conditions include musculoskeletal disorders (back, spine, knees, and shoulders), cancers, and injuries.

Some disability insurance only covers a person for a specific type of disabling condition. Some policies only cover accidental disability; they do not cover disabling illnesses. Occupational policies cover someone if the disability is job related, and non-occupational policies only cover non-work-related disabilities. (The theory is that workers' compensation insurance pays for occupation-related disabilities. However, this amount is entirely inadequate for most dentists.)

If someone becomes disabled, they should not assume that the insurer or agent is a friend. It can often be a nightmare getting the insurer to agree that the person is, in fact, disabled and not just trying to defraud the company. The dentist may need to prove to the insurer, through letters from physicians and medical test results, that they are genuinely unable to practice. The policyholder must keep excellent paperwork (and copies), including all medical reports, correspondence, and phone conversations with insurers and physicians. They must be sure to use a physician knowledgeable about the disabling problem (e.g. a general practitioner should not certify an orthopedic disability). Sometimes the insurer will even require that the policyholder see a particular physician for evaluation. The dentist needs to get the best board-certified orthopedic surgeon in the area. Some people have had to sue their disability insurers to get the insurance company to pay benefits.

SOURCES OF INCOME IF DISABLED

Several sources of income will be available to a practicing dentist during a disability:

- Suppose a practice owner and accounts receivable provide an initial income flow. This flow lasts for 30–60 days before it dwindles. However, the dentist will have an additional cash-flow problem when they return to work after the disability is over, and it takes a while to get the cash flowing through the practice. They need to have savings or an emergency fund established for this possibility. This is the perfect use and justification for having such a fund.

- Social Security provides some disability income. This is not significant for most professionals, and it is limited to people who have 40 quarters of payments into the system and also who are permanently disabled. Payments are meager compared to the lifestyle of most professionals.

- A dentist in a group practice may have arrangements built into a contract that protects each person in case of a disability.

- A spouse or other family member can support the family without the practitioner's income being replaced.

- Depending on the disability, a dentist may continue to own and manage the practice. For example, assume that a dentist suffers a compound fracture of their right (dominant) arm in a skiing accident and they cannot pick up a handpiece. However, they can hire an associate dentist to keep the practice going. The owner–dentist can then come to the office to conduct staff meetings, meet and greet patients, and perform other ownership duties. Most insurers consider any profit earned from these activities to be income and will decrease payments by this amount.

- Disability income insurance will provide the bulk of a lost income stream. Because this income replacement is necessary, a dentist must understand their policy and review it annually.

FACTORS IN CHOOSING A POLICY

Many factors affect the individual policy's limitations and benefits (and therefore cost):

- **The definition of disability**
  A stricter definition of the term disability means that fewer people will become disabled. This lowers the insurer's payout, and therefore the cost of the policy, but it decreases protection. Is someone disabled if they cannot practice dentistry or if they cannot do any meaningful work? If someone loses a hand in an automobile accident but can pull cans of peas across the laser scanner at the local grocery store, are they disabled? Some policies will pay benefits if someone cannot perform the duties of their occupation (so-called own-occupation or "own occ" policies). This means that if someone is a practicing periodontist and cannot perform the duties of a practicing periodontist, they are disabled. Other policies require that a person be unable to do the duties of any occupation ("any occ" policies) to be disabled. If the person can work in any occupation (such as at the local grocery store), they are not disabled. Own occ policies have been abused by practitioners, but many occupational policies do not offer enough protection. Most insurers now have language that defines disability in terms such as "substantially similar occupations," "occupational specific," or "work in which a person is qualified by education, training, and experience." This protects someone from having to dig ditches, but does not allow them to claim that they are a periodontist, not a general dentist. Many policies also allow for the insurer to provide retraining. For a practitioner, this means that under the insurance policy provisions, the insurer might retrain them to review insurance claims or teach in a dental school. The policy will declare this.

- **Amount of monthly benefit**
  The more a benefit someone receives, the more the policy will cost. Practitioners must be realistic about how much income is insured, and it is possible to be overinsured. As mentioned, insurers will generally only pay for income that they can show that they have lost (i.e. the amount they made before the disability). This is to prevent fraudulent disability claims. (If someone can make more income while disabled, why work?) It also prevents malingering or someone being exceedingly slow to return to work.

- **Length of elimination period**
  The time before the insurer's payments begin (the elimination period) affects the cost of the policy. The shorter the elimination period, the more likely it is that the policyholder will collect from the policy at some time, and the higher the cost. Someone may recover from a disabling condition when a longer elimination period takes effect. They are much less likely to collect if they must wait 90 or 120 days than if they must wait 30 or 60 days. Someone could theoretically buy a policy that covers them from the first day of disability, but it would be prohibitively expensive. Some people buy a short-term disability policy to cover the elimination period.

- **The length of the benefit payment**
  How long someone continues to collect benefits if they are totally or permanently disabled affects the policy. Standard periods include lifetime, until age 65 or 70, and for 5 or 10 years. The longer the potential payout for the insurer, the higher the cost of the policy (premiums).

- **Guaranteed renewability and non-cancellability**
  If someone contracts a potentially recurring disease (such as a heart condition or cancer), they want to be sure they can renew the disability policy when renewal time comes. Otherwise, the insurer might claim that person is now a poor risk and cancel the policy or refuse to insure them. Other insurers would also refuse to insure that person based on their history, or charge such high rates that the insurance would not be affordable. Dentists should be sure that a policy is guaranteed to be renewable to age 65 or 70. This means that the policy cannot be canceled if they continue to make payments. Premiums can rise if they rise for everyone (contingent on state approval). A more favorable policy is a non-cancellable policy. In this type, the insurer cannot increase the premium over the term of the policy. A non-cancellable, guaranteed renewable policy provides the most protection, but at an added cost.

- **Inflation rider**
  This factor helps someone maintain purchasing power if they become disabled for an extended period

by increasing benefits at the same rate as inflation. These are often called cost of living adjustment (COLA) policies.

- **Residual or "back-to-work" clause**
These clauses protect both the insured and the insurer. A residual clause allows the insured to continue to receive partial benefits when they return to work part-time. For example, assume that someone had a heart attack. After six months of total disability, the physician clears that person fir to return to work two days per week, to build gradually until they are back five days per week as before the illness. A residual clause pays partial benefits while that person is working part-time. Without this clause, benefits end when the person returns to work, even part-time, although their income is much less than before the illness.

- **Guaranteed purchase option**
This is the right to buy additional insurance as income rises without new medical examinations or tests. This option allows someone to purchase additional insurance at specified times (e.g. every three years) if their income warrants it. This is important for dentists because their incomes often increase because of inflation and practitioner maturity.

- **Exclusions**
Disability income policies do not cover every disabling condition. An exclusion is a condition that is not a covered disabling condition. Many are the result of individual choice. Typical policy exclusions include:
  ○ Self-inflicted injuries.
  ○ Attempted (unsuccessful) suicide.
  ○ Illegal drug use.
  ○ Injuries that happen while flying in a non-commercial airplane.
  ○ Injuries that happen because of a war.
  ○ Conditions that existed before a person was eligible for coverage (preexisting condition).

GUIDELINES FOR CHOOSING A DISABILITY POLICY

Given the apparent complexity of these policies, what ought someone look for in a disability income policy? There are several general rules to consider:

- A dentist should plan for disability as if it will happen tomorrow. In this way, they will be prepared when it does happen. The practitioner should plan with a group of local practitioners to cover each other's practices in case one individual has a disability. They need to let family and advisors know where the policies are and who the agents are.

- Group plans are usually cheaper than individual policies. If there is coverage via a group policy through work, the dentist should participate in that. The coverage may not be ideal, and they may need to supplement it with another policy, but these group policies are usually a good starting place.

- A dentist should plan to replace 60–80% of pretax income. Because the benefits received will usually be tax free, they do not need to replace the income that would have been spent on income taxes. However, retirement plan contributions need to be included with a policy that ends at age 65 or 70. Most insurers will limit the benefit based on proven income, which is tough on beginning practitioners (who can show little income). Nevertheless, many insurers will write beginning policies to gain someone as a customer for the firm.

- Dentists need shorter elimination periods and more extended payment periods early in a dental career than later in their career. Unfortunately, this is also when a practitioner can least afford the higher premiums that come with this type of insurance. A practice owner needs to look at accounts receivable and the emergency fund to decide how long an elimination period they can weather. Initially, they may need a short (30–60-day) elimination period, which they may lengthen when they build up funds. A 90- or 120-day elimination period policy will save someone a substantial amount of money in lower premium payments.

- Dentists should review policies every year. A person's needs change as their income and assets change. They need to carry enough insurance but not overinsure; both are costly mistakes.

- A practitioner should have a residual or return-to-work clause. Many people become disabled by illness and return to work gradually; they should be sure that insurance reflects this.

- Most practitioners would like a non-cancellable policy to lock in premiums until age 65 or 70.

- Disability income insurance covers income for personal family budget needs; a separate office overhead policy helps defray the costs of office expenses. A business-reducing term disability (BRTD) insurance policy remains in place for a specific time to cover a particular need. For example, if someone buys a practice that requires a monthly loan payment of $4000 for five years, BRTD insurance is an excellent low-cost way to ensure the need. A personal disability income replacement policy is more expensive and is required for *personal* income needs.

- A practitioner should skip any riders that are intended to feed a retirement plan while they are disabled. The riders cost a lot and often require the policyholder to invest only with the insurance company's affiliates. A dentist needs adequate disability income coverage to contribute to their retirement plan.

- Some insurance advisors suggest sticking with a company that has the endorsement of professional organizations (such as the American Dental Association, ADA). They are easier to deal with if a large portion of their business is from a single, tight-knit profession. These "association policies" are packages that are not as flexible as an individual policy. However, if they meet someone's needs (they are designed to meet the needs of typical association members), they can provide significant cost savings.

ACCIDENTAL DEATH AND DISMEMBERMENT INSURANCE

Accidental death and dismemberment (AD&D) policies, although common, serve a limited need for independent dental practitioners. Their purpose is to provide a lump-sum payment if someone dies or loses a limb in an accident. Some policies require that the limb be severed for payment; others only require loss of use or function to pay the benefit. Most policies cover the policyholder whether the accident was at work or not. The policies will not cover if someone dies or loses a limb from an illness or disease (these are not accidents). Some policies have additional discriminators that qualify the accident for coverage.

Most dental practitioners do not need AD&D policies. They should have adequate disability and life insurance to cover their unique financial needs. AD&D policies are less expensive to cover some of those needs, but most practitioners need a more comprehensive insurance plan. Some practitioners have AD&D policies in an insurance package for staff members as an employee benefit. An employee dentist eligible for this insurance needs to coordinate it with a disability income policy.

LIFE INSURANCE

Like disability insurance, life insurance is a bit of a misnomer. People do not insure against death, and everyone will die eventually. Instead, someone buys life insurance to guard against premature death or death before they have had a chance to build assets to provide for a given financial need. They will lose if life insurance is viewed as a bet or a game of chance. They will also lose if they do not collect because their actuaries have determined premiums to profit the company. They will certainly lose if they collect, because they will be dead and unable to enjoy the benefits. This is not to say that people never need life insurance. Instead, they ought to buy it for a specific purpose.

The terminology of life insurance is like other types of insurance. Someone buys a contract or policy that offers specific coverage, and they pay premiums to the insurer. If that person dies, the person named as the beneficiary receives the benefits or payout of the policy.

Insurance sales agents are good at making people feel obligated to buy life insurance or guilty if they do not have any. First, it is essential to consider why someone would buy life insurance, its potential purpose. If someone does not fit into one of the categories outlined shortly, they do not need life insurance and should not feel guilty about not having any.

PURPOSES OF LIFE INSURANCE

The purposes of life insurance include the following:

- Someone may want to provide money after they are gone to maintain a standard of living for their family. Suppose that person is the sole support or provides a significant contribution to the family budget. In that case, they need to plan to replace that income if they die prematurely (before adequate savings and assets have been built up). On the other hand, if a spouse is an employed professional who can earn an adequate family income if that person dies, they may choose not to carry life insurance. Life insurance is not winning the lottery for the family. Practitioners should plan a specific amount to replace income.

- Lending agencies may require a person to carry life insurance to secure business assets. A banker may require a life insurance policy, naming the bank as beneficiary, to the amount of a practice loan. If the insured person dies prematurely (before the loan is paid off), the insurance policy will pay the remainder of the loan to the bank. Practice assets go to the person's estate for heirs' handling.

- Life insurance can fund cross-purchase agreements for practice purchases in estate planning. If someone is a member of a group practice, they and their partners may carry life insurance on each other. (One person carries a policy on their partner; the partner carries one on the first person.) If one of them dies, the other has the money (and a contractual obligation) to buy out the other's portion of the practice. (Hence the name, cross-purchase agreement.) The person's estate, and therefore the family, benefits by having a previously agreed purchase price and not having to sell the person's portion of the practice at the time of death. The partner(s) benefits by knowing that the other person's heirs will not sell their portion of the practice to a stranger, who may not fit into the practice style that the group has developed.

- Someone may have specific financial needs for which to plan. A spouse might provide for the family budget but cannot contribute to certain family benefits, such as paying for children's higher education. Others may be paying off business start-up costs or paying a mortgage on vacation property.

- Life insurance has been touted as a savings and retirement planning mechanism. As a rule, there are much better savings and retirement planning techniques. Someone might want to use life insurance as a savings mechanism if they are a terrible money manager and cannot budget a savings plan any other way.

- Life insurance can be used as an estate planning technique, saving estate taxes. Most people will not need these techniques until late in their careers. When someone gets to this point, they will have tax advisors to help.

TYPES OF LIFE INSURANCE

There are two basic types of life insurance and several hybrid or combinations of the basic types.

- **Term life insurance**
  Term insurance is also known as pure life insurance. This type of policy is valid only for a specific period. Someone may have a term life insurance policy effective from July 1 through June 30 of the following year. If they die at 12:01 a.m. on July 1 of the following year, the death is not covered, and the beneficiaries receive no benefits. If that person dies two minutes earlier, at 11:59 on June 30, the beneficiary receives the policy's full benefit. Many policies are renewable, which means that the policy owner can pay an additional premium and extend coverage for another period. Other policies, especially those that cover a specific event, such as a practice purchase, are non-renewable and exist only for the insurance period. Term insurance is pure insurance because, unlike whole-life policies, no cash value accumulates in the policy. A person cannot save money or borrow against a term life policy. Nevertheless, term policies are much cheaper than other types of policies for comparable levels of insurance coverage.

- **Whole-life insurance**
  Whole life is also known as "ordinary," "permanent," or "cash value" insurance. Unlike term policies, whole-life policies last for an entire lifetime. They allocate part of each payment to pure life insurance (like a term policy) and a portion to a savings account within the policy. The policyholder can then borrow against the value accumulated within the policy or cash it in after payments at maturity (e.g. retirement). The value accumulates tax free within the insurance policy. This makes whole-life insurance a combination of a pure insurance product and a tax-advantaged savings vehicle. Before rushing to buy this type of insurance, consider the following. Insurance executives are conservative investors. (As well they should be: people do not want them squandering their insurance payout by investing in risky ventures.) The return within the policy is safe but low. The company charges the policyholder interest to borrow on the account, essentially charging interest to borrow their own money. Moreover, whole-life policies are so profitable for insurers that they generally give 50–75% of the first two years' premium payments as commission to the agent selling the policy. That is quite an incentive for agents to sell whole-life policies.

- **Hybrid policies**
  To solve problems associated with whole-life policies, insurers have developed a group of hybrid insurance products. These have characteristics of term policies, whole-life policies, and actual investments. Variable life policies take the savings portion of a whole-life premium and invest it in a mutual fund or another investment vehicle that pays (potentially) more than a traditional whole-life policy. The cash value that builds up varies as the underlying investment return varies. Depending on the policy, the amount of insurance may also vary. Universal life policies are like whole-life policies, except they pay a competitive interest rate. The underlying investment portion of the payment is tied to the money market or US Treasury Bill interest rates. Endowment life policies pay dividends as annuity or regular payments. These policies can supplement retirement income once someone has fully funded their retirement plan.

GUIDELINES FOR CHOOSING LIFE INSURANCE

If a person is considering buying life insurance, they need to answer several before they sign any contracts or checks. These include the following:

- The person must know the reason for buying it and decide what specific financial goal will be accomplished by buying insurance. They must determine their insurance needs based on their income replacement needs. They might not need any life insurance at all. If someone is buying insurance because an agent called on the phone and said that a young dentist needs insurance, they should reconsider.

- The person must decide how much insurance they need. The answer to the first question will help to answer this one. They should estimate the cost of a college education or family income needs, but they should only buy enough insurance to provide for the family's benefit. If buying insurance to provide a family income, the purchaser must buy approximately six to eight times the annual net income. This is an amount that, if invested at 8%, would replace lost income.

- The person needs to decide when to buy life insurance. If they have identified the need, they buy the insurance when required, not before and not after. If someone becomes a poor health risk (because of a disease or condition), they may have difficulty buying life insurance at any cost. This is the one valid reason for buying insurance before it is needed.

- The person needs to decide when the insurance ends. They should end the coverage when the need ends. Insurance to cover a practice loan can end when the loan has been paid off. Insurance to provide a college education can end when a college fund is funded, or the child completes college. As a person ages, they usually need less insurance. As they move through their professional career, they pay off debts and build assets. These assets can provide income in case of death. Insurance provides for loss of income if someone dies before they have had a chance to build an asset base. Many professionals find renewable term policies ideal for this insurance coverage.

- The person needs to decide what type of life insurance they should buy. The type of policy they buy should depend on the needs identified previously. A five-year decreasing term policy would be most appropriate to secure a five-year practice loan. The insurance ends after five years, but the loan is paid by then. The benefit decreases each year, but so does the remaining principal. A whole-life policy, in this case, would be financial overkill and obligate someone to premium payments for years after the loan is paid.

- People should not buy life insurance when purchasing automobiles or other large items. Sales agents try to sell this insurance as "mortgage protection" or "loan protection" insurance that will pay off the loan if the person dies without "burdening" the family. This is simply an expensive term policy. The purchaser should say "no" and mean it.

- The person should not buy insurance from anyone who calls on the phone soliciting business. These callers are generally starting agents whose sole purpose is to sell policies, regardless of someone's needs.

- The person should not buy whole-life insurance. Whole-life policies are expensive, and relative term policies cost about 50% as much as a whole-life policy. The person ought to buy term insurance and invest the difference. If someone can manage a dental practice, they can manage the finances involved in insurance.

- Be sure to name a specific beneficiary (individual or trust) on the policy, not the estate. The beneficiary is the person who will get the proceeds of the policy if a policyholder dies. There can be enormous adverse estate tax consequences if a person does not do this.

AUTOMOBILE INSURANCE

Automobile insurance is an area in which many professionals can save significant amounts of money. Most people keep the same automobile insurance year after year, yet dentists spend more money on this insurance annually than on malpractice insurance. Automobile insurance policies follow a standard procedure, so comparing one policy with another is easy.

As a rule, the auto owner is responsible for ensuring the auto. If someone grants another person permission to use their car, then the owner's insurance generally will cover the other person. Some states have different rules, and some policies have specific exclusions, so the auto owner needs to check with the agent and policy to ensure coverage.

NO-FAULT INSURANCE

Some states have a "no-fault" auto insurance system. In these states, auto owners' insurance covers their driver and passengers' injuries, regardless of who caused the accident. Other coverage (such as collision or uninsured motorists) remains the same.

No-fault insurance intends to reduce the number of auto accident-related lawsuits. In most states, if someone is in an accident, the insurance companies try to determine who caused the accident or who is at fault. Once that is decided, the other driver can file a claim against the accident-causing driver's insurance for damages or injuries that resulted. In no-fault states, it does not matter who was at fault. Instead, each driver files a claim with their insurance company, which then pays damages for the losses their driver sustained. (The other driver's insurance pays for their losses.) In these states, a person cannot sue for injuries, damages, or pain and suffering unless the damages go beyond a threshold set by the state. No-fault policies generally require coverage for bodily and property liability and personal injury protection (PIP). The individual state sets limits, requirements, and benefit payments for these kinds of coverage.

No-fault insurance is mandatory in some (currently 12) states. In these "pure" no-fault states, the driver's insurance pays benefits to their driver and passengers, regardless of who is responsible for the accident. The trade-off for this is that drivers are restricted in their rights to sue the other driver (and their insurance company) for damages. Several (currently three) states give residents the option of either a pure no-fault or traditional auto policy that allows the driver to sue. Several other states have hybrid (or "add-on") policies where the primary insurer pays its driver's benefits, but the driver still has the right to sue. To add to this confusion, states change their insurance laws from time to time, either enacting or eliminating no-fault provisions. An experienced agent in the state of residence will help clear up the confusion.

TYPES OF CAR INSURANCE COVERAGE

Auto insurance is a package of coverage that protects the car owner from risks. Different states may require these kinds of coverage, and others may be optional. The insurance agent will help sort through the needed coverage, including the following:

- Collision coverage pays to repair damage to the car if it is in a crash. Often banks, leasing companies, and rental car agencies require this coverage.

- Comprehensive coverage handles damage to a car that is not caused by accident. Examples include stone chipping the windshield, car theft, or a tree falling on the car.

- Liability coverage for property damage pays for repairs to someone else's car if the policyholder cause an accident, and does not cover damage to the policyholder's vehicle.

- Liability coverage for bodily injury helps pay medical expenses for drivers and passengers in someone else's car if the policyholder causes an accident. It does not cover the policyholder or their passengers.

- Uninsured (and underinsured) motorist coverage helps to protect the policyholder if someone who does not have any (or adequate) insurance causes a wreck.

- In states that have no-fault insurance, PIP helps pay for injuries to a driver or passengers of the insured's car. Depending on the policy, it may also pay for lost wages or required household help. This coverage is only found in states with no-fault insurance laws, and it only covers passengers in the insured's car. Liability coverage still pays for injury to people in the other car.

- In states that do not have no-fault insurance, medical payments coverage pays for injuries to the driver or passengers in the insured car due to an accident.

Components

Auto policies consist of four areas of insurance, and some policies may not include all four areas.

- **Part A: Liability** covers a policyholder if they cause an accident. This person also may be required to pay for fixing someone else's property (such as their automobile) or paying them for injuries.

- **Part B: Medical payments** provides medical payments to the policyholder or someone in their car injured in an accident. These medical payment amounts are low, and the policyholder should have health and liability insurance to help cover these expenses.

- **Part C: Uninsured motorists** covers the policyholder if an uninsured motorist causes an accident that damages the policyholder's car or causes the policyholder or the passengers of the policyholder harm.

- **Part D: Damage to covered autos** pays to fix the policyholder's car if it is damaged. Comprehensive coverage includes damage not caused by a collision (e.g. windshield cracks because of a stone). Collision coverage pays (less the deductible) to repair the policyholder's car if they damage it in a collision.

Cost Factors

Several factors affect the cost of an auto policy, including the age and sex of the drivers. Young males have more accidents and therefore cost more to insure. The use of the automobile changes rates. The more miles and more frequently a person drives, the more likely they will be to have an accident. The rates go up accordingly. Some areas, especially large cities, are more prone to accidents and theft. Higher rates are the norm in these areas. The operators' driving record is essential. If a person has had several accidents or received several tickets for unsafe operations (speeding, etc.), that person is a bad risk.

Their rates will probably go up. New cars have devices that can record someone's driving habits. Many insurers will give customers better rates if one of these reporting devices is installed and linked to their system. These customers give up considerable personal privacy for lower rates.

One point to note: a practitioner's automobile policy does not cover employees driving the dentist's car for business reasons. So, if a staff member runs to the bank in the dentist's car, the practice owner, not the staff member, runs the risk of being personally liable if the employee has an accident. The practitioner needs to be sure that the office liability policy has a rider to cover employees if they regularly use the dentist's vehicle. If a practitioner deducts a portion of auto expenses as a business expense, they need to inform the insurance agent. It could change the insurance classification, making it more expensive but complete coverage.

GUIDELINES FOR CHOOSING AUTO INSURANCE

If someone is considering buying automobile insurance, they need to investigate several issues before they sign any contracts or checks. These include the following:

- Auto insurance requirements vary significantly from state to state. Almost every state requires car owners to have basic liability coverage, although the amount is different in each state. Some states have no-fault provisions and others do not.

- Auto owners need to coordinate liability coverage with other insurance carefully. Often an "umbrella" liability coverage will be like auto, homeowner's, and personal liability. If someone owns a business (such as a dental practice), they should be sure that their business use of the car is adequately insured.

- As in all insurance, a higher deductible leads to lower premiums.

- Be sure to have coverage for uninsured motorists. About 10% of drivers do not have insurance, despite laws requiring every car owner to have coverage.

- Consider whether to purchase collision insurance. If a car is not valuable and someone has assets to cover that loss, it is cheaper not to buy the collision portion and to self-insure.

- Look for discounts. These include good student discounts, driver's training, low mileage, safety, anti-theft devices, and good driver history. Different states and companies may have these discounts.

Section I: Property coverage
    Dwelling
    Other structures
    Personal property
    Loss of use

Section II: Liability and medical
    Personal liability
    Medical payments to others
    Damage to property of others

HOMEOWNER'S INSURANCE

GENERAL AREAS OF COVERAGE

Homeowner's insurance protects the policyholder against losses: loss of property and the liability arising from owning the property. Box 8.2 shows the general areas of homeowner's coverage. Like auto insurance, homeowner's insurance policies follow standard formats.

Loss of Property

If someone's house catches fire and burns down, they have lost their property and not only the house structure but the contents. Homeowner's insurance covers those types of incidents and other structures on the property, such as sheds or detached garages. If someone's house is damaged and cannot live in it (loss of use), the insurance will generally pay for them to live somewhere else while their home is being repaired.

BOX 8.2	GENERAL AREAS OF HOMEOWNER'S COVERAGE

Section I: Property coverage
Dwelling
Other structures
Personal property
Loss of use

Section II: Liability and medical
Personal liability
Medical payments to others
Damage to property of others

There are three ways in which the insurer may define (and therefore cover) a loss:

- **Actual cash value**

  Actual cash value is the current cost of the house and the occupants' belongings, and it is the original value minus the property's depreciation (wear, tear, and aging). It does not matter how much was paid for them or how much it would cost to replace or repair them, and this may lead a homeowner to be underinsured in the event of a significant loss.

- **Replacement cost**

  Replacement value policies cover the actual value of the home and possessions without considering depreciation. Owners could repair or rebuild their homes and contents up to the original value.

- **Guaranteed (or extended) replacement cost/value**

  This is the most comprehensive way to determine the value of the property. This type of policy pays whatever the cost to repair or rebuild a home, accounting for inflation of the cost of rebuilding or replacement. Some insurers even offer extended replacement, which offers more coverage than the homeowner purchased. These are generally the most expensive types of policies.

There are several everyday riders (special provisions) that policies may contain. A "replacement cost provision" obliges the carrier to replace the damaged property. Inflation can dramatically escalate the value of a home and its contents over a few years. This rider protects the policyholder from being underinsured by rising costs. Losses to personal property are limited. If someone has expensive personal property (such as jewelry, a stamp collection, expensive guns, or fine art), they must document the property and inform their insurance agent. The agent will write a special rider to cover the expensive property in case of loss or theft. This is an extra cost for the insured. The same applies to personal "toys," such as boats. Property and liability resulting from such toys are limited if the policyholder has not informed their insurance agent and made coverage provisions.

This insurance generally does not cover widespread disasters. Examples include war, nuclear disasters, earthquakes, civil unrest, and flooding. If someone is in an area prone to earthquakes, they should get a rider to cover this. Flooding is a particular case that is covered by federal flood insurance. Many hurricane victims have found they were covered for wind damage but not adequately insured for the flood damage that resulted from the storm. Homeowners need to check their policy to see what it covers before they need the insurance. These additional forms of coverage are extra costs for the insured.

Liability from the Property

If a neighbor's child injures themselves while in the policyholder's yard, the homeowner may be liable for damages the child sustains. Most policies have liability exclusions. The homeowner generally will not be covered if the injury or damage occurred because the home was being used for business purposes. If a spouse gives piano lessons in the home and a pupil is injured there, the homeowner's insurance may not pay the claim because it was business related. A separate business liability insurance is needed for that coverage. Another frequent exclusion is if the homeowner intentionally harms someone. Liability coverage may be limited if the property includes a swimming pool or other dangerous equipment. Having a dangerous dog (e.g. a pit bull) or other dangerous animals as a pet may require additional coverage. Policyholders should check their policies before a bad occurrence to ensure they are adequately covered.

TYPES OF COVERAGE

The coverage someone requires depends on what type of home they live in and what they feel they need to cover. There are eight types of homeowner's coverage, standard coverage that applies to all homeowner insurance policies across the United States. The purpose of requiring standard types of coverage is so that the consumer can compare the coverage of different policies and the cost of each policy for the given coverage. The types of coverage are shown in Box 8.3. An insurance agent will help decide which coverage is best for the situation.

GUIDELINES FOR CHOOSING HOMEOWNER'S INSURANCE

If someone is considering buying homeowner's insurance, they need to answer several questions before they sign any contracts or checks. These include the following:

- The homeowner must decide what they need in coverage. Most people think of just their home, but they should be sure to include the contents, including special items (such as artwork or jewelry). If someone has recreational vehicles (such as a boat, motorcycle, or airplane), they need additional coverage for these toys and their increased liability.

- The homeowner must be sure to protect against inflation. A policy should include an inflation protection feature or rider that automatically raises the coverage to reflect annual increases in home values. An extended replacement type of policy helps to solve this problem.

BOX 8.3	**TYPES OF HOMEOWNER'S COVERAGE**
Homeowner's 1 (basic)	Fire, lightning, extended coverage, vandalism and mischief, theft, glass breakage on dwellings and personal contents, and comprehensive personal liability
Homeowner's 2 (broad form)	All primary and additional extended coverage for other specific causes Homeowners 3: "All Risks" on buildings and Broad Form on personal property (i.e. everything is included unless the policy expressly excludes it)
Homeowners 3 ("all risks")	"All risks" on buildings and broad form on personal property (i.e. everything is included unless the policy expressly excludes it)
Homeowner's 4	Personal property only (broad form); for tenants
Homeowner's 5	"All risks" on buildings and personal property
Homeowner's 6	Personal property and loss-of-use coverage (broad form); for condominium unit owners
Homeowner's 8	Coverage on buildings and personal property is somewhat more limited than basic; for homes that may not meet underwriting requirements

- The homeowner should decide whether to bundle their insurance. Many companies give discounts to clients who have more than one type of insurance (homeowner's, auto, excess liability) through them. This also makes it easier to ensure there are no gaps or overlaps in coverage and makes payment and record-keeping easier. Compare the cost of these multipolicy discounts with the cost of individual policies.

- The homeowner needs to check their liability protection. Most personal liability protection begins with homeowner's insurance, which needs to be coordinated with auto and excess liability protection. The professional should increase this limit as their asset base grows.

- The homeowner should raise their deductible. Like any other insurance, a higher deductible leads to a lower premium. Increasing the homeowner's deductible from $500 to $1000 will lower the annual premium substantially. Be aware that minor damage, such as broken windows or damage from a broken pipe, may not raise the cost of meeting the deductible.

- The homeowner should tell their insurer about improvements to their home. Any improvements the homeowner makes that lower the likelihood of a claim may lead to a lower premium. Examples include a sprinkler system, a new roof, an alarm system, carbon monoxide detectors, or removing dry brush or other fire hazards around the home.

PERSONAL EXCESS LIABILITY INSURANCE

The final type of personal insurance a person ought to have is a personal excess liability policy. This type of policy is also known as an "umbrella liability" policy. Its purpose is to ensure that the policyholder has adequate personal liability insurance. Homeowner's and automobile insurance have liability protection, but these are limited policies, often set to $50 000–$100 000 per occurrence. It is not unusual for liability cases to be settled for much more than these amounts. The excess liability policy coordinates other liability coverage and extends it to a maximum amount.

For example, suppose someone has a $100 000 homeowner's liability policy. The neighbor's child falls off the homeowner's deck, sustaining a severe head injury. In the subsequent lawsuit, the jury awards the child $3 million in damages. The homeowner's policy has a limit of $100 000, which is all that the insurer must pay. Homeowners must pay the rest from their assets, savings, and future earnings. If the homeowner has an umbrella liability policy, it will pick up where the other (homeowner's) policy ends and pay damages up to the limits of the liability in the umbrella policy (perhaps $3 or $5 million).

Umbrella policies are relatively inexpensive. They must be carefully coordinated with other insurance policies to ensure there are no gaps or duplications in coverage. This is for personal liability only. Office liability and professional liability require different insurances. A personal liability policy will not cover someone in the event of a business-related lawsuit. Since dentists are often seen as rich members of society (and therefore able to pay large liability settlements), they need to protect themselves and their families with this type of coverage. The amount that is right for a particular person changes with inflation and as they build personal assets.

TAX CONSEQUENCES OF PERSONAL INSURANCE

The following relates to current (2023) tax laws. As a rule, insurances for a business are a tax-deductible cost of doing business; insurances for personal affairs are not tax deductible. Most small business people want to make their insurance premium tax deductible because that decreases the total cost of the insurance. However, simply wanting them to be tax deductible does not make them so. The practitioner must know the IRS rules regarding insurance premium payments to make informed decisions about insurance premium deductibility. These rules and their interpretations change frequently. The dentist needs to check with an accountant or tax advisor concerning the current tax consequences of insurance.

MEDICAL INSURANCE

If someone (or their spouse) is given medical insurance as an employee benefit, the cost of the premium is tax deductible to the employer and tax free to the employee. This lowers the apparent cost of insurance coverage because the government essentially pays for some of it through tax savings. Medical insurance premiums that a dentist provides for themselves and their family through the practice are tax deductible, regardless of the form of business (corporation, proprietorship, partnership, or limited liability company). If a practice is a corporation or has a flexible benefit (cafeteria-style) plan, the rules get complex. Again, the practitioner should check with their accountant or tax advisor.

LIFE INSURANCE

In "normal," individually purchased life insurance policies, the policyholder pays the premium with after-tax money, and a beneficiary receives the benefit free of any income taxes. The rules get more complex when someone gifts someone else a policy or pays the premiums, and a tax advisor needs to be consulted in these cases.

Employer-sponsored life insurance policies are different. The employer may provide up to $50 000 per year of term life insurance as an employee benefit. Premiums for additional insurance provided by the employer are included in income, based on IRS rules and tables. If a practitioner incorporates the practice (and is therefore an employee), they qualify for this benefit. The tax rules get complex regarding additional or whole-life policies. The rules become even more complex when the corporation purchases life insurance for cross-purchase or other arrangements. An accountant, financial advisor, and insurance agent should work out the best arrangement for the particular practitioner's circumstances and follow the tax rules in force.

DISABILITY INSURANCE

Any benefits received will be tax free if a person pays premiums with after-tax dollars. If the practice (or employer) pays the premiums, then any benefit would be taxable income to the recipient. The dentist will need a higher level of coverage in this case. Therefore, paying for the insurance personally with after-tax money is generally better, and receiving the benefits is tax free.

AUTOMOBILE INSURANCE

All costs associated with the use of an automobile for business purposes (including the cost of insurance) are ordinary costs of doing business and therefore tax deductible. The costs associated with using an automobile for personal purposes are not tax deductible. The problem is deciding the proportion of business use to personal use. The practitioner must keep a log of use (as described in Chapter 17) to justify the percentage of total automobile costs allocated for business purposes.

HOMEOWNER'S INSURANCE

Homeowner's insurance is generally not tax deductible. If part of a home is used as a qualifying home office, a proportional amount of homeowner's insurance premiums may be allocated to business use. The rules on home office deductions are strict.

Retirement Planning

CHAPTER 9

If I'd known I was going to live so long, I'd have taken better care of myself.

Leon Eldred

GOAL

This chapter emphasizes the general and financial planning aspects of retirement.

LEARNING OBJECTIVES

At the completion of this chapter, the student will be able to:

- Discuss the major financial factors involved in retirement planning.

- Discuss the essential components of retirement plans for dentists.

- Discuss the principles of retirement saving for dental practitioners.

- Discuss factors affecting dentists' ability to meet retirement goals.

- Identify the various retirement plans available to the dentist.

KEY TERMS

401(k) plans	IRA individual retirement account	SIMPLE plans
annuity	IRA back-loaded	SEP plans
composition of net worth	IRA Roth	Social Security
compounding	IRA traditional	tax-deferred annuity
contribution limits	qualified plans	tax sheltering
defined benefit plans	retirement plan savings	vesting
defined contribution plans	risk–return relationship	

Most dentists realize that they will not be able (or want) to practice their entire lives. Private dental practitioners do not have pensions or retirement income plans funded by a large employer. Instead, they are responsible for funding their retirement savings. When they retire, they draw down their retirement savings as they withdraw funds for living expenses. The obvious fear is that retirement will last longer than the retirement funds. Retirement planning then becomes a critical personal financial planning task. Fortunately, dentists are relatively highly paid professionals. This makes it easier than for many other vocations to set aside money for retirement planning. For the more straightforward plans described in this chapter, a dentist can work with the office accountant

Business Basics for Dentists, Second Edition. James L. Harrison, David O. Willis, and Charles K. Thieman.
© 2024 John Wiley & Sons, Inc. Published 2024 by John Wiley & Sons, Inc.

or financial planner to select and carry out a plan. For the more complex plans, practitioners will need to use a specialist in retirement plans. Fortunately, if a dentist starts a plan early and funds the simpler plans with the maximum amount permitted, they should not need the more complex (and more expensive) plans. A dental practice owner might use several types of retirement plans. Congress and the Internal Revenue Service (IRS) change the tax implications of these plans frequently. Practice owners must check with an accountant or tax advisor for the current tax laws before establishing or contributing to a plan.

This chapter describes the principles of retirement planning for dental practitioners (Box 9.1). For many, retirement implies a gold watch and a porch swing. But people are living longer and healthier lives than in the past. Many dentists are retiring at a younger age than in years past. Some of them leave work entirely. Some pursue a hobby or a second career. This leads to more years of retirement and a more active (and expensive) retirement. Others continue to work well into their later years, working part-time. For these reasons, many financial planners prefer to call this process planning for financial independence rather than for retirement. Financial independence is the time in life when someone can work or not. They have adequate resources to support themselves and their family in their chosen lifestyle.

Retiring from dental practice involves significant personal self-examination and planning. Many private practitioners have so much of their self-esteem committed to their practice that it becomes difficult for them to walk away. This, after all, has been a large part of their professional and personal identity. Successful retirees develop projects and interests that extend well into retirement. These tasks provide emotional and intellectual challenges that lead to high self-esteem. Playing golf every day sounds wonderful when someone works every day. After playing every day for a month, golfing may lose some of its luster.

Sometimes people think only about the financial aspects of retirement planning. Personal emotional preparation is as essential and often inadequately addressed. However, this chapter examines *only* the financial bases of retirement planning.

COMPONENTS OF A RETIREMENT PLAN

Retirement planning for dentists is like a three-legged stool: each component is necessary for the system to work, but none of them can work alone. The three components of retirement plans are Social Security, private savings and assets, and retirement savings and pensions.

SOCIAL SECURITY

Self-employed dentists pay into the Social Security system through the SETA self-employment tax. If a dentist is employed by someone else or their own corporation, then the employer pays half the Federal Insurance Contributions Act (FICA) Social Security payments. (If dentists own their corporation, they pay both halves.) Given the aging of the US population, Congress continually grapples with the problem of funding Social Security. Social Security retirement payments are not large to begin with. In the future, higher-income earners will pay more (both while working and in retirement) to help keep the system solvent. This effectively decreases their return. So, although Social Security will probably not end in the future, most dentists should not plan for Social Security to be a significant part of their retirement income. They need to plan as if Social Security will not exist. Any payments received from Social Security will then be a bonus. Practitioners ought to keep up with the news and the changes that Congress makes in the Social Security system.

Everyone should regularly check their Social Security status and benefits on the Social Security website (www.ssa.gov). The Social Security Administration provides an online "Personal Earnings History and Benefits Statement." This is a history of reported earnings (throughout a person's lifetime) and an estimate of benefits at retirement. (The statement also shows estimated benefits for disability and for a surviving spouse and children.) It shows benefits in today's dollars, although actual benefits are indexed for inflation so that the amount will be higher.

PRIVATE SAVINGS AND ASSETS

Private savings are those made with after-tax money. Examples include a dental practice, a home, and most investments. Financial assets (investments) are a valuable component of the total retirement asset base. Someone can turn these assets into immediate income by selling them (stock, etc.) or using any income (such as dividends) for personal income. Private savings and investments are generally used for non-retirement purposes. Some assets, such as a home or an automobile, should not be included as a component of a retirement plan because they will be needed in retirement.

Many dental practice owners plan on selling their practice to fund their retirement plans. This is a risky strategy. They may be unable to sell the practice when they want to sell or at the price they hoped to get. Taxes then eat up a sizable portion of the proceeds, which may leave them with too small a remaining asset base to fund retirement adequately. Many practitioners then find that they cannot afford to sell the practice and retire.

RETIREMENT SAVINGS AND PENSIONS

The essential component of most dentists' retirement plans is their retirement plan savings. These are funds specifically earmarked for retirement savings purposes and are designed to be a retirement savings method, not a personal savings plan. If someone withdraws money from retirement plan savings for other uses (e.g. to buy a boat), they will face significant taxes and penalties. "Qualified" plans receive favorable tax treatment for both employer and employee because they comply with specific IRS code requirements. Overall, these requirements protect employees through non-discrimination and fiduciary responsibility rules. Retirement savings are good investments because people fund them with pretax money, and they grow tax free until withdrawn (possibly in a lower tax bracket). However, this advantage only comes with specific stipulations, the largest of which is that the dental practice owner (the employer) must also fund their employees' retirement plans. As a rule, a practice owner funding their tax-advantaged retirement plan to the maximum amount permitted is still advantageous. (Details about retirement plans are found later in this chapter.)

Some dentists will have a pension to provide retirement income. A pension is a set income that the retiree receives each month. This may be indexed for inflation, and it may be for their life and the life of their spouse. Large corporations and government organizations more commonly provide pensions. A dentist generally only sees a pension if they have been employed by the military or other branch of government for many years. They are being phased out as a business retirement plan in favor of one of the Individual Retirement Account (IRA) or defined contribution types of plans described later.

BOX 9.2   RETIREMENT SAVINGS

	20 years	30 years	40 years	50 years
5%	2653	4321	7039	11467
10%	6727	17449	45259	117390

This chart shows $1000 invested, once, at various rates and times. If a person invests at 5% and gets X in return, then if they invest at 10%, they will get X times 2. In addition, the effect of compounding more than doubles their return.

Retirement plans allow someone to save money with many tax advantages. When they retire, they live off these savings. If they have adequate savings, they live off the investment increase (interest and gain), leaving the principal intact. If the savings are inadequate for this strategy, they must gradually erode the principal or lower their retirement income expectations (Box 9.2).

PRINCIPLES OF RETIREMENT SAVINGS

The following principles apply to all investments, especially tax-advantaged retirement plans.

TIME

The longer the time until retirement, the more the investment will grow. The rule of 72 is an excellent method for determining how quickly an investment will double (see Box 9.3). This rule says that the time for an investment to double equals 72 divided by the investment rate of return. For example, if someone earns 6% on an investment, it will double in about 12 years (72/6). This can also estimate any compounding value. For example, a person may expect inflation to be 3%. Prices for goods and services then will double in approximately 24 (72/3) years. A financial advisor has calculators that are more exact, but the rule of 72 is a good estimator for how quickly an investment can grow.

BOX 9.3   THE RULE OF 72

$$\text{Years to double} = \frac{72}{\text{Interest rate}}$$

Where interest rate = investment rate of return

COMPOUNDING

Compounding is one of the most powerful concepts to understand in retirement planning. Compounding occurs when someone earns interest on the interest they have already earned. The value of an investment then mushrooms as the portion they contributed decreases. Compounding needs time (many years) to work, which is another reason to begin retirement plan contributions as early in a career as possible (Box 9.4). The sooner someone begins retirement plan contributions, the more compounding helps, and the healthier the retirement plan will be.

BOX 9.4	HOW TO BUILD RETIREMENT SAVINGS

Beginning age	One-time contribution	Monthly contribution
20	$6098	$46
25	$10748	$84
35	$33378	$283
40	$58823	$527
59	$506631	$9456

This chart shows the *investment* needed to earn $1 million by age 65, assuming a 12% return.

TAX SHELTERING

Retirement savings gain their advantage because they are sheltered from taxes. Tax sheltering means that a person gains an immediate tax deduction for the contribution (tax deductible), and the investment grows tax free until they draw it out of the fund (tax deferred). This allows for a higher return (the money grows tax free) and a possibly lower tax rate when they withdraw the money. Note that these plans defer taxes until retirement; they do not altogether avoid or eliminate income taxes.

Tax Deductibility

Qualified retirement plans use pretax money for funding. If someone is in the 33% marginal tax bracket, that means that for each $1000 they contribute, they get a total of $1000 going toward retirement savings. A posttax (taxable) contribution means that for each $1000, the person must first pay 33% in taxes ($333) and then invest the remainder ($667). The total return will be less. Box 9.5 shows the difference between using a tax-deductible retirement plan and not using one.

Tax Deferral

Qualified retirement plans also grow with tax deferred. That means the owner does not pay income tax on the earnings until they withdraw them at retirement. Assume someone is in a 25% marginal tax bracket and earns 8% on an investment (i.e. a $10000 investment yields $800 per year). If the investment is in a tax-advantaged retirement

BOX 9.5	TAX DEDUCTIBILITY – TAX SAVINGS WITH AND WITHOUT A RETIREMENT PLAN

	No retirement plan	With retirement plan
Gross income	$100000	$100000
– Exemptions	$8000	$8000
– Itemized deductions	$10000	$10000
– Retirement plan (13%)	$0	$13000
Taxable income	$82000	$69000
– Tax due (25% taxable income)	$20500	$17250
Posttax income	$61500	$51750
Tax savings		$3250

The calculations assume 25% income tax and a 13% retirement plan contribution.
The immediate tax savings ($3250) means the retirement plan contribution only costs $9750 ($13000 – $3250).
This is an immediate return of 25% on the investment.

plan, they keep the entire $800. Next year, that person earns 8% of $10 800 (the initial $10 000 plus $800 earned last year) and so on (i.e. compounding). The same investment in a taxable account would only yield a $60 return. A person would earn the same $800 but pay 25% ($200) in taxes. Compounding is slowed significantly under this later scenario. Box 9.6 shows the power of adding tax deferral to tax deductibility.

BOX 9.6	TAX DEFERRAL – THE EFFECT OF DEFERRING TAXES

	Taxable	Tax deferred
Initial amount	$10 000	$10 000
– Tax	$2 500	0
– Investment	$7 500	$10 000
ATIR	6%	8%
Future value before tax	$57 645	$147 853
– Tax (25%)	0	$36 963
Future value after tax	$57 645	$110 890

Assumptions:

- Initial amount $10 000
- Tax rate 25%
- Non-taxed investment return 8% per year
- After-tax investment return (ATIR) 6% per year (8% – 2%)
- Term 35 years

This chart shows the difference between putting $10 000 into a taxable account and a tax-deductible, tax-deferred account.

RISK–RETURN RELATIONSHIP

A general rule of investing is that the higher the risk, the higher the return required to get people to invest in the project. Risk is a measure of the variability of the return on investment. Figure 9.1a shows that lower-risk investments tend to have lower total returns and lower swings from high to low. Higher-risk investments (Figure 9.1b) have greater long-term returns and "ups and downs." The timing of when the person needs the investment plays a key role. The practical effect of this principle is that early in a career (and a retirement plan), someone can tolerate more risk (and gain a higher return) than later in the plan. At this later point, people generally want to preserve their gains as they begin to draw money from their funds.

FACTORS THAT DETERMINE PEOPLE'S ABILITY TO REACH RETIREMENT GOALS

As a rule, a person will need 75–80% of their preretirement income as a level for their retirement income. This can vary depending on the situation. Most retirees have lower monthly costs due to not buying work clothes, traveling to work, or other costs (such as meals) resulting from work. At this time in their careers, most people have also paid off their house mortgage and other loans. They have fewer purchases as the children grow and leave home. On the other hand, they may have higher expenses in some categories, such as travel and entertainment, as they act on their retirement dreams.

Several factors determine whether someone can meet their retirement income goal.

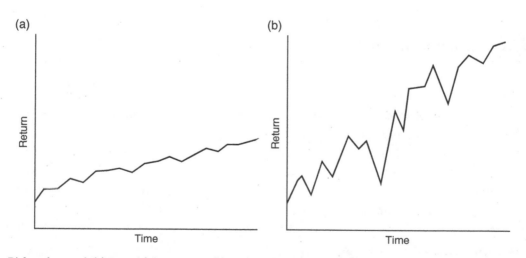

FIGURE 9.1   Risk and reward. (a) Low-risk investment. (b) High-risk investment.

INCOME LEVEL DESIRED

The higher the income someone requires in retirement, the more retirement savings they require. This makes intuitive sense. The tricky part is to quantify how much is enough. As with all investment decisions, estimating based on expected returns and inflation is the best thing to do. One significant problem early in a career is estimating what inflation will be by the end of that career. An income level of $20 000 per month today may be paltry when the effects of 25 years of inflation are considered.

ESTIMATED LENGTH OF TIME IN RETIREMENT

How long a person will be in retirement depends on their age at retirement and an estimate of the longevity of that person and their spouse. If they retire when they are 55 years old, they need to plan for a longer retirement than if they retire at age 80, all things being equal. The longer the time in retirement, the longer that person needs to be concerned about inflation eroding the buying power of their retirement income. Each person needs to look realistically at their family history, personal health, and habits when estimating life expectancy. (An honest appraisal of an expected lifetime is an important exercise.) If someone has a family history of heart disease and does little to address it, they can plan to have a shorter time in retirement than otherwise. They must also plan for their spouse's lifetime income in retirement if that spouse depends on them for income. As a rule, everyone needs to plan on living until the age of 90 if they have no significant health problems. This allows for a complete retirement for about 90% of Americans.

PRESENT RETIREMENT SAVINGS PATTERN

A person who only saves $1 per year will not realize their retirement goals. Although saying that people should increase their retirement plan contributions is easy, each person must evaluate their personal budget to identify areas of possible savings. To do this, they must first have a budget and know where they spend money. They must rank retirement savings along with other long- and short-term goals. (Once they earn money, it can only be saved or spent.) These priorities will change as stages of life and family circumstances change.

COMPOSITION OF NET WORTH

Two people may have the same net worth but have different income-generating potential from their assets. In Box 9.7, both dentists have the same net worth. However, Dentist 2 has more assets in their home, which does not produce retirement income. Dentist 1 has a more significant value in their retirement plan and, therefore, a more considerable monthly income in retirement.

INVESTMENT RATE OF RETURN

Risk is a measure of the variability of an investment. There is always some risk that the underlying company, country, or other entity will become insolvent. Then investors will lose their entire investment. That occurrence is rare with mainstream US Wall Street investments. Instead, the greater risk is from the normal fluctuations of the economy. The primary risk is that the value of an investment will decline just when someone needs the investment. How

---

BOX 9.7   COMPOSITION OF NET WORTH

	Dentist 1		Dentist 2	
	Book value	Income-producing value	Book value	Income-producing value
Home equity	$250 000	$0	$400 000	$0
Retirement plan	$425 000	$425 000	$225 000	$225 000
Practice	$225 000	$150 000	$225 000	$150 000
Personal investments	$150 000	$100 000	$150 000	$100 000
Total	$1 000 000	$675 000	$1 000 000	$475 000
Estimated income		$2 250/mo		$1 583/mo

Assumption: 4% per year withdrawal of retirement assets.

BOX 9.8   IMPORTANCE OF THE INVESTMENT RATE OF RETURN

Years	Investment rate					
	1%	3%	6%	9%	12%	15%
10	$1 105	$1 344	$1 791	$2 367	$3 106	$4 406
20	$1 220	$1 806	$3 207	$5 604	$9 646	$16 367
30	$1 348	$2 427	$5 743	$13 268	$29 960	$66 212
40	$1 489	$3 262	$10 286	$31 409	$93 051	$267 864
50	$1 645	$4 384	$18 420	$74 358	$289 002	$1 083 657

Hypothetical one-time $1000 investment.

assets are allocated within the retirement plan becomes essential for an adequate return.

Early in a retirement plan, a person can tolerate more risk to gain higher returns. A few percentage points can make a tremendous difference over the long haul (Box 9.8). As a person is near to and enters retirement, they need to decrease their risk exposure to protect the assets they have built along the way.

DESIRE FOR LEGACY

Some people want assets left over so they can pass money or property to their heirs or a favorite charity. They will need more assets than a person who does not feel the need to do that. Some people may need to leave money to heirs. For example, if a disabled adult child depends on the parent for income, the parent may need to provide income for the child's continued support. (They can also do this through life insurance, trusts, or other methods.) They may want to leave money to some or all of their children. If so, they will need to accumulate more in a retirement account and other assets than if they do not. Many want to spend all their retirement savings, so they spend the last dollar saved with their final dying breath. They believe that providing their children with a solid moral, ethical, and educational foundation early in life serves them more than an inherited handout later in life.

COMMON TYPES OF RETIREMENT PLANS

There are three general categories of retirement plans that most small businesses use. These are IRAs, defined contribution plans, or defined benefit plans. Larger organizations (governmental agencies, large corporations) often use variations of these basic plans that meet their needs better. These other plans may be more expensive to establish and

maintain, so smaller businesses do not use them. Most financial institutions have one or more of these retirement plans preapproved by the IRS, making it easy for small business owners to set them up. The solo practice owner will have different retirement planning needs and constraints than an employee dentist working for the government or extensive corporate practice. In this discussion, we will concentrate on standard plans for smaller businesses. Congress and the IRS frequently change amounts and specific rules about retirement plans to encourage participation by groups or businesses. We present general information about these plans. The dentist should check with their accountant or financial advisor concerning specific eligibility, contribution limits, and other plan requirements.

INDIVIDUAL RETIREMENT ACCOUNT– BASED PLANS

IRAs are retirement accounts that individuals set up and contribute to on their own. However, employers can help set up and fund these accounts. The amount of retirement income that an IRA generates depends upon the amount of money contributed along the way and the account's investment return (gain or loss).

Individual Retirement Account-Based Plans

Individual retirement plans are not office plans. As the name implies, an individual establishes the plan. Many new dentists use these plans to begin their retirement savings because they do not have the added expense of funding staff plans, and their income is lower, so the saving amounts are less. As the practice becomes more profitable, they may switch to a practice-based plan. These individual plans come in two general varieties: traditional and back-loaded (Roth). There are limits up to which an individual may contribute to an IRA annually.

Traditional Individual Retirement Accounts

An IRA is an investment account that the person tells the IRS is their IRA. They can then invest in stocks, bonds, mutual funds, or other investments within that account. IRAs can be set up through banks, mutual fund companies, or security brokers. IRAs are easy to set up: talk to a banker or stockbroker and they will establish one. A more popular method is to contact any of the families of mutual funds and ask for an IRA application.

Money that someone contributes to an IRA is tax deductible (they do not pay income tax on the money they contribute), and the account grows on a tax-deferred basis (they do not pay income tax on it until they withdraw it during retirement). A person and their spouse may each have an IRA, even if they do not work and earn income.

Traditional IRAs are for individuals. Their advantages are ease of use, tax deductibility, and tax deferral. There are several disadvantages, including the limited amount that can be contributed, income phase-outs for high-income individuals, and penalties for early withdrawals or loans. IRAs can be invested in almost any legitimate investment. These include stocks, bonds, or mutual funds, but not art or other personal-use assets.

Back-Loaded (Roth) Individual Retirement Accounts

A Roth IRA is like a traditional IRA, with the significant differences that contributions to the plan are not deductible, and qualified distributions during retirement are not taxable. Earnings on the account still grow tax free and are taxed only when a distribution is not qualified. (Qualified distribution includes retirement and taxpayer death or disability.) A person who has earned income may contribute to a Roth IRA, provided their income does not exceed certain limits. Annual contributions are limited, but both taxpayer and spouse may contribute to their own Roth IRAs even if one of them did not work. As a rule, if someone has several years until retirement, the Roth IRA is a better retirement investment because it essentially allows more money to be sheltered. This is because after-tax money is used for contributions, and future withdrawals are not taxed.

Office-Based Individual Retirement Accounts

Several types of IRA plans are designed for small business owners. The general advantage of these plans over individual IRAs is the higher contribution limits. (That is, a person can shelter more income each year.) The downside (financially) to these plans is that if dental practice owner uses them for themselves, they must include staff members at their expense, which can significantly drive up the plan's cost. When a practice owner can effectively use these plans, they will be making enough money to fund an employee plan with minor pain, using it as a staff recruitment and retention tool.

Payroll Deduction Individual Retirement Accounts

Employers who do not want to adopt a formal retirement plan can encourage employees to contribute to an IRA through payroll deductions. This is a simple way to help employees save for retirement. In this arrangement, the employee always decides whether, when, and how much to contribute to the IRA. (The IRS sets annual limits.) Some individuals wait until the end of the year to set aside the money and then find that they do not have sufficient funds. These payroll deductions eliminate this problem by withholding small amounts each pay period. Payroll deduction contributions are tax deductible by the employee to the same extent as other IRA contributions. Once the contribution is made, it is treated like any other IRA.

Simplified Employee Pensions

Simplified employee pension (SEP) plans are like traditional IRAs. The significant differences are in the contribution limit and employees' participation. If an employer makes contributions for themselves, they must make similar percentage contributions for all eligible employees. These contributions are 100% immediately vested in the employees and are treated like IRAs for the employee. They are tax deductible for the business owner. The exact amount or same percentage does not have to be contributed every year, so an owner can tie contributions to practice profitability. An employer does not have to make a contribution in any given year and can skip a year. An employer can contribute up to 25% of each employee's compensation. Self-employed dentists can contribute for themselves up to a maximum earned income.

SEP plans are simple to establish, much like an IRA. Financial institutions have prototype plans, which are popular because of the higher contribution limits and ease of establishment. Even with eligible employees, they are relatively inexpensive. For example, a $20 000 per year employee with a 5% contribution receives $1000 in the plan for the year. An owner can establish a SEP without paying large amounts for professional advice from actuaries and high-profile financial planners. The practice owner should involve an accountant or financial planner to ensure the plan complies with tax rules.

SIMPLE Individual Retirement Account Plans

A SIMPLE (Savings Incentive Match Plans for Employees of Small

Employers) plan allows employees to contribute a percentage of their salary each paycheck and requires employer contributions. Employees set aside money by payroll deduction. The employer then must contribute funds for employees to individual SIMPLE IRAs by one of two methods:

- A 100% match of the first 3% contributed by each employee.

- A 2% contribution for all eligible employees.

This plan allows employees to contribute to their own retirement accounts, up to $10 000 pretax contribution per year. All employee contributions, employer matches, and earnings are immediately and fully vested in the employee. Like with a SEP, all contributions go into an IRA for the employee. SIMPLE plans are common in dental practices and easy to set up. Like other small business plans, most financial institutions have basic prototype plans for businesses to adopt. There are contribution and eligibility rules that the business owner needs to follow, but these are described in the plan documents. SIMPLE plans are flexible, allow employee participation, and offer a relatively high contribution limit, with the most significant contribution going to the practice's owner(s).

DEFINED CONTRIBUTION PLANS

Defined contribution plans are employer-established plans. Like an IRA-based plan, they do not promise a specific income at retirement. Employees or their employers (or both) contribute to employees' accounts under the plan. The contributions to the plan are sometimes at a set rate (such as 5% of salary annually). Other times the defined contribution may be variable. Like an IRA, the amount of retirement income depends upon the amount of money contributed along the way and the account's investment return (gain or loss). If good investment decisions are made, retirement assets will grow much more than if poor decisions are made. Retirement income is unknown until someone begins to take it out. It varies depending on how much money is in the plan at retirement, how long they will need the income (life expectancy), and whether they want to leave any assets to heirs upon death. Most retirement plans are presently defined contribution plans.

Profit-Sharing Plans

Profit-sharing plans vary significantly in their complexity. The employer makes contributions to employees' accounts based on a set formula, and each employee must account for funds separately. Because of administrative complexity, few dental offices have these plans.

401(k) Plans

Some incorporated dentists have a type of retirement plan known as a 401(k). These plans were more popular before Congress established SEP and SIMPLE plans. They have similar eligibility and vesting rules to SEP and SIMPLE plans. Employees can choose to defer a portion of their salary until their retirement. The employees contribute to a 401(k) plan sponsored by their employer. These deferrals are accounted for separately for each employee. They are more complex, so usually an advisor is needed (at an additional cost) to establish and administer them. Generally, large, high-income practices can take advantage of 401(k)s. Most dental practitioners can easily manage their retirement plans with one of the more straightforward plans.

DEFINED BENEFIT PLANS

Defined benefit plans, on the other hand, do not define the amount contributed but define a specified benefit at retirement. The amount needed to contribute along the way to reach that amount varies. The retirement benefit is generally based on a percentage of pay multiplied by the years of employment, and actuarial calculations set the employer's contribution to funding the future benefit. Defined benefit plans are more complex and expensive to establish and maintain than other plans. They are seen mainly in government and large corporations; these entities have documents and employee training to help understand them.

RULES FOR OFFICE RETIREMENT PLANS

Several laws (such as the Employee Retirement and Income Security Act, ERISA) govern the conduct of any tax-advantaged retirement plan. Several plans can be chosen, but some rules apply to all the tax-advantaged plans. Generally, employees cannot be required to participate in the plan or fund all or part of their retirement plans. There may be a minimum required participation by employees or a minimum percentage of employees to be covered. There are "top-heavy" and "highly compensated employee" rules limiting the amount owners may contribute to their own retirement plans. Because these complex rules were limiting participation by small business owners, Congress developed several types of simplified plans (e.g. SEP, SIMPLE) to induce small business owners to develop retirement plans for themselves and their employees. Those rules cover the following issues.

REQUIREMENT FOR A PLAN

A business owner is not legally required to provide retirement plans or funds to employees. (They must provide Social Security, which contains an essential retirement component.) However, most qualified retirement plans (those that are tax advantaged) require that if an owner develops a qualified plan for the business, then they must include employees (at the owner's expense). The advantages of tax deferral and tax deductibility usually make it worthwhile financially to implement the plans. From an employee management perspective, many career-oriented employees understand and value retirement plans, which helps motivate and retain valuable employees. In this sense, providing a retirement plan for employees becomes a cost of doing business for the progressive dental practice.

CONTRIBUTION LIMITS

For defined contribution plans, an owner is limited in the amount they can contribute to their own and employees' plans. The owner generally cannot fund their plan at a higher rate (percentage of income) than they fund the employee's plans. There is a limit to what someone can contribute to their plan, and complex tax formulas change this number somewhat. Congress has also indexed the amount for inflation, so the maximum contribution limit changes every year with inflation and the whims of Congress.

ELIGIBLE EMPLOYEES

Depending on the specific plan, an owner might define certain employees as ineligible for participation in the retirement plan. Any employee who is 21 years old, works full-time, and has at least one year of service (two years if there is a 100% vesting schedule, see the next paragraph) is eligible for any qualified retirement plan. Because many dental office employees do not stay in long-term employment, these rules often result in decreased employee participation and contributions.

VESTING

Vesting describes whether the employee has control over the assets contributed to them. A fully vested employee takes their retirement assets with them if they leave (for any reason). Depending on the plan, an employer can choose several vesting schedules. Most IRA-type plans require immediate 100% vesting of all funds contributed for employees; others have graduated vesting over three or five years. Any assets that are not vested return to the contributor in the event the employee leaves.

SOURCE OF CONTRIBUTION

Some plans require that all the contributions come from the employer. Others allow a matching employee–employer contribution. Matching plans are helpful when not all employees want to participate in a plan and they may self-exclude themselves. There are rules about how much of the contribution can go to owners or highly compensated employees, so the employer should check with an accountant to be sure a plan will comply with the regulations.

NON-TAX-ADVANTAGED PLANS

A tax-advantaged plan should be funded to the maximum amount possible. If someone have money left for additional retirement savings, they can use another tax-advantaged investment or an after-tax investment account.

A tax-deferred annuity is one type of investment that is halfway between a retirement plan and personal savings. An annuity is a series of regular payments. In a sense, a loan payment is an annuity for the bank or other mortgage holder. Retirement annuities are contracts purchased through insurance companies in which a person makes a series of regular payments into the annuity. (Payments should be made into the annuity with after-tax money.) At retirement, that person then receives a series of regular payments from the savings and investment growth. The advantage of annuities is that the money inside the investment grows on a tax-deferred basis. (Taxes are paid on the money when it is withdrawn.) The disadvantage of annuities compared with tax-advantaged plans is that the payments into the plan are not tax deductible. Also, the person is generally limited in their investment options within the plan.

Some insurance sales agents claim that variations in whole-life policies can replace traditional tax-advantaged retirement plans. The IRS and tax courts have consistently struck down most of these schemes. Life insurance may be a method to increase tax-deferred savings once someone maximizes a tax-advantaged plan, but it must not be used as a primary retirement planning method.

TAKING MONEY AT RETIREMENT

When it comes time for someone to withdraw retirement assets, they must follow IRS rules. These change frequently, so only a primer is given here. It is important to check with an accountant or tax advisor when that time comes.

Retirement income can be taken in two significant ways: withdrawing from accumulations (either in a tax-advantaged plan or after-tax savings) or buying an annuity contract from an insurance company.

HOW MUCH IS ENOUGH?

The first question that most people ask is "How much money do I need?" The answer depends on many factors, as described earlier. The most obvious is the income needed in retirement. If someone needs more to live on, they need a larger cache of savings. As a rule, most people live on about 80% of their preretirement income. This is because of less need for clothing, transportation, lunches, and other work-related expenses. Generally, the house has been paid for by this time, and the kids are grown. Therefore, day-to-day expenses are less. Some people's retirement income needs will increase if they have expensive hobbies or plan to travel frequently. Those of others may not be as great if they continue to work part-time to supplement their retirement income. People eligible for Social Security retirement benefits will need less than those not yet eligible.

The investment rate of return on retirement assets during retirement is another deciding factor. If someone earns 13% consistently on retirement assets during retirement, then the money will last much longer than if the person makes 3%. However, most people become more conservative investors as they near and enter retirement, and rightly so. They do not want to take on unnecessary risks for the money on which they will be living. However, people also do not want to be too conservative with retirement assets, experiencing almost no growth. Not only does the principal shrink quickly, but as withdrawals increase with inflation, the shrinkage accelerates. To stay even, a person needs to grow the principal at least at the inflation rate. Box 9.9 shows approximately how much investment someone needs for given lengths of retirement and rates of return.

Inflation is the general increase of prices in an economy. Inflation eats away at the buying power of money. A dollar in the future will not buy as much as a dollar will buy today because of inflation. Because of this, we will need more money in the future to equal money today. But how much more? That depends on the inflation rate and how far into the future we look. Box 9.10 shows how much someone would need in the future to equal $1 000 000 today. Economists say that inflation averages about 2.5–3% a year. Some years it is higher and some lower, but the

BOX 9.9	HOW MUCH IS ENOUGH?			
Years in retirement	6%	8%	10%	12%
15	$11 910	$10 534	$9 383	$8 415
20	$14 028	$12 035	$10 449	$9 173
25	$15 598	$13 043	$11 096	$9 590
30	$16 763	$13 719	$11 490	$9 819
35	$17 626	$14 173	$11 729	$9 945

The chart shows the amount needed to withdraw $100 per month in retirement, given the investment rate of return and a 4% withdrawal *rate*.

BOX 9.10	EFFECTS OF INFLATION				
Inflation rate	10 years	20 years	30 years	40 years	50 years
1%	1 104 622	1 220 190	1 347 849	1 488 864	1 644 632
2%	1 218 994	1 485 947	1 811 362	2 208 040	2 691 588
3%	1 343 916	1 806 111	2 427 262	3 262 038	4 383 906
4%	1 480 244	2 191 123	3 243 398	4 801 021	7 106 683
5%	1 628 895	2 653 298	4 321 942	7 039 989	11 467 400

A person estimates they need $1 000 000 in retirement savings (in today's money) to give them enough income. How much will that be in the future? The chart shows how much they will need in the future to equal today's $1 000 000, given different time horizons (across the top) and inflation rates (down the left side). For example, if they estimate that to retire comfortably they will need $1 000 000 in 40 years with average inflation of 3%, they will need $3 262 038 in the future to equal the buying power of that $1 000 000 today.

long-term historical average is in that range. If someone believes they need twice that amount to live on ($2 000 000), they must multiply the result by two. While that future number may seem significant, investments should grow at several percentage points above inflation.

A financial planning professional can run different investment and withdrawal scenarios that estimate how much money someone needs at retirement, given the various inputs and the investment portfolio that will safely achieve that objective. For rough planning estimates, there are several quick "rules of thumb" for the income retirement assets can provide.

- **Rule # 1**
  A person can take about 4% of the value of their retirement plan per year. This assumes that they earn 7% per year on their investments, of which 3% goes to keep up with inflation, leaving 4%. Withdrawing this amount ought to mean they will never run out of retirement money and leave a nest egg for heirs. If someone has $2 million in retirement savings, they can take $80 000 per year to live on, leaving the principal intact. Real-world fluctuating returns and inflation can make this scenario attractive or not.

- **Rule # 2**
  For every $1000 (pretax) of monthly income they want, the person needs to have retirement savings of $240 000. Remember, unless the money is in a Roth IRA, it will be taxed when it is withdrawn. The math works the same as in the preceding scenario but focuses on income requirements. Both rules assume a moderate investment strategy of 60% growth stocks and 40% income-producing stocks and bonds (giving the 8% annual return).

SOCIAL SECURITY

Social Security pays retirement income to people who have paid into the system (through Social Security or self-employment taxes) for at least 40 quarters. It also pays surviving spouse benefits, even if the spouse did not work. The amount someone receives depends on the amount they paid in along the way. (The benefit amount is adjusted annually for inflation.) Even if a person pays the maximum amount each year, the top retirement income will not be enough to support most retirees.

To qualify for benefits, a person must have reached a minimum age. That age changes (upward) at the whim of Congress. There is an age at which someone receives full benefits. If they opt to take benefits earlier, they receive reduced benefits. There is a choice, but it is a one-time choice. The present law calls for total payments at age 70. People can receive reduced payments (80%) at age 65. These ages will increase as Congress tries to reduce payments to keep the system solvent.

One other quirk of Social Security payments involves earned income. If someone has earned income while collecting Social Security retirement benefits, their benefits are reduced. That reduction is about $1 for every $3 earned for people younger than 70. Older than age 70, there is no reduction. The notion is to keep people from "double-dipping" and collecting Social Security while working. The effect is to make retirees decide if it is financially worthwhile to work, even part-time, during retirement.

TAX-ADVANTAGED PLAN WITHDRAWAL RULES

For defined contribution plans, the rules are like IRA withdrawals. Most people place their funds into an IRA and make withdrawals from it. These are called rollover IRAs, although there is no difference between them and other IRAs; the money is rolled over into one fund. Any money that someone puts into a tax-advantaged plan is not taxed when they put it into the plan, but any earnings are taxed when they take them out of the plan. The exception to this rule is that Roth (back-loaded) plans are funded with money on which tax has previously been paid. So, money in this type of plan is not taxed when it is withdrawn.

The IRS rules currently state that a person cannot withdraw funds until they reach the age of 59½ and must begin to withdraw them when they reach 72, even if they are still working. The IRS has tables that detail these required minimum distributions (RMDs). A person may take more than the minimum but not less. Any money not distributed at death goes to the named "beneficiary" of the fund, and that person then pays income taxes when they withdraw the money.

The IRS has many other rules that govern retirement plans. Besides the RMDs, there are excess contribution, excess distribution, premature distribution, and lump-sum death payment rules. There is no need to know these rules, just that they exist, and that a tax advisor or tax study is needed when retirement time comes.

ANNUITY

As mentioned previously, an annuity is a series of regular payments. When someone retires, they can buy an annuity contract from an insurance company, with a one-time, lump-sum payment into the annuity. These annuities are like a whole-life insurance policy, only in reverse. A person makes a lump-sum payment into the contract and receives a monthly payment out of the contract. The annuity can be set up so that they receive payments for a certain number of years (period certain), for a lifetime (single life), or for the lifetime of the policyholder or spouse, whoever lives longer (joint and last survivor). Insurance companies use actuarial tables that estimate how long a person will live in combination with expected investment returns to decide the pay-out. The contacts will have different pay-out and cost numbers depending on age, health status, spouse age, and contract provisions.

The purpose of an annuity is to guarantee an income for a particular period. People can probably receive a higher retirement income if they properly manage their tax-deferred retirement assets. However, these assets must be actively managed and are not guaranteed. When someone buys an annuity for retirement income purposes, they forego some monthly income for the security of known payments and an income that they cannot outlive. In this sense, an annuity becomes like a pension. This may be valuable for a spouse who is not financially savvy or for a disabled retiree or dependent. People are betting the insurance company that they will live longer than the insurance company actuaries estimate that the policyholder will live.

STAGES IN RETIREMENT PLANNING

The following discussion is based on a "typical" dentist's professional financial life cycle. Each individual is going to be different. One person, for example, may have a working spouse who can contribute to the family and retirement budgets. Another person may enter a salaried position with a retirement plan in the compensation package. Regardless, the principles involved in the life cycle remain. The cycle itself is described in Chapter 7.

The sooner someone makes maximum contributions to a tax-advantaged retirement plan, the better. However, there is an apparent trade-off between present income needs (or wants) and savings. Early in a career, there is often a need to pay off debt. A dentist may have large monthly payments for a practice buy-out or start-up loan plus student debt and personal debt for housing and other needs. The cash flow for the family budget is very tight. During this phase, they ought to start a retirement plan to develop the savings habit and to take advantage of compounding over time. An IRA (back-loaded) is perfect for this stage. If cash flow permits, they can develop a SEP or SIMPLE plan, although the more important issue is to pay

down the enormous debt load and build personal assets. Retirement assets can be placed in more aggressive investments during this early stage

Once they pay down the initial debt, the dentist enters the second, or middle, career stage. During this stage, the concern is to make the practice more efficient and profitable. The dentist can apply a large portion of the previous practice loan payment to a tax-advantaged plan for the office. They use the time to advantage for compounding the account's value. With increased cash flow, they can now comfortably make the maximum contribution to the plan. SEP and SIMPLE plans can be used to the best advantage. The dentist may also contribute to an annuity to build retirement income further. Here, they can still hold a reasonably aggressive portfolio, but as the retirement accounts grow they will probably become a less aggressive investor.

As a person nears retirement, they should not need to change retirement plans, but continue to fund the existing plan. If that person decides the plan is underfunded, they need to consider an age-weighted, defined benefit, or a target income type plan. They should not need these plans if they have planned properly along the way. As the person nears retirement, they will probably use less aggressive (less risky) investments to protect their retirement account balances.

EXAMPLE STRATEGIES

Table 9.1 shows the results of several different strategies for timing retirement savings. The results for these hypothetical practitioners assume that they begin retirement savings at age 25 and retire at age 65. They earn an 8% average annual return on investment and are in a 35% marginal tax rate. The average return means that some years the investor earns 12%, and some years they lose 3%, but on average they gain 8%. The marginal tax rate is constant over the investor's life. At retirement, these examples assume that the investor takes money out of the plan in a lump sum and pays 35% income tax. Most investors take only as much as they need, leaving the rest to continue to grow on a tax-deferred basis.

These examples show the value of early retirement savings, using tax-deductible and tax-deferred investment accounts, and continuing to fund the retirement plan throughout a career. Saving for retirement is a slow and steady process. Through proper planning and implementation, a dentist can accumulate retirement savings that will allow them to choose how to spend time later in their career.

Table 9.1 Example Individual Retirement Account (IRA) strategies.

Tax Rate = 35.0% Annual Investment Return = 8.0%

Age	Dr. Adams Dr. Adams pays tax on $5,000, then invests it in a taxable account			Dr. Boyd Dr. Boyd puts $5,000 in a tax-deferred IRA and pays taxes at withdrawal			Dr. Clark Dr. Clark waits until age 34, then puts $5,000 per year in a tax-deferred IRA			Dr. Dent Dr. Dent begins an IRA immediately, then stops contributions at age 34			Dr. Eden Dr. Eden begins an IRA early and continues contributions until retirement age		
	Annual payment	Total payments	Posttax value	Annual payment	Total payments	Total value	Annual payment	Total payments	Total value	Annual payment	Total payments	Total value	Annual payment	Total payments	Total value
25	3,250	3,250	3,419	5,000	5,000	5,400	0	0	0	5,000	5,000	5,400	5,000	5,000	5,400
26	0	3,250	3,597	0	5,000	5,832	0	0	0	5,000	10,000	11,232	5,000	10,000	11,232
27	0	3,250	3,784	0	5,000	6,299	0	0	0	5,000	15,000	17,531	5,000	15,000	17,531
28	0	3,250	3,981	0	5,000	6,802	0	0	0	5,000	20,000	24,333	5,000	20,000	24,333
29	0	3,250	4,188	0	5,000	7,347	0	0	0	5,000	25,000	31,680	5,000	25,000	31,680
30	0	3,250	4,405	0	5,000	7,934	0	0	0	5,000	30,000	39,614	5,000	30,000	39,614
31	0	3,250	4,634	0	5,000	8,569	0	0	0	5,000	35,000	48,183	5,000	35,000	48,183
32	0	3,250	4,875	0	5,000	9,255	0	0	0	5,000	40,000	57,438	5,000	40,000	57,438
33	0	3,250	5,129	0	5,000	9,995	0	0	0	5,000	45,000	67,433	5,000	45,000	67,433
34	0	3,250	5,396	0	5,000	10,795	5,000	5,000	5,400	0	45,000	72,827	5,000	50,000	78,227
35	0	3,250	5,676	0	5,000	11,658	5,000	10,000	11,232	0	45,000	78,654	5,000	55,000	89,886
36	0	3,250	5,971	0	5,000	12,591	5,000	15,000	17,531	0	45,000	84,946	5,000	60,000	102,476
37	0	3,250	6,282	0	5,000	13,598	5,000	20,000	24,333	0	45,000	91,742	5,000	65,000	116,075
38	0	3,250	6,609	0	5,000	14,686	5,000	25,000	31,680	0	45,000	99,081	5,000	70,000	130,761
39	0	3,250	6,952	0	5,000	15,861	5,000	30,000	39,614	0	45,000	107,007	5,000	75,000	146,621
40	0	3,250	7,314	0	5,000	17,130	5,000	35,000	48,183	0	45,000	115,568	5,000	80,000	163,751
41	0	3,250	7,694	0	5,000	18,500	5,000	40,000	57,438	0	45,000	124,813	5,000	85,000	182,251
42	0	3,250	8,094	0	5,000	19,980	5,000	45,000	67,433	0	45,000	134,799	5,000	90,000	202,231
43	0	3,250	8,515	0	5,000	21,579	5,000	50,000	78,227	0	45,000	145,582	5,000	95,000	223,810
44	0	3,250	8,958	0	5,000	23,305	5,000	55,000	89,886	0	45,000	157,229	5,000	100,000	247,115
45	0	3,250	9,424	0	5,000	25,169	5,000	60,000	102,476	0	45,000	169,807	5,000	105,000	272,284
46	0	3,250	9,914	0	5,000	27,183	5,000	65,000	116,075	0	45,000	183,392	5,000	110,000	299,466
47	0	3,250	10,429	0	5,000	29,357	5,000	70,000	130,761	0	45,000	198,063	5,000	115,000	328,824
48	0	3,250	10,971	0	5,000	31,706	5,000	75,000	146,621	0	45,000	213,908	5,000	120,000	360,530
49	0	3,250	11,542	0	5,000	34,242	5,000	80,000	163,751	0	45,000	231,021	5,000	125,000	394,772
50	0	3,250	12,142	0	5,000	36,982	5,000	85,000	182,251	0	45,000	249,503	5,000	130,000	431,754

Age															
51	0	3,250	12,773	0	5,000	39,940	90,000	5,000	202,231	45,000	0	269,463	5,000	135,000	471,694
52	0	3,250	13,438	0	5,000	43,136	95,000	5,000	223,810	45,000	0	291,020	5,000	140,000	514,830
53	0	3,250	14,136	0	5,000	46,586	100,000	5,000	247,115	45,000	0	314,301	5,000	145,000	561,416
54	0	3,250	14,872	0	5,000	50,313	105,000	5,000	272,284	45,000	0	339,446	5,000	150,000	611,729
55	0	3,250	15,645	0	5,000	54,338	110,000	5,000	299,466	45,000	0	366,601	5,000	155,000	666,068
56	0	3,250	16,458	0	5,000	58,685	115,000	5,000	328,824	45,000	0	395,929	5,000	160,000	724,753
57	0	3,250	17,314	0	5,000	63,380	120,000	5,000	360,530	45,000	0	427,604	5,000	165,000	788,133
58	0	3,250	18,215	0	5,000	68,451	125,000	5,000	394,772	45,000	0	461,812	5,000	170,000	856,584
59	0	3,250	19,162	0	5,000	73,927	130,000	5,000	431,754	45,000	0	498,757	5,000	175,000	930,511
60	0	3,250	20,158	0	5,000	79,841	135,000	5,000	471,694	45,000	0	538,657	5,000	180,000	1,010,352
61	0	3,250	21,206	0	5,000	86,228	140,000	5,000	514,830	45,000	0	581,750	5,000	185,000	1,096,580
62	0	3,250	22,309	0	5,000	93,126	145,000	5,000	561,416	45,000	0	628,290	5,000	190,000	1,189,706
63	0	3,250	23,469	0	5,000	100,576	150,000	5,000	611,729	45,000	0	678,553	5,000	195,000	1,290,283
64	0	3,250	24,690	0	5,000	108,623	155,000	5,000	666,068	45,000	0	732,838	5,000	200,000	1,398,905
65	0	3,250	25,973	0	5,000	117,312	160,000	5,000	724,753	45,000	0	791,465	5,000	205,000	1,516,218
Pretax		**3,250**	**25,973**		**5,000**	**117,312**	**160,000**	**5,000**	**724,753**	**45,000**		**791,465**	**205,000**		**1,516,218**
Taxes		0				41,059			253,664			277,013			530,676
After taxes		$25,973				$76,253			$471,090			$514,452			$985,541

- **Dr. Adams**

  Dr. Adams makes a one-time investment. She earns $5000 and then pays 35% income tax, leaving her $3250. She invests this in a taxable account (neither tax deferred nor tax deductible). Each year, she pays 35% income tax on her earnings, which essentially decreases her earnings to 5.2% per year (8% reduced by 35% tax). At the end of the 40 years, she has earned $25 973 and owes no taxes because she has paid them each year of the investment.

- **Dr. Boyd**

  Dr. Boyd earns $5000 and puts it into a traditional IRA. Because IRAs are tax deductible, he does not have to pay income taxes on the initial investment, putting the entire $5000 to work for him. The earnings are also tax deferred, meaning he gets the total value of the 8% annual investment return. He earns $117 312 from his initial $5000 investment, pays taxes of $41 059, and still has three times as much ($76 253) as Dr. Adams. This shows the dramatic advantage of using a tax-advantaged retirement plan over a taxable investment account.

- **Dr. Clark**

  Dr. Clark believes he cannot afford to put money into a retirement plan early in his career. His current family budget will not allow it, so he waits nine years until age 34 to begin a retirement savings program. He then puts $5000 per year into a tax-advantaged retirement plan, such as an IRA. At age 65, his IRA is now worth $724 753 from a total investment of $160 000. After paying income tax, his plan is worth $471 090.

- **Dr. Dent**

  Dr. Dent takes the opposite strategy to Dr. Clark. She puts $5000 per year into a tax-advantaged (tax-deductible, tax-deferred) IRA. However, she only invested for the first nine years. At age 65, her retirement account is worth more ($791 465) than Dr. Clark's. This result is from a minor total investment ($45 000). Her strategy shows the advantage of early retirement savings, so the investor has more time for the assets to compound as they grow.

- **Dr. Gardner**

  Dr. Gardner combines the strategies of Drs. Clark and Dent. He starts putting $5000 per year into a tax-advantaged retirement plan and continues until age 65. His account is worth more than $1.5 million before taxes and almost $1 million after taxes. It is the sum of those of Drs. Clark and Dent.

Personal Taxes

The only thing that hurts more than paying an income tax is not having to pay an income tax.

Lord Thomas R. Duwar

GOAL

This chapter is a general discussion of personal income taxes. The discussion focuses on dentists who are practice owners (proprietors or partners) and employees. The chapter also discusses personal tax planning strategies.

LEARNING OBJECTIVES

At the completion of this chapter, the student will be able to:

- Describe the organization of federal Form 1040.

- Define the purpose of the various supporting federal forms and schedules:
  - ○ Schedule A: Itemized Deductions.
  - ○ Schedule B: Interest and Dividend Income.
  - ○ Schedule C: Profit or Loss from Business.
  - ○ Schedule D: Capital Gains and Losses.

- Differentiate between deductible and non-deductible personal expenses.

- Apply the principles of basic tax planning to the personal tax return.

KEY TERMS

adjusted gross income (AGI)
adjustments to income
alternative minimum tax (AMT)
earned income
federal income tax
filing status
itemized deductions
marginal tax rate
net tax liability
occupational taxes
progressive tax rate

proprietorship
regressive tax rate
Schedule A: Itemized Deductions
Schedule B: Interest and Dividend Income
Schedule C: Profit or Loss from Business
Schedule D: Capital Gains or Losses
Scheduled SE: Self-Employment Tax

self-employment tax (SECA)
standard deduction
tax audits
tax credits
tax-free income
tax rate
taxable income
tax rate
unearned income

Business Basics for Dentists, Second Edition. James L. Harrison, David O. Willis, and Charles K. Thieman.
© 2024 John Wiley & Sons, Inc. Published 2024 by John Wiley & Sons, Inc.

Taxes are a fact of life in the United States. As the government provides more services for the population, it requires more money to do those services. Government services may primarily be considered entitlements (such as welfare and Social Security), probably because those items are often in the news. However, governments at all levels provide many other services used by everyone, including military protection, the road system, primary education, the university system, air traffic safety, and restaurant safety inspections. Because of these varied services, taxes to pay for them are also varied and substantial. Box 10.1 shows how much someone might pay in total taxes (actual and hidden). Given this considerable tax liability, dentists must manage their tax liability effectively.

The single most significant item of tax expense for most Americans is the personal income tax. This chapter discusses personal income taxes, how the taxes are calculated, and what can be done to reduce this tax burden. The federal government levies the most significant portion of income tax. Many states also have separate income taxes. As a rule, states with income taxes follow the format of federal forms reasonably closely. Some states use the same form, applying different percentages for the taxes. Most states have a few differences in state-specific municipal bonds and other state-specific initiatives. Some cities, counties, and other municipalities also have income taxes. These vary tremendously. Some cities call them "occupational taxes"; some call them "sinking fund taxes" (because they often retire sinking fund debt). Regardless of the name, they are a form of income tax.

BOX 10.1   EXAMPLE OF TOTAL TAX PAYMENT

Type	Percentage
Federal income tax	28%
Social security tax	7%
State income tax	7%
City income tax	2%
Sales tax	5%
Property tax	3%
Total	52%

The chart shows both actual and hidden taxes. Additional (hidden) taxes include real estate transfer taxes, licenses, excise tax, gasoline tax, personal property tax, recording fees, inheritance tax, airport departure fees, corporate income tax, entertainment tax, hotel room tax, and transportation tax.

Remember, tax laws frequently change as different political parties with different agendas are elected. This chapter is intended as a general primer on personal taxes, and we present information that we believe will not change significantly soon. Each state (and many municipalities) taxes income and property in addition to the federal government, and we cannot cover all of those in this book. Practitioners should check with their accountant or tax advisor concerning current federal and state tax laws and their application to their situation.

Most dentists have their accountants "do their taxes" (calculate and prepare reporting forms). If dentists understand the basics of tax law, they can give their accountant complete information and make more informed decisions regarding their tax status.

FEDERAL INCOME TAXES

Federal income taxes are due on any money someone makes during the year. This income can be earned income or from investments (unearned income). Dentists in a proprietorship business determine their profit or loss from operating their business on a separate form (Schedule C) and then bring that profit or loss to the personal tax form (Form 1040). If someone owns a corporate or partnership practice, they must file returns for those entities, bringing their taxes owed to their personal tax form. If someone is a non-owner employee of a practice, they will have a simpler time computing personal taxes because they do not have to report the practice information.

INCOME

The Internal Revenue Service (IRS) develops and implements tax laws for the federal government. The IRS has a simple rule concerning whether money made is income or not for tax purposes. It considers any money made to be taxable income unless there is a specific waiver for that type of income in the tax codes.

Taxpayers are generally taxed on available income, regardless of whether it is actually in their possession. This means that someone pays tax when the value changes hands. The income is available to them if they have received a check, regardless of whether they cash it. By the same reasoning, a dentist pays no income taxes on accounts receivable because they are not income until the money is received.

Taxes are owed only when the income is realized. For example, someone buys 100 shares of XYZ stock at $10.00 per share. If the price goes to $25.00 in the first year and $35.00 per share in the second year, they pay no tax until they sell the stock. If the stock is sold in the fourth year for $55.00 per share, they pay tax on the appreciated value (55.00 − 10.00 = $45.00 per share) in the fourth year.

The IRS has many ways to check that someone reports all their income. Be sure to report all income. However, a few specifically designated types of income are exempt from income taxes. Some common sources that are non-taxable income include:

- Inheritances and gifts.

- Scholarships and grants (for tuition and fees, not living expenses).

- Disability insurance payments (if the premiums were paid with taxed money).

- Many employer-provided insurances.

- Life insurance payouts.

- Municipal bond interest.

Earned Income

Earned income is money that comes from personal effort. It is also called ordinary income. This may be through a 9–5 job, consulting, or freelancing. It can be wages, salary, commission, tips, many benefits, or self-employment. This is usually the primary income for working people.

The form of the income is immaterial. (It does not have to be cash.) If a dentist barters a crown for a house-painting job, they have received income, according to the IRS. That person should record as income the value of the house-painting job, and the painter should similarly include the value of the crown in their income.

Taxpayers must pay two types of taxes on earned income: income taxes and Social Security/Medicare (also called FICA, payroll, or SETA). They pay income taxes on all earned income, and Social Security taxes (currently 12.4%) are paid yearly on earned income up to a specified limit, which changes yearly. The Medicare tax portion (currently 2.9%) applies to all wages (no upper limit). If someone is employed, their employer pays half of this tax, but a person must pay the total amount if they are self-employed.

Unearned Income

Unearned income is any money that someone does not earn from their active work. It is often called passive income since they do not actively work to earn it. They may make money through investments, savings, rental property, or a business in which they do not actively participate.

Unearned income is taxed differently from earned income, depending on the type. The IRS still considers it as income and usually taxes it at the standard rate. However, certain types (dividends and capital gains) are taxed at lower rates. Unearned income is not subject to Social Security/Medicare taxes. However, as a rule, the unearned income also does not qualify as compensation that someone can contribute to a tax-advantaged retirement plan (such as an Individual Retirement Account, IRA). Alimony is an exception to this rule.

The characterization of income (and therefore its tax treatment) gets very complex when someone owns a business and works for the business (as in a dental practice). They must work closely with their accountant or tax advisor to comply with current laws and regulations.

Some common sources of unearned income include:

- Interest in savings accounts.

- Capital gain when investments are sold.

- Dividends from investments.

- Rental (property) income.

- Distributions from most retirement accounts.

PERSONAL DEDUCTIONS

Deductions are IRS-defined expenses subtracted from income before calculating the tax owed. Some deductions are personal, and some are for business. (In this chapter we only discuss personal deductions.) The IRS has a rule similar to the "income rule" for deductions, and it considers no expense to be deductible unless it has expressly granted deductibility in the tax codes. (Just because someone believes an expense should be deductible does not make it so.) A dentist may need to prove the amount and necessity of this expense to the IRS, so keeping excellent records that include a description of the deduction, a receipt, and a canceled check or another payment record for the item is always a good idea. A canceled check, by itself, is not enough documentation.

BASIC PERSONAL TAX FORMULA

Box 10.2 provides a basic tax formula. Dentists need to understand the components of this formula to understand how to reduce tax liability. This is for personal (not business) tax, which will be covered in Chapter 17. Net income from the practice becomes personal gross income for tax purposes.

- **Total (gross) income**
  Gross income is all the money someone makes in a year. It includes income and wages, tips, profits from a

BOX 10.2   PERSONAL INCOME TAX FORMULA

Gross income

− Adjustments to income

= Adjusted gross income

− Standard or itemized deductions

= Taxable income

<<Calculate Tax>>

− Tax credits

= Net tax liability

business, such as a dental practice, tax refunds, rental income, or any other form of income. Earned income (from working) and unearned income (from investments) are both income for tax purposes, although the IRS treats them differently in specifics of the tax code.

- **Adjustments to income**
  The tax code allows someone to adjust (or subtract) amounts that they paid for some specific items. Those include IRA and other retirement contributions (for themselves), moving expenses if they moved to take a new job, half of the self-employment tax (SECA; if they are self-employed), and any alimony (but not child support) that they paid. Adjustments are essential because they decrease income and how much tax someone will pay later.

- **Adjusted Gross Income**
  Adjusted gross income (AGI) is simply gross income less any adjustments to income. AGI is important because it determines the minimums for Schedule A deductions, phase-outs for exemptions, and other tax matters.

- **Standard or itemized deduction (whichever is greater)**
  Taxpayers then may deduct useful tax deduction items from the AGI. Two methods can determine this adjustment, and either one can be used. There is a choice, but taxpayers should use the larger one because it reduces their apparent income more, resulting in a lower tax liability. The two methods are:
  - **Standard deduction**. A person may take a standard amount, regardless of the number of their actual deductions. This amount changes depending on the filing status. There are four possible filing statuses. As a rule, if a couple is married, they should file jointly. The exception is if one spouse has high itemized

deductions that could not be used if using a joint filing status because of AGI limitations. The standard deduction is an amount the IRS estimates typical filers would show. If someone owns a home or has significant medical or employee expenses, they may be better off itemizing deductions.
  - **Itemized deduction**. The second method that may be used to calculate deductions is to itemize personal deductions. (Business deductions are itemized on a different form, Schedule C.) If a person itemizes their deductions, they must have receipts and payment proof for each deduction. Several of these items are tied to the AGI. This means that someone may only deduct that portion of those expenses that exceed a certain percentage of the AGI, and the rest is lost as a deduction. The specific items, amounts, and conditions change frequently.

- **Taxable Income**
  Taxable income is AGI minus exemptions and deductions. This is the number that someone uses to calculate their tax liability (or how much tax they owe). From a tax planning perspective, they want this number to be as low as it can legally be. A person can do this by lowering income, raising adjustments, or increasing deductions and exemptions.

- **Calculate tax**
  The next step in the formula is to calculate how much tax is owed by applying a tax rate or table to the taxable income figure calculated.

- **Tax credits**
  A credit is an allowance that Congress has provided, and is a one-to-one reduction of tax liability. (For every dollar of a tax credit, taxes go down by a dollar.) Therefore, credits are much more valuable than deductions because they reduce tax (not just taxable income) dollar for dollar. Credit is available for child and elder care expenses, foreign taxes paid, and other targeted expenses. A person subtracts tax credits from the tax owed.

- **Net tax liability (total tax due)**
  The balance is the net tax liability. At this point, the IRS requires that a person adds other non-income taxes, such as SECA and Alternative Minimum Tax (AMT). When these are added in, this becomes the net tax liability – the total amount of tax owed for the year. Any estimated payments made or amounts withheld during the year offset this tax liability. At this point, these amounts are reconciled. If someone has paid too much through the year, they get a refund. If they have not paid enough, they owe additional money to make up the difference.

TAX RATES

Every tax-paying entity has specific tax rates, and Congress alters these rates frequently to meet changing fiscal and social moods and responsibilities. It also change the rules regarding income exclusion, deductions, and many other tax-sensitive issues. Therefore, only concepts are discussed in this chapter, not specific numbers or rates.

A personal income tax rate is a specified percentage that the law stipulates an individual will pay on taxable income. Some taxes (such as federal income taxes) are "progressive," which means that the rate increases by a series of percentages as the taxable income increases. Other taxes are "flat" because the rate remains flat despite the income. Still others are "regressive" taxes that tax higher incomes at a lower rate than lower income levels.

The tax system developed in the United States is graduated or progressive. The more someone earns, the higher the rate of tax they pay. This increased rate is only for the amount above the particular threshold. When income takes a person into the next higher bracket, they do not pay the higher percentage on all of the income, only on the amount above that bracket cut-off. This marginal tax rate is one of the more powerful concepts for the taxpayer to learn. The marginal rate is the tax someone will pay on the next dollar earned. If they earn enough to qualify for the next higher tax bracket, only the amount above it is charged the higher rate, not all of the income. For example, using the fictional tax table in Box 10.3, if a dentist earned $250 000, they would pay 10% on the first $100 000 of income ($10 000), 20% on the next $100 000 of income ($20 000), and 25% on the remaining $50 000 of income ($12 500) for a total of $42 500. They would be in the 25% marginal tax bracket, which means that if they earned an additional $25 000 this year, they would pay 25% (or $6250) in additional tax. Their total tax rate is 17% ($42 500/$250 000).

BOX 10.3	A FICTIONAL ILLUSTRATION OF PROGRESSIVE TAX RATES

Taxable income	Marginal tax rate
$300 000 and above	30%
$200 000–$300 000	25%
$100 000–$200 000	20%
$0–$100 000	10%

Note that the actual tax rates are different.

BOX 10.4	MARGINAL RATE AND TAX SAVINGS

Amount of deduction	Marginal tax rate	Cost	Tax saving
$1000	15%	$850	$150
$1000	35%	$650	$350

The marginal rate is also significant because it determines the value of the tax savings that result from tax planning strategies. If someone has a business deduction that costs $1000 and they are in the 15% marginal tax rate, the after-tax cost is $850. (There is a $150 saving on taxes.) If someone is in the 35% marginal tax bracket, the after-tax cost is only $650 because there is a $350 savings on taxes (Box 10.4).

COMPONENTS OF FORM 1040

Form 1040 is the basic tax form that all individuals must file with the federal government. It reports their income for the previous year, allowable deductions, taxes already paid, and the tax owed. If someone uses certain items or lines on Form 1040, they may need to complete a supporting schedule or form that gives the details of the transactions on that line. For example, suppose a person operates a sole proprietorship business, such as a dental office. In that case, they report the profit or loss from operating that business on one line of Form 1040 (business income or loss). They then attach a completed Schedule C: Profit or Loss from Business that details all income and expenses from running a business. Form 1040 comes in several levels of complexity. Most dentists complete the full Form 1040 rather than the abbreviated Form 1040-EZ.

TAX FORMS AND SCHEDULES

Some common forms and schedules that many dentists use are described here.

Schedule A: Itemized Deductions

This form is used to detail allowable personal deductions. If someone does not have enough personal itemized (specific) deductions, they may take the standard deduction if it is larger. If someone is an employed (non-owner) dentist, they must take professional expenses as miscellaneous deductions on this schedule. This is a problem, because there is a threshold amount these deductions must meet before they can be used.

Schedule B: Interest and Dividend Income

A person with an investment portfolio usually receives interest and dividends from those investments. That income is itemized on Schedule B and entered into the "Income" section of Form 1040.

Schedule C: Profit or Loss from Business

This form will be used to report business income for a sole proprietor. Business-related expenses are subtracted from gross income to arrive at a net income for the business, and this amount is carried over to Form 1040 in the "Income" section.

Form 4562: Depreciation and Amortization

A business owner must keep a running tally of equipment age and depreciation status to determine the amount of that value that they claim as a depreciation expense in any given year. This form determines the amount of that deduction, which is entered as a business expense on Schedule C.

Schedule D: Capital Gains or Losses

Like Schedule B, this schedule is generally used when someone has an investment portfolio, and a dentist may also need this form when selling a dental practice. The gain (or loss) amount is detailed on this sheet and then carried to the "Income" section of Form 1040.

Schedule SE: Self-employment Tax

This schedule determines the amount someone must pay in SETA self-employment tax (FICA and Medicare; see the later section). Because the self-employed person had to pay their own matching Social Security, they can deduct half this amount from taxable income. (Other wage earners did not have to pay tax on that amount either.) This is done by entering half of this tax as an "Adjustment to Income" on Form 1040. If the dentist practices as a corporation, the corporation takes the deduction for matching Social Security and Medicare taxes, the employee equivalent of the self-employment tax.

Schedule K-1

If a practice files taxes as a partnership, the partnership will file a form for the entity and give each partner a Schedule K-1 to help them report their income from the partnership. Because a partnership is not a separate taxable entity, these are information-only forms for the IRS. The K-1 is not filed with Form 1040 but kept with the individual's records. The amounts on K-1 may be carried to several places on Form 1040, depending on the type of income or expense.

Form 1120: Corporate Tax Return

If a practice is a corporation, the corporation will file this return. A dentist will be an employee of the corporation and receive a W-2 for services like any other employee (entered on Form 1040). If the dentist is an owner or part-owner, they may also have dividends from the corporation to report.

ALTERNATIVE MINIMUM TAX

The tax laws give special treatment to certain types of income and deductions. In the past, taxpayers who used these special rules aggressively could substantially (or completely) avoid paying income tax. Some people saw this as unfair and tantamount to abusive use of the system. To ensure everyone pays their "fair share," Congress developed the AMT. It is intended to ensure that everyone pays a certain minimum amount in taxes, even if they have used the rules correctly to reduce their tax burden. The AMT calculations require a person to figure out tax the standard way and then refigure it without particular income and deductions (so-called tax-preference items). The person then must pay income tax based on whichever method leads to higher taxes.

AMT often hits start-up dentists who have relatively high incomes (because of the high depreciation) and mid-career high-income dentists (because of the loss of exemptions and deductions). Dentists need to be aware of the problems of AMT and work with an accountant to reduce the impact on taxable income. (A dentist might, for example, not accelerate depreciation deductions if it causes them to be subject to AMT.)

ISSUES FOR THE SELF-EMPLOYED DENTIST

Several tax issues relate especially to self-employed dentists.

ESTIMATED TAX DECLARATION AND PAYMENT

Anyone whose income does not have tax withheld by their employer must estimate income for the upcoming year and make four equal quarterly payments instead of withholdings. This includes proprietors, partners, and employees who receive dividends and other forms of unearned income. The dates that these federal payments are due are:

- April 15 – Declaration and first payment.
- June 15 – Second payment.
- September 15 – Third payment.
- January 15 – Fourth payment.

Many states that impose state income taxes have similar rules about prepaying estimated income taxes. There would be penalties and interest if someone underestimated their tax liability too much. An accountant will help calculate estimated tax payments.

SELF-EMPLOYMENT TAX (SOCIAL SECURITY AND MEDICARE TAX)

An additional tax that the federal government levies on all earned income is the Social Security and Medicare Tax, also known as the Federal Insurance Contributions Act (FICA). This is composed of two taxes, one on the employee and an equal one on the employer. Together, they fund Social Security benefits and the Medicare program. Everyone who has earned income pays this tax: employees pay it as Social Security and Medicare taxes, and self-employed individuals as SECA. Self-employed individuals must pay not only the employee portion of the tax but also their own matching portion. They get some deduction for their SETA on Form 1040, and SECA is calculated on Schedule SE and attached to Form 1040.

TAX PLANNING FOR THE INDIVIDUAL

Tax planning is a lifetime work for many individuals, so this section barely begins the process. The business taxes and planning section interweaves with this section for practicing dentists.

Most accounting firms send their clients a tax information organizer at the end of the year. This contains the information from the previous year's tax returns and gives prompts for the current year's information. Sometimes they have separate organizers for personal and office information. This should not be a huge burden if the individual has done proper bookkeeping along the way. If they get the information to the accountant well before the deadline, the accountant can examine the upcoming return and make suggestions to lessen the tax burden for the current and next year.

Many firms also distribute a tax planning workbook that summarizes current tax laws. These are excellent sources to begin learning about individual tax planning. These workbooks point out that there are only five strategies to (legally) reduce the tax burden. Tax planning goals are to increase spendable, after-tax income and wealth. (Business taxes are covered in Chapter 17.) The strategies are tax elimination or reduction, recharacterizing income, shifting income, postponing taxes, and using business expenses judiciously.

TAX ELIMINATION OR REDUCTION (AVOID OR REDUCE THE TAX)

The most important thing someone can do here is to know the tax laws to communicate effectively with an accountant or tax preparer. If a person does not take a deduction to which they are entitled, the IRS generally does not call it to their attention. The federal tax code is so complex and ever-changing that it is not worth someone's time to know all of the laws' details, amounts, and nuances. By learning about and using the general rules, such as the proper filing status, personal deductions, and charitable giving, a person can keep taxes as low as possible. They can earn some income that is free from federal income tax, such as municipal bond income.

RECHARACTERIZING INCOME (TURN EARNED INCOME INTO UNEARNED INCOME)

All income is subject to income tax and only earned income is subject to FICA or SECA. If a person can take some earned income and make it unearned, they can save themselves the FICA or SECA. Unearned income includes rent (for the office), lease income (for equipment), and corporation dividends. By establishing separate tax entities for these activities, they can often take income that would be earned and make it unearned, with the associated tax savings.

SHIFTING INCOME (INCOME TAXED AT A LOWER RATE)

A person can shift income to family members in lower tax brackets, thereby decreasing the tax the family unit owes. They can employ family members through the practice or establish a family entity that earns and distributes some income that a dentist would typically earn, taking it from their high tax bracket to family members' lower tax bracket. These strategies are sometimes red flags for IRS audits. A dentist needs advisors to establish that these plans to meet current tax laws.

POSTPONING TAXES (WEALTH ACCUMULATION WITHOUT CURRENT INCOME TAXES)

The most common way of using this strategy is for someone to fund a tax-deferred retirement plan for themselves. This takes money out of current taxable income and allows it to grow without paying taxes until it is withdrawn at retirement. If a dentist hires family members in the practice, they can contribute to their retirement plan, increasing the value of this strategy. A person can also postpone taxes by using some forms of life insurance, annuities, and family gifting programs.

USING BUSINESS EXPENSES JUDICIOUSLY (SHIFTING EXPENSES TO THE BUSINESS UNIT)

The IRS does not allow some expenses as full deductions for an individual. However, the same expense is deductible from a business if it is a reasonable cost of doing business, so as many of these costs as possible should be shifted to the business to take the full deduction. Examples here include continuing education courses, business use of the car, and professional dues. If the dentist does not own a practice, they might consider moonlighting or setting up a consulting business to ensure that these expenses are fully deductible.

TAX AUDITS

The IRS examines (audits) tax returns to verify that the tax reported is correct. It has two intentions for the audit process. First, it recovers taxes that are owed but unreported. Some large cases make significant sums for the treasury. Secondly, the IRS also scares people into reporting accurately. With sizable penalties and interest, everyone needs to take this threat seriously. If a return is selected for examination, this does not necessarily mean that the taxpayer has made an error or been dishonest. Often the IRS needs additional information to verify numbers. Other audits may be more onerous.

The IRS levies significant penalties and fines for cheating on taxes if they catch someone doing so. If a person makes a simple mistake, they will probably only have a fine, back taxes, and interest on the unpaid taxes to pay. If they knowingly cheated the government (e.g. not declaring income or not filing taxes), they may be found guilty of tax evasion and spend time in prison, as well as having to pay the fines, interest, and back taxes due.

HOW RETURNS ARE SELECTED FOR AUDIT

There are several reasons a return may be chosen for an audit. The most common are computer scoring, large corporations, information matching, related examinations, and taxpayer compliance audits.

Computer Scoring

Most returns are selected for examination based on a computer scoring system. A computer program (the Discriminant Function System) compares a return to accepted averages or norms for the same return type. (It compares dentists' offices to other dentists, not physicians' offices or hair stylists.) The program scores every individual and many corporate tax returns. IRS agents then review the highest-scoring returns. It selects some for an audit based on which it feels are most likely to need review and which items are commonly misreported. It calls these audit triggers. Common audit triggers include office expenses, meal and entertainment expenses, and home office deductions. If a return is out of line with norms for the same type of return, the IRS may contact that person.

Large Corporations

The IRS examines many significant corporate returns annually. Dental professional service corporations (PSCs) are not part of this program, but may be subject to audit through any of the other programs.

Information Matching

The IRS examines returns when payment reports, such as W-2 forms and bank interest statements, do not match the income reported on the tax return. This often happens to dentists because insurance companies report to the IRS how much money they pay each dentist each year. If income numbers do not match the numbers reported by the insurers, the dentist will likely get a call (or a letter) from the IRS. This is especially a problem in group practices where insurers may make payments in one doctor's name but credit them to another's.

Related Examinations

Returns may be selected for an audit when they involve issues or transactions with other taxpayers, such as business partners or investors, whose returns were selected for examination.

AUDIT METHODS

The IRS may conduct an audit by mail or through an in-person interview and review of the taxpayer's records. The IRS conducts most audits (at least initially) through the mail. If a person receives a letter from the IRS, the letter will generally claim that it has recomputed their tax based on the enclosed reasons or information. Generally, the tax will be higher as a result, although occasionally it may be reduced. The letter then states that the person should reply within a specific time if they want to dispute the IRS's findings. (The IRS takes its deadlines seriously.)

At this point, contact an accountant and reply quickly to the letter. If the IRS requires an interview, the problem may be more serious. These interviews may be at an IRS office (an office audit), the taxpayer's home, a place of business, or the accountant's office (a field audit). Regardless, the dentist will need to have records to prove their claims.

Estate Planning

CHAPTER 11

A man's dying is more the survivor's affair than his own.

Thomas Mann

GOAL

This chapter examines the basic principles of estate planning.

LEARNING OBJECTIVES

At the completion of this chapter, the student will be able to:

- Describe the purposes of estate planning.

- Identify the primary techniques of planning an estate.

- Discuss common methods of estate transfer.

- Discuss the use of a testamentary letter.

- Discuss issues of personal competency and standard methods of addressing competency problems.

KEY TERMS

advance directive
agent
beneficiaries
community property
estate planning
estate taxes
executor
federal unified gift and estate tax

general power of attorney
intestate
joint tenants with rights of
    survivorship (JTWROS)
letter of instruction
lifetime transfers
limited power of attorney
living will

powers of attorney
present power of attorney
probate court
springing power of attorney
testamentary letter
trustee
wills

Most people do not think of estate planning as a pleasant task. After all, it forces them to face their mortality. It is, however, a valuable and necessary task and can also be personally satisfying. Estate planning is not about the person doing the planning because they will not be around to know the difference. Instead, estate planning is a task done for family, heirs, and those who that person loves and cares about. An estate plan can be as simple as a

Business Basics for Dentists, Second Edition. James L. Harrison, David O. Willis, and Charles K. Thieman.
© 2024 John Wiley & Sons, Inc. Published 2024 by John Wiley & Sons, Inc.

will or involve a will, trusts, contracts, and named beneficiaries. It depends on how much the person owns and how complex their wants are.

People should probably dust off their estate plan every three to five years or whenever they have a significant life change. As their estate gets more valuable and complex, they will seek out lawyers who deal with estate planning issues. People often forget what they put into their plans. Circumstances also change quickly. Retirement savings or the value of the practice may have blossomed over the past several years. They may have had additional children, got divorced or remarried, received another inheritance, or changed their insurance significantly. All these can affect how a will and estate plan are structured.

PURPOSE OF ESTATE PLANNING

Planning an estate will accomplish several purposes.

TO BE SURE WHO GETS WHAT

A person may have a unique gold watch or Aunt Tillie's flower vase that they want to go to a particular child. Although not trivial (in fact, these decisions are often the most contentious), the decision takes on added importance when significant amounts of money are involved. This money may be from assets owned, insurance policies, retirement plan proceeds, a practice sale, inheritances, or countless other sources. If a person correctly plans their estate, they will resolve conflicts, reduce squabbles between family members, and ensure that assets will be distributed the way they intend.

TO GIVE BENEFICIARIES PROTECTION AND GUIDANCE

The person doing the planning may be the primary source of family income and financial expertise. If they die, beneficiaries may need help managing family finances or other affairs. They may want to appoint a banker or other trusted advisor as the trustee until family members are old enough to manage their affairs. Through estate planning, they can ensure that beneficiaries are protected from fraudulent advisors and kept from squandering the money earmarked for a particular purpose.

TO PROVIDE FOR THE WELFARE OF MINOR CHILDREN

If someone has minor children, they have a particular estate planning problem. If the spouse is still alive, they will generally take care of any minor children. However, if both die

(e.g. in an accident), the problem suddenly becomes enormous. Not only does the child or children have to cope with the parents' deaths, but they also must forge new parental ties. A parent needs to ensure that someone will be the child's or children's guardian until they reach the age of majority when they can legally manage their affairs. If someone is not selected ahead of time, then the state will appoint someone. That may not be someone in whom the parent would have had trust or confidence. The person chosen needs to provide the emotional and financial guidance the parent would have customarily provided. (The potential guardian should be asked before being named.) Unmarried siblings or couples may not be the best choice if they are not tuned into raising children. Elderly parents may want the responsibility, but may not be physically able to parent children until the youngest child is 18. If a person is divorced, remarried, or part of a blended family, additional legal problems develop concerning visitation and support. The more that can be decided ahead of time, the more service will be provided for the family.

TO HELP GUIDE THE EXECUTOR (ADMINISTRATOR)

An executor (sometimes called the administrator or personal representative) is responsible for collecting information, paying bills and expenses, seeing that assets are appropriately distributed, and generally marshaling an estate through probate. Being an executor is a thankless job, and relatives and creditors try to influence the executor. In addition, there is much hard work to do, including selling assets, having other assets appraised, paying bills, closing credit cards and other accounts, and keeping everyone informed of the process. Executors can be paid (from the estate) for their work. The executor is named in the will. The estate planner should consider who would do these duties best and ask that person ahead of time.

TO ELIMINATE DELAYS AND THE EXPENSE OF PROBATE ADMINISTRATION

A probate court is responsible for seeing that estates are adequately distributed after someone's death. Probate administration takes many months, or even years, to complete. This happens especially when the estate is not well planned. Lawyers then bicker over who gets what and who deserves which assets. A well-planned estate reduces these delays and expenses. When the estate is in probate, the assets are essentially "locked up" until they are distributed. This can be a problem if family members or other heirs need that money. In this case, a person needs to provide sufficient liquid assets outside the probate process for their support. If a large portion of the estate assets is non-liquid (not cash or near-cash), then the estate may have to sell some crucial assets to pay the estate taxes. Many professional people have large estates that trigger significant estate taxes. Proper planning will reduce those taxes and allow the maximum amount for the heirs' support and enjoyment.

TO PLAN FOR THE BUSINESS TRANSITION

If the person owns a dental practice or other business, they have another special estate planning problem. This problem is that the value of the practice drops quickly if the owner is not present seeing patients. An owner should have a plan for what would happen to the practice in case of death or disability. If they are in a group practice, they may have cross-purchase agreements to cover the eventuality. If they are a solo practitioner, they should have an accountant or other trusted advisor with a plan for continuing and selling the practice. A spouse, significant other, executor, or agent should have enough information to deal with the practice immediately. Any delay can be financially devastating. Often the spouse does not even know how to get into the office, much less how to look for a buyer or sell the practice. This should be taken care of for their peace of mind and financial security (Box 11.1).

TO REDUCE ESTATE TAXES

Depending on the value of an estate, taxes can take a significant amount that might otherwise go to heirs. The estate pays any taxes that are due and then distributes the assets. Whoever receives the asset then receives it

BOX 11.1	ITEMS TO CONSIDER DURING A BUSINESS TRANSITION

- Location of the office keys.

- How to use the office security system.

- Computer security codes.

- Home phone numbers of office staff.

- Names and numbers of major suppliers and labs.

- Combination of the safe.

- Name of doctor to refer patients to.

- Plan for practice continuation.

- Plan for practice sale.

free of income tax because taxes have already been paid (by the estate). However, if the estate contains many non-liquid assets (e.g. real estate), the estate may have to sell some of those critical assets to pay the estate taxes. Proper planning will reduce those taxes and allow the maximum amount to flow through to the heirs.

THE ELEMENTS OF AN ESTATE PLAN

An estate plan is a collection of documents that outline a person's plans for when they die or if they become incapacitated (unable to make decisions). If someone dies or becomes incapable of making decisions, decisions will be made for them, often by the court system in a long and cumbersome process. Some estate plans are more complex than others. However, at a minimum, the following elements are strongly recommended.

WILL

A will is a written instrument or legal document that takes effect on a person's death. It disposes of the person's rights to real or personal property that they own at death. It also names someone as the executor (or administrator) to execute the will in the probate court. A will may give specific money or items to specific heirs or direct or allow the executor to distribute funds and property in a specified way. It may set up trusts to hold money or property, naming a person (or institution) to manage the trust according to the person's directive. A will becomes a compelling document that ensures that a person's wishes regarding their property are followed after their death.

Everyone has a will. Some are written by the person who owns the property; the state defines others through the probate court. If a person dies without their own written will, they have died *intestate*. This means that the state will determine who receives their property. These "state-made" wills vary tremendously from state to state. They allocate assets to various family members. These may include a spouse, surviving children, parents, brothers and sisters, and grandparents. The estate is generally turned over to the state if the person has no heirs. Many states have a "surviving spouse exemption," which declares that if someone dies intestate, a certain amount (such as the first $10 000) of the personal property goes to the surviving spouse (ahead of all creditors and funeral expenses). Some states also have "dower and curtsey" rights. This antiquated term says that the surviving spouse is entitled to one-half the real and personal property as a "dower" and not an heir. The intelligent thing is to write a will to avoid all these legal problems. There is more information on wills later in the chapter.

A DURABLE POWER OF ATTORNEY

A power of attorney allows a particular person (the agent named in the document) to make certain decisions and actions for others. The person holding power does not hold title to any property but acts or decides for the other person. Powers of attorney come in several types. A limited power of attorney allows the agent to act only in a particular area, for example selling a house or paying bills for a dental practice. A general power of attorney gives the agent broad authority to transact almost any matter that the original person could, such as selling personal property and financial assets or filing tax returns. A present power of attorney takes effect immediately. A springing power of attorney lies dormant until it "springs" into action, generally when the person becomes disabled. (Often, a physician or third party must certify that the principal lacks capacity.) A durable power of attorney allows another to handle an incapacitated person's financial and business affairs. Traditionally, powers of attorney end when the incapable person dies or becomes competent again. Formalities of establishing a durable power of attorney vary from state to state. Some states require that they be filed with the register of deeds.

A durable power of attorney is essential when someone becomes disabled because it allows the agent access to bank and investment accounts. It is imperative if the person is the owner of a business (such as a dental practice) and they have exclusive access to the business's finances.

ADVANCE DIRECTIVES

Advance directives, also known as end-of-life documents, help to ensure that a person's wishes for medical care are carried out if they are incapable of making or communicating those wishes. This may happen, for example, when someone is near death, in a coma, or suffering from severe dementia. These documents include proxies, living wills, do-not-resuscitate (DNR) orders, and organ donor cards. Most states have prepared forms that someone can fill out to be sure they are valid, and some states have a single document that combines several of these other documents. Be sure to talk with a lawyer from the resident state to ensure that the advance directive is valid.

Healthcare Proxy

A healthcare proxy is often called an advance medical directive. A person names someone to act on their behalf (an agent) to make medical (not financial) decisions for them if they become incapacitated. In most states,

healthcare providers are bound to follow the agent's decisions as if they were their own. If someone wants (or does not want) extraordinary life-saving treatments, this document should clearly state that. It helps loved ones and medical providers to make difficult end-of-life decisions, knowing that the decision is what the person wants.

A Living Will

A living will describe someone's wishes for life-extending treatments. This is especially important if they become permanently in a coma or vegetative state or are dying from an illness. The living will outline the conditions under which they want to be kept alive or allowed to die. If a person does not have a living will, doctors and hospitals often do all they can to keep them alive. That could mean, for example, keeping someone in a long-term vegetative state. Some of these medical treatments may include being put on a respirator or feeding tube, having cardiopulmonary resuscitation (CPR) performed, or having emergency surgery. States vary somewhat in their interpretation of the validity of such living wills. So, if someone spends significant time in more than one state, they may need more than one.

HIPAA Release

The Health Insurance Portability and Accountability Act (HIPAA) laws or advance medical directives will include a document that states what medical information can be released and to whom. There are many stories of family members who could not get information from a doctor about a loved one's condition because of HIPAA. While HIPAA does not keep this information from being shared in many cases, to avoid any confusion it is a good idea to include a HIPAA release as an additional document.

LETTER OF INSTRUCTION (TESTAMENTARY LETTER)

A letter of instruction, or a testamentary letter, is not a legal document. It is a convenience for the person who is the executor of the will (or the administrator of the estate). The outline gives specific information that the executor will need to properly process and probate the estate, including whom to contact, the location of critical documents, and any specific wishes. The letter should be prepared as if for someone totally unfamiliar with the writer's personal situation, which makes the process easier for an outside person who does know the writer. A testamentary letter should include the following information:

- **Personal Information**
  Social Security number, birth certificate location, etc.

- **Lists and locations of documents**
  Assets, real estate, stocks, automobiles (title location), mortgage information, retirement accounts, safe deposit (lock) boxes, and combinations to safes.

- **Practice information**
  Accountant, location of deeds, leases, computer back-ups, buy-out provisions, security passwords, etc.

- **Names of and contact numbers for advisors**
  Attorney, accountant, investment advisor, insurance agent, and stockbroker

- **Personal wishes**
  Burial/cremation, funeral wishes, distribution of personal property, etc.

- **Insurance policies**
  Company, agent, policy number, and location, especially for life insurance policies.

- **Liquidity**
  Where money is available for taxes, expenses, and living costs until the distribution of the estate.

METHODS OF PROPERTY TRANSFER

There are three basic methods of transferring property: wills, estates, and lifetime transfers (gifts and trusts). A person can also transfer some property outside the probate process. This is done through jointly held property (which passes to a survivor) and through life insurance or pensions, which pass directly to a named beneficiary.

WILLS

Wills are the primary and most common form of asset transfer. They are legal documents, although many states do not require that a lawyer write them. A person should have several copies of their will. One should be kept at home, one in a safe deposit box (in case of a house fire), and one with a lawyer as a back-up. When the person dies, a probate court will settle the will. These are special courts that handle estate cases. They establish the will's validity, "read the will," and distribute assets according to the will or intestacy law.

Each state has requisites for a valid will, which vary by state. Some more common requirements include the following:

- The will must be in writing and signed by the will writer.

- The will must show testamentary intent (i.e. the person recognizes this as their will).

- The person must have testamentary capacity (18 years old or older, sound mind, not acting under fraud or influence, etc.).

- Credible witnesses must witness the will.

- Some states allow handwritten (in the testator's handwriting) or "holographic" wills.

Because each state's requirements are different, having a lawyer draft the will is a good investment. Lawyers can help ensure that the will complies with the relevant state's rules. They can also be sure that the estate plan has been designed to meet the person's needs and desires.

Wills may be revoked. This revocation may be intentional (on the person's part) or unintentional. Reasons for revocation include physical destruction, writing a subsequent will, or through the operation of law (such as marriage or divorce). If someone gets married or divorced, they should be sure to write a new will. A codicil is simply a written modification to an existing will. A codicil does not revoke the original will; it just amends it.

TRUSTS

There are two kinds of trusts: living (revocable) and non-revocable.

LIVING TRUSTS

A living (or revocable) trust is a legal entity into which someone can transfer assets during their lifetime. The will can also stipulate that specified assets should be transferred into a living trust at death. The trust takes ownership of the assets. However, the owner can cancel or change (or revoke) the trust any time before death. The person retains control (but not ownership) of the assets.

Individuals can use a revokable trust, much like a will, by instructing how assets in the trust will be distributed after death. These assets are distributed outside the probate process so that they will be distributed more quickly and less expensively. The owner can also name a bank or financial advisor as the trustee (the person who "runs" the trust), or they can act as a trustee while they are still alive. Revocable trusts do not present any tax advantage that cannot be achieved in a will because the owner still has control of the assets in the trust.

NON-REVOCABLE TRUSTS

Non-revocable trusts are, as the name says, not revocable. That means that the owner cannot get the assets back once they set a trust up and place assets within it: the trust takes ownership of the assets, and the individual does not retain either control or ownership of the assets.

Non-revocable trusts have a distinct tax advantage over revocable trusts. Because the individual does not retain any control, the assets placed into the trust are removed from their estate for tax purposes. Depending on how the trust is set up, a person may gain a tax deduction for the contribution. These trusts get complex, and a lawyer and tax planner will be needed to maximize their effect.

LIFETIME TRANSFERS

A person can arrange for estate transfers by gift or sale during their lifetime.

JOINT TENANTS WITH RIGHT OF SURVIVORSHIP

This transfer method says that two people are equal asset owners. Upon the death of one of the owners, the asset passes to the other owner. There is no testamentary control. Therefore, these properties are not included in the person's estate or probate. However, when establishing the account, the person must be sure that it is listed as joint tenants with right of survivorship (JTWROS).

COMMUNITY PROPERTY

Some states have community property laws. This means that spouses have a one-half vested interest in all property owned in the marriage.

GIFTS

Anyone may give up to $17000 annually (2023 figure) to any other person without incurring a tax liability. More than this triggers a gift tax liability. This means that a husband and wife may each give (through gifts) to each of their children a total of $34000 each year. These lifetime transfers can decrease the amount of an estate, and the transfers can be in cash, securities, property, or other items of value. The combined Gift and Estate Tax rules apply if more is gifted during a year.

GENERAL ESTATE PLANNING ISSUES

The Federal Unified Gift and Estate Tax is of most concern in estate planning. Most states have additional taxes on estates. The federal limit on estates is presently (2023) about $12.92 million. (Congress can change that amount at any time. It also has been scheduled to change yearly for inflation.) There are also generation-skipping taxes, excess retirement accumulation taxes, and sometimes transfer taxes. If someone's estate is more than the unified gift and tax limit, they must plan carefully to avoid taxes as much as possible. The more the estate grows above this cut-off point, the more the person needs professional estate planning help.

Each estate situation is unique. A person's will and estate plan will also be unique. There are computer programs that can generate basic wills. Most dentists, especially practice owners, have complex estates and would face potential problems if the estate is not properly planned and structured. The practitioner probably needs a lawyer to draft a will and to ensure that the estate plan gives the heirs maximum benefit. They should review the estate plan any time they have a significant life event, such as a family birth or death, a divorce or marriage, or a practice purchase or sale. Other than that, they should review the estate plan every year or two to ensure it still meets current needs.

Life insurance has been called the "poor man's estate." The policyholder should name a beneficiary for life insurance proceeds. This payout goes directly to the named beneficiary, not through the probate court. Whoever receives those benefits receives them tax free. If the decedent does not name a beneficiary, the proceeds will be included in the estate for tax purposes and distributed by the administrator. A person can split beneficiaries, naming several people, each to receive a part of the insurance benefit.

Any pension, profit-sharing, IRAs, or other retirement accounts should have named beneficiaries. The funds in these accounts will pass directly to the named beneficiary, and the probate court will not distribute them. There are special tax rules about withdrawing money from these accounts.

The owner of a dental practice should ensure that their survivors know that time is essential in terms of what happens to it after the owner's death. The longer the survivors wait to sell the practice, the less valuable it becomes. They should not be surprised if dentists call inquiring about the practice soon after the news of the death. The survivors should take names and return the calls as soon as possible. The planner should have a detailed plan to sell the practice (who the advisors are, who will value the practice, who will run the practice until it sells, etc.) and arrange for someone to maintain the practice until the sale is completed.

There is currently an unlimited marital deduction for estate taxes. This means that a person can give their spouse the estate tax free. However, there may be a huge tax liability when the second spouse dies. It is possible to avoid many of these taxes with proper planning.

Business Foundations

A dental practice is a small business that sells dental services. As such, it is subject to the same laws, community forces, and business principles as any other business. Business owners and operators have studied, applied, and refined these principles over the years. There is a common language of business; some words carry specific meanings that are different from common usage. Businesses act and report information to interested outsiders (such as bankers or the Internal Revenue Service) in commonly accepted ways. These all become the foundation or building blocks of a successful business.

A dental practice exists in the social environment of the community in which its people are practicing. Patients come from the community. Staff members live and raise their children in the community. Dentists are visible, active, and esteemed members of the community. So, the entire fabric of the practice is drawn from the community it serves. The two become inseparable. This is not only the immediate community but also the larger state and national communities. Many external factors influence practitioners and small business operators, but some of these factors can be controlled. Others, such as the economy, are factors that cannot be controlled, only responded to. Dentists must therefore learn to be members of the community if they are to prosper. They should not define their job as sitting in an office fixing teeth. Instead, they must see themselves as important providers of care and purchasers of goods and services in the community.

Some dentists believe that applying hard business logic to professional practice is unprofessional or undignified. However, there is nothing sinister about establishing an efficient business framework in which a person practices the art of patient care. Certainly the two intersect in many places, but by keeping patient care as the focus of every patient interaction, the two can be equally served.

CONCERNS OF THE BUSINESS FOUNDATIONS SECTION

Businesses do not operate in a vacuum. They operate within a community and must respond to the wants, needs, and norms of the community. This business foundations section relates to three major goals:

- **Make the practice responsive to the community**
  A dental practice owner must understand the forces in the community that affect small businesses and use the same forces to improve the dental practice.

- **Make the practice act like a business**
  A dental practice owner must understand basic business principles so that they can make the dental practice efficient and effective.

- **Make the practice act legally**
  The regulatory environment demands that all businesses, especially those delivering personal or medical services such as dentistry, act legally and keep patient care and safety as their top priority.

OBJECTIVES OF THE BUSINESS FOUNDATIONS SECTION

Given these three main goals, this section discusses the blocks that are used to build the foundation of a strong business:

- **Chapter 12: Basic Economics**
  Dentists need to understand how the economy affects their practice so that they can respond appropriately. By making correct decisions that depend on the economic environment, they can maximize profit and their net worth.

- **Chapter 13: Business Entities**
  Dentists should establish a business entity that protects and enhances their business purpose.

- **Chapter 14: The Legal Environment of the Dental Practice**
  Dentists need to be sure that the practice operates according to the laws that regulate businesses.

- **Chapter 15: Financial Statements**
  Financial statements are part of the common language of business. Dentists need to understand these statements so that they can converse effectively with their bankers and advisors.

- **Chapter 16: Basics of Business Finance**
  Businesses borrow and use money. The entire banking system is based on the time value of money and its outgrowths. If dentists understand this building block, they can maximize their return.

- **Chapter 17: Business Taxes and Tax Planning**
  As part of the greater community, everyone must pay taxes. Dentists need to know which taxes to pay and how to plan legally to reduce the tax burden and increase profitability.

- **Chapter 18: Management Principles**
  When dentists structure a business, they need to address several common areas.

- **Chapter 19: Planning the Dental Practice**
  Dentists should develop an effective plan to help guide themselves to a successful practice.

Basic Economics

If you teach a parrot to say "Supply and Demand," you can get him a PhD in economics.

Thomas Carlyle

GOAL

This chapter aims to make students aware of the economic factors that affect contemporary practicing dentists.

LEARNING OBJECTIVES

At the completion of this chapter, the student will be able to:

- Discuss the economics of dental care delivery, specifically supply-and-demand issues related to practicing dentists.
- Discuss the factors that influence the supply of dental services.
- Discuss the factors that impact the demand for dental services.
- Discuss the effect of managed care on the economics of dental practices.
- Discuss the role of technology in the economics of dental practices.
- Discuss the use of dental auxiliary personnel and the economics of dental practices.

- Discuss the predominant social trends that impact the economics of dental practice.
- Differentiate between public and private consumption goods.
- Discuss gross domestic product and its effect on dental practices.
- Discuss the business cycle and its effect on dental practices.
- Discuss inflation and its effect on dental practices.
- Discuss how the Federal Reserve Bank influences dental practices.
- Discuss how the federal budget influences dental practices.

Business Basics for Dentists, Second Edition. James L. Harrison, David O. Willis, and Charles K. Thieman.
© 2024 John Wiley & Sons, Inc. Published 2024 by John Wiley & Sons, Inc.

Economics deals with human wants, needs, behaviors, and responses. As such, economists can never "prove" anything. That is, there are always confounding factors in real-life economics that make all economic ideas "theories" that must be applied in individual circumstances.

Dental services respond to the laws of economics like any other good or service. Therefore, practitioners need to understand the basic notions of supply-and-demand economics to respond to changing economic conditions. The study of economics is usually broken into two general areas: *macroeconomics* and *microeconomics*. The difference between the two is a difference in scope. Macroeconomics looks at the whole economy and the forces that affect it. Suppose forces that affect the entire dental industry, such as national economic policies, changing demographic patterns, bank interest rates, inflation, and labor supply issues, are examined. In that case, this is a macro view of economic conditions. Microeconomics looks at the individual business, person, or practice and how they respond to changing conditions. It examines how prices are determined and how many goods and services each individual produces and consumes. Each of these areas has significant implications for how someone practices dentistry.

LAWS OF SUPPLY AND DEMAND

The primary issue of economics is choice-making. Both a society as a whole and individuals within that society decide what to produce and consume. How people use their limited resources determines the supply and demand for goods and services within a market economy. This free choice leads to the US capitalistic, market-driven economy. Other systems (communism and, to a degree, socialism) plan the economy and determine how much of each good and service is provided and at what price.

DEMAND

To the economist, *demand* means the quantity of a good or service that individuals can buy at every possible price. Demand then defines a relationship between the price of a commodity and the number of units the buyer is willing to purchase. It implies that consumers both want the product and can pay for it. The resulting law of demand states that "as the price of any good decreases, the quantity of that good that consumers are willing and able to purchase will increase. As price increases, consumers will demand a smaller quantity of the good." This is an inverse relationship: the other gets smaller as one factor increases. Evidence of this law can be seen by looking at everyday buying habits. Clothing stores lower the price at the end of the season to clear their racks of goods. Unscrupulous contractors and building suppliers increase prices after a natural disaster when demand is high. Automobile dealers stimulate demand through rebates and other discount offers.

Demand has the important characteristic of elasticity. Very elastic demand means that the quantity demanded (and bought) is sensitive to price. Here, the demand curve is much flatter. For example, as the price of coffee rises, consumers buy less and less coffee and instead buy substitutes, such as tea and colas. Inelastic demand means that the quantity demanded is insensitive to the price of the good or service. For example, people with diabetes will buy the same amount of insulin despite the price, their demand for the good is inelastic, and the curve is steeper.

A demand curve is a graphical representation of the relationship between price and quantity demanded. A demand curve can be drawn for any good or service in the market, and the curve always slopes down and to the right. Although many actual demand curves have been determined for various products, they are more helpful in understanding economics concepts. Figure 12.1 shows a typical, hypothetical demand curve, in this case for crowns. As the price of crowns increases, fewer people are willing and able to afford this service; the quantity demanded then decreases. Any individual buyer will reach a point where they refuse to buy any additional units because they have fulfilled their needs or because their opportunity costs are too high. Their demand is essentially satiated. However, as the price decreases, more buyers come into the market and are willing to purchase the good, although other consumers may have dropped out of the market.

An individual consumer's demand for services will vary depending on income level, future expectations, and personal wants and desires. Demand curves are generally determined for the entire market, and market demand is equal to the sum of all individual demands. This realizes that some consumers will never buy the product (e.g. gold crowns) at any price, others may buy many products at an unlimited price, and most fall on a continuum between the two extremes.

SUPPLY

To this point, only one side of the economic exchange, the buyer, has been examined. The behavior of the seller or producer (the "supplier") is equally essential to the transaction.

To the economist, *supply* means the quantity of a good or service the supplier can sell at every possible price. Suppliers are usually thought of as those who own factories, shoe stores, or dental offices. These are the suppliers in the product market for final goods and services. However, there is a similar market for resources to produce the goods. Producers must compete in the open market for wheat for bread, steel for cars, and an hour of the hygienist's time.

Supply then defines a relationship between the price of a commodity and the number of units the seller is willing to supply. The resulting law of supply states that "as the price of any good increases, the quantity of that good that suppliers are willing and able to offer for sale will increase. Suppliers will supply a larger quantity of the goods as price increases." This is a direct relationship: as one factor gets larger, so does the other. Supply displays the characteristic of elasticity similar to demand. Elastic supply means that a change in the price of the good leads to a large change in the quantity supplied.

A supply curve is a graphical representation of the relationship between price and quantity supplied. A supply curve can be drawn for any good or service in the market, and the curve always slopes upward and to the right. Figure 12.2 shows a typical, hypothetical supply curve, in this case also for gold crowns. As the price of gold crowns increases, dentists are willing to work harder and produce more products; the quantity supplied then increases. Any individual seller will reach a point where they refuse to produce any additional units because they have fulfilled

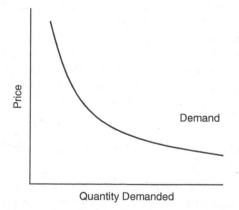

FIGURE 12.1   A demand curve.

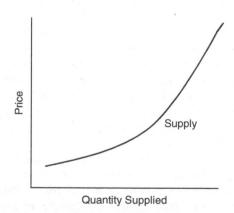

FIGURE 12.2   A supply curve.

their needs or because their opportunity costs are too high. Their supply is essentially satiated.

An individual producer's supply of services will vary depending on factors such as the cost of production, degree of profitability, future expectations, and personal wants and desires. Supply curves are also determined for the entire market. A market supply is equal to the average of all the individual supplies. The obtainable profits mainly determine the market supply. If supplying the good or service is lucrative compared with other forms of income generation, then more people will attempt to become suppliers. The size of the market, social climate, and barriers to entry limit the number of successful suppliers. Dentistry, for example, has steep barriers to entry in that there are academic dental school entrance requirements, a limited number of dental school places, licensure requirements, and high start-up costs. These barriers keep the supply curve for dentistry stable.

There is mixed support for the idea that having more health service providers lowers public costs. The opposite may be the case. It is well established that the number of surgeons in an area determines how much surgery is done there. Dentistry may follow a similar pattern. Rather than competition stimulating price reductions, it may increase prices in an area. One explanation for this apparent paradox is that practitioners may need to generate a certain amount of money to meet expenses and have a targeted income for themselves. According to this "target income hypothesis," fees in an area will increase until practitioners meet those needs.

MARKET EQUILIBRIUM IN DEMAND AND SUPPLY

A "market" occurs when suppliers and demanders (consumers) exchange value (money). In a dynamic market, changes are expected to take place in both supply and demand for services as the underlying conditions change. When the forces of supply interact with the forces of demand, a market price is established, an equilibrium point where the supply and demand for those same goods are equal. Graphically, this occurs where the upward-sloping supply curve and the downward-sloping demand curve intersect (Figure 12.3). The equilibrium point for the quantity demanded is shown at point A on the graph; the equilibrium point for the price is shown at point B.

A market is never in exact equilibrium. Instead, there is fluctuation as producers and consumers adjust to changing conditions. A market shortage is a condition in which the demand for a good or service is greater than the supply of that good or service. The price then rises as consumers bid up the price. More dollars then chase fewer goods until

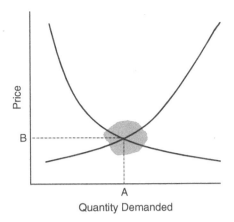

FIGURE 12.3　Market equilibrium.

suppliers produce more goods or services or more suppliers enter the market (increasing production) to take advantage of excess profits. A market surplus is a condition in which the supply of a good or service is greater than the demand for that good or service. Prices drop as suppliers accept less to sell products. Profits for producers decrease as the price falls. Eventually, inefficient producers are forced from the market as profit margins decrease.

If a good is freely traded, shortages and surpluses do not last. The forces of market competition cause a readjustment of prices, and that establishes a new equilibrium. Those willing to pay more will get what they want, pushing up prices and eliminating the shortage. Those willing to sell for less will gather sales, driving down prices and eliminating surpluses.

Resource markets behave similarly to final goods and services. Businesses become the demanders, and households (and the people who make them up) are the suppliers. Dentists compete not only with each other for staff services but also with alternative forms of employment. A shortage will occur if dentists, as a group, do not pay a wage comparable to similar forms of employment, given similar backgrounds, training requirements, and working conditions. This drives the price of staff members up. Suppose an individual dentist wants to hire a hygienist at less than the market rate for hygienists. In that case, they probably cannot hire one unless other non-wage factors (e.g. benefits, time off, convenience) balance the hygienist's opportunity cost of a lower wage.

MICROECONOMICS: THE INDIVIDUAL BUYER AND SELLER

Microeconomics examines the individual firm (or practice) and individual consumers who purchase goods and services from those firms. It attempts to answer why people buy, at what price they will buy, and what producers can do to influence their buying decisions. Several microeconomic theories and their effects on dental practices are described.

PUBLIC AND PRIVATE GOODS

Any time economists speak of economic "goods," they are referring to anything that is both desirable and limited and to obtain which people will give up something else. Goods may be physical items for sale (e.g. cars, televisions, or shampoo) or services that consumers buy and use immediately (e.g. haircuts, dance lessons, or massages). Dentistry sells physical products such as dentures, partials, and restorations and less tangible service "goods" such as prophylaxes, endodontics, whitening procedures, or extractions. Some people even view intangible items such as leisure time and health as goods because people are willing to sacrifice to "buy" these commodities.

Economists often speak of public or private consumption goods. Private consumption goods are purchased and consumed by individuals rather than the whole society. (A whole group may individually purchase and consume the good, but that is not done as an act of the whole, rather as acts of individuals.) When individuals purchase DVD players, vacations, automobiles, and food, they consume those goods privately. If someone cannot pay the price required, they are excluded from having the use and benefit of the good. Public consumption goods benefit the whole of society or at least many people. National defense, the road system, and police and fire protection are examples of public goods enjoyed equally by most people. Society cannot legitimately exclude those who cannot pay from enjoying the use and benefit of these goods.

Because private suppliers cannot exclude non-payers from enjoying public consumption goods, they generally will not provide these goods on a for-profit basis. Instead, the government provides public consumption goods. (Government may contract with private suppliers to provide the good or service, but the government is still ultimately responsible.) There is a significant ongoing debate in the United States over what a public good is and what level of those services the government should provide. People believe that healthcare, medical care, and dental care "fit" as private or public goods. Depending on the answer, a different set of financing, access, delivery, and pricing policies will result.

Presently, US society considers dentistry a private consumption good. People will purchase as much of the service as they want and can afford. Although the government provides some dental services, people do not have unlimited and equal access to the service. Because dentistry is a private consumption good, it follows the economic laws of supply and demand.

ECONOMIC CHOICES

Economists believe that all economic resources are limited. That is to say that everything people use to produce or purchase the economic goods and services that they desire is limited or scarce. Because these resources are limited, people must choose between alternatives that provide satisfaction. The choice not taken is lost and therefore sacrificed. This sacrifice is called an "opportunity cost." For example, a family may have a given income. They want to purchase both a new car and a larger home. Because of their income limitations, they cannot purchase both goods (the car and the home). Instead, they must decide between the two. If they choose to buy the car, they lose the enjoyment of the new home (an opportunity cost). However, if they decide to make a down payment on a new home, they forgo the satisfaction of the car.

The notion of economic choice applies to both producers and consumers. Different people weigh the values of goods and services differently, and therefore the opportunity cost of forgoing those goods. A consumer with limited resources may need to decide between a vacation and extensive dental work, and the opportunity cost associated with forgoing each option will help to decide. As a producer, a dentist must decide the value of economic goods such as leisure and recreational time. Although a person may have the opportunity to make additional income by working longer hours, they will weigh the opportunity costs associated with forgoing time for personal and family enjoyment.

THE MICROECONOMICS OF DENTAL SERVICES

Since dentistry is a private consumption good, it should react to the marketplace's forces of supply and demand like any other consumer good. Moreover, that is what happens, and these macro forces occur through an aggregation of individual micro choices. When thinking about the overall demand for services, more (but not all) dental patients respond as the macro theory predicts.

Demand for Dental Services

Demand for dental services follows the classic downward-sloping demand curve. However, many social factors affect the shape of the demand curve, and these are called the determinants of demand.

Price Price is, by definition, one primary determinant of demand. Equally crucial to the actual price is the apparent price for the consumer. Third-party plans, in effect, reduce the apparent price to the consumer by 50, 80, or even 100%. If a patient's insurance pays 50%, the procedure, which costs $300, only costs $150. Consumers will buy many more services at this lower price. Someone's higher income lowers the opportunity costs because they will not have to forgo as many purchases as a trade-off for dental services. The person with the higher income then buys more dental services because their out-of-pocket expense appears smaller. On the other hand, physicians' services are not nearly as sensitive to family income, and lower-income families use physician services more than their wealthy cohorts.

Non-price Considerations Many non-price considerations affect demand for dental services. An individual's tastes, wants, needs, and desires play a role in the individual's demands. Society generates tastes and wants as trends, fads, and fashions. To the extent that these trends affect the core of the business of dentistry or alternative forms of discretionary spending, they will affect the demand for dental services. If, for example, society values preventive health behaviors or esthetics more highly over time, then logically, the demand for related dental services would be expected to increase. The great demand for tooth whitening and other cosmetic services indicates this increase. Consumers also place a value on attributes of the product or service other than the face attributes. These extended features, such as guarantees, convenience, or availability, can also increase demand. If a practitioner stays open for extended hours, this convenience may generate additional demand for their services.

Availability of Substitutes If lower-priced substitutes exist, consumers will migrate to those substitutes as the price of the good increases. Tea is a good substitute for coffee. As the price of coffee increases, more consumers drink tea. When the price of coffee declines, those tea drinkers migrate back to their original drink of coffee. People with diabetes have a more difficult time finding substitutes for insulin. Their dependence makes the demand for insulin almost perfectly inelastic. If the price of insulin increases, they will pay for it because there are no reasonable substitutes. There are no legal substitutes for dentistry. The only people who can legally "sell" dental services are dentists. However, to the extent that dentists compete with each other, other dentists act as substitutes. Dentists who can differentiate themselves from other dentists in the area have few substitutes. Their patients are more reluctant to leave to find substitutes if prices rise. This loyalty may be generated by specialty work or by the interpersonal skill and behaviors of the dentist and their staff members.

General Economic Prosperity Primary industries are those that bring money into a region. This is generally in wages paid for workers or natural resources used. Examples include manufacturing plants, mining and forestry, agriculture, and tourism. Secondary industries, such as computer support and subassembly plants, support the primary people who work in those industries. Tertiary industries provide services for workers in higher-level industries. Grocery stores and dental offices are examples. General economic prosperity affects personal incomes. Personal income, in turn, affects the individual's demand for discretionary services, such as dentistry. If the economy is robust, workers have more money as producers compete for workers, bidding up the price. The workers, in turn, spend their wages at automobile dealerships and shoe stores. Automobile dealers and shoe salespersons have higher incomes and buy more discretionary services, such as dentistry. A dollar often flows through the economy as workers purchase goods and services from neighboring businesses.

Demographics of the Demand for Dental Care Several factors point toward long-term growth in demand for dental services. The increasing educational level of the population and increasing disposable income, caused partly by the increase in two-wage-earner families, leads to higher demand. An increase in third-party dental coverage leads to a lower apparent cost for the service and higher demand. The public has an increased awareness of dental health caused partly by professional efforts and partly by advertising messages for dental care products such as toothpaste. The overall health consciousness of the population is increasing, as evidenced by fitness centers, dietary changes, and a decrease in alcohol consumption. There is an increase in the senior segment of the population who have higher disposable incomes and more teeth at risk for a longer time. Prime users are young adults with above-average incomes living in suburban metropolitan areas. Usage patterns have begun to merge over various demographic groups (e.g. age, sex, income, and census tracts).

Supply of Dental Services

The supply of dental services follows the classic upward-sloping supply curve. However, like the demand side, many social factors affect how the supply curve acts, which are called the determinants of supply.

The Number of Producers Is Limited The dental profession holds a monopoly in the dental care market, including steep barriers to entry (e.g. educational requirements, licensure). The cost of starting dental schools and the pressure from the profession work to hold the number of new practitioners stable in the future. New dental schools and increasing enrollment of existing schools work to increase the number of practitioners. Given an aging population of practitioners, no one is sure what to expect regarding the supply of dental services in the future.

The Productivity of Producers Varies The productivity of individual producers varies tremendously depending on the dentist's age, educational currency, business interests and skills, personal tastes and desires, use of auxiliary personnel, and use of new technology. There is presently a small excess capacity in the system, which is more pronounced in some areas. Many experts expect the excess capacity to decrease over the next several years as more practitioners retire or decrease practice size.

Technological Improvements Changing technologies are increasing how much dentistry can be produced. They are also increasing the number and types of services provided. Changing the types of services provided increases the demand for those services. Changing technology affects the materials that dentists use, making more materials available and also materials that are easier and faster to use, leading to more services being provided. Technological improvements also allow the office to process the paperwork associated with treatment more quickly and efficiently. Computerized, electronic claim processing, for example, frees up receptionist time.

Regulations Regulatory bodies can significantly affect the supply of dental services. Licensing of independent paraprofessionals (such as denturists and hygienists), state regulations regarding delegation of intraoral duties, foreign-trained dentists, and corporate ownership of practices all affect the aggregate supply of dental services. Significant regulatory pressures exist to maintain the existing supply patterns of dentists. Although the government will not pay to increase the number of dental schools, entrepreneurs see a market for developing private dental schools. However, there may be pressure from practitioners and the public to change the laws regarding the delegation of duties, allowing dentists to leverage their time, energy, and knowledge more efficiently.

Demographics of Supply for Dental Services Most dental practitioners in the United States are individual general dentists. The supply of new practitioners is stable and under the general influence of dental practitioners through various accrediting and licensing bodies. The population of dentists is aging, with a large group in the 45–60-year-old cadre. As dentists age, their productivity decreases significantly, and they often continue to practice part-time or reduce their hours as they enter retirement.

ECONOMIC CHARACTERISTICS OF THE DENTAL CARE MARKET

Given the previous discussion, the following can be said regarding the dental care marketplace in the United States.

- The purchase of dental care follows traditional supply-and-demand economics, and dentistry is a private consumption good.

- Not all consumers purchase dental services for the same reasons, at the same prices, or with the same convictions.

- The supply of practitioners does not change abruptly but instead ebbs and flows as conditions change. Significant barriers to entry exist for dentistry, and no one expects this to change significantly soon. The supply of dental practitioners is relatively steady, and demand fluctuates more quickly.

- Demand for dental services is tied closely to disposable income. As such, it varies with general economic conditions, third-party coverage, and alternate forms of spending. Presently, demographic factors indicate increasing demand for dental services across all population groups.

- Increasing demand for services with relatively tight constraints on the supply of services leads to higher service prices and higher income for providers. Recent trends show dental incomes to be steadily rising, both on a current dollar and an inflation-adjusted basis.

MACROECONOMICS: THE BIG PICTURE

Macroeconomics looks at the economy in total. It is not concerned with how the individual consumer, firm, or business acts, except as it contributes to the whole. Individual differences may exist (companies may grow during an economic slowdown). Regional, local, sector, or specific products may not follow the overall national trend. Economic effects ripple through the economy. If a business slows production, its suppliers and the suppliers' suppliers (and all of their employees) also feel the slowdown. So, all parts of an economy are interconnected and interdependent. Dentists depend on a stable economy to give consumers spendable income and employee benefits to help pay for dentists' services. What follows is a primer on macroeconomics and how economic changes affect dental practices.

GROSS DOMESTIC PRODUCT

Gross domestic product (GDP) is a measure of general economic prosperity for a country for a given period. It is the sum of the market value of all goods and services produced. When GDP is increasing, the economy is growing. People then produce more goods and services, and more have jobs and can afford to purchase those goods and services. Money ripples through the economy as it passes from hand to hand. General economic prosperity is increasing.

Conversely, when GDP is decreasing, the production of goods and services slows. Unemployment increases and paychecks lower as businesses lay off workers to keep costs in line with lower production. This general economic slowdown spreads through the economy as fewer people have extra money to spend on goods and services.

Composition of GDP

GDP is composed of four large categories. Consumption by individuals is the most significant single component of GDP, accounting for approximately 68% of the US economy. The confidence consumers have is a primary driver of consumption in the economy. If they believe their jobs are secure and economic prosperity will continue, they buy more goods and services, often borrowing money to finance their purchases. The consumer confidence index (CCI) measures these consumers' attitudes. It is often used as a leading indicator of consumer purchases. Investment in inventory, plant, and equipment (and houses) is the second-largest component of GDP at 18%. When businesses purchase equipment for their factories (or dental practices), they do not consume that equipment. However, they expect it to contribute to the firm's productive capacity for many years. Businesses buy business assets in anticipation that they will need additional products to sell; that is when they believe the economy will improve (or remain strong). When GDP is decreasing, businesses do not invest in new plants and equipment, exacerbating the decline until they believe the economy is ready to improve. Houses are long-term assets that individuals purchase, similar to businesses' equipment and plant purchases. At the federal, state, and local levels, government spending is the third component of GDP, at 18%, which is approximately the same as the investment category. Government spending comes from the taxes that it collects. The federal government may also borrow money to spend more than it brings in through taxes. (This is known as deficit spending.) State and local governments cannot issue money, so by law most must operate in a

| BOX 12.1 | COMPOSITION OF GDP |

GDP = C + I + G + NE

Where:

C = consumption by individuals of durable and non-durable goods and services

I = investment in inventory, plant, equipment, and new homes

G = government (federal, state, and local) spending

NE = Net Exports

balanced budget mode, spending only what they bring in. The final component of GDP is net exports. This is the difference between total exports (all goods and services sold to or in foreign countries) less all imports (foreign goods and services sold in the United States). If the nation imports more goods and services, net exports are negative, decreasing GDP. If the nation exports more than it imports, then the difference raises the GDP of the country (Box 12.1).

Gross national product (GNP) is similar to GDP but does not include net imports. Most economists believe that the inclusion of net imports makes GDP a better indicator of a national economy than GNP, although they commonly report both. Increasing GDP is different from inflation. Inflation is a general increase in the prices of goods and services, and GDP is an increase in the number of goods and services produced. (Real GDP is adjusted to remove the effects of inflation.) So, the economy can experience rising GDP without inflation, inflation without rising GDP, or even deflation (a general decrease in prices) with rising or falling GDP. However, as a rule, inflation increases as GDP rises.

Why GDP Is Important for Dental Practices

Dentistry is primarily a discretionary service. That is to say, people (in total) have the option of purchasing dental services or not. If they have extra discretionary income, they may spend it on elective (and expensive) dental services, keeping dentists busy with high-margin services. When the economy slows (decreasing GDP), then people have less money and are less willing to spend what they have on expensive, elective services. The dental marketplace slows; dentists' services are often less complex, less expensive, and therefore lower-margin items. So, a dentist may end up working harder but making less profit.

THE BUSINESS CYCLE

The business cycle is a way of describing the typical increases and decreases in economic prosperity. It is also

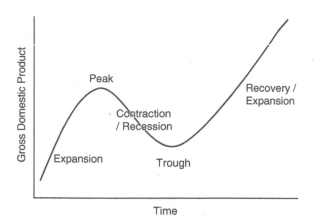

FIGURE 12.4 The business cycle.

used to decide when to purchase certain investments and when many business decisions are appropriate. Although the idealized cycle is shown in Figure 12.4, no cycle perfectly fits the curve. Slight changes occur because of regional economic differences, different responses of the government and the Federal Reserve System (the "Fed"), and different expectations of consumers and business leaders. Given these caveats, the business cycle still provides a valuable framework for understanding economic change.

An entire cycle may take between a few and many years to complete. The United States recently (1992–2000) went through a prolonged period of economic expansion, followed by a period (2001–2005) of slowing GDP growth. Predicting the cycle's future direction is vital to any rational business decision. To help their predictions, economists use a series of indicators that usually lead the actual economy by several months to years.

Expansion Phase

During the expansion phase, GDP increases. Businesses buy more raw goods, parts, and supplies. Employment is high as companies hire more people to keep up with the increasing demand for goods and services. Workers' incomes increase as they demand higher wage rates. Inflation then begins to rise as wealthy workers buy more goods and services at higher and higher prices. Business capacity use nears a high point. Loan demand is strong as families buy houses and companies borrow to finance their expansion plans. The Fed then tightens the money supply to keep inflation in check, causing interest rates to rise. The higher cost of borrowing, in concert with the decreasing profits from higher wages and supply costs, causes GDP growth to slow, forming a peak. Investors bail out of stocks as expected company profits decline, often buying tangible assets or commodities, hoping for stable values in these markets.

Contraction (Recession) Phase

As the economy enters a contraction phase, GDP growth slows or declines. The government increases its spending to offset the private sector's slowdown. It often must finance this spending with deficit spending (borrowing) because tax revenues also fall as profits and incomes decline. Because of lower demand and high inventories generated during the expansion phase, businesses buy fewer parts and supplies, leading to slowdowns in those suppliers' industries. Unemployment rises as businesses lay off idle workers. Even those working are reluctant to spend much money as their confidence in the future economy wanes – business and personal borrowing decline, along with consumer and business purchases. Inflation subsides as consumers become much more selective shoppers. The Fed expands the money supply, lowering interest rates to promote borrowing. Eventually, the economic recession ends as consumers and businesses take advantage of lower interest rates and begin to gear up for the upcoming expansion. (A recession occurs when GDP declines for two consecutive quarters. Depression is a severe and prolonged recession.) The trough formed becomes a new base for the economy's next round of recovery (or expansion).

Recovery Phase

During the economic recovery, consumers begin to spend on goods and services that are at depressed prices. This drives GDP higher. Businesses spend down their previously built-up inventories. Unemployment is high but steadily declining as businesses begin to hire back workers. Business profits recover sharply – demand for credit and borrowing increases. However, the Fed keeps monetary policies steady as inflation and interest rates remain low. Investors begin to buy stocks in anticipation of future profits. As the general economic recovery continues, the economy enters a new phase of expansion, leading to higher levels of GDP.

The Effect the Business Cycle Has on Dental Practices

Dental practices are businesses and are therefore subject to the same economic forces as other, larger businesses. Although the economic climate cannot be controlled, dentists can respond appropriately. Remember, there are overall trends. Some people will buy the finest dentistry even during a profound depression, and others will not, even when the economy is expanding rapidly.

During the expansion phase of the business cycle, more patients are ready and willing to purchase more complex care. Often workers receive better benefits packages (including dental benefits), which further help them to pay for extended dental care. The mature practice can tighten credit and collection policies as demand for services remains strong. (Growing practices do not have as much discretion in their policies and tend to be locked into the convention for the area.) Staff will expect higher raises as alternative employment opportunities bid up the price of labor. Inflation means that a dentist needs to manage fee increases aggressively to keep up with rising costs and general price increases. Before the Fed tightens the money supply, the dentist should lock variable-rate loans into fixed rates, anticipating higher interest rates.

Consumer spending will decline as the economy peaks and enters a contraction phase. Patients generally will be more reluctant to spend large amounts of money on "big-ticket" items, such as reconstructive work. Instead, many will be more cautious, buying essential and less costly services such as routine prophylaxes and fillings. Often even established practitioners find that they need to extend easier credit terms to patients, prolong the duration of treatment, or offer discounts as inducements to have more expensive work completed. Costs remain steady. Staff members want to keep their jobs and are not in a strong bargaining position for wages or benefits packages. Suppliers have inventory to sell down. If a dentist has a ready supply of money as the economy nears a trough, they can find and negotiate significant major equipment bargains. Interest rates begin to fall, lowering the cost of financing a purchase and stimulating the dentist to invest in plant and equipment. Stock investors move away from growth stocks to stable consumer products, such as food, clothing, and cleaning products, that people continue to buy instead of discretionary products.

During the early part of the recovery, if a dentist plans to expand the practice physically, they should set the facility up to be ready for the coming turnaround. As pent-up consumer spending begins to pick up, they need to have the capacity to see the additional patients and do the additional work. This is easy financially because interest rates continue to be low, but competition for suppliers may lead to a wait to complete the work. Once the recovery is in full swing, the practice responds to the cycle's expansion phase.

INFLATION AND DEFLATION

Inflation

Inflation is a general increase in the price of goods and services. Inflation occurs in a healthy economy when "too many dollars chase too few goods," thereby bidding up the prices of those goods. Modest (1–2% per year) inflation is acceptable if GDP growth leads to inflation. Inflation raises the prices of goods and services that are purchased and produced. It also makes borrowing easier because people will pay off future loans with dollars worth less than today's dollar. Suppose prices rise faster than the economy expands (inflation is greater than GDP growth). In that case, economic planners will generally try to cool off inflation while maintaining growth, a tricky proposition at best.

Deflation

Deflation is a decrease in the general price of goods and services. The United States has not experienced a significant period of deflation since the Great Depression in the early 1930s. Although falling prices sound good from a consumer's perspective, several collateral problems arise when prices fall. Businesses do not make as much money because they now sell their goods at lower prices. They have produced them with the expectation of higher margins, so money is lost on each item sold. Businesses then have trouble making debt payments, so investors dump stocks, decreasing the value of individual portfolios and the companies themselves. Layoffs then result, and the economy spirals downward. Deflation is a more significant worry for economic planners than hyperinflation. (Disinflation means inflation but at a decreasing rate, which is different from deflation.)

Two economic indices are often used to gauge inflation. The Consumer Price Index (CPI) is the cost of a representative "market basket" of urban consumer goods (including food, clothing, and energy costs). The federal government has tracked and reported the change in the price of this market basket monthly. (It also have variations of the CPI, such as for healthcare-related costs.) A second index is the Producer Price Index (PPI). This is similar to the CPI but looks at the cost of raw materials and labor for producers. It is conducted and reported similarly to the CPI. Although both are leading indicators (i.e. they predict future economic trends), the idea is that the PPI leads more than the CPI.

The Effect Inflation and Deflation Have on Dental Practices

People cannot control inflation but they can monitor and respond to it. If prices are rising rapidly, dentists should raise fees to keep pace. (If underlying GDP is not growing, dentists may not have much freedom to raise fees because patients will not purchase the same amount of dental services at the higher fees.) Otherwise, the cost of materials and labor will rise, decreasing the dentist's profitability. Lower inflation means that dentists need more modest increases to keep profitability up.

Inflation usually means that the Fed and member banks will raise interest rates. Higher rates mean that people will pay more to the bank and take less home as profit, squeezing the family budget. Dentists may be priced out of the market for borrowing money if rates rise too much. This is especially common with new practitioners with a poor credit risk (because of high existing student loans, low net worth, and low demonstrated income). Dentists who have a fixed-rate loan will pay with inflated dollars (a good thing). If dentists have a variable-rate loan, the interest rate (and therefore payments) will soon rise (a bad thing).

FISCAL AND MONETARY POLICY

The federal government and the Federal Reserve Bank (the US national bank) influence the economy differently. They often work together to affect the economy. However, politicians and bankers may have different opinions of what should be done to stimulate or slow down the economy. They have a set of tools to bring about this change (Box 12.2).

FISCAL POLICY

Fiscal policy is the combined action the federal government uses to help manage the economy. A combination of Congress and the President initiates fiscal policy. Despite

BOX 12.2	**FISCAL AND MONETARY POLICY**	
Issue	Fiscal policy	Monetary policy
Who is responsible	Congress and the President	Federal Reserve Board
Authority	Congress passes legislation; President signs into law	Federal Reserve Board acts independently and implements decisions
Tools available	Changes in tax laws	Change reserve requirements for banks
	Increase or decrease in government spending	Change the discount rate
	Finance deficits through borrowing by issuing new government securities	Conduct open-market operations

political rhetoric, it takes both sides to have any effect. Congress passes legislation (such as tax cuts) and the President signs them into law. The President may propose tax changes (such as decreasing the capital gains tax rate). However, the proposal can never become law if Congress does not pass the enabling legislation. Neither side can act unilaterally, so for either side to blame the other is pure nonsense but makes good political fodder.

The purpose of fiscal policy is threefold, namely to (i) maintain full employment, (ii) keep prices stable, and (iii) continue economic (GDP) growth. Because this is to do with politicians, they will often use these actions to promote social and purely fiscal (financial) goals. For example, Congress decided that helping existing businesses to make their facilities more accessible to disabled individuals was important. So, it passed a law signed by the President that created tax credits for small business owners who spend money remodeling their facilities to make them more accessible (part of the Americans with Disabilities Act). Here, Congress did not intend a change in tax law to stimulate the economy, but rather to meet a socially desirable goal.

The government only has three tools at its disposal in initiating fiscal policy: tax law changes, government spending, and government borrowing. Congress and the President use these tools to keep the economy strong and to get reelected.

Tax Law Changes

Changes in tax law can stimulate expansion or contraction. Any change that leaves more money in the hands of private businesses or the public is considered expansionary. For example, suppose the government increases depreciation deductions for businesses or adds a tax credit for children. In that case, more money will remain in the hands of individuals and businesses for them to spend, thereby boosting the economy. (This also means that less tax revenue is in the hands of the government, and it must either cut its spending or borrow to maintain current expenditures.)

Tax changes are often viewed from the supply-and-demand perspective. A tax cut stimulates demand, moving the demand curve to the right. More people buy more goods and services at higher prices. Depending on the amount of increased demand, this may lead to inflationary pressures.

Tax cuts can also lower business costs, stimulating the supply curve to move upward (an increased quantity at lower prices). Supply-siders believe this stimulates further demand for these lower-priced goods and services. Tax increases move the supply and demand curves in the opposite direction as tax cuts.

Changes in tax law come in many forms. They may be across-the-board rate reductions or changes targeted at particular groups or business sectors. Remember that politicians who want to reward their cronies and get reelected bring tax changes. Issues of tax fairness always enter these decisions. Should changes favor the "fat cats" and businesses (where most of the money is) or be spread across the board? Tax cuts for higher-income individuals often go to savings or investments. Cuts for lower-income individuals are usually spent immediately. If so, who benefits more and less, and is that fair? Political rhetoric on the issue increases with the proximity to elections.

Government Spending

When consumer and business spending is low, such as during a contraction or recession, the government tries to stimulate the economy by spending more. Although the government sector cannot fully compensate for the lack of consumer and business spending, it tries to "prime the pump," hastening economic recovery. Often this spending surpasses revenues from taxes. When this occurs, it must finance the deficit through government borrowing or actions by the Fed. As an economic expansion occurs, the government can reduce its spending, paying down its deficit. This hardly ever occurs because politicians are running this system.

Government Borrowing

When the federal government spends more than it takes in through taxes, it must finance the difference by borrowing money. It does this by issuing Treasury bonds, bills, and notes. (These differ based on the length of maturity). In these, the Treasury borrows a certain amount of money, promising to pay it back in a certain period at a given interest rate. This interest rate (called the "risk-free" rate) is low because the full faith and confidence of the federal government back it. (If the federal government defaults on its loans, the financial markets would be chaotic.) This borrowing increases the nation's total deficit, which must be paid back in the future from tax revenues. (Inflation helps to soften the cost of payback by the government.)

There are several side effects of government borrowing. Issuing federal debt securities causes a general increase in interest rates because lenders are lending money to the federal government. Increases in interest rates lead to decreased borrowing, decreased buying, and therefore decreased economic activity. Borrowers that are riskier than the federal government must pay higher rates to offset the increased risk. This "crowding-out" of businesses in the debt security market leads to a decrease in corporate borrowing and a resulting decrease in economic activity.

MONETARY POLICY

Monetary policy is concerned with the amount of US money that is in circulation. The Federal Reserve system (the US central bank) controls the money supply. Its customers are not consumers like ordinary people but are instead the country's banking system and the federal government.

The Federal Reserve System

The Fed comprises a board of governors, the Federal Open Market Committee (FOMC), and 12 Federal Reserve district banks. The Fed is an independent branch of government; it is not a profit-making institution and must periodically report its actions and plans to Congress. The Fed controls the monetary policy and, therefore, the money supply of the United States. It is not the US Treasury, but it does issue debt securities for the government to finance budget deficits. The Federal Reserve bank issues money (Federal Reserve notes) and makes loans to commercial banks, lending money to US businesses and individuals.

The Federal Reserve system has four functions. It conducts the nation's monetary policy, regulates the banking industry, supervises the financial system and markets, and provides financial services to the US government. The Fed uses three tools to accomplish its functions. It can set the reserve requirements for banks, change the discount rate to banks, and buy (or sell) US government securities on the open market (Box 12.3).

The Federal Reserve's Tools

The Fed requires member depository institutions (banks, savings, and loans) to keep a certain percentage of the money deposited on "reserve." This means that they may not lend that reserved money. The higher the required

BOX 12.3	THE FEDERAL RESERVE'S MONETARY POLICY ACTIONS
Desired effect	**Federal Reserve Board action**
Expansionary (expand the money supply)	Purchase government securities
	Lower reserve requirement
	Lower discount rate
Contractionary (reduce the money supply)	Sell government securities
	Increase reserve requirement
	Raise discount rate

reserve, the less there is to lend out, and the higher the interest rates rise in response. (Supply and demand dictate that more borrowers push the rate on low loans.) The Fed requires banks to reserve 8–14% of transaction (checking) accounts and 0–9% of savings (certificate of deposit [CD] and savings) accounts. Changing this requirement by a few percentage points (within the range) can profoundly affect how much money is available to borrow. The Fed does not change this often, so it is unimportant daily. If the Fed does change the reserve requirement, something big is happening in the economy.

The discount rate is charged to member banks for them to borrow money to issue loans. By changing this discount rate, the Fed encourages (or discourages) banks from lending money, affecting the liquidity in the banking system. The discount rate is for short-term loans only, and long-term interest rates consequently change. Changing the discount rate also affects stock and bond prices because required rates of return change in response to changing interest rates.

The most powerful tool that the Fed uses to accomplish its purpose is open-market operations. The Federal Open Market Committee (FOMC) meets periodically (usually monthly) to assess and change its policy. These meetings are so important that the daily and financial press report them. Open-market operations consist of selling or purchasing government securities (bonds, bills, and notes), which then expand or contract the nation's money supply. If the Fed sells securities, it receives cash, which it removes from the banking system (therefore, there is less to lend or invest), slowing the economy. When the Fed buys securities, it pays cash, which is added to the banking system (therefore there is more to lend or invest), stimulating the economy. Because the Fed prints money, it can never run out.

The Fed has a target (sustained, non-inflationary) for GDP growth. Growth above this target is considered inflationary, so the Fed steps on the "brake," slowing the economy. Below the target, the Fed presses the "accelerator," trying to stimulate the economy. In the past several years the Fed has tried to smooth out the business cycle from a boom-or-bust mode to one of slower growth and "soft landings" by using a gentler foot on both the brake and the accelerator.

Box 12.4 shows the difference in a monthly payment on a $100 000 loan over seven years, based on different interest rates. Over the seven-year loan term, the difference in payments between the lowest rate (3% = $110 964) and

BOX 12.4	EFFECT OF INTEREST RATE ON LOAN PAYMENTS	
Annual interest rate	Monthly payment	Total payments
3%	$1321	$110 964
6%	$1461	$122 712
9%	$1609	$135 148
12%	$1765	$148 283

Assumptions:

Principal = $100 000

Term = 7 years

the top rate (12% = $148 283) is $37 319. This shows how the Fed's decisions on interest rates can affect the cost and affordability of loans to small businesses.

In the real world, the economy is a complex system to manage. Politicians (who control fiscal policy) want prosperity (people employed) just before an election. They want aggressive, expansionary monetary policies. The Fed, on the other hand, wants to keep economic stability. It wants slow, steady (even unspectacular) growth. If the growth is too rapid, the country may face an economic crash. Consumer confidence affects spending and therefore GDP. Politicians, the news media, and world events affect consumer confidence, consumer spending, and the economy. Finally, economic policy is established based on forecasts (such as leading economic indicators). The policy is only as good as the forecasts.

The Effect of the Federal Reserve on Dental Practice

The Fed's actions do not affect a dental practice directly, but their indirect effects make them an essential component of the economic environment. The Fed indirectly sets the interest rate someone pays for a loan, profoundly affecting the growth in GDP and the business cycle.

Interest rates have a dramatic and immediate effect on new dentists. When a dentist borrows money to establish a practice, buy into or buy out an existing practice, or purchase a new home, car, or another consumer good, the prevailing interest rate will determine their monthly payback and, therefore, the amount that they can borrow.

Business Entities

Any business arrangement that is not profitable to the other person will in the end prove unprofitable for you. The bargain that yields mutual satisfaction is the only one that is apt to be repeated.

B.C. Forbes

GOAL

Make students aware of the various business arrangements that are available to dentists. The student should be able to define their own desires regarding participation in such an arrangement.

LEARNING OBJECTIVES

At the completion of the chapter, the student will be able to:

- Understand the various forms (business entities) of dental practices:
  - Proprietorship
  - Partnership
  - Corporation
  - C corporation
  - S corporation
  - Limited liability company.

KEY TERMS

board of directors
business entity
C corporation
corporation
dividends
employee status
joint and severable liability

limited liability company (LLC)
ownership interest
partnership
partnership agreement
pass-through entity
piercing the corporate veil

professional service corporation (PSC)
S corporation
shareholders
sole proprietorship
stock

Business Basics for Dentists, Second Edition. James L. Harrison, David O. Willis, and Charles K. Thieman.
© 2024 John Wiley & Sons, Inc. Published 2024 by John Wiley & Sons, Inc.

Business entities in dentistry can take any of several forms. There is no "right" business arrangement for dentists. Many physical, financial, managerial, and legal considerations will influence their decision. Because each dentist's circumstances are unique, their resolution of these issues will be similarly unique. Understanding the differences between these arrangements will help match a dentist's needs with the type of entity selected. Any business arrangement should maximize factors that are important in someone's situation. A practitioner will work with an accountant, lawyer, and management consultant to decide which business entity is best for their situation.

The business entity that a practice owner chooses has almost no bearing on the practice's day-to-day operations. A dentist still sees patients, hires staff, collects payments, and pays expenses regardless of the type of business.

ENTITY DECISION POINTS

Dentists should consider four main factors when deciding which business entity to use for a practice.

- The tax liability can differ among the various entities. Because each circumstance is unique, some practitioners can take advantage of taxes differences that others cannot.

- Business entities also differ in liability protection. Some entities provide general liability protection (though not professional protection) that others do not. Along with adequate insurance protection and a personal risk tolerance level, the business entity's choice contributes to the office risk management plan. As with taxes, each circumstance is different, so no one business entity is best for all dentists.

- Some entities limit the number of owners, and some require owners to be US citizens.

- Finally, some entities (mainly corporations) require additional administrative burdens in tax forms, meeting minutes, and officer elections. Dentists who are unwilling to put in the extra time and effort to comply with the regulations must choose a different, less burdensome entity.

The owner(s) of the practice must understand and evaluate the advantages and disadvantages of each form of business, given their circumstances. Lawyers, accountants, and management consultants can give valuable advice, but it is up to the practice's owners to decide the form of business the practice should take.

TYPES OF BUSINESS ENTITIES

A general business (such as a hardware store or building contractor) can take any of the five types of general business entities listed in Box 13.1. Each state defines these types of businesses (or entities) in state laws and tax codes, and the federal government also has tax rules regarding the entities. These primary business forms have a unique combination of advantages, disadvantages, ownership, and compensation issues.

There are special rules for health professionals and others who perform professional services for the community (e.g. architects, accountants, and lawyers). These businesses (including dental practices) must take one of the four types of business entities for professionals listed in Box 13.1: sole proprietorship, general partnership, PC, or PLLC. State laws generally require incorporated healthcare providers to use a particular form of corporation. Different states have different names for them (professional corporations, professional service corporations, professional service associations, or professional associations). Each state has a professional association act that governs these entities. Some states require that only practicing providers be shareholders; others allow corporate or non-provider ownership of PCs. Dentists must check with an attorney to be sure of the state's rules on the entity types for a professional business.

SOLE PROPRIETORSHIP

A sole proprietorship is the simplest form of business. It exists any time an individual earns money on their own. In this form of business, the owner is the business. Profits and losses are therefore personal. The person who has

---

BOX 13.1   TYPES OF ENTITIES

Types of general business entities
Sole proprietorship
General partnership
Limited partnership
Corporation
Limited liability company (LLC)

Business entities for professionals
Sole proprietorship
General partnership
Professional service corporation (PC)
Professional limited liability company (PLLC)

day-to-day responsibility for running the business usually owns the business. There are advantages and disadvantages to a sole proprietorship (Box 13.2).

Advantages

Proprietorships are easy and inexpensive to establish. If someone operates a business and does not declare another type of entity, they are, by default, a sole proprietorship. There are no special accounting rules except general Internal Revenue Service (IRS) rules and rules of good accounting practice.

Disadvantages

Because the person is the business in a proprietorship, they are not isolated from the business's legal or financial responsibility and liability. They must sign personally for loans, pledging personal assets as collateral, and they may have to use personal assets to satisfy any debts or judgments against the business.

Ownership

As the name implies, sole proprietors are the business's only (sole) owner (proprietor). If there are two or more owners, the business is not a proprietorship but a partnership (or another form of business).

Compensation

Because a sole proprietor is an owner rather than an employee, they do not pay themselves a salary or a wage. Instead, they take a draw from the assets of the business or practice.

Taxation

A sole proprietorship is not a separate tax entity. The owner reports all profits or losses on their tax return on a federal Schedule C. They must estimate their income tax liability and prepay it quarterly. A sole proprietor must also pay self-employment taxes – the equivalent of Social Security (FICA) and Medicare taxes. From a tax perspective, it does not matter how much someone takes out of the business as a draw, and taxes are paid on how much money (profit) the business makes.

Dental Practice Implications

Proprietorships are the most common form of individual dental practice because they are so easy and inexpensive to set up, and dentists typically protect themselves from liability through adequate insurance.

GENERAL PARTNERSHIP

A partnership is a business entity in which two or more people have a common interest and share ownership, profits, and losses from a business. Although the partnership is a separate legal entity from its owners, it is conceptually like a multiowner proprietorship. If two people join in owning and operating a business, they are a partnership unless they explicitly state (and file papers stating) that they are establishing another business. This arrangement combines each participant's abilities, energies, and financial risks. Partnerships have no limit as to the number of partners (although there must be at least two). From a practical standpoint, large groups often take a corporate structure for reasons discussed in that section. There are advantages and disadvantages to a partnership (Box 13.3).

Advantages

A partnership is perhaps the most versatile method of group dental practice organization. It allows varying degrees of ownership, income distribution, and cost allocation. Compensation, for example, may be based on fixed dollar amounts or percentages of production or collections. Partnerships can make allowances for including new partners or for partners who leave the partnership. A partnership agreement must be prepared for the entity. Start-up costs and technicalities are low. The combined creditworthiness of the partners may make securing loans easier.

Disadvantages

Several significant disadvantages exist to the partnership form of a group practice. First, partners share "joint and severable liability" for partnership debts. That means that each person is personally liable for the debts of the partnership or the acts of the other partners. For example, if one of the partners acting for the partnership buys a piece of property, other partners are responsible for the debt as if they had purchased it themselves. If a partner is guilty of malpractice, the court may require other partners to help pay any judgments not covered by insurance. Another disadvantage is that if an adequately constructed partnership agreement is lacking, ownership in the partnership may be more difficult to transfer if one partner decides to leave. Finally, management of the partnership may be more complicated because each partner has a voice in the decision-making. A well-written partnership agreement that lists the responsibilities, provisions, and requirements of the group members helps to overcome these problems.

Ownership

Partnerships involve more than one owner, but these do not need to be equal owners. One person can provide more of the start-up capital and have more say in the operation of the business. Because partnerships can take so many forms and can even exist on a handshake, dentists should always have a written partnership agreement when entering a partnership. A written partnership agreement clarifies each partner's role and identifies the rights and responsibilities of each partner. The written agreement compels the partners to define their relationship in advance. This exchange of ideas gives partnerships a greater chance of success. Most states have enacted some form of the Uniform Partnership Act that defines the rules of a partnership for that authority. For these reasons, consult an attorney familiar with the law in this area before completing an arrangement.

Compensation

Partners are compensated like proprietors and they draw on the partnership's assets. Partners do not necessarily need to divide income from the business evenly, but whatever the income distribution method decided on, the partnership agreement should state it clearly. For example, dentist partners may decide to divide income according to production levels for the month or may allocate specific payments to specific dentists.

Taxation

The partnership is like a proprietorship from a tax perspective. The IRS does not tax the partnership itself, but the partnership must still determine its profit or loss and file an information tax return. Like a proprietorship, a partner must estimate individual income taxes, prepay them quarterly, and pay self-employment taxes. Once the partnership determines the profit or loss, this is passed through to the individual partners based on their partnership agreement for taxation purposes. For example, if someone has a 50/50 partnership with an income of $10 000, each partner would receive and pay tax on $5000 in compensation. If losses occur, these also apply to the individual partners' tax returns. The partnership files a tax return (Form 1065) with the IRS that states how much income each partner has for the year (Form K-1). The IRS then runs a computer match to ensure each partner has reported their income correctly.

Dental Practice Implications

Partnerships are not common in dentistry. Most practitioners prefer the independence of an individual practice or the protection of a corporation or LLC.

CORPORATIONS

A corporation is the third common business form a dental practice may take. Incorporated dental practices operate similarly to other business corporations. Owners establish corporations under applicable state law. They issue stock or shares in the ownership of the corporation. They may issue one or millions of shares. The number of shares that someone owns is proportional to their ownership interest. People who buy stock buy a share in the assets of the company. If the company's value increases or decreases, each share of stock also changes. If the corporation makes a profit, the board of directors may elect to pay out some (or all) of the profits to the stock owners as dividends. Changing the ownership of a corporation is easy: a person sells shares of stock. There are places where someone can buy or sell shares of publicly traded stock called stock exchanges

BOX 13.4	ADVANTAGES AND DISADVANTAGES OF CORPORATIONS FOR DENTISTS

Advantages
    Limited shareholder liability
    Separate entity for tax purposes

Disadvantages
    Time and cost of set-up
    More paperwork and legal formalities
    Federal and state securities law compliance
    Possible double taxation

(e.g. New York Stock Exchange (NYSE), Nasdaq). No one publicly trades shares of individual dental practices, so the sale occurs between two or more private citizens. (In the real world, dental practice transfers get more complex.) Some of the more extensive networks of dental practices may trade on the public stock exchanges.

A corporation functions as a separate legal entity. It has an unlimited lifetime unless the shareholders dissolve it. It pays tax on its profits. A corporation owns the practice assets and hires staff and dentists. The individual dentists may be the corporation's owners, employees, or both. Those who are employees receive a salary or other compensation that they pay tax on individually. If the dentists are also owners (stockholders) in the corporation, they also pay tax on any profit (earnings) the corporation distributes to its shareholders. There are advantages and disadvantages to corporations (Box 13.4).

Advantages

Corporations provide the primary benefit of liability protection for the owner(s). Liability is of two types: professional liability (malpractice) or general business (slip and fall) liability. Because the corporation is a separate entity, the owners are not *personally* responsible for acts of negligence by other shareholders or employees. Owners can only lose the money they have invested in the corporation. Therefore, they protect their assets in case of a shareholder's professional negligence but not from acts of their negligence. If a corporate shareholder is guilty of professional negligence, someone may sue them both as an individual practitioner (personally) and as an owner of the corporation. The plaintiff may also sue another shareholder but only as an owner of the corporation. They can only recover what the shareholder has invested in the corporation, not their assets.

Corporate practices have less frequent tax audits. Accountants complete most corporate returns; individual dentists complete many Schedule C forms. Some auditors may assume that a Schedule C (proprietorship) return may hide many personal expenses not found in a corporate return. Although this may or may not be true, the result is a lower audit rate for corporations (based on IRS audit statistics).

Disadvantages

Corporations are more costly to set up and require significant paperwork to maintain. The owners of a corporation must be sure to act as a corporation (hold annual meetings, formally elect officers, have minutes, etc.). Otherwise, during a legal action, the courts may rule that if a group has not acted like a corporation, it should not be treated as a corporation and will remove corporate protection. Because a corporation is a separate business entity, a dentist may pay income tax twice, once on the corporation's earnings and again when dividends are paid to the shareholder(s). As an employer, the corporation must also pay FICA, federal, and state unemployment taxes on an employee, including a dentist employee. FICA taxes are like self-employment taxes. Transfer of the shares in case of a dental practice sale can cause tax problems because the stock is neither depreciable nor deductible to the buyer.

Ownership

In corporations, the shareholders are the owners of the corporation. They own the individual shares (or ownership rights) of the corporation. The shareholders elect a board of directors that makes the major management decisions for the corporation. These people serve at the pleasure of the stockholders, and the stockholders can remove them under the articles of incorporation and bylaws. The board elects officers (such as a president) to manage the corporation's day-to-day operations. The officers then hire employees to work for the corporation. Dentist shareholders elect people, usually themselves, to serve on the board of directors. The board then appoints the corporate officers, including the corporation's president. In an individual-incorporated practice, the dentist is usually the sole stockholder, the board chairperson, the corporation president, and the dentist–employee all at the same time. Only "qualified professionals" (dentists) can be shareholders in a PC in some states. Being an owner does not necessarily mean being an equal owner. For example, a dentist may only own 5% of the stock of an incorporated practice and, therefore, only have a minority (5%) say in management decisions.

Compensation

Two forms of compensation exist in a corporation. First, someone earns money for the work they do as an employee of the corporation. This is the more common compensation method and may take the form of a salary, commission, or wage. The corporation withholds FICA, federal income, state income, and any local taxes from the wages, the same as for other corporate employees. This person, therefore, generally does not have to estimate income taxes and file them quarterly as in a partnership or sole proprietorship. In the second form, a shareholder earns money for the ownership of the corporation's stock and is sometimes paid dividends.

Taxation

Corporations take two forms (or "flavors") from a tax perspective: the regular (or "C" corporation) and the pass-through (or "S" corporation). The IRS assumes that a corporation is a C corporation unless the owners elect or declare themselves to be an S corporation. These other forms affect how the IRS taxes the corporation's profits, but do not affect the corporate structure or day-to-day functioning.

Dental Practice Implications

Several good reasons exist for incorporating a dental practice. In group practices, especially high-risk groups, liability shielding is worth the incorporation costs. Suppose a dentist is practicing in a group that does many high-risk procedures (such as surgeries and implants). In that case, the corporation shields its assets from the professional negligence of other providers in the corporation. Practice transfers become easy in corporate practices, especially in large groups in which owner–dentists may enter or leave the practice frequently. Special ownership rules (such as no foreign owners) apply to S corporations.

Types of Corporations

PCs may take one of two types; the only difference between them is how the owners elect to be taxed.

C Corporations A C corporation has many advantages and disadvantages (Box 13.5). If the C corporation chooses to pay dividends, it pays them from after-tax profits. Dividends are taxable income for the individual who receives them. Therefore, dividends are taxed twice, once at the corporate level and again at the individual level. PCs generally must pay a flat (non-graduated) rate (currently 21%) on all profits retained in the corporation. Prudence dictates that PCs pay out all their annual profits as bonuses to the

---

| BOX 13.5 | ADVANTAGES AND DISADVANTAGES OF A C CORPORATION FOR DENTISTS |

Advantages

Maintains liability protection

Disadvantages

Possible double taxation of corporate profits

Must follow corporate rules and regulations

Losses are not passed through to the shareholder

---

providers and owners, showing no corporate profit for the year (and therefore declaring no dividends).

In the C corporation, the dentist files their wages and earnings on their personal Form 1040 based on the W-2 provided by the corporation. Employees of the corporation are eligible for many employee benefits offered by the corporation that pass-through owners are not. These may include cafeteria plans, dependent care allowances, or specific insurance. Depending on a person's needs, this may be an important decision factor.

Most of the disadvantages of the C corporation can be overcome with proper planning. A double tax on annual corporate earnings can usually be avoided by reducing the corporation's profit to zero. Paying end-of-year bonuses to owner–dentists and making retirement plan contributions usually help to accomplish this. However, it is essential to note that tax preference items (such as losses or specific tax credits) do not pass through to the owner(s) so they do not reduce the tax liability.

S Corporations S corporations are formed under applicable state law and are subject to Subchapter "S" of the Internal Revenue Code. That is to say, the corporation follows all the regular corporation rules about incorporation, shareholders, and liability protection. However, the owners have elected to be treated like a partnership for tax purposes, so the S corporation becomes a hybrid tax entity. There are many advantages and disadvantages to S corporations (Box 13.6). These corporations do not pay a tax on their corporate profits. Instead, the corporation's income, expense, and credit items pass through to the shareholders. The shareholder(s) then report the flow-through items on their income tax returns. This election allows business expenses, such as depreciation, tax credits, and losses, to flow through to the owners, just like a partnership.

Like a partnership, the S corporation files an informational return for the IRS (Form 1120S). The individual

BOX 13.6

ADVANTAGES AND DISADVANTAGES OF AN S CORPORATION FOR DENTISTS

Advantages
Maintains liability protection
Profits are passed through without double taxation
Losses are passed through to the shareholder

Disadvantages
Must follow corporate rules and regulations
Profits are taxable based on ownership percentage

owners receive a Form K-1 from the corporation that describes how much income they should declare on their taxes. Owners (shareholders) may also receive a distribution of profits of the corporation. Unlike the C corporation, the S corporation does not pay taxes but passes tax items to the owners. So, the S corporation does not pay a tax profit. When the individual receives a dividend (distribution) payment, this payment is unearned because they earned it through investment, not sweat and toil. Because this income is unearned, the individual does not pay Social Security or Medicare taxes on the dividend payment as they would have on earned income. The IRS rules require that the corporation compensate owner–dentists for the dentistry they do at a "reasonable" level. (Owners cannot claim all income as dividends.) However, some tax savings may be available for S corporation owners who use this strategy.

Form 2553 must be completed and filed with the IRS to elect S Corporation status. As a rule, this election is especially valuable for start-up corporations with many deductions and a loss for tax purposes. This loss can offset the "ordinary" income of the shareholders up to the amount they have invested in the corporation ("basis"). (The accounting for this is complex, so the dentist should check with an accountant.) Tax credits flow through to the owners' returns as well. The IRS taxes all the income of S corporations, whether from earnings or the sale of assets, directly to the shareholders in proportion to their interest, even if the income is not distributed. This can lead to "phantom income" that shareholders must pay income tax on.

Piercing the Corporate Veil

Piercing the corporate veil is a legal doctrine that allows the courts, when justified, to ignore the corporate structure. The courts then hold the corporation's shareholders personally responsible for the actions carried out in the corporation's name. States differ somewhat in their interpretation of this doctrine. Generally, piercing the corporate veil can happen when someone does one or more of the following:

- Undercapitalizes the corporation.

- Fails to deposit taxes withheld from employees' wages.

- Fails to observe the formalities of corporate existence, such as annual meetings and minutes.

- Intentionally does something fraudulent, illegal, or reckless that causes harm to the company or someone else.

To protect a professional corporation from being "pierced," dentists should practice good preventive business practices. They should maintain adequate insurance and corporate assets and follow all corporate formalities. Shareholder and director meetings should be held as required, and directors and officers should be elected as called for in the charter. Dentists should keep accurate and timely minutes of all corporate meetings, noting all personnel issues, such as changing salaries or benefits, in the corporate minutes. Each state views this differently, so the dentist should check with a lawyer and an accountant for local preventive business practices.

LIMITED LIABILITY COMPANY

LLCs are a form of business organization that possibly combines the best aspects of the corporate entity (i.e. limited liability) and the partnership entity (i.e. pass-through tax flow). LLCs are becoming common in the dental practice world. Like the corporate form, professional practices are generally PLLCs, subject to those state laws.

Advantages

LLCs are flexible. One of many (even an unlimited number of) owners may be known as a member. It is a separate legal entity from its members. LLCs are easy to establish. Like a corporate entity, the LLC has an unlimited life unless dissolved, and LLC members have limited personal liability. Members set the level of these requirements through the LLC's operating agreement. They can run the business themselves or elect or appoint one (or more) of the members to operate the business. The members may elect the tax status of the LLC (Box 13.7).

Disadvantages

There are a few disadvantages to the LLC form of business. An LLC's operating and legal documents can be very confusing and difficult to understand. Also, some states have a nominal annual fee for LLCs.

<table>
<tr><td>

BOX 13.7

</td><td>

ADVANTAGES AND DISADVANTAGES OF LIMITED LIABILITY COMPANIES FOR DENTISTS

</td></tr>
</table>

Advantages
    Maintains liability protection
    Ability to choose a tax status

Disadvantages
    Legal documents required are confusing

Ownership

The owners of the LLC are the "members." There may be one or many members. Each may own equal or different shares in the LLC. The operating agreement, like a partnership agreement or corporate bylaws, defines how the LLC operates. The members may operate the LLC or have a manager to manage the entity.

Compensation

Members receive compensation according to the LLC's operating agreement, which leads to great flexibility in compensation methods.

Taxation

Taxation for LLCs is flexible, and the members elect how they want the LLC to be taxed.

Single-member LLCs, by default, are treated as sole proprietors for income tax purposes. In this form they are considered a "disregarded entity," so the individual does not have to file a separate LLC return, only a personal federal Schedule C. The member may elect to be treated as a corporation (either C or S corporation) and file appropriate tax forms and information.

Multimember LLCs, by default, are treated as general partnerships for income tax purposes and must file informational returns similar to a partnership. The members may elect the LLC to be taxed as a corporation (either C or S corporation) and file appropriate tax forms and information.

WHEN TO USE THE VARIOUS ENTITIES

There are common instances when dentists use each of the various business entities for their practice formation, depending on the characteristics that suit their circumstances (Box 13.8).

PROPRIETORSHIP

Proprietorships are the simplest form of business, so they are often used for start-up practices. Many established individual practitioners who do not use tax planning strategies (such as renting space or equipment from themselves) use this simple form of business for their entire professional careers.

PARTNERSHIP

Partnerships are not joint in dentistry because of shared liability. They are often seen in family-limited partnerships that lease space or equipment to the practice. These are frequently set up to have different ownership and management rights (limited partnership) in the family situation. Limited partnerships in real estate ventures, where one partner (the general partner) has the expertise that the contributing (limited) partners do not, are also frequently seen.

C CORPORATION

A C corporation is the only entity not considered a "pass-through" entity. They are sometimes used for group practices to shield the owners from liability, but the tax advantages of the S corporation or LLC often make them today's preferred choice.

S CORPORATION

Practices can enjoy the flow-through of start-up deductions and losses while keeping the liability protection of the corporate entity. High netting practices can distribute some profit, reducing Social Security and Medicare taxes.

Limited Liability Company

LLCs are becoming very common both in dental practice and in practice-related entities. Rules for LLCs vary by

BOX 13.8	CHARACTERISTICS OF DIFFERENT BUSINESS ENTITIES

Characteristic	Sole proprietor	General partnership	C corporation	S corporation	Limited liability company
Separate entity?	No	Yes	Yes	Yes	Yes
Pass-through?	Yes	Yes	No	Yes	If elected
Number of owners	One	Two or more	Unlimited	Limited to 75; limited foreign ownership	Unlimited
What a person owns	Assets	Partnership interest	Shares of stock	Shares of stock	Membership interest
Required documentation	None	Should have a partnership agreement (not required)	Articles of incorporation, bylaws, minutes of the annual meeting, employment agreements	Articles of incorporation, bylaws, minutes of the annual meeting, employment agreements	Operating agreement
Personal liability of owners	Unlimited	Unlimited, joint, and severable	Limited, except for an individual's professional errors	Limited, except for an individual's professional errors	Limited, except for an individual's professional errors
Management	Owner	Managed by partners	Board of directors and officers of the corporation	Board of directors and officers of the corporation	Managers or members, by agreement
Taxation level	Individual reports on Schedule C	Individual reports share of income/expenses (Form K-1); partnership tax return (Form 1065)	Individual earnings taxed as wages/salaries and possibly dividends (Form W-2, 1099-Div); corporate income tax on corporate profits (Form 1120)	Individual reports share of income/expenses (Form K-1); corporate tax return (Form 1120-S)	Single owner: withhold or estimate depending on election Multiowner: tax return depending on election
Individual taxes	Quarterly estimates	Quarterly estimates	Corporation withholds taxes as an employee	Corporation withholds taxes as an employee, quarterly estimates on distributions	Depends on election

state, so the value of setting one up may change depending on specific state rules. Generally, they are easy to establish, and they hold the limited general liability of the corporate form without many administrative requirements. They are a separate business entity, so dentists may set up both the practice and a real estate or leasing company as LLCs so they can do business with the separate entity.

An LLC has the benefit of limited liability, similar to a corporate entity, and provides the flexibility to choose the desired tax status.

The Legal Environment of the Dental Practice

CHAPTER 14

What do I care about the law? Hain't I got the power?

Cornelius Vanderbilt

GOAL

The aim of this chapter is to familiarize students with the common legal issues faced by dental practitioners.

LEARNING OBJECTIVES

At the completion of this chapter, the student will be able to:

- Describe the sources of laws.

- Describe the common methods of resolving legal disputes.

- Define criminal law and give examples of both felonies and misdemeanors.

- Describe the principal elements of contracts.

- Describe the common types of contracts seen in dental practices.

- Define torts and give examples of intentional torts.

- Differentiate between negligence and liability.

- Describe the common labor laws and describe how they affect dental practice.

- Describe the common consumer protection laws and describe how they affect dental practice.

- Describe elements commonly found in state dental practice acts.

KEY TERMS

absolute or strict liability
administrative regulation
Americans with Disabilities Act
antitrust laws
arbitration
attractive nuisance
bankruptcy

breach of contract
capacity of the parties
Chapter 13
Chapter 7
child labor laws
common law
comparative negligence

consumer protection
contracts
contributory negligence
court precedent
creditors
criminal law
debtor protection laws

Business Basics for Dentists, Second Edition. James L. Harrison, David O. Willis, and Charles K. Thieman.
© 2024 John Wiley & Sons, Inc. Published 2024 by John Wiley & Sons, Inc.

Employee Retirement Income Security Act (ERISA)
employment at will
Equal Employment Opportunity Commission (EEOC)
exempt employees
Fair Credit Billing Act
Fair Credit Reporting Act
Fair Debt Collection
Fair Labor Standards Act (FLSA)
Fair Trade Commission (FTC)
Federal Unemployment Tax Act (FUTA)
felonies
intentional torts
lawyer's inquiry

legality of purpose
legislative mandates
legislatively enacted statutes
liability
litigation
mediation
minimum wage laws
misdemeanors
negligence
Occupational and Safety Health Administration (OSHA)
overtime laws
plaintiff
Practices Act
principal–agent relationship
punitive damages

respondeat superior
secured creditors
Social Security
Stark Law
state Dental Practice Acts
State Unemployment Tax Act (SUTA)
strict liability
torts
Truth-In-Lending Act
unemployment compensation Insurance
unjust (or unfair) dismissal
vicarious liability
workers' compensation system

This chapter gives the new dentist an overview of common legal issues that affect dental practices. It is intended only as an introduction. Any time a dentist faces legal issues they should gain competent legal advice, preferably from a lawyer who is knowledgeable about the specific concern. Laws exist for many aspects of people's daily lives, from operating motor vehicles to divorce. This chapter concerns laws as they relate to the small business owner. Dental malpractice law specifically will be covered in another chapter.

THE SOURCE OF LAWS

Governments make laws to protect citizens or to help settle disputes between them. The US Constitution is the "supreme law of the land." Along with state constitutions, it sets the framework for how governments are formed and how they exercise their powers.

The method most people think of in forming laws is a legislatively enacted statute. In this type of law, a legislative body (either local, state, or national) passes a statute or law for the jurisdiction they cover. There are often additional hurdles to pass before the statute carries the true force of law (e.g. executive branch endorsement), but the basic form of the law originates in the legislative branch. Legislatures often pass legislative mandates, which arc not laws but carry the same force as a law. For example, by law employers must carry unemployment and workers' compensation insurance on all of their full-time employees. This mandate results in an added expense to the employer, equivalent to a tax on employees. Although the employer does not pay the government directly through a tax, the mandate has the equivalent force of law as if they did.

Laws may also be enacted by administrative regulation. Legislatures may establish agency boards and commissions to oversee and enforce particular legislation. For example, Congress has not written specific workplace rules and regulations but instead established the Occupational Safety and Health Administration (OSHA). Congress then charged that organization with developing and implementing rules and regulations to guide workplace safety. These regulations carry the same force and effect as a legislative statute.

The final way laws are formed is through the court system or court precedent. Legislatures cannot pass laws to cover every possible circumstance. The courts may judge the legality of a certain action or who should prevail in a certain circumstance. Future courts may then use that initial ruling as a precedent and apply that ruling as a basis for making a new ruling. The gradual accumulation of these rulings and precedents becomes part of the common law of the land.

RESOLVING DISPUTES

Often people have differing opinions concerning how to apply the law in a particular case. This may result from different views of facts or circumstances or varying notions of guilt or innocence, right or wrong. Nevertheless, the dispute must be resolved. Two common methods exist for resolving disputes: litigation and some form of alternative dispute resolution (ADR). Litigation occurs when one person (or government) takes another person to trial in a court of law. The person who initiates the proceeding (sues or takes the other to court) is the *plaintiff*; the person they take to court to defend against the suit is the *defendant*. The trial may be decided by a trial judge or jury, depending on the type of dispute and the desires of the participants. Many contracts may call for ADR through mediation or arbitration to avoid the cost and time involved in trials. Mediation and arbitration happen when both sides agree to present their case to a knowledgeable third party. In mediation, the mediator tries to resolve the problem through discussions and assisted negotiation. Mediation is a voluntary process: either side may still take the other to court if they are not satisfied with the results. In arbitration, the arbitrator makes a decision that is binding: the decision of the arbitrator is final.

CRIMINAL LAW

Criminal law is concerned with wrongs against society. These wrongs may be violent acts, deceit, concealment, or wrongful use of force. They are prosecuted by an agent of the government, such as the district attorney (DA), on behalf of the state, not the victim. Criminal law is divided into felonies and misdemeanors. This classification is based on the severity of the punishment. Felonies, the more serious crimes, are punishable by death, fine, and imprisonment for more than one year. Misdemeanors, the less serious crimes, are punishable by fines and jail sentences of less than one year. Some lawyers add the classification of petty offenses, for minor violations of traffic ordinances, building codes, or other municipal ordinances. Punishment for criminal conduct is imposed for two reasons: to punish the guilty person and to deter others from committing similar crimes. Box 14.1 gives some common examples of crimes.

CIVIL LAW

Civil law concerns rights, duties, and wrongs against individuals rather than against society. If someone wrongs a person, they are entitled to a "day in court." Civil law defines the legal relationship between individuals in three general areas: contracts, torts, and property. This chapter discusses the first two, which contain the bulk of issues important for practicing dentists.

CONTRACTS

A contract is a legally enforceable agreement involving the mutual promises of two or more parties. Most states require that some contracts (e.g. real estate contracts) be in writing to be enforceable. As a rule, all contracts *should* be in writing to record the true understanding among or between the parties. People hear what they want to hear and understand what they want to believe. Their perception of an agreement may be entirely different from someone else's. Oral or verbal contracts are usually enforceable. The problem is to define what either party truly said. Written contracts avoid this problem. A contract does not need to be written by a lawyer to be legally binding, but a person should be careful if they try to negotiate and enter a contract without competent legal advice. They can be bound to a bad contract as easily as a good one.

A contract states the rights and responsibilities of the parties. It has five principal elements:

- **Offer**
  An offer is a specific promise to do something in exchange for the other party doing something in return. For example, the buyer will promise to pay the seller $300 000 for the assets of the seller's dental practice if the seller promises to sell them to the buyer.

- **Acceptance**
  The acceptance says that there is an agreement to the terms and conditions of the offer. In the preceding example, the seller agrees to sell the buyer the seller's practice assets according to the terms of the buyer's offer.

- **Consideration**
  Consideration is the value exchanged between the parties to perform their mutual promises. For example, the buyer and seller exchange $300 000 as consideration (or value) for the assets.

BOX 14.1	COMMON CRIMINAL ACTS

Felonies	Misdemeanors
Assault	Battery
Arson	Gambling
Bribery	Petty larceny
Burglary	Littering
Embezzlement	Prostitution
Forgery	Public disturbance
Grand larceny	Simple assault
Kidnapping	Traffic violations
Manslaughter	Trespass
Murder	
Price-fixing	
Rape	
Robbery	

- **Capacity of the parties**

  All parties must have the mental and legal capacity to enter into a contract. Someone who is under age or mentally impaired cannot enter contracts without their guardian's consent.

- **Legality of purpose**

  A contract must have a legal purpose to be enforceable. For example, an employment contract made with an unlicensed person in a regulated profession (dentistry) would be void because one person cannot legally employ another with no license.

Some contracts may be assigned, meaning one party has the right to transfer the promise to a third party not part of the original agreement. For example, a person might assign the lease for office space to another person. Most personal contracts cannot be assigned.

Common contracts in dental practice include the following:

- Office lease

- Employment (associate) agreement

- Insurance (managed care) plan participation contracts

- Promissory note

- Partnership agreement

- Buy–sell agreement

- Bill of sale

- Contract for practice purchase.

As stated previously, a contract is a promise by two or more parties to do something. If one party fails to fulfill the contractual obligations, a breach of the contract has occurred. The non-breaching party can attempt to receive monetary damages to compensate for their loss because the contract was not fulfilled. When someone breaches a contract, there are four common alternatives for reaching a remedy: negotiation, arbitration, mediation, or litigation. Some contracts state how any disputes will be handled.

TORTS

A *tort* is a civil wrong, other than a breach of a contract, committed against a person or their property for which the law gives the right to recover damages. Torts differ from crimes, which are wrongs against society (Box 14.2). Some acts, such as assault, may be both a wrong against a person (a tort) and a wrong against society (a crime). Intentional

BOX 14.2	COMMON TORTS
Assault	Placing another in fear for their physical safety
Battery	Illegal touching of another person
Libel	Written defamation of another to ridicule their character
Slander	Verbal defamation of another to ridicule their character
False arrest	Unjustified confinement of a non-consenting person
Trespass	Entering another's property without consent or refusing to leave

torts involve deliberate actions that cause injury. Unintentional torts are not deliberate.

Negligence is a tort that involves an injury that results from the failure to use "reasonable care." Negligence is the most commonly discussed tort in dentistry. The four elements needed to prove negligence are given here. (Professional negligence is a special type of negligence discussed later in the chapter.) One critical element of this tort is duty. Without a duty (or obligation or relationship) to another person, one does not owe that person reasonable care. The duty arises from a person's conduct or activity.

Someone who is doing something has a duty to use reasonable care so as not to injure others. Whether a person is driving a car or practicing dentistry, they have a duty not to injure others through unreasonable conduct. Usually, people do not have a duty to avoid injury by non-conduct. A member of the public has no obligation to warn someone else of a possible problem, even if they have seen the problem. (There may be a moral call to warn the other but no legal requirement.) A sunbather has no legal obligation to warn swimmers of a shark in the area. However, the situation changes if there is a special relationship between the parties. A business that rents surfboards has a special relationship with the renter and probably does have a legal responsibility to warn of sharks in the area. The business is potentially liable if it negligently rents the board without proper warning. Consequently, many professional office buildings are justifiably concerned with security and other protection measures.

Negligence is the failure to behave as a reasonable and prudent person in a similar situation would behave (Box 14.3). A person has a duty not only to recognize a

---

| **BOX 14.3** | **ELEMENTS OF NEGLIGENCE** |

- The existence of a duty of care owed by one person to another.
- Unreasonable care that breaches the duty.
- The defendant's behavior caused the plaintiff's injury.
- There was an actual injury.

---

potential problem, but also to do something to prevent the problem (a duty to act). This is not an absolute differentiation. Instead, the individual's actions (or inactions) must be compared to a norm that changes over time and for which different people may have different values. For example, assume a person has a dental office in a northern state with steps leading to the front door. If it snows, most people would say that a reasonable and prudent person would sweep the snow from the steps and apply salt to melt any remaining ice to prevent people from slipping and injuring themselves. If the dentist fails to sweep the snow, they have probably not acted as a reasonable and prudent person would have acted in a similar situation. If a patient or anyone else who has a reason for being there slips on the ice or snow and gets injured, they would probably sue the dentist for damages (and win), claiming that the dentist was negligent in not sweeping the snow and ice from the steps. This example is obvious. The problem comes when juries are asked to decide on cases in which it is not clear whether or not a prudent person would have recognized a danger in a similar circumstance and acted to prevent the accident. Lightning strikes a golfer. Should the golf course superintendent have warned the golfers (by sirens or other devices) that there is lightning in the area and to take cover, or should the golfers have known, without warning, to take cover during a thunderstorm? A doting elderly patient trips on the door threshold while entering a dental office and sustains injuries. Was the threshold loose or in another way hazardous or a potential problem? If so, would a reasonable and prudent person have previously fixed the threshold? Did the person's impaired condition contribute to the accident? Obviously, juries need to make judgments concerning both the degree of hazard presented by a problem and what is a reasonable and prudent response to a potentially hazardous situation.

There are several instances in which the law further defines negligence. Contributory negligence says that the failure to use reasonable care by the plaintiff (or injured party) in a negligence suit contributed to the

injury. In the past, cases in which the plaintiff's own actions contributed to the injury "in any degree, however slight," were dismissed. The trend today, however, is to move from this strict interpretation toward one that compares how much of the fault is the plaintiff's and how much is the defendant's. Juries award damages based on the proportionality found. Comparative negligence then allocates the plaintiff's and defendant's fault (and damages).

Vicarious liability is imputed liability. The negligence of one person makes another liable. A common example is the legal doctrine of *respondeat superior* ("let the master reply"). This doctrine assumes that if an employee is liable for acts committed while performing their job, then the employer (or business owner) is also liable. This results from the principal–agent relationship, which says that the employee is advancing the employer's interests. Once the employee is found negligent, the owner is strictly liable. Warning a staff member to be careful when driving cases to the lab does not prevent the owner from being vicariously liable when the employee runs a red light and has an accident while doing so. Or consider a case in which a hygienist drops an instrument in a patient's eye, causing significant and permanent visual damage to the patient. The hygienist is personally liable for professional negligence. Similarly, the dentist is personally negligent for failing to supervise the hygienist adequately, and the employer is liable to the full extent of its assets under the doctrine of respondeat superior. As a rule, the corporate structure does not protect a person from professional negligence caused by that person or one of their employees. The limited liability purportedly given to shareholders of professional service corporations is illusory. Any liability protection is for business liability only, not professional liability.

Absolute or strict liability assesses negligence without fault. Juries award damages, although there was nothing wrong with what the liable person was doing. This is the one case given in which negligence does not need to exist for there to be a liability. Besides the one in the preceding paragraph, a common example is in workers' compensation cases. The juries assume that the owner is liable, although the employer may not have been negligent. The worker then collects compensation from the business owner's workers' compensation insurance carrier. In these cases, this is the sole remedy: the worker cannot sue the owner for any damages above those compensated by the insurance carrier, even if the owner was negligent or had an unsafe workplace or work practices. This is the trade-off for requiring employers to carry state-approved workers' compensation insurance.

An attractive nuisance is an event or item that might attract and injure someone, especially a child. The owner or occupier of the property must use due care to discover children on the property and then warn them or protect them from injury or death. A swimming pool in a crowded neighborhood will attract many children who live nearby. Besides using reasonable protection methods, such as non-climbable fences, the owner should find children and warn them against the dangers of being around an unsupervised pool. Pets, especially wild animals, can attract children, with dangerous consequences.

Liability is the legal responsibility to make good a loss or damage that has occurred because of a person's negligent actions or inactions. It is important to note that, except in strict liability cases, liability occurs only if negligence is proven. If someone is found negligent and therefore liable, the courts will require that person to compensate the injured party for repairing the injuries suffered. (To indemnify is to make whole or make good for a loss.) These compensatory damages include the following general categories:

- Past and future medical expenses.

- Past and future economic loss, including loss of property and loss of earning power.

- Past and future pain and suffering.

Determining the actual amount awarded for each category creates significant problems and many horror stories from those who love to bash the legal system. Often juries decide by sympathy as much as true financial loss.

Courts and juries may also require punitive damages from liable individuals. They levy these punitive damages to punish the defendant for grossly negligent or "willful and wanton" behavior. A key element of punitive damages is deciding the defendant's motive. If the jury determines that the motives were malicious or intentionally damaging, then punishment is in order. The amount and appropriateness of punitive damages are presently being debated in US courts and Congress.

EMPLOYMENT (LABOR) LAW

Congress has developed many statutes that address the relationship between owners of businesses and their employees. Most of these laws are intended to protect workers from unfair practices by a business. They give few privileges to the owners of businesses.

WORKERS' COMPENSATION ACTS

The workers' compensation system was designed to provide a way to pay workers or their families if the worker is accidentally injured, killed, or contracted an occupational disease because of employment. Two simple tests determine whether an employer must pay workers' compensation:

- Was the injury accidental? Although the laws apply only to accidentally injured workers, proving that employers acted intentionally to injure a worker is difficult. Most states have an exclusive remedy rule, which states that these compensation laws are the only remedy for a worker against an owner for injuries on the job. They may not sue the owner separately for negligence in the workplace.

- Was the injury during employment? The courts have broadly interpreted the meaning of the term "in the course of employment." Generally, if the injury was in any way related to work, it might be a workers' compensation issue. An employee might have a heart attack or chronic fatigue syndrome, claiming the cause was a stressful job. Because the states are involved heavily in administering the workers' compensation system, there is a wide variation in qualifications and awards nationally.

The effect of the Workers' Compensation Act on dental practice is seen when an employee is injured while on the job. These injuries may be physical, such as a cut or an eye injury; they may be infectious, such as contracting hepatitis through an inadvertent needlestick; or they may be mental or emotional. (Each state administers its own workers' compensation system and has different definitions of qualification for these injuries.) The injured worker will generally receive medical care for the injury, compensation for lost wages while recuperating, and often disability payments if the injury causes long-term disability. Because this program is "insurance," a person pays for these benefits indirectly through insurance premiums.

WAGE AND HOUR LAWS

The Fair Labor Standards Act (FLSA) is a federal law that is administered by the states. It defines the rules regarding wages and hours in the workplace. Because each state administers the laws, there is some variation in their interpretation. However, these all have some provisions for the following issues.

The FLSA has significant effects on dental practice through minimum wages, overtime rules, and exempt employee status. Dentists should keep excellent time records for accurate wage determination and to guard against claims by disgruntled present or former employees.

- **Minimum wage laws**

  Minimum wage laws define the minimum hourly rate an employer may pay an employee. Congress periodically changes this base rate. Although technically this applies only to businesses in "interstate commerce," nearly all firms have a customer or supplier in another state and therefore fall under these rules. If Congress increases the minimum wage rate, firms often raise the wage rates of all employees as they try to maintain pay differences among classes of jobs and employees. Many states and municipalities have minimum wage laws that dictate a minimum wage higher than the federal minimum.

- **Overtime laws**

  Overtime laws describe how the employer must treat overtime work. Overtime is considered all work more than 40 hours per week. Note that this is not based on 8 hours per day or 80 hours per two-week pay period, but on a 40-hour workweek. (A few states define overtime as more than 8 hours of work per day.) If an employee works more than 40 hours in a workweek, the law requires the employer to pay the employee's base pay plus a 50% premium (i.e. "time and a half") for all hours worked beyond the basic 40-hour workweek. The employer may not offer or require compensatory time the following week to make up for the overtime worked.

- **Exemption from overtime laws**

  Certain employees may be exempt from overtime laws. They are generally professional or managerial people. Owners do not have to pay these exempt employees overtime, which is why entry-level managers at the local fast-food restaurant may work 60- or 80-hour workweeks. Few dental office employees qualify as "exempt" employees. Associate dentists are professional personnel and therefore exempt. True office managers (who supervise several people and have hiring authority) probably would qualify as exempt employees. Dental assistants, hygienists, and receptionists are not exempt from overtime laws in most states. If the employer pays them a "salary," the employer must still pay overtime if the employee works more than 40 hours a week.

- **Child labor laws**

  Child labor laws define how many hours a child (younger than 18 years of age) can work and the types of jobs they may hold. As a rule, children may not work in any physically demanding or dangerous occupation. The hours for which they may work are also limited. The number of hours allowed is often based on whether or not schools are in session.

UNEMPLOYMENT COMPENSATION

The government requires that employers carry unemployment compensation insurance on all their employees. This joint federal–state program is composed of the Federal Unemployment Tax Act (FUTA) and a State Unemployment Tax Act (SUTA). Although this is technically a tax, from an employer's perspective unemployment compensation behaves more like insurance. The more claims former employees collect on an employer's "account," the higher the premium the employer will be charged.

Unemployment compensation is designed to help people who have lost their job through no fault of their own. They must actively look for another job while they are collecting unemployment compensation, and the government limits the length of time for which a person can collect unemployment. The laws usually disqualify an employee from collecting any unemployment compensation if any of the following three events happen:

- The employee refuses other similar work.

- The employee was discharged for proper cause.

- The employee quit employment voluntarily.

If a former employee files for unemployment compensation listing an employer as a former employer, the employer will receive information regarding the claim. If an employer wants to dispute the claim, they should initially complete the paperwork without delay. A hearing may be held, where the employer, former employee, and a hearing officer sit together. The hearing officer may ask for records (such as timesheets) or other documentation from the employer. After hearing from both sides, the hearing officer makes a decision. Without proper documentation, an employer does not stand a chance of winning. Even with proper documentation, hearing officers often lean toward the side of the former employee. The moral of this story is that an employer should always keep excellent employee records.

OCCUPATIONAL SAFETY AND HEALTH ADMINISTRATION

The federal government requires that employers provide a safe workplace for their employees. The way they enforce this requirement is through OSHA. Congress established OSHA under then-President Richard Nixon. Congress has expanded it from high-risk industries, such as construction and mining, to incorporate nearly all employment situations, including dental offices and other healthcare settings. OSHA works closely with other governmental organizations, such as the Centers for Disease Control and Prevention (CDC), when it establishes regulations that pertain to its particular area of expertise.

OSHA is concerned only with worker safety. It does not have authority over patient safety in the dental office. If a dentist practices as a corporation, the dentist is an employee of the corporation (although also an owner), and then OSHA regulations apply to the dentist in the workplace. If a dentist is a proprietor or a partner owner of a dental practice, OSHA has no regulatory authority over the dentist in the workplace (because they are an owner, not an employee), but the regulations apply to all other office employees regardless of the form of business. However, other regulatory organizations (such as the state board of dentistry) may apply standards (such as the CDC standards) to a healthcare provider.

In the dental office, OSHA is concerned with three general areas:

- Infectious diseases and their spread to workers.

- Hazardous chemicals in the work environment.

- General work conditions, including problems such as fire safety, office ventilation, and ergonomics.

OSHA standards are discussed in more detail in Chapter 28.

AMERICANS WITH DISABILITIES ACT

The Americans with Disabilities Act (known as "the other ADA" in the dental profession) is intended to ensure that disabled people are not discriminated against in the US commercial world. The ADA defines a disability as "a physical or mental impairment that substantially limits one or more major life activities." The law stipulates that disability includes hearing and visual impairments, paraplegia, epilepsy, past drug use, alcoholism, HIV, and AIDS. The law does not define what "major life activities" are. The ADA has the potential to affect dentistry in several ways.

Businesses may not discriminate against customers or patrons based on any disabling conditions. The provisions of this part of the law apply to all places of "public accommodation," which includes dental offices. It is, therefore, illegal to treat any person with a disability differently (from a dental standpoint) than a dentist would treat a non-disabled person. Any new building or major remodeling must be prepared to allow people with disabilities access to the office. If a dentist treats a person with a disability, they must make reasonable accommodations for that person's treatment and ensure that the disabling condition does not compromise the quality of the care provided. If a person with hearing impairment is a patient, a dentist must ensure that the person understands the treatment options and fully consents to the treatment. This may require the use of written notes, sign language, or a professional signer. (Dentists must bear the cost of this unless they have made other provisions with the patient.)

Businesses must also make reasonable accommodations to protect the rights of individuals with disabilities in all aspects of employment. There is no absolute rule about what makes an accommodation reasonable. It depends on the size of the employer, the cost of any changes, and the impact on others. Possible changes may include restructuring jobs, altering the layout of workstations, modifying equipment, or providing special equipment. Employment aspects include the application process, hiring, wages, benefits, and all other aspects of employment.

Presently, dental practices that employ fewer than 15 people are exempt from two federal statutes: Title VII of the Civil Rights Act of 1964 (which prohibits discrimination based on race, religion, etc.) and the ADA (which prohibits discrimination based on disabling conditions). Most individual dental offices are therefore exempt from the federal legal statute. Whether a dentist chooses to abide by the moral imperative of the federal statute is a personal choice, if the dentist has fewer than 15 employees. Be aware, however, that many states and local governments have similar laws that apply to smaller employers. In addition, many lawyers will attempt to hold a business to the standard despite the number of employees. So, the best strategy is to follow the law, even if the dentist does not think that it applies. A job description and open communication (and documentation) should be used during the interview process.

SOCIAL SECURITY

Social Security provides income when a family's earnings are reduced or stopped because of disability, death (survivor protection), or retirement. The government requires an employer to participate in the Social Security system by matching contributions to employees' wages. This is covered in more detail in the Chapter 17.

PENSION PLAN INCENTIVES AND PROTECTION

To participate in most tax-deferred, tax-deductible ("qualified") retirement plans, an employer must include employees in the plan and fund their retirement contribution if eligible. The Employee Retirement Income Security Act (ERISA) has set guidelines for participation and contribution. Because there are so many types of plans and because this area of tax law changes frequently, it is only mentioned here that there are law provisions that affect how a person can structure a retirement plan. Retirement planning is discussed in more depth in Chapter 9.

UNJUST DISMISSAL

In the United States, people generally practice the doctrine of "employment at will," which states that the employer hires the employee at the employer's will, and the employee works at their own will. Either can end the relationship at any time (unless a contract states otherwise). (The converse is the fire-at-will doctrine, which states that the employer may fire an employee "for good cause, for no cause, or even for cause morally wrong" unless prevented by agreements or contracts.) However, the days when an employer can exercise the fire-at-will doctrine and fire an employee without fear of retribution are quickly fading into the history books. Unjust (or unfair) dismissal occurs when an employee is forced to accept employment termination in harsh, unreasonable, or unjust circumstances. Examples of unreasonable firings include firing a person because they are pregnant, because they will soon be vesting in a pension plan, or because of a discriminating factor, such as race, age, or religion. An unfairly dismissed employee may seek reinstatement or compensation from the previous employer through the courts. (Firing issues are dealt with in more detail in Chapter 26.)

An employer might face consequences for firing an employee despite the justness of the firing. The employee may collect unemployment compensation, affecting the employer's unemployment tax rates. The former employee may attempt to retaliate, through either legal or illegal methods. A former employee with a key to the office can easily cause havoc by disrupting utilities, and disturbing materials, records, or computer files. They may cause problems by calling OSHA, the IRS, the Wage and Hour Cabinet, the board of dentistry, or other regulatory agencies claiming that an employer has acted illegally. Although

these organizations all understand employee retaliation, the laws require many of them to investigate all complaints brought to their attention.

There is no single law that regulates the dismissal of employees. But the effect of this concept on the dental office is that an employer should be careful when firing an employee. They should check the date when the employee vests in a pension plan (if any) and be aware of any other potential reason for a former employee to sue (e.g. pregnancy, race, age), claiming *that* was the reason for the dismissal rather than their job performance. If the employee falls into any of these protected groups, the employer should be sure to have excellent documentation before firing. Otherwise, it may appear, on the face of it, that the employer is firing this employee unjustly (because of the discriminating factor). It would be up to the employer to prove this is not so.

DISCRIMINATION AND THE EQUAL EMPLOYMENT OPPORTUNITY COMMISSION

The Equality Employment Opportunity Commission (EEOC) enforces federal laws prohibiting employment discrimination based on an individual's race, religion, sex, gender, national origin, age, or disability. The EEOC coordinates the enforcement of several different laws related to employment discrimination. These include Title VII of the Civil Rights Act of 1964, the Age Discrimination Employment Act of 1967, Title I of the ADA, and the Equal Pay Act (EPA) of 1963.

Overall, these laws prohibit hiring discrimination, workplace harassment, or firing preferences based on any of the listed discriminating factors. (In this sense, sexual harassment in the workplace is a form of unlawful sex discrimination.) In fact, most of these laws apply only to larger employers (15 or more employees). However, as with the Americans with Disabilities Act, many states and municipalities have similar laws that apply to all employers. Just because a law does not apply, this does not absolve anyone of the moral imperative to treat people fairly and equally, no matter their external characteristics.

CONSUMER PROTECTION LAWS

Another body of law concerns the relationship of the business with its consumer and the public as a whole. These can be grouped under the general heading of consumer protection and include debtor protection, antitrust laws, and price-fixing–related laws. Consumer protection is an idea that has really only emerged since the end of the Second World War. Although there were limited consumer

BOX 14.4	CONSUMER PROTECTION LAWS

Law	Duty
Truth-in-Lending Act	Requires lenders to fully disclose all credit terms before a loan is made or an account is opened
Fair Credit Reporting Act	Regulates the consumer credit reporting industry
Fair Debt Collection Practices Act	Prevents debt collection agencies from abusive or deceptive collection practices

protection laws in force before this time, the rise in consumerism accompanied by an increase in the number of consumer protection laws has blossomed as the US consumer has become wealthier (Box 14.4).

The Federal Trade Commission (FTC) was created in 1914 as an independent regulatory body aimed to protect consumers and keep competition free and fair. The FTC enforces competition through the various antitrust laws and enforces consumer protection through trade practice regulations. In fact, these two charges overlap considerably.

DEBTOR PROTECTION LAWS

Fair Credit Reporting Act

Congress designed the Fair Credit Reporting Act to ensure that credit bureaus and clearinghouses keep accurate credit histories. Credit histories are important for consumers because businesses use them to qualify individuals for loans, mortgages, and other forms of credit. They also are often used in insurance ratings and even job decisions. A bad credit history may mean that an individual pays higher interest rates or does not qualify for a loan or credit card. Because a credit bureau posts information given to it by lenders and other creditors, it is unaware if inaccurate and potentially damaging information is placed on someone's credit history. The Fair Credit Reporting Act requires that credit bureaus allow an individual to challenge the completeness and accuracy of the information in their credit file. If the credit reporting agency cannot verify a disputed item, it must delete or correct it. If a reinvestigation does not resolve the dispute, the Fair Credit Reporting Act permits the consumer to file a statement of up to 100 words to explain their side of the story.

In the dental office, the effect of this Act is most noticeable if the employer is a credit bureau member and regularly verifies clients' credit history before extending credit to them. If a practitioner uses a collection agency to help collect overdue accounts, they will find that the agencies will inform the various credit reporting agencies of the patient's poor payment history. This then affects the patient's creditworthiness. Individuals, even dentists, should check their credit history regularly. (The process for that is given in Chapter 7.)

The Truth-in-Lending Act

Congress designed the Truth-in-Lending Act to ensure a meaningful disclosure of credit terms so that consumers can compare various sources and forms of loans. This Act does not limit the charges imposed, but requires that the lender fully show all charges before the completion of the credit. The lender accomplishes this disclosure through the finance charge and the annual percentage rate (APR). The finance charge is the sum of all charges by the debtor (or someone else) to the creditor as a condition of credit extension. These include interest charges, service charges, loan fees, points, credit report fees, and any other charges for extending credit. The law also requires that the lender show the finance charge, expressing it as an APR, and even specifies how this rate should be computed. The finance charges and lending rates must be shown to the borrower on a financing statement, including any delinquency charges, late payment charges, and securities.

In dental practice, this law requires a business owner to make full disclosure any time they plan to charge interest for any unpaid balances. The owner may be subject to civil and criminal penalties for violating this law. It is perfectly within their right to charge interest on unpaid balances. However, if the practice owner does so, they must be sure to abide by the spirit and the letter of the truth-in-lending laws. (Model disclosure forms will help keep a business owner on the fair side of the law.) An owner's confidence in following the law will partly make this decision. The rest is what similar practitioners in a particular community customarily do. If no other dental practitioners charge interest on unpaid balances, from a marketing perspective it becomes problematic for one practitioner to charge interest. Service charges (a fixed amount per month rather than a percentage of the remaining balance) are not interest and, therefore, are not included in this law.

THE FAIR DEBT COLLECTION PRACTICES ACT

Congress designed the Fair Debt Collection Practices Act (FDCPA) to prohibit debt collection agencies from using abusive or deceptive collection techniques (Box 14.5). The Act applies only to agencies and individuals whose primary business is to collect debt for others, unless a person represents themselves to be a debt collector or makes the debtor believe that the person is. Creditor collections (such as a dentist or the dentist's staff collecting on their own accounts) are exempt from the Act. It assumes that most creditors will want to maintain the goodwill and patronage of the patron (or the patient) besides collecting the amount owed. However, many people assume that these collection requirements apply to all collection efforts and will try to hold the individual creditor to the same standards.

The effect of this law on dental practice is twofold. First, a dentist should understand the limitations placed on a debt collection agency's effort to collect money owed to the dentist. If a dentist has conducted "in-house" collection efforts effectively, a collection agency cannot do much more to collect the debt. Secondly, although no one holds a dentist to the FDCPA standard, consumers may hold the dentist to this standard in their minds. Many states also have laws that place creditors (dentists) on the same ground as collection agencies regarding collection practices. So, it is a good idea when a dentist or staff attempts to collect overdue accounts to follow the same rules as collection agencies must follow.

BANKRUPTCY

Bankruptcy is a common and confusing occurrence in modern US society. Bankruptcy laws apply to both consumers and incorporated businesses. The intent of bankruptcy is to give the debtor some protection from creditors to make a fresh start and to treat creditors fairly. This discussion limits itself to individual consumers' bankruptcy, the type that a dentist might encounter if a patient files for bankruptcy.

Bankruptcy proceedings begin upon filing either a voluntary (filed by the debtor) or involuntary (filed by one or more creditors of the debtor) petition to a special bankruptcy court. Two outcomes are possible in bankruptcy proceedings against an individual. This is the individual's decision, not the creditor's. The first option (called Chapter 7) occurs when the individual's non-exempt property is liquidated (sold), and the money realized goes to pay off as many debts as possible. The court then discharges or eliminates all of the debts (paid and unpaid). The second option (called Chapter 13) occurs when the individual's finances are reorganized. The debts will be adjusted, not eliminated. In this latter case, the court will rearrange the amount and repayment schedule of the debts to allow the debtor to pay them off. Most debtors choose to have their debts discharged (wiped off the books) and their property liquidated, rather than seek an adjustment, because they would remain obliged to pay some of the debt. Even when an individual's property is liquidated, federal and state laws allow them to exempt certain portions of their property from the process. This often includes the person's personal house and certain retirement accounts.

The effects of bankruptcy laws on dental practice are minor. (If a dentist declares bankruptcy, the effects are obviously major, and an attorney experienced in bankruptcy law is needed.) When a patient files for bankruptcy and owes a dentist money, they will list the dentist as a creditor. There is a hierarchy or priority for paying debts off from liquidation proceeds. If a patient files for Chapter 13 bankruptcy, general (or unsecured) creditors (like a dentist) are the last group paid, after secured creditors such as business creditors, governments (taxes), estate administrators, and others. The best cure for patient bankruptcy is active prevention. Be sure to qualify patients financially before doing large cases on them.

ANTITRUST LAWS

Antitrust laws began in the United States in the late nineteenth and early twentieth centuries. The purpose of this series of laws is to promote healthy economic competition

BOX 14.5	FAIR DEBT COLLECTION PRACTICES

The collector may *not*:

- Physically threaten the debtor.
- Claim to be an attorney if they are not.
- Use obscenities.
- Telephone before 8:00 a.m. or after 9:00 p.m.
- Telephone repeatedly, in an attempt to annoy.
- Place collect calls to the debtor.
- Threaten with arrest or garnishment, unless a person can legally and intends to do so.
- Use any "unfair or unconscionable means" to collect the debt.
- Continue collection efforts after written notification to stop by the debtor; the sole remedy is to sue.
- Limits contact with third parties.

and all of the benefits supposed to result from that competition. Congress aimed the original laws at large corporations that formed "trusts" or conglomerates to gain monopolistic control over a given industry. Once they gained monopolistic control, they eliminated competition, established common business policies, and controlled territories and price levels to prohibit any new competitors from gaining a start in the market. Consumers paid higher prices and lost control of markets as a result.

Many different laws are collectively known as antitrust laws. They deal with price-fixing, exclusive contracts, mergers, acquisitions, and interlocking directorates. The Federal Trade Commission (FTC) and the Department of Justice ensure a competitive marketplace by enforcing these various laws. The important fact to note in antitrust laws is an attempt by more than one person or firm to influence the marketplace. Nothing prohibits a person from setting any price they choose for fees or participating (or not) in any managed care plan. However, if a dentist gets together with other practitioners and agrees to make similar business decisions to influence the marketplace, there are potential antitrust violations in that scenario. If guilty, fines are large. Guilty or innocent, legal fees are huge. The simple solution is to avoid any group or association activity attempting to influence the marketplace.

Antitrust laws do not affect dentistry often, but the effect can be profound when they do. The following are general categories and examples of possible antitrust violations in dentistry:

- Agreeing with competitors not to participate in a certain reimbursement program is a restraint of trade.

- Forming a trade group with an exclusive contract (such as an Independent Practice Association, IPA) would be a restraint of trade if that group controls the local marketplace.

- When there are price discussions with competitors and parallel pricing decisions result, price-fixing is assumed to have happened.

- Any attempt by organized dentistry to limit participation in or eliminate a third-party payer (such as a managed care plan) is strictly illegal, even if the restriction is based on a professional ethical standard.

STARK LAW AND ANTI-KICKBACK STATUTE

The Stark Law and the Anti-Kickback Statute only apply to dentists who participate in Medicare, Medicaid, TRICARE, or other federally funded plans. The Stark Law prohibits doctors from referring patients to providers of "designated healthcare services" with whom the referring doctor has a financial relationship. An example in the dental field would be referrals between a physician and a dentist for an oral appliance, if the two have a financial relationship. These referrals demand scrutiny to ensure that such referrals would not be prohibited under the Stark Law. Violations of the Stark Law carry significant monetary penalties.

The federal Anti-Kickback Statute provides criminal penalties for any dentist who knowingly and willfully accepts or offers remuneration of any kind with the intent to influence the referral of Medicare or Medicaid services. Illegal remuneration includes, but is not limited to, gifts or below-market rent or lease arrangements. For example, a financial relationship between an orthodontist and the referring dentist could create a kickback issue under the Anti-Kickback Statute.

LAWS REGULATING THE DENTAL PROFESSION

Each state has its own set of laws that regulate the practice of dentistry in that state. They are known as the Dental Practice Act for the particular state. Note that no national law governs the practice of dentistry. Because it is left to each state, each state's laws will be unique. Each state's Dental Practice Act is unique. However, most have many common legal issues for dentists that they discuss. Many consist of a shell of the law, followed by an interpretation by the regulatory agency responsible for interpreting and administering the law. Different states give different amounts of authority in these areas to the representative board.

DEFINITIONS

Most state Dental Practice Acts begin with a series of definitions. What is "practicing dentistry" or "dental hygiene?" What is a dental laboratory, a dental student, or a university? What is the Board of Dentistry, and where does it gain its power? The answers to these questions affect the interpretation of the rest of the law that follows.

BOARD OF DENTISTRY

Often the next section of the law discusses the board of dentistry. It details the source of the board's authority, powers, and duties. A section on membership, qualifications for members, and terms of office follows.

LICENSING FOR DENTISTS AND DENTAL HYGIENISTS

Generally, the Acts have separate sections describing the laws and regulations for licensing dentists and dental hygienists.

Practicing without a License

A person may not practice dentistry without a valid and current license. This section of the Act describes the fines and other punishments levied against someone who breaks this portion of the law. It is intended to protect the public from unlicensed practitioners.

Student Licenses

Students must learn to do dentistry. But they are unlicensed and, therefore, cannot do dentistry. This section of the law grants students the privilege of doing dental procedures. There are strict requirements, such as enrollment in an accredited program, not gaining personal financial benefit from the procedure, and being under the direct supervision of a licensed instructor.

Qualification for License

Each state has qualifications for gaining an initial dental license. There may be reciprocal licensing agreements with other states. Many states accept licenses by credential. This means that if a person has practiced in another state for a certain number of years, this state will review their record and grant a dental license. Generally, the dentist must have a "clean" record and show a history of taking continuing education courses. Reciprocal agreements will allow a dentist in another state to gain licensure in this state if the other state grants the same privilege to dentists from this state. Many states may grant special licenses. These may be for educators, dentists who are working in charitable or public health settings, or residents in postgraduate educational programs. There are often special agreements that they have contracted with these licenses.

Renewal of Dental License

All states have requirements for license renewal once the dentist or hygienist has gained initial licensure. Many states have continuing educational requirements, and all have fees associated with renewal. This section may also detail grounds for refusal of relicensure.

Revocation or Suspension of License

All states have grounds for revoking or suspending a dental license. This Act carries significant financial implications for the dentist, so these sections are usually specific in granting authority to the board. It will usually describe the procedure it will follow and what records (public and private) it will keep. It will describe the method and procedure of appeal as well.

AUXILIARY PERSONNEL

Each state Dental Practice Act declares what a dentist may legally delegate to auxiliaries within the practicing state. Some states allow hygienists to practice independently, but others require general supervision. (This means that a dentist must have seen the patient and have given written orders, but does not have to be physically present while the hygienist does the procedure.) Other states require direct supervision, meaning that the dentist must be physically present when the hygienist (or another auxiliary) works on a patient. Some states allow assistants to function in an expanded role. They often call these auxiliaries expanded duty dental assistants (EDDAs) or expanded function dental auxiliaries (EFDAs). Some states require formal training. Different states allow EDDAs to do different intraoral procedures, from taking intraoral radiographs, rubber cupping a patient's teeth, placing fillings, and constructing temporaries to filling endodontics. Because each state is different, the dentist must carefully review the state Dental Practice Act to learn what procedures auxiliaries are allowed (positive law) or not allowed (negative law) to do.

ANESTHESIA, DEEP SEDATION, AND CONSCIOUS SEDATION

Many states have regulations concerning who can put patients under general anesthesia and deep sedation. They often impose additional education and certification requirements on those dentists who do these procedures. Many states have educational requirements that they must meet before a dentist may use conscious sedation (e.g. nitrous oxide–oxygen analgesia).

COMPLAINT PROCEDURES

If someone has a complaint against a practicing dentist, this section of the Dental Practice Act describes how they should handle the complaint. It will tell if an investigation is allowed or required, what the procedures are, and what the possible outcomes of a hearing are.

SPECIALTIES

All states define who may act, advertise, and promote themselves to be a dental specialist. This section of the Act will also describe the educational and experience qualifications required, the limits of practice for declared specialists, and the examination procedures required for designation.

DENTAL LABORATORIES

Some states set limits on dental laboratories, requiring registration and certification. Dentists may then only use registered and certified dental laboratories. This section of the law describes that process.

WHAT TO DO IF SUED

There are several levels of legal maneuvers that people may call "being sued," including personal inquiries, legal inquiries, and a summons and complaint. Most legal inquiries will relate to patients and a person's role as a dentist. However, other issues, such as general business liability, may trigger legal inquiries. Whatever the legal problem, the most important line of defense is to contact a lawyer as soon as practical.

If the problem involves professional liability, the dentist should also contact their malpractice carrier when they are aware of a potential problem. Besides providing coverage for certain claims made against the dentist, most policies have provisions for paying for all or part of the legal fees involved in defending the suit. The specific carrier and policy determine whether they allow a dentist to choose (or contribute to the choice of) a defense attorney. If the carrier is not notified of a problem in a "timely" manner, this may allow the carrier to refuse coverage for loss or defensive costs. If a person has a question about whether to report a particular issue, they should err on the safe side and inform the carrier. It is in the carrier's interest to ensure that the person does not get hit with a loss.

PERSONAL INQUIRY

A patient may make a personal inquiry, asking to see or copy "their" record. The dentist owns the physical record, but the patient owns the information contained in the record. The Health Insurance Portability and Accountability Act (HIPAA) requires that a dentist provide the patient with a record copy (free of cost to them). Any additional copies may carry a reasonable fee for copying and handling. A dentist should never give up the original record and should only give copies of paper or radiographs. The dentist needs to keep the original in the event of a malpractice suit. The dentist should never make up, alter, or forge paper or computer records.

An obvious question for a dentist (or staff) is to ask the person who requested a copy of their records why they want these. If the patient is dissatisfied, the dentist might satisfy the patient then and defuse a developing problem. If the action is a malpractice action, the dentist should immediately contact their carrier whenever they become aware of a potential malpractice action. If the

issue is as simple as the patient moving and needing to transfer records to a dentist out of town, then there is no problem.

LAWYER'S INQUIRY

A lawyer may request information or a copy of a patient's record. A HIPAA release form should always be included with the request. This is generally a more serious matter than a patient making an inquiry. If a lawyer contacts a dentist, the dentist should find out the information requested and the reason, and then agree to contact the lawyer later. This allows the dentist to gather their thoughts, contact a lawyer, make appropriate copies of the information, and gather other material. Besides contacting a lawyer, a dentist should immediately contact their liability insurance carrier.

SUMMONS AND COMPLAINT

A dentist may be served with a summons and complaint either in person or through the mail. (The summons says that someone has sued, and the accompanying complaint gives the allegations against the person and begins the suit.) Generally, the dentist would only have 20 days to file an "Answer" or formal response to the complaint. Failure to meet this deadline often results in a default judgment against the person who was served. Time is critical in this situation.

Immediately upon receiving a summons, the dentist should contact an attorney. The dentist should never try to answer the complaint because they do not know the law and may cause problems, such as making a procedural error, giving the other side unnecessary information, or unknowingly admitting facts alleged.

The dentist should also begin immediately to collect any documentation related to the issue. (As stressed earlier, the dentist should never make up, alter, or forge paper or computer records.) They should also list anyone who may have information about the lawsuit, although the dentist should not speak to anyone other than an attorney or insurer about the suit. All this information will be useful to an attorney in the defense of a suit.

A lawsuit is never a pleasant experience for anyone involved. The dentist should contact a lawyer and liability carrier early in the process and keep excellent records and notes. The dentist should not tell the opposing lawyer or patient any more than their lawyer says to do, and they should not talk with staff or other people about the suit. By following these guidelines, the dentist will help to ensure that the legal process is as easy as possible.

Financial Statements

In business a reputation for keeping absolutely to the letter and spirit of an agreement, even when it is unfavorable, is the most precious of assets, although it is not entered in the balance sheet.

Lord Chandos

GOAL

This chapter aims to define the common financial statements that are used in dental practice and describes the information that they contain and how dentists use the statements.

LEARNING OBJECTIVES

At the completion of this chapter, the student will be able to:

- Differentiate between the following financial tools:
  - Family budget
  - Business balance sheet
  - Business profit-and-loss (income) statement
  - Cash-flow statement
  - Personal net worth statement
  - Personal cash-flow statement
  - Pro-forma statements.
- Describe how to use each financial statement in dental practice.
- Describe cash flow and its importance to the dental practice.
- Describe working capital and its use in the dental practice.

KEY TERMS

assets
balance sheet
budget
cash-flow statement
financial statement expenses

income statement
liabilities
net worth
operating statement
pro-forma statements

profit-and-loss statement
statement of financial position
variance

Business Basics for Dentists, Second Edition. James L. Harrison, David O. Willis, and Charles K. Thieman.
© 2024 John Wiley & Sons, Inc. Published 2024 by John Wiley & Sons, Inc.

Business has a vocabulary that is as specific and descriptive as any other written or spoken language. Words have meanings in the language of business that business people the world over recognize. The first set of those words are the different types of financial statements.

Financial statements are the way in which businesses commonly express their financial transactions and history. They take the same, standard format, regardless of the type or size of the business. In this way, banks and other financial institutions can easily assess financial health and compare one operation to other, similar organizations. Dentists need to understand how to develop these statements, what each component is, and how to use them. Bankers will probably call a dental practitioner to develop each of these forms if they request a loan for a practice purchase or start-up.

Two forms of financial statements, personal and business, are shown in this chapter. Because most dentists must personally guarantee loans and other practice finance options, bankers generally require a personal financial statement for these guarantees. The proprietor–practitioner is inseparable from the practice, so personal statements are especially appropriate for them. With large or networked practices, bankers may request the business form of these statements because the personal involvement of a dentist is less critical for their success. The format of the forms is similar, though not exactly the same.

The forms discussed are:

- Personal forms:
  - Personal cash-flow statement
  - Personal net worth statement.

- Business forms:
  - Business income statement
  - Business balance sheet
  - Business cash-flow statement

PERSONAL FINANCIAL FORMS

Personal financial forms show the state of someone's personal financial health. If a dentist owns a dental practice, they may find it difficult to separate themselves financially from the businesses. These financial forms will help to examine that difference.

PERSONAL CASH-FLOW STATEMENT

The personal cash-flow statement is a moving picture of someone's personal cash inflows and outflows (Box 15.1). The cash-flow statement examines money flows over a specific period, generally a month or a year. It is often used

| BOX 15.1 | PERSONAL CASH-FLOW STATEMENT |

$$Income - Expenses = Cash - Flow$$

as the basis for developing a budget, which aims to use past income and expenditures to plan for the future.

This statement looks at the sources and uses of personal family money. The exact categories of income and expense will differ depending on the person's situation. If, for example, someone is not married, then a spouse's income is meaningless. If they are divorced, a line for alimony or child support payments might be added to the income or expense section (depending on whether they are paying or receiving these payments).

Expenses are usually grouped by type on the cash-flow statement. Savings and investments are really payments that someone makes to themselves. The payments still represent cash flowing through to the savings or investment vehicle, so they must be accounted for. They then appear on the personal net worth statement, making that statement more positive. Fixed expenses are those that generally cannot be changed over the short term. Someone can buy a smaller home, decreasing the payment in the future, but for the immediate concern they cannot change a home mortgage payment. (Most debt service is a fixed expense.) The person may have some control over expenses such as food (buying hamburgers instead of steak), but they still must spend money on these fixed expenses. Discretionary, or variable, expenses are those that someone consciously chooses to make. They do not *need* to go out to a restaurant for dinner. They can save money by staying in and cooking, so the dining experience is a discretionary financial decision. (There is an obvious personal choice in deciding which of these expenses are discretionary and which are fixed.) The difference between income and expenses tells whether someone lives within their means.

Many people use the personal cash-flow statement as the beginning point for developing a budget for personal financial planning. A budget is a statement of how they have spent money in the past and an estimate of future income and expenses. Budgets are used for planning the financial needs of a family by setting expected goals for income or expense by explaining and evaluating spending patterns. As such, they become a target for day-to-day financial living. Budgets are most frequently used when a family is having a financial problem. They then help set targets for spending and let everyone know why spending is limited in one area or another. A budget can help coordinate savings and improve living standards by identifying areas of waste. Bankers may require that a dentist develops a personal cash-flow statement or family budget when borrowing money to set up or buy out a dental practice. The bank wants to ensure that the person has assessed how much money is needed for family living expenses so that the bank can evaluate whether the business can support all of the cash needs (operating, tax, financial, and personal).

EXAMPLE PERSONAL CASH-FLOW STATEMENT

The sample statement in Box 15.2 shows a personal cash-flow statement for John and Mary Doe for the year given. It shows family income from Mary's practice, John's work, and other sources. The total of each category is in the next column to the right of the last entry for the category. Family expenses for the Does are divided into three categories: savings, fixed, and variable. In the example statement, John and Mary are close to living within their income. They are making substantial deposits into savings, investments, and retirement plans. Most of their discretionary expenses are well under control, allowing a high savings rate.

PERSONAL NET WORTH STATEMENT

The statement of financial position (net worth statement) shows what someone owns (assets) and what they owe (liabilities) at a specific point in time (Box 15.3). The net worth statement is a "snapshot" of the person's financial position at a declared date. It will be different tomorrow as assets change in value and as loans are paid off. In fact, bankers and financial planners like to examine changes in a net worth statement to learn how well someone is doing financially. (Total net worth should be growing.)

The net worth statement should become more positive over time. This shows that someone is accumulating wealth and paying off loans. There are really only two ways for net worth to grow (Box 15.3). A person can increase assets by either saving money or increasing the value of an asset. Or they can decrease liabilities by paying off debt. If they borrow and then use the money to purchase an asset, their net worth remains unchanged. This happens, for example, when someone buys a dental practice. They take on debt but also now own an asset of equal value. Their net worth remains unchanged. As the debt is paid down or the value of the practice increases, their net worth becomes more positive.

It is possible to have a negative net worth. This happens to young professionals who have significant educational debt and few assets. Their total liabilities (educational

BOX 15.2	EXAMPLE PERSONAL CASH-FLOW STATEMENT

Personal cash-flow statement
John and Mary Doe
for the year January 1–December 31, 202X

Income		
Practice income (after taxes)	$99338	
Spouse's income	$67200	
Investment income	$2570	
Other income	$1250	$170358

Expenses			
Savings and investment			
Credit union savings account	$5800		
Stock investments	$4067		
Retirement plan contribution	$10000	$19867	
Fixed expenses			
Home mortgage note payment	$18250		
Practice note payment (practice buy-in)	$28500		
Student loan payment	$12000		
Auto note payment	$4800		
Credit card payments	$800		
Food	$6400		
Medical	$1600		
Insurances	$6500		
Utilities/household	$8000		
Dependent care	$6000		
Taxes	$29000	$121850	
Discretionary (variable) expenses			
Entertainment/dining	$3900		
Clothing/personal care	$5500		
Stewardship/donations	$3000		
Auto expenses	$5200		
Miscellaneous	$6000		
Cash	$5200	$28800	$170517
Cash-flow			(159)

BOX 15.3	NET WORTH STATEMENT EQUATION

Assets – Liabilities = Net Worth

and other debts) are more than the total of what they presently own (assets). Although not an enviable position, this is common.

Bankers generally ask a person to prepare a personal net worth statement when they apply for a loan or borrow money for a business or personal purchase. It is also good practice for the person to prepare one each year to assess their financial status. If someone is a proprietor, they will use a personal net worth statement (because all assets and debts are personal) and include the practice as an asset on the statement. If they own an incorporated business, they may need to develop two statements, one for the practice (a business balance sheet) and the other a personal statement of financial position. Often banks have specific forms that need to be completed. These forms are usually the bank's particular versions of the generic balance sheet.

EXAMPLE PERSONAL NET WORTH STATEMENT

Box 15.4 is a personal net worth statement for John and Mary Doe. These are things that they own as husband and wife. The net worth statement is for the date given. It will be different as the Does' investments change in value or as they pay off loans or buy new assets. Each type (or class) of asset or liability is grouped together. The value of each asset is in the first column, and the sum of the value of the assets in the class is in the second column, next to the last individual asset value. The assets class values are then summed similarly to develop a total of all assets (in the third column).

The first asset class is "Cash" (or items we can quickly convert into cash). Cash is needed for routine, daily purchases and for an emergency. Investments are not considered "near-cash" because someone might lose a large portion of their value if they were forced to sell the investments at the "wrong time." Personal-use assets are not important from a financial planning perspective. For example, most people will not sell their house or car when they retire, so these assets are not used for retirement or investment planning purposes. Business-use assets should generate income at a level that gives a reasonable return on the investment. These assets are often sold at retirement and can become a part of the retirement portfolio. The personal net worth statement shows personal items owned and amounts owed. One of those business assets may be a dental practice. Investments are long-term assets that should generate a reasonable return (over time). They become the backbone of retirement, personal, and business planning efforts.

BOX 15.4	EXAMPLE PERSONAL NET WORTH STATEMENT

Statement of personal financial position
John and Mary Doe
as of December 31, 202X

Assets

Cash/cash equivalents

Checking account	$3050	
Credit union savings	$4000	
Money market account	$7500	
Life insurance cash value	$8000	$22550

Personal use assets

House	$135000	
Automobiles	$28000	
Personal property	$52000	$215000

Business use assets

Dental practice	$467500	$467500

Investments

Stock portfolio	$7800		
Mutual funds	$6500		
Simplified Employee Pension/Individual Retirement Account	$18980	$32280	$738330

Liabilities

Short-term liabilities

Credit card balances	$950	$950

Long-term liabilities

Auto note balance	$4920		
Home mortgage balance	$87900		
Student loans	$175000		
Dental practice	$270300	$537820	$538770

Net worth			$199560

Liabilities are similarly grouped. Short-term liabilities are debts someone owes that are due in one year or less. In Box 15.4, credit card balances are due immediately. This might include signature loans, bridge loans, or other short-term borrowings. Long-term liabilities are debts that will take more than one (or many) years to pay off. The example shows an auto loan, a home mortgage, a student loan, and a practice loan. Each of these long-term liabilities should have a capital (or other large) asset on the list for which the liability is paid. The auto, home, and dental practice notes are each associated with an obvious asset. The one questionable item is the "student loan" entry. The student loan payment purchased a "hidden" asset that does not appear on the net worth statement (a dental degree), but the associated liability must be included. In a sense, people have invested in their human capital when they borrowed money for education. Unfortunately, the Internal Revenue Service (IRS) does not allow this as a depreciable asset for tax purposes.

Box 15.4 shows a total of $738 330 in assets (things that the Does owned) and $538 770 in liabilities (or things that the Does owed). The difference ($199 560) is their net worth. In other words, if they sold everything they owned and paid off all of their debts, they would have (less commissions, sales fees, and taxes) $199 560. As they build their asset base and repay loans, their net worth will become more positive.

HOW THE PERSONAL FINANCIAL STATEMENTS ARE RELATED

The easiest way to understand how personal financial statements are related is to look at the previous examples. On the cash-flow statement, someone earns money through work or investment return. One of two things can be done with that money: spend it and it goes away, or invest it and purchase an asset that the person then owns. Some of the money has to be spent. People need food, utilities, and clothing. Other items may be required by contract or facts. People need to provide daycare for the children so that they both can work. Taxes and student loan payments are required by law or contract. The financial value of these payments evaporates when they are paid. If someone "spends" $1000 in savings however, they now have an additional $1000 as a financial asset on the net worth statement.

Using debt is a little more complex. Assume that someone purchases an automobile. If an automobile is purchased for cash, the net worth statement is unchanged. The person has decreased cash but increased the personal-use asset by an equal amount. As the car ages and decreases in value, the net worth statement declines by an appropriate amount. If the automobile is purchased with debt (borrowing the money for the purchase), the net worth statement will remain unchanged. Payments for the automobile loan are part interest, which goes away to the bank, and part principal, which decreases the loan

liability, improving the net worth statement. However, the asset decreases in value as it ages, canceling out most of the decrease in liability.

BUSINESS FINANCIAL FORMS

Business financial forms describe the financial condition of a business entity. The entity may be a proprietorship, corporation, partnership or limited liability company.

PROFIT-AND-LOSS STATEMENT

The profit-and-loss (P&L) statement is similar to the personal cash-flow statement used for personal financial analysis (Box 15.5). One is personal and one is business related. This statement shows income and expenses and the resulting net income or net loss for a specific period. In business forms, it is commonly called a P&L statement or an operating statement because it shows the results of the business operations over a given period. If the income items that flow in are more than the expense items that flow out, there is a profit. If the outflows are greater, then a loss is registered.

The income statement forms the basis of income taxes. If someone is a sole proprietor, they report taxes on the IRS's Schedule C, which is nothing but a modified P&L statement. Many income statements are arranged according to this Schedule C format (where the expenses occur alphabetically). Others attempt to organize the information better by categorizing expense items for analysis. Both types are given as examples.

Sample Income Statement (Schedule C Format)

Box 15.6 is a P&L statement because the bottom line (literally and figuratively) is the profit or loss from operating the business. The form lists income, then expenses, by category. This format lists those expense items alphabetically because the IRS tax form Schedule C lists them this way. It makes year-end tax accounting easier. The income statement shows depreciation that is not a cash expense but a calculated amount. Loan payments consist of part interest and part principal. The interest

BOX 15.5	PROFIT AND LOSS EQUATION

$$Income - Expenses = Profit(Loss)$$

BOX 15.6 SAMPLE INCOME STATEMENT (SCHEDULE C FORMAT)

Business profit and loss (income) Statement
(Schedule C format)
for the year ending December 31, 202X

Income

Gross collections	$298723	
Returns and allowances	$875	
Net collections		$297848

Expenses

Advertising	$854	
Auto expense	$1928	
Commissions	$0	
Depreciation	$23047	
Employee benefit program	$3640	
Insurance	$1650	
Interest expense	$12487	
Legal and professional	$1790	
Office expense	$3817	
Pension/profit sharing	$3048	
Rent or lease	$12000	
Repairs and maintenance	$270	
Taxes and licenses	$9108	
Meals and travel	$139	
Utilities	$8955	
Wages	$60950	
Other expenses		
Temporary services	$340	
Bank charges	$120	
Office supplies	$1000	
Office cleaning	$3055	
Dental supplies	$17010	
Dental lab	$29754	
Dues and publications	$1050	
Continuing education	$1808	
Postage	$690	$198510
Profit (Loss)		$99338

portion is an expense, but the principal portion is not. Instead, the principal is accounted for through the depreciation of the underlying asset purchased. The statement includes neither a cash infusion from a loan nor a loan principal payment because these are not generated from business operations.

Box 15.6 shows that Dr. Mary Doe collected $298723 in the dental practice last year. She wrote return checks for $875, leaving a net collection of $297848. She recorded a total of $198510 business expenses for the practice. She categorized them as shown. (Chapter 17 gives details about these tax expense categories.) Because income was greater than expenses, Mary showed a profit of $99338 for the calendar year.

Sample Income Statement (Categorized Format)

Box 15.7 shows the same information as in the previous statement (Box 15.6). The difference is that this form collects the information into logical categories. These forms can better analyze the business than a simple alphabetical listing. For example, total staff costs include wages and benefit plans, temporary services, pension plan contributions, and any commissions paid. Although this number seems large, it represents 23% of collections, which is within the normal range for a general dental practice. By grouping similar items, the form shows more easily where expenses occurred.

BUSINESS BALANCE SHEET

The business balance sheet is different from the personal net worth statement because there is no net worth. Instead, the balance sheet lists the owner's equity, which is, in a sense, the net worth of the business. From an accounting perspective, a business is the sum of its liabilities and assets. After liabilities are subtracted from the value of the assets, the remainder is the equity in the business (Box 15.8). Business balance sheets show assets in one section, and liabilities and equity in the other. The two sections must be equal ("balance").

Sample Business Balance Sheet

Dr. Doe's business balance sheet (Box 15.9) shows the practice's financial position as of December 31, 202X. It lists total assets of $467500. Current assets are those that are liquid. That is to say, they are cash or can be quickly and easily converted into cash. Long-term assets are physical equipment and real estate and the intangible asset of goodwill. Liabilities are similarly broken into current and long-term categories. Current liabilities are due immediately or within one year. Long-term liabilities are due in more than a year. They are generally used to buy long-term (capital) assets.

BOX 15.7	SAMPLE INCOME STATEMENT (CATEGORIZED FORMAT)

Business Profit-and-Loss (Income) Statement (Categorized Format) for the year ending December 31, 202X

Income

Gross collections	$298 723	
Returns and allowances	$875	
Net collections		$297 848

Expenses

Staff costs

Commissions	$0	
Employee benefit program	$3 640	
Pension/profit sharing	$3 048	
Wages	$60 950	
Temporary services	$340	$67 978

Office space costs

Depreciation	$23 047	
Rent or lease	$12 000	
Repairs and maintenance	$270	
Utilities	$8 955	
Office cleaning	$3 055	$47 327

Office expenses

Insurance	$1 650	
Office expense	$3 817	
Postage	$690	$5 157

Marketing expenses

Advertising	$854	$854

Bank expenses

Interest expense	$12 487	
Bank charges	$120	$12 607

Variable (production) Expenses

Dental supplies	$17 010	
Dental lab	$29 754	
Office supplies	$1 000	

Professional expenses

Legal and professional	$1 790	
Taxes and licenses	$9 108	$10 898

Owner's expenses

Auto expense	$1 928		
Meals and travel	$139		
Dues and publications	$1 050		
Continuing education	$1 808	$4 925	$198 510

Profit (Loss)		$99 338

BOX 15.8	ASSETS EQUATION

Assets = Liabilities + Equity

BOX 15.9	BUSINESS BALANCE SHEET

Business balance sheet
Dr. Mary Doe, PLLC
December 31, 202X

Assets

Current assets

Cash accounts	$32 000		
Accounts receivable	$53 500		
Inventory (supply)	$6 000		
Prepaid expenses	$2 000	$93 500	

Long-term assets

Equipment	$85 000		
Goodwill	$130 000		
Real estate	$160 000	$375 000	$467 500

Liabilities

Current liabilities

Accounts payable	$15 000	$15 000	

Long-term liabilities

Mortgages	$240 300		
Other debt	$15 000	$255 300	$270 300

Owner's equity			$197 200
Total liabilities and owner's equity			$467 500

BOX 15.10	BUSINESS CASH FLOW

Inflows – Outflows = Change in cash position

BUSINESS CASH-FLOW STATEMENT

The cash-flow statement shows the cash receipts and disbursements for a specific period and the resulting cash balance changes (Box 15.10). It essentially describes the office checkbook.

The cash-flow statement shows cash changes. The P&L statement shows net income.

Box 15.11 gives an example of a cash-flow statement for a start-up practice.

BOX 15.11   SAMPLE CASH-FLOW PROJECTION

Cash-flow projection

	Month 1	Month 2	Month 3	Month 4	Month 5	Month 6	Month 7	Month 8	Month 9	Month 10	Month 11	Month 12	Year #1
Doctor production	$7621	$8764	$10079	$11590	$13329	$15328	$17627	$20271	$23312	$26809	$30830	$35455	$221016
Hygiene production	$1732	$2078	$2494	$2993	$3591	$4310	$5172	$6206	$7447	$8937	$10724	$12869	$68553
Total production	$9353	$10842	$12573	$14583	$16920	$19638	$22799	$26478	$30759	$35746	$41554	$48324	$289569
Total cash receipts	$4676	$7946	$11084	$12855	$14912	$17304	$20086	$23322	$27088	$31473	$36580	$42531	$249859
Dental laboratory	$842	$976	$1132	$1312	$1523	$1767	$2052	$2383	$2768	$3217	$3740	$4349	$26061
Clinical supplies	$561	$651	$754	$875	$1015	$1178	$1368	$1589	$1846	$2145	$2493	$2899	$17374
Office supplies	$187	$217	$251	$292	$338	$393	$456	$530	$615	$715	$831	$966	$5791
Total variable costs	$1590	$1843	$2137	$2479	$2876	$3338	$3876	$4501	$5229	$6077	$7064	$8215	$49227
Staff wages	$5265	$5265	$5265	$5265	$5265	$5265	$5265	$5265	$5265	$5265	$5265	$5265	$63183
Employment taxes	$684	$684	$684	$684	$684	$684	$684	$684	$684	$684	$684	$684	$8214
Total staff costs	$5950	$5950	$5950	$5950	$5950	$5950	$5950	$5950	$5950	$5950	$5950	$5950	$71397
Office rent/lease	$1500	$1500	$1500	$1500	$1500	$1500	$1500	$1500	$1500	$1500	$1500	$1500	$18000
Utilities	$800	$800	$800	$800	$800	$800	$800	$800	$800	$800	$800	$800	$9600
Repairs	$100	$100	$100	$100	$100	$100	$100	$100	$100	$100	$100	$100	
Total office space costs	$2400	$2400	$2400	$2400	$2400	$2400	$2400	$2400	$2400	$2400	$2400	$2400	$28800
Office expenses	$317	$317	$317	$317	$317	$317	$317	$317	$317	$317	$317	$317	$3800
Insurance, business	$416	$416	$416	$416	$416	$416	$416	$416	$416	$416	$416	$416	$4992
Total office costs	$733	$733	$733	$733	$733	$733	$733	$733	$733	$733	$733	$733	$8792
Bank charges	$50	$50	$50	$50	$50	$50	$50	$50	$50	$50	$50	$50	$600
Mortgage payment (practice)	$3041	$3041	$3041	$3041	$3041	$3041	$3041	$3041	$3041	$3041	$3041	$3041	
Total bank costs	$3091	$3091	$3091	$3091	$3091	$3091	$3091	$3091	$3091	$3091	$3091	$3091	$37098
Marketing and promotion	$583	$583	$583	$583	$583	$583	$583	$583	$583	$583	$583	$583	$7000
Total marketing costs	$583	$583	$583	$583	$583	$583	$583	$583	$583	$583	$583	$583	$7000
Management consulting	$0	$0	$0	$0	$0	$0	$0	$0	$0	$0	$0	$0	$0
Accounting	$200	$200	$200	$200	$200	$200	$200	$200	$200	$200	$200	$200	$2400
Total professional costs	$200	$200	$200	$200	$200	$200	$200	$200	$200	$200	$200	$200	$2400
Draw	$4000	$4000	$4000	$4000	$4000	$4000	$6000	$6000	$6000	$6000	$6000	$6000	$60000
Personal insurances paid	$300	$300	$300	$300	$300	$300	$300	$300	$300	$300	$300	$300	%3600
Continuing education	$50	$50	$50	$50	$50	$50	$50	$50	$50	$50	$50	$50	$600
Professional dues and journals	$83	$83	$83	$83	$83	$83	$83	$83	$83	$83	$83	$83	$1000
Total owner's costs	$4433	$4433	$4433	$4433	$4433	$4433	$6433	$6433	$6433	$6433	$6433	$6433	$65200
Total cash outflows (costs)	$18981	$19234	$19528	$19870	$20267	$20729	$23266	$23892	$24620	$25467	$26455	$27606	$269913
Net cash flow	($14304)	($11287)	($8444)	($7015)	($5355)	($3425)	($3181)	($570)	$2469	$6006	$10126	$14925	($20054)
Cumulative cash position	($14304)	($25591)	($34035)	($41050)	($46405)	($49830)	($53011)	($53580)	($51111)	($45105)	($34980)	($20054)	($20054)

Several important differences exist between the cash flow represented by the checkbook and the P&L statement. The major differences are:

- Depreciation is a non-cash expense on the P&L statement. It does not occur in the checkbook.

- A loan payment is composed of part loan principal and part interest. The entire payment (principal and interest) is recorded in the checkbook, but only the interest portion is on the P&L statement.

- When someone borrows money, cash flows into the checkbook but does not show on the P&L statement. Likewise, an amount for savings paid from the office checkbook is a cash event but does not show on the P&L statement.

- When someone pays the money back (principal on a loan), cash flows from the checkbook but does not show on the P&L statement.

- A draw is a cash flow from the checkbook but does not appear on the P&L statement. The same is true for any money for personal use taken from the checkbook. (It is also considered a draw.)

Three major sources of cash flow into or out of the practice. Cash flow from operating activities is the result of daily practice operations. That is to say, these are payments from patients, insurance companies and credit cards for the dental services done. Offsetting this is money spent to pay suppliers and employees, which decreases cash from operating activities. Bankers are interested in operating cash because it shows the cash flow from the core business. The cash flow from investment activities relates to money spent on property, plant, equipment, and other capital assets.

Note that some outflows (such as savings) is "taking money from one pocket and putting it in the other." In reality, savings are an asset that increases on a balance sheet. This improves a person's overall financial position. Cash-flow statements are often used to decide if someone has enough money flowing through the practice to make recurring mortgage and other loan payments. Any excess cash can pay down the principal on a loan. Any cash shortage must come from savings or borrowing.

Cash flow is important because it shows someone's liquidity and solvency (ability to pay immediate bills). These include regular office expenses, payroll and loan payments. Banks are concerned that a person can make these payments. If they cannot pay them from operating income, then that person should plan to borrow enough money to pay them while the practice is growing to the point where it can sustain the payments. The only way to decide this is to prepare a cash-flow projection.

The practice owner should leave enough cash in the office checking account for two to three months' expenses. This changes over time as cash flows into and out of the account. A dental practitioner needs enough cash for the following:

- All monthly expenses (bills paid, credit cards paid, salaries).

- Routine purchases (lab, rent, etc.).

- An unexpected loss of income (office closed, vacations, etc.).

- Annual ebb and flow of business.

- Minimums required by banks (for no fees).

- Future obligations (employee taxes withheld, personal tax payments, insurance owed, etc.).

- Special needs (injury, disability, savings).

The cash-flow projection shows how the person expects the cash to flow through the practice for a given time, often the critical first year. When a procedure is done on a patient, a dentist may not receive the entire amount as a cash payment. Instead, some may come in the future as payment from an insurance company or from a patient who did not pay a bill in full at the time of the service. This accumulates over many patients and many procedures. Accounts receivable is the cumulative amount that patients owe a dentist for services already done. The dentist's expenses (owed) to suppliers, landlords, and staff are due immediately. However, if the dentist has not received full payment for those dental services billed, this leads to a "cash-flow problem" or "cash-flow crunch," in which the office will be profitable, but cash is flowing in so slowly from patients that immediate bills for suppliers, staff, and other expenses are unable to be made. The solution is to borrow money (called "working capital") to cover these cash-flow shortages. The cash-flow projection estimates how large the cash shortage is and, therefore, how much working capital someone will need. Typically, dentists need from three to six months' expenses as working capital for a start-up practice in a moderately competitive environment. If the area is more competitive, growth and cash flow will be slower, and therefore the working capital needs will be more.

Sample Cash-Flow Projection

Box 15.11 shows an example cash-flow projection for the first year of Dr. Doe's dental practice. It gives good-faith estimates of how much the doctor and hygienist will produce for each of the first 12 months and an estimate of how much the resulting collections will be. (Obviously, these are only as good as the estimates that form the basis of the projection.) The projection contains cash expenditures, including a "draw" and personal expenses like insurance and continuing education expenses. Because it is a cash statement, it contains loan payments but not depreciation.

The most important lines are at the bottom of the form. "Net cash flow" shows how much cash can be expected to flow through the practice each month. In the first month, collections of $4676 and cash expenses (actual checks written) of $18 981 for a cash deficit of $14 304 are estimated. In the second month, the cash deficit is $11 287 for the cumulative total of the two months of $25 591. Monthly cash flow is expected to be negative through month 8, when a total cumulative deficit of $53 580 is expected. It is not until month 9 that the monthly cash flow is projected to be positive, and the cash deficit starts getting paid down. Using this analysis, more than $53 500 of working capital is needed to get through the first year of practice. If the cash inflows with outflows were balanced, the necessary cash from loan proceeds would be entered as an inflow similar to collections.

HOW THE BUSINESS STATEMENTS ARE RELATED

The business balance sheet lists what Dr. Doe's practice owns and owes. The P&L statement shows the result of operating her practice. The cash-flow statement shows the actual cash transactions for the year.

PRO-FORMA STATEMENTS

Pro-forma statements are projected statements. They can be any of the four types described in this chapter. The essential element of a pro forma is that it is a guess at what the statement will be at a given time in the future. If someone is preparing a pro-forma income statement for the practice, they need to estimate the number of patient visits, average charges, number and pay rate of staff, and many other items of expense. Obviously, a pro-forma statement is only as accurate as an educated guess about the future. Often, banks will ask their customers to develop a pro-forma cash flow (to assess whether they have adequate cash to meet expected expenses) and an income statement (to determine expected income and tax situations).

Basics of Business Finance

The safest way to double your money is to fold it over once and put it in your pocket.

Frank McKinney (Kin) Hubbard

GOAL

This chapter present concepts of business finance, with specific examples of how these ideas are used in dental practice.

LEARNING OBJECTIVES

At the completion of this chapter, the student will be able to:

- Describe how the time value of money affects dental practice management decisions.

- Use the time value of money formulas to solve common dental office finance problems.

- Describe the elements of loan amortization.

- Describe common lease–purchase decisions in dental practices.

- Describe the advantages and disadvantages of leasing assets.

- Discuss common issues in leasing office space.

- Discuss common issues in leasing automobiles.

- Discuss common issues in leasing office equipment.

KEY TERMS

amortization	IRS useful lifetime	principal
amortization schedule	leasehold improvements	property lease
compounding	leverage	residual value
down payment	loan conditions	sublease
economic useful lifetime	money factor	term of a loan
equipment replacement plan	net lease	time value of money
future value	operating lease	triple net lease
future value of a present amount	payment	value of an annuity
gross lease	present value	
interest	present value of a future dollar	

Business Basics for Dentists, Second Edition. James L. Harrison, David O. Willis, and Charles K. Thieman.
© 2024 John Wiley & Sons, Inc. Published 2024 by John Wiley & Sons, Inc.

Business finance looks at how dentists use money in dental practice to gain or improve profitability. Dentists use money to purchase equipment and materials, hire staff members, and pay the costs of the business. Applying finance principles properly maximizes the profit from the practice.

TIME VALUE OF MONEY

A basic premise of finance is that money has a time-associated value and time has a money-associated value. A dollar in the future will be worth less than a dollar received today, just as paying a dollar in the future is less costly than paying a dollar today. There is a psychological reason for this, given that most people prefer the certainty of having a dollar now to the uncertainty of having a dollar in the future. That future dollar will be worth less because of the likelihood of inflation eating away at its buying power. In addition, a dollar invested wisely will bring a positive return, increasing the value of that present dollar in the future. Time value of money calculations let someone evaluate how much less that future dollar is worth so they can make informed financial decisions. This is done by bringing cash flows to a present value for comparison. The higher the assumed interest rate, the more important these calculations become.

These calculations all depend on the idea of compounding. This is the financial process in which someone earns interest on the principal amount, and then they earn interest on the interest and the principal. That person thus earns interest on an increasing amount over time. The total amount compounds as the interest portion becomes larger and larger.

For example, someone feels they need $3 million (in today's money) to retire comfortably in 30 years. If 3%

annual inflation is assumed, how much will they need to save each year to meet the goal? Or say someone agrees to buy a dental practice for $350 000 after a five-year associateship. How much is that in today's money? The answers to these questions have an obvious, important financial impact.

These numbers can easily be calculated with a financial calculator (e.g. HP 12-C), a spreadsheet with financial functions (Excel), or the tables included in this chapter. Although these tables do not give the precise results that a banker may have available, they are more than adequate for planning purposes. Throughout the chapter, several common examples of using these important techniques are given.

FUTURE VALUE OF A PRESENT AMOUNT

The future value of a present amount is the future amount of an initial deposit when compounded for a given number of periods at a given rate. This calculation is important when planning future expenditures or savings. To compute this amount, the first three of the four values are needed:

PV Present value, the amount in today's dollars

i Interest rate, the compounding rate for each period

n Number of periods, number of compounding periods

FV Future value, the amount in future dollars

Using Table 16.1, find the future value factor (FVF) for the given i and n. Multiply the PV by the FVF to figure out the FV:

$$PV \times FVF = FV$$

Table 16.1 Future value of a single present amount.

	2%	3%	4%	5%	6%	7%	8%	9%	10%	12%	15%	20%
1	1.0200	1.0300	1.0400	1.0500	1.0600	1.0700	1.0800	1.0900	1.1000	1.1200	1.1500	1.2000
2	1.0404	1.0609	1.0816	1.1025	1.1236	1.1449	1.1664	1.1881	1.2100	1.2544	1.3225	1.4400
3	1.0612	1.0927	1.1249	1.1576	1.1910	1.2250	1.2597	1.2950	1.3310	1.4049	1.5209	1.7280
4	1.0824	1.1255	1.1699	1.2155	1.2625	1.3108	1.3605	1.4116	1.4641	1.5735	1.7490	2.0736
5	1.1041	1.1593	1.2167	1.2763	1.3382	1.4026	1.4693	1.5386	1.6105	1.7623	2.0114	2.4883
6	1.1262	1.1941	1.2653	1.3401	1.4185	1.5007	1.5869	1.6771	1.7716	1.9738	2.3131	2.9860
7	1.1487	1.2299	1.3159	1.4071	1.5036	1.6058	1.7138	1.8280	1.9487	2.2107	2.6600	3.5832
8	1.1717	1.2668	1.3686	1.4775	1.5938	1.7182	1.8509	1.9926	2.1436	2.4760	3.0590	4.2998
9	1.1951	1.3048	1.4233	1.5513	1.6895	1.8385	1.9990	2.1719	2.3579	2.7731	3.5179	5.1598
10	1.2190	1.3439	1.4802	1.6289	1.7908	1.9672	2.1589	2.3674	2.5937	3.1058	4.0456	6.1917
15	1.3459	1.5580	1.8009	2.0789	2.3966	2.7590	3.1722	3.6425	4.1772	5.4736	8.1371	15.4070
20	1.4859	1.8061	2.1911	2.6533	3.2071	3.8697	4.6610	5.6044	6.7275	9.6463	16.3665	38.3376
25	1.6406	2.0938	2.6658	3.3864	4.2919	5.4274	6.8485	8.6231	10.8347	17.0001	32.9190	95.3962
30	1.8114	2.4273	3.2434	4.3219	5.7435	7.6123	10.0627	13.2677	17.4494	29.9599	66.2118	237.3763

Box 16.1 presents several example problems (#1, 2, and 3) for this calculation and their solutions.

PRESENT VALUE OF A FUTURE DOLLAR

The present value of a future amount is how much must be deposited today to have a given amount in the future when compounded for a given number of periods at a given rate. This calculation is not used as much as the other calculations, but it is still important when planning future expenditures. To compute this amount, the first three of the four values are needed:

FV Future value, the amount in future dollars

i   Interest rate, the compounding rate for each period

n   Number of periods, number of compounding periods

PV Present value, the amount in today's dollars

Using Table 16.2, find the present value factor for the given interest and number of periods. Multiply the FV by the PVF to figure out the PV:

$$FV \times PVF = PV.$$

Box 16.2 presents an example problem using this calculation.

ANNUITIES

An annuity is a series of regular, periodic payments. When someone buys a car and sets up a loan, the repayment is an annuity. If a savings plan is established in which a certain amount is set aside each month, an annuity has been established. Because an annuity compounds (i.e. earns interest on the interest earned), a table is needed to determine how much the annuity earns or costs. Two annuity tables will be used. One (Table 16.3) determines how much a regular savings plan will be worth in the future. The other (Table 16.4) determines how much the payment on a loan will be.

Determining Payments

When someone repays loans as an annuity, the loans are usually compounded monthly. Table 16.3 determines a monthly payment based on compounding the interest monthly. If the interest is 12% per year compounded monthly, the actual interest rate is 12.68% (1% compounded monthly). This amount will be more than an annual compounding amount, but it is more accurate. (Tables 16.3 and 16.4 have this conversion built into them.)

To compute the payment amount, the first three of the four values are needed:

PV   Present value, the amount of the loan principal

i   Interest rate, the annual interest rate charged on the loan

n   Number of years, number of years you will pay on the loan

PMT Payment, amount of the periodic payment

BOX 16.1	FUTURE VALUE OF A SINGLE PRESENT AMOUNT

Example problem 1

A person invests $2000 in a certificate of deposit (CD), earning 8% interest, compounded annually. What will the CD be worth when it matures in 5 years?

PV = $2000
FV = ??
i = 8%
n = 5

Looking at Table 16.1, find the FVF at the intersection of 8% and 5 periods (1.4693). Multiply this FVF by the PV ($2000) to find the FV = $2938.60.

Example problem 2

A person needs $3 million (in today's money) to retire comfortably in 30 years. If 3% annual inflation is assumed, how much will they need in today's dollars to meet the goal?

PV = $3 000 000
FV = ??
i = 3%
n = 30

Looking at Table 16.1, find the FVF at the intersection of 3% and 30 periods (2.4273). Multiply this FVF by the PV ($3 000 000) to find the FV = $7 281 900.

Example problem 3

A person wants to start a college fund for a newborn daughter. They believe that $120 000 ($30 000 per year × 4 years) in today's dollars is needed, and this money in will be needed in 20 years. Assuming 3% annual inflation, how much will be needed in today's dollars for the daughter's college fund?

PV = $120 000
FV = ??
i = 3%
n = 20

Looking at Table 16.1, find the FVF at the intersection of 3% and 20 periods (1.8061). Multiply this FVF by the PV ($120 000) to find the FV = $216 732.

Table 16.2 Present value of a future amount.

	2%	3%	4%	5%	6%	7%	8%	9%	10%	12%	15%	20%
1	0.9804	0.9709	0.9615	0.9524	0.9434	0.9346	0.9259	0.9174	0.9091	0.8929	0.8696	0.8333
2	0.9612	0.9426	0.9246	0.9070	0.8900	0.8734	0.8573	0.8417	0.8264	0.7972	0.7561	0.6944
3	0.9423	0.9151	0.8890	0.8638	0.8396	0.8163	0.7938	0.7722	0.7513	0.7118	0.6575	0.5787
4	0.9238	0.8885	0.8548	0.8227	0.7921	0.7629	0.7350	0.7084	0.6830	0.6355	0.5718	0.4823
5	0.9057	0.8626	0.8219	0.7835	0.7473	0.7130	0.6806	0.6499	0.6209	0.5674	0.4972	0.4019
6	0.8880	0.8375	0.7903	0.7462	0.7050	0.6663	0.6302	0.5963	0.5645	0.5066	0.4323	0.3349
7	0.8706	0.8131	0.7599	0.7107	0.6651	0.6227	0.5835	0.5470	0.5132	0.4523	0.3759	0.2791
8	0.8535	0.7894	0.7307	0.6768	0.6274	0.5820	0.5403	0.5019	0.4665	0.4039	0.3269	0.2326
9	0.8368	0.7664	0.7026	0.6446	0.5919	0.5439	0.5002	0.4604	0.4241	0.3606	0.2843	0.1938
10	0.8203	0.7441	0.6756	0.6139	0.5584	0.5083	0.4632	0.4224	0.3855	0.3220	0.2472	0.1615
15	0.7430	0.6419	0.5553	0.4810	0.4173	0.3624	0.3152	0.2745	0.2394	0.1827	0.1229	0.0649
20	0.6730	0.5537	0.4564	0.3769	0.3118	0.2584	0.2145	0.1784	0.1486	0.1037	0.0611	0.0261
25	0.6095	0.4776	0.3751	0.2953	0.2330	0.1842	0.1460	0.1160	0.0923	0.0588	0.0304	0.0105
30	0.5521	0.4120	0.3083	0.2314	0.1741	0.1314	0.0994	0.0754	0.0573	0.0334	0.0151	0.0042

BOX 16.2	**PRESENT VALUE OF A FUTURE AMOUNT**

Example problem 4

A person wants to save $30 000 in 5 years for a down payment on a vacation home. How much should they deposit today to have $30 000 in 5 years? They believe they can earn 8% after taxes on the investment.

FV = $30 000
i = 8%
n = 5
PV = ??

Looking at Table 16.2, find the PVF at the intersection of 8% and 5 periods (0.6806). Multiply this PVF by the FV ($30 000) to find the PV = $20 418. That is to say, if they deposit $20 418 in an account and earn 8%, after five years it will be worth $30 000.

Use Table 16.3 to determine the annuity monthly payment (AMP) factor for the loan's annual interest rate and term (number of years). Multiply the resulting AMP by the number of thousands of dollars of loan principal. Remember, this is a monthly payment per $1000 borrowed. Be sure to multiply by 12 for an annual amount.

Box 16.3 presents two problems (#5 and 6) that ask how to determine the amount of a payment for a loan.

Determining Savings

When a regular savings plan is established, an annuity is essentially being set up. A series of regular payments are made into an account. That account earns interest on the money deposited each period and earns interest on interest earned in the account.

To compute the payment amount, the first three of the four values is needed:

i   Interest rate, the annual interest rate earned on the annuity

n   Number of years, number of years you will pay into the annuity

PMT   Payment, amount of the annual payment into the annuity

FV   Future value, the future amount the annuity will be worth

Use Table 16.4 to determine the future value annuity (FVA) factor for the annuity's annual interest rate and term (number of years). Multiply the resulting FVA by the amount of the regular annual payment (in dollars).

$$PMT \times FVA = FV$$

Box 16.4 presents three problems (#7, 8, and 9) that use this calculation.

Table 16.3 Annuity monthly payment factor.

	2%	3%	4%	5%	6%	7%	8%	9%	10%	12%	15%	20%
1	84.24	84.69	85.15	85.61	86.07	86.53	86.99	87.45	87.92	88.85	90.26	92.63
2	42.54	42.98	43.42	43.87	44.32	44.77	45.23	45.68	46.14	47.07	48.49	50.90
3	28.64	29.08	29.52	29.97	30.42	30.88	31.34	31.80	32.27	33.21	34.67	37.16
4	21.70	22.13	22.58	23.03	23.49	23.95	24.41	24.89	25.36	26.33	27.83	30.43
5	17.53	17.97	18.42	18.87	19.33	19.80	20.28	20.76	21.25	22.24	23.79	26.49
6	14.75	15.19	15.65	16.10	16.57	17.05	17.53	18.03	18.53	19.55	21.15	23.95
7	12.77	13.21	13.67	14.13	14.61	15.09	15.59	16.09	16.60	17.65	19.30	22.21
8	11.28	11.73	12.19	12.66	13.14	13.63	14.14	14.65	15.17	16.25	17.95	20.95
9	10.13	10.58	11.04	11.52	12.01	12.51	13.02	13.54	14.08	15.18	16.92	20.03
10	9.20	9.66	10.12	10.61	11.10	11.61	12.13	12.67	13.22	14.35	16.13	19.33
15	6.44	6.91	7.40	7.91	8.44	8.99	9.56	10.14	10.75	12.00	14.00	17.56
20	5.06	5.55	6.06	6.60	7.16	7.75	8.36	9.00	9.65	11.01	13.17	16.99
25	4.24	4.74	5.28	5.85	6.44	7.07	7.72	8.39	9.09	10.53	12.81	16.78
30	3.70	4.22	4.77	5.37	6.00	6.65	7.34	8.05	8.78	10.29	12.64	16.71

Table 16.4 Future value of an annuity.

	2%	3%	4%	5%	6%	7%	8%	9%	10%	12%	15%	20%
1	1.000	1.000	1.000	1.000	1.000	1.000	1.000	1.000	1.000	1.000	1.000	1.000
2	2.020	2.030	2.040	2.050	2.060	2.070	2.080	2.090	2.100	2.120	2.150	2.200
3	3.060	3.091	3.122	3.153	3.184	3.215	3.246	3.278	3.310	3.374	3.473	3.640
4	4.122	4.184	4.246	4.310	4.375	4.440	4.506	4.573	4.641	4.779	4.993	5.368
5	5.204	5.309	5.416	5.526	5.637	5.751	5.867	5.985	6.105	6.353	6.742	7.442
6	6.308	6.468	6.633	6.802	6.975	7.153	7.336	7.523	7.716	8.115	8.754	9.930
7	7.434	7.662	7.898	8.142	8.394	8.654	8.923	9.200	9.487	10.089	11.067	12.916
8	8.583	8.892	9.214	9.549	9.897	10.260	10.637	11.028	11.436	12.300	13.727	16.499
9	9.755	10.159	10.583	11.027	11.491	11.978	12.488	13.021	13.579	14.776	16.786	20.799
10	10.950	11.464	12.006	12.578	13.181	13.816	14.487	15.193	15.937	17.549	20.304	25.959
15	17.293	18.599	20.024	21.579	23.276	25.129	27.152	29.361	31.772	37.280	47.580	72.035
20	24.297	26.870	29.778	33.066	36.786	40.995	45.762	51.160	57.275	72.052	102.444	186.688
25	32.030	36.459	41.646	47.727	54.865	63.249	73.106	84.701	98.347	133.334	212.793	471.981
30	40.568	47.575	56.085	66.439	79.058	94.461	113.283	136.308	164.494	241.333	434.745	1181.882

CAPITAL BUDGETING

Capital assets are things that the practice owns that last for several to many years. Examples include dental chairs, computers, curing lights, and furniture. These long-term assets are usually purchased with a loan that also lasts for a long time. In fact, most corporate finance officers try to match the term of the loan with the approximate expected lifetime of the asset. They do not want to extend the term of the loan for a longer period than the useful lifetime.

(No one wants to be still paying for a piece of equipment after it has been disposed of.) Capital assets are usually large, expensive pieces of equipment. The decisions about financing these assets carry a large price tag. So, planning for the purchase of these assets becomes an important managerial function.

There are several reasons someone might make capital purchases in a dental practice. When buying an existing practice, the person buys the assets of the practice. These

BOX 16.3	DETERMINE THE PAYMENT AMOUNT

Example problem 5

A person is buying a new car. The price of the car is $28 000. A $2000 down payment is made and the loan is at 9% for 4 years. What is the monthly payment?

PV = $26 000 ($28 000 to $2000)
i   = 9%
n   = 4
PMT = ??

Looking at Table 16.3, find the AMP at the intersection of 9% and 4 years ($24.89). Multiply this AMP by the number of thousands borrowed (present value/1000 = 26) to find the monthly payment amount, $24.89 × 26 = $647.14 per month ($7766 per year).

Example problem 6

A person is buying a dental practice. The price of the practice is $350 000. The entire amount will be financed. The loan is fixed at 10% for 7 years. What is the monthly payment for the practice?

PV = $350 000
i   = 10%
n   = 7
PMT = ??

Looking at Table 16.3, find the AMP at the intersection of 10% and 7 years ($16.60). Multiply this AMP by the number of thousands borrowed (present value/1000 = 350) to find the monthly payment amount = $5810 ($69 720 per year).

BOX 16.4	DETERMINE SAVINGS AMOUNT

Example problem 7

A person is saving for a down payment on a vacation home. The home will be purchased in 5 years and they can save $1000 per month. They believe that 8% can be earned in the market (after taxes) on the investment. How much will the person have for a down payment in 5 years?

i   = 8%
n   = 5
PMT = $12 000 (this is $1000/month × 12 months)
FV = ??

Looking at Table 16.4, find the FVA at the intersection of 8% and 5 years (5.867). Multiply this FVA by the annual payment amount ($12 000) to find the value of the annuity at the end of the time = $70 404.

Example problem 8

A person is saving for retirement. They can put $15 000 per year into a tax-deferred retirement account, and they estimate earning 12% in the market on the investment. How much will accumulate in 30 years?

i   = 12%
n   = 30
PMT = $15 000
FV = ??

Looking at Table 16.4, find the FVA at the intersection of 12% and 30 years (241.333). Multiply this FVA by the annual payment amount ($15 000) to find the value of the annuity at the end of the time = $3 619 995.

Example problem 9

A person previously decided they needed $400 000 in 20 years for a newborn daughter's college fund. If this person believes they can reasonably earn 9% (after taxes) in the market, how much will they need to save each year to fully fund the daughter's college savings?

i   = 9%
n   = 20
PMT   = ??
FV   = $400 000
PMT × FVA = FV
PMT   = FV/FVA

This problem is different because the future value is known and the payment must be solved. Looking at Table 16.4, find the FVA at the intersection of 9% and 20 years (51.160). Divide the FV ($400 000) by the FVA to figure out the annual savings needed to fund the plan fully = $7751.

may be hard assets (such as dental equipment) and soft assets, such as goodwill and ongoing concern value. The equipment will need to be replaced in a practice periodically as older equipment wears out. A facility might need to be modernized as newer equipment and technology becomes available. An existing facility might need to be expanded. Each of these should be done with a definite plan and timetable for paying for them.

ASSET TYPES

Supplies are things that the practice buys and uses up quickly, typically in less than a year. The practice buys assets that last for more than a year (often many years). These assets are usually broken into soft and hard assets and are then further categorized by their expected useful lifetime. Two types of "useful lifetimes" are used. The IRS declares a useful lifetime for tax purposes. This determination states how many years must be used to determine the asset's tax depreciation. Economists are interested in establishing an "economic useful lifetime," which estimates how long the asset is expected to serve its function for the business before it needs to be replaced. So, although the IRS may state that a dental chair should have a useful lifetime of 7 years (meaning the chair should be depreciated over 7 years), in fact a dental chair should last for 15–20 years if it is well cared for and well maintained. Its economic useful lifetime (for practice planning purposes) is probably 20 years.

MORTGAGE TYPES

A mortgage is an installment loan (a series of equal payments) secured by a hard asset that it has been used to purchase. Many corporate finance managers will match the term of the loan to the expected lifetime of the asset purchased. The business owner wants to be sure that the term of the loan is no longer than the lifetime of the asset so that they are not paying for the asset when it has no more value. Box 16.5 shows the typical term for loans for various types of assets.

The term of the loan then has a large impact on cash flow. This allows the lowest safe cash requirements to pay off the loan before the asset completely depreciates, increasing how much cash is freed for other purposes. This keeps the cash needed for the payment at the lowest possible amount.

EQUIPMENT REPLACEMENT PLAN

If assets lasted forever (or an entire professional lifetime), they would be purchased once and forgotten about. In fact, assets wear out from use. New and better equipment

becomes available. Developments in the industry make some equipment obsolete. Other equipment continues to be useful. To prepare for large asset purchases, many practices budget a certain amount of income for equipment updates and replacement. In this way, they can be assured of modern methods and techniques. Especially with the reliance on computers and software (which are expensive and have relatively short economic useful lifetimes of 3–7 years), an equipment replacement plan becomes a near necessity. During the practice pay-off phase, most dentists spend 8–10% of gross revenues on a loan pay-off (capital and interest). Although not usually necessary in the mature practice, it is prudent to budget half this amount (2–4% of revenue) for replacing and updating equipment.

BORROWING MONEY

Almost every business borrows money to purchase equipment or expand facilities. The business usually pays this off through the process of loan amortization. This becomes an important topic for financial managers.

When someone borrows money and purchases a large asset (e.g. a car, house, or dental practice), they own it. It is titled in their name, which means that they must pay for its upkeep and repairs and can (with certain restrictions) sell it whenever desired. The banker (or another lender) will file a lien with the county in which the asset resides. This legal document says that the lender has an interest in the property (they have lent money to buy it), and it cannot be sold until the loan is paid in full. If all payments are completed as agreed, then the lender will "release" the lien so that the owner has no more restrictions. If someone wants to sell the asset while still owing money, they must use the sale proceeds to satisfy the loan. The lender will then release the lien on the property.

LEVERAGE

Financial leverage occurs when someone takes out a loan and then reinvests the proceeds with the intent of earning a greater rate of return than the cost of the loan (interest). That asset may generate money (a dental practice or piece of dental equipment) or may be sold later (real estate or other investment). If the rate of return on the assets purchased is higher than the interest rate on the loan to purchase the asset, then the return on equity will be higher than if it had not been borrowed. However, if the return on the asset is lower than the interest rate, then the return on equity will be lower than if it had not been borrowed. Leverage allows greater potential returns but greater potential losses to the investor. If the investment declines

BOX 16.5	MATCHING THE TERM TO THE TYPE OF LOAN

Type of debt	Term of loan
Credit card debt	Immediate
Auto purchase	5 years max
Dental practice	5–7 years
Dental equipment	2–5 years
Dental building	20 years
Home mortgage	30 years
Education loans	20 years

significantly or becomes worthless, the loan principal still needs to be paid to the lender.

LOAN SECURITY

A banker makes a "secured" loan when the borrower pledges, or promises, certain assets or things of value if the borrower defaults on the loan. An automobile loan is secured by the automobile. If the borrower defaults on the loan, the lender can repossess the automobile, selling the car to satisfy the unpaid portion of the loan. Here, the borrower pledges the automobile as "collateral" for the loan. When the bank (or other lending agency) lends the money to purchase the automobile, it files a lien in the local courthouse. Therefore, the loan is secure from its perspective. Unsecured loans have no assets pledged as collateral. These are obviously more risky loans for the banker, so they generally carry a higher interest rate. A "signature loan" is guaranteed only by someone's signature guaranteeing to repay the loan. It is obviously in a person's best interest to repay the loan so they can borrow again with an unblemished credit history. The banker can still take that person to court to satisfy an unsecured loan, but if the person has no assets (or has lost them all), the bank probably could not collect. A person may use signature loans to pay tax bills or other short-term obligations if they are short of immediate cash. These loans are often found among borrowers who have developed excellent relationships with their bankers.

A loan may be secured in several ways. As previously mentioned, the borrower may pledge certain assets as collateral. This might include the car for a car loan, business assets for a practice loan, or stocks for an investment account. A cosigner can secure a loan by pledging specific assets (e.g. their house, stocks, or bonds) or may take on a general obligation by signing and personally guaranteeing that the borrower will pay the loan. (The banker will obviously investigate the cosigner carefully before doing this!) Young professionals may not qualify to borrow money alone but may gain financing if a parent or relative cosigns the loan, often pledging specific assets. If the loan payment goes as planned, the cosigner has no cost from cosigning the loan. On the other hand, if the primary borrower defaults on the loan, the bank can (and generally will) institute legal proceedings to ensure payment from the cosigner.

PRINCIPAL AMOUNT

The principal of a loan is the amount borrowed. It is the value of the asset or property, less any down payment, with fees possibly added. A down payment is the amount of money someone pays as an initial, upfront portion of the total amount due. It is usually given in cash at the time of completing the loan. The larger the down payment, the lower the amount financed. Bankers often require some loan value (often 10–25%) as a down payment. This does several things. It qualifies the person as having enough money to participate in the venture. It makes the person more interested in the success of the venture because they have some of the money at stake in the deal. That person, therefore, has an interest in seeing that the asset remains in good repair and condition. It protects the banker, to a degree, from default. For example, assume someone makes a 25% down payment. If the asset's cost declines by 10% and it is sold, the banker gets all of their money back. The 10% loss comes from the owner's portion. Because little of the initial payment goes to reducing the principal, the asset can decrease in value faster than it is paid off, resulting in "negative equity," in which the borrower owes more than the asset is worth. (This is known as being "upside-down" in the loan.) If the owner tries to sell the asset, they must pay the difference ("bring money to the table") to sell. If the owner defaults ("walks away from the loan"), the value lost comes first from the owner (down payment) and then from the lender (borrowed capital). It protects the lender if the asset does not decrease in value more than the down payment.

INTEREST

Interest is the money that the borrower pays the lender for the privilege of using the principal. Interest is usually expressed as an annual percentage. This is then applied to the remaining loan principal to decide the interest owed. Although the rate is expressed as an annual amount, it is usually compounded monthly. For example, a 12% per year compounded monthly rate is the same as 1% per month. However, 1% compounded 12 times is actually 12.68%. The difference in these two rates applied to a $100 000 loan is more than $682 in the first year.

An interest rate might be a fixed rate. This means that the percentage charged during the loan will remain fixed throughout the loan. If the borrower negotiates the loan for 6%, then 6% it remains. Lenders have often lost money by charging fixed rates for their loans. For example, if a loan is at 4% fixed and the inflation rate climbs to 8% per year, the bank is losing money by lending it. If it could offer that loan to someone else instead, it would now get 8%, or twice the interest it is presently charging. Most lenders have variable, or "floating," interest rate loans to solve this problem. In these types of loans, the interest rate changes depending on some agreed-on economic indicator. If the economic indicator rises, the loan's interest rate goes up. Conversely, if the indicator drops, the loan's rate decreases. This protects the bank and the borrower (especially the bank) from locking in unfavorable interest rates.

As a rule, banks use the "prime interest rate" in determining the specific variable rate for business loans. "Prime" is the rate the biggest banks charges to their best customers (e.g. Ford, General Electric, etc.). The prime rate is published daily in the business press and most metropolitan newspapers' business section. The banks often charge an additional 1½–2% points above prime for a new professional's loan. So, if a loan has an interest rate of "prime + 2," that person pays 2% points above the prime interest rate. For variable-rate loans, the rate is usually recomputed annually based on changes in the prime rate. There are often limits to the frequency of change or the amount of increase or decrease in the rate that can be applied.

Some banks and most mortgage lenders offer the choice of either a fixed- or variable-rate loan. The fixed-rate loan usually carries a higher nominal interest rate to protect the lender from the possibility of rising rates. All the loan factors, not just the interest rate, must be considered if the bank offers a choice of fixed- or variable-rate loans (Box 16.6). What are the rates? How often are the variable rates adjusted? Are there maximum or minimum rate changes? Are there different closing costs or other hidden costs of a particular loan? What is the estimate of the future economy? Will interest rates will be rising or falling soon? Does the higher fixed rate lead to unacceptable payment schedules?

TERM OF A LOAN

The term of a loan is the number of payments required to pay off the principal under normal conditions and with no changes in any other loan factors. Most dental business (start-up or buy-out) loans have terms of five to seven years.

There is a trade-off between the term of the loan and the payment amount. The longer the term (the greater the number of payments), the lower the regular payment, but the higher the total amount of interest paid. As a rule, a shorter term is desired so the loan will be paid off sooner. However, someone may not be able to afford the higher regular payment required by the shorter-term loan and may need to lengthen the term of the loan to decrease the payment to a manageable amount. If a dentist has a large student debt load, some bankers will allow them to stretch the practice loan out to 10 years. This lowers the practice loan payment amount so that the person can more easily

BOX 16.6		AMORTIZATION SCHEDULE		
Year	Payment	Principal	Total interest	Principal remaining
1	$54 773	$9 773	$45 000	$490 227
2	$54 773	$10 653	$44 120	$479 574
3	$54 773	$11 612	$43 162	$467 962
4	$54 773	$12 657	$42 117	$455 306
5	$54 773	$13 796	$40 978	$441 510
6	$54 773	$15 037	$39 736	$426 473
7	$54 773	$16 391	$38 383	$410 082
8	$54 773	$17 866	$36 907	$392 216
9	$54 773	$19 474	$35 299	$372 742
10	$54 773	$21 226	$33 547	$351 516
11	$54 773	$23 137	$31 636	$328 379
12	$54 773	$25 219	$29 554	$303 160
13	$54 773	$27 489	$27 284	$275 671
14	$54 773	$29 963	$24 810	$245 708
15	$54 773	$32 659	$22 114	$213 049
16	$54 773	$35 599	$19 174	$177 450
17	$54 773	$38 803	$15 970	$138 647
18	$54 773	$42 295	$12 478	$96 352
19	$54 773	$46 102	$8 672	$50 251
20	$54 773	$50 251	$4 523	$0
	$1 095 465	$500 000	$595 465	$119 093

Assumptions:

Principal = $500 000
Term = 20 years
Rate = 9.0% per year

In this example, Dr. Jones buys a house, securing a mortgage for the amount shown. Her annual payments are given. (This loan would be compounded monthly but the chart would be too large to show.) Over the 20-year life of the loan, Dr. Jones pays a total of $595 465 in interest, and the principal of $500 000.

meet all cash needs. However, more in total interest cost is paid by using the longer term.

The loan decision is a balancing act between the interest rate and the term to keep the payment amount (cash flow) within the budget. Because interest rates are less negotiable, many people extend the term of the loan to get the payment down to a level that fits their budget. The problem with this approach is the higher debt cost through increased total interest payments. Box 16.7 shows the effect of interest rates and terms on a loan principal of $100 000.

BOX 16.7	COMPARISON OF TERM AND RATE FOR A LOAN

COMPARISON OF TERM AND RATE FOR A LOAN

		8%	9%	10%	11%	12%
5-year term	Annual payment	$24332	$24910	$25496	$26091	$26693
	Monthly payment	$2028	$2076	$2125	$2174	$2224
7-year term	Annual payment	$18703	$19307	$19921	$20547	$21183
	Monthly payment	$1559	$1609	$1660	$1712	$1765

Assumption:

Principal = $100000

The payment amount is related to the term and the interest rate. The longer the term, the lower the payments. The lower the interest rate, the lower the payment.

PAYMENT SCHEDULES

When a banker decides on a loan, they will develop a schedule for the borrower to make payments. These payment schedules may take any of several basic forms. There are, of course, hybrids and combinations of the basic forms. As a rule, borrowers must make monthly payments unless specifically negotiated otherwise. If additional payments or payments that are larger than required by the loan contract are made, the extra amount should go toward reducing the principal. Make certain in the negotiation that this is the case.

AMORTIZATION SCHEDULE

A typical loan is paid off or amortized over time in a series of regular, equal payments called installments. An amortization schedule shows these installments and the amounts that are allocated to principal and interest within each payment. (Box 16.6 is an example of an amortization schedule. Amortization schedules are usually done on a monthly basis. Because of space constraints, an annual report is shown.) The amortization schedule points out several important things. The interest portion of a business loan is deductible as a normal business expense in the year in which it occurs. During the initial payment portion of the loan, most of the payment satisfies the interest needs rather than the principal. This creates a much larger tax benefit early in the amortization. As the borrower moves through the lifetime of the loan, a higher proportion of the payment is applied to the principal. The principal portion is not directly deductible. It is an asset that improves the balance sheet. The value of the asset can generally be deducted through depreciation. (To the extent that the principal represents the value of the asset purchased, the entire cost of the loan is deductible, either directly through the interest deduction or indirectly through depreciation of the asset.) Most depreciation methods load more of the depreciation expense earlier in the asset's lifetime. So, tax deductions decrease while a loan is amortized, although cash flow remains steady.

INTEREST ONLY

Some loans require interest-only payments for a certain period. Bankers often offer this facility to professionals and other new business owners. The bankers realize that it may take several months to get the business (or practice) up and running so that it is producing enough cash to pay the bills and the start-up loan. New practitioners frequently negotiate to pay the interest portion only of the normal payment for the first several months to a year to solve this problem. They still eventually pay the entire principal, but the principal has been put off until the borrower is, hopefully, better able to afford the cash flow needed for the entire payment. Box 16.8 show the effect of paying only the interest for the first year of a loan.

BALLOON PAYMENT

The second type of payment schedule is called a balloon payment. In this schedule, the borrower pays the entire principal at the end of the loan period. Often they must still pay interest monthly. Using a balloon payment allows the borrower to keep the payments as low as possible, although there is an additional risk at the end of the term that the borrower cannot make the entire balloon payment.

ACCELERATING DEBT PAYMENTS

As a rule, the faster debt is paid off, the fewer interest payments are made. Therefore, on the face of it, it is always a good thing to pay off debt as quickly as possible. However, there are several times when this rule of thumb may not be valid. Someone may need to stretch a debt payment out (thereby lowering each payment) to have an adequate cash flow for other budget expenses. Or they may have an incredibly low interest rate or generous terms on a loan that makes it attractive to keep.

A small additional payment makes a huge difference in the total loan payout. Box 16.9 shows what happens to the number of payments when the amount paid each month is increased. By simply adding $50 per month to a

BOX 16.8	EXAMPLE OF INTEREST ONLY FOR FIRST YEAR

Year	Total payment	Principal	Interest	Principal remaining
Interest-only in the first year option				
1	$27 000	$0	$27 000	$300 000
2	$77 128	$50 128	$27 000	$249 872
3	$77 128	$54 639	$22 489	$195 233
4	$77 128	$59 557	$17 571	$135 676
5	$77 128	$64 917	$12 211	$70 759
6	$77 128	$70 759	$6 368	$0
	$412 640	$300 000	$112 639	

Normal payment option

Year	Total payment	Principal	Interest	Principal remaining
1	$77 128	$50 128	$27 000	$249 872
2	$77 128	$54 639	$22 489	$195 233
3	$77 128	$59 557	$17 571	$135 676
4	$77 128	$64 917	$12 211	$70 759
5	$77 128	$70 759	$6 368	$0
	$385 640	$300 000	$85 639	

Assumptions:

Principal = $300 000
Term (1) = 1 year (interest only)
Term (2) = 5 years (normal schedule)
Interest rate = 9.0%

Dr. Jones buys a dental practice, securing an installment note for the amount shown. She has the option to pay interest only during the first year. Her annual (estimated) payments are given. (This loan would actually be compounded monthly.)

BOX 16.9	ACCELERATING DEBT PAYMENTS

		Additional principal payment			
		+$50	+$100	+$200	+$500
Normal payment	$1267	$1317	$1367	$1467	$1767
Years	10.0	9.4	8.9	8.0	6.2

Assumptions:

Principal = $100 000
Term = 10 years
Interest rate = 9%

The chart shows the effect of making a larger payment on the length of the loan. By adding additional principal to each payment, the loan is paid off much faster.

for the investment, invest rather than pay off the loan. If the after-tax interest rate of the loan is higher, then pay off the loan. There are several times when this rule does not apply. If someone needs to save for a particular purpose, then save or invest rather than pay off the loan. For example, if a person has adequate cash flow, they should establish an emergency fund, even if they have remaining debt on which payments are being made. A solid emergency fund is more important. They may be saving for a down payment on a house or other cash needs. Here the person may make the savings/investment rather than extra debt payments. Although many people have the admirable goal of being debt free, balancing the value of readily available cash assets and more debt with the position of no ready cash and less debt is more important. As a rule, one is better off with the available cash.

LEASE–PURCHASE DECISIONS

If a practice needs an asset (e.g. a new piece of equipment, office space, or an automobile), there are several ways to pay for it. It may purchase the asset outright with existing cash, replenishing the cash through lower future earnings. It can borrow money to buy the asset and then pay back the lender over time, or the asset can be leased, often with an option to purchase it at the end of the lease period. Each carries advantages and disadvantages.

If an asset is leased, the total cost of leasing is usually more than purchasing the same asset. The landlord or leasing company must borrow money, buy the asset, and then charge a higher interest rate to make a profit. If someone leases (or rents) the asset, the entire lease payment is (with certain exceptions) a tax deduction. The

10-year loan, the number of payments made is halved. (The principal paid remains the same, but it is paid more quickly, so less interest is paid.) Greater savings are seen with larger monthly additions. Most loans (especially mortgages) do not have prepayment penalties associated with paying all or a portion of the principal early. If the cash flow will support it, the borrower will come out ahead financially by making an extra principal payment as often as possible.

PAYING OFF DEBT EARLY OR INVESTING

To solve this problem from a purely financial perspective, the borrower should compare the after-tax interest rates of the loan and the investment. If the interest rate is higher

person does not own the asset at the end of the lease (unless they then purchase it).

If money is borrowed to purchase the asset, the person owns it, but they also incur a balancing liability (debt) to purchase the asset. The asset value may grow, remain the same, or decrease while the loan is being paid off. The cost of the interest for the loan is deductible. The cost of the asset is deducted through depreciation. If someone has enough cash to purchase the asset outright, they do not have any finance charges (interest) to pay, but they lose any investment gain that they could have made with the money. For example, assume someone can reasonably expect to make 10% after taxes on an investment, and a loan to buy the asset costs 6% after taxes. In this scenario, the person should borrow the money, earning the difference of 4% (10% – 6%). If, on the other hand, they are earning 4% on investments and a loan is at 10%, they are better off buying the asset outright and avoiding the interest charges.

Nearly half of all assets used by businesses today are leased. Dental practices lease equipment less frequently than general businesses do. The decision of whether to lease or buy is obviously one that astute business owners need to understand. There are both financial and nonfinancial reasons for someone choosing to lease or buy assets for the practice.

There are several types of leases, depending on what is being leased. A property lease occurs when a property owner allows a tenant to use a property for a defined rent payment for a defined time. This does not occur often in dentistry (except in office space leases). The entire lease payment is tax deductible if the property is used for business purposes. An operating or true lease is similar to a property lease (the equipment is rented). In operating leases, the lessee can deduct the full value of the lease payments, but because they do not own the asset, they cannot claim depreciation on the asset. Maintenance, upkeep, and often taxes on the equipment must still be paid, although they do not own the asset. A financing or capital lease is a method of paying for an asset more closely akin to gaining a bank loan. In this arrangement, a leasing company buys the asset someone wants and then leases it to them. Because the person owns the asset or equipment, they cannot claim the entire lease payment amount (only the interest portion) as a tax deduction. However, because they own the asset, they get to claim depreciation. There is no buy-out option at the end of the lease because they already own the asset. There are usually stiff prepayment penalties and even larger penalties if the person wants to break either an operating or a financing lease. Tax rules for leases can be complex and changing, so the practitioner should consult their accountant before signing any lease. The advantages and disadvantages of leasing and purchasing equipment are outlined in Box 16.10.

LEASING BY ASSET TYPE

There are three common areas in dentistry where the lease-or-buy decision occurs. This section discusses each of those.

Automobiles

Leases and purchase loans are two different methods of automobile financing. Each has its own benefits and drawbacks, depending on the person's circumstances, wants, and needs. A loan may finance the purchase of a vehicle. The borrower owns it and can drive it for as many miles as desired, with only the cost of additional maintenance and wear and tear to consider. The loan is based on the interest rate negotiated, generally based on the borrower's credit history. They can sell the vehicle at any time for its depreciated resale value, taking the gain or loss.

A lease finances only the use of a vehicle for a specified time. In a sense, the lessee only pays for the portion of the cost they use during the lease term. They pay a financial rate (the money factor or lease rate) similar to a loan's interest. It is generally a couple of percentage points higher than a comparable auto purchase interest rate, so the leasing company can profit from the difference. Credit requirements for leasing (e.g. credit score) are somewhat stricter than for purchase loans because of higher risks to the finance company. At the end of the lease, the automobile can be returned to the leasing company or it can be purchased for its depreciated resale (residual) value.

For example, if someone leases a $30 000 car with an estimated resale value of $20 000 after 24 months, they only pay for the difference, $10 000 (depreciation), finance charges, and fees. If, on the other hand, they purchase the same automobile, they pay the entire $30 000, finance charges, and possible fees (Box 16.11). This is the reason that leasing offers much lower monthly payments than buying. Leasing does not build equity; buying does. Leasing has lower monthly payments but no equity. In the short term, someone is better off financially leasing. In the long term, they are better off buying.

When an automobile is leased, there are several considerations. The lessee still pays for routine maintenance and any major repairs (such as wrecks) not covered by the automobile's warranty. (Therefore, the lessee must keep insurance on the vehicle.) The lessee may have to make a down payment (an origination fee) and other start-up costs for the lease. Leasing companies allocate a

BOX 16.10	ADVANTAGES AND DISADVANTAGES OF LEASING EQUIPMENT VERSUS PURCHASING EQUIPMENT

Option	Advantages	Disadvantages
Purchase		
	You own the asset	Asset may decrease in value
	Less expensive (in long run)	Uses up free money
	Depreciation and interest expense appears on balance sheet	Uses up borrowing ability
Buy with cash	No finance charges	Lose alternative use of money
Borrow and buy	Uses leverage (other people's money)	Interest expense (finance charge) may require down payment
Lease		
	Lower monthly expense	More total expense
	No down payment	
Property lease	Appears on profit-and-loss account (not balance sheet)	Do not own the asset
	Less initial expense	Have to make leasehold improvements
Operating lease	Payment is deductible	Do not own the asset
	Appears on profit-and-loss account (not balance sheet)	
	Option to purchase (often)	
Capital lease	Appears on balance sheet (not profit-and-loss account)	
	Depreciation and interest expense	
	May have favorable terms	

BOX 16.11	LEASING VERSUS BORROWING FOR AN AUTOMOBILE

	Lease	Loan
Car price	$30 000	$30 000
Down payment	$2 000	$2 000
Residual value	$18 000	N/A
Amount financed	$10 000	$28 000
Months	36	36
Interest rate	7.5%	6.0%
Monthly payment	**$311.06**	**$851.81**

A person wants a $30 000 automobile. They can lease it for three years (7.5% money factor) with an $18 000 residual value or can purchase it at 6% interest.

certain number of miles to the lease, for example two years and 25 000 miles. That means if the lessee drives more than 25 000 miles during the two-year lease, they pay a hefty penalty (generally 15–25 cents per mile above 25 000 miles) when the lease ends. If they drive less, they do not get a rebate. A lease cannot generally be canceled early without substantial penalties. If the person does not like the car, too bad; they are stuck with it for the term of the lease. Even if their needs change or they decide the car is junk, unless they are willing to pay substantial penalties, the car is theirs for the term of the lease. New cars are generally the only ones leased. Automobiles that hold their value as used cars are better lease candidates than those that depreciate quickly. (The leasing company has less residual value to sell at the end of the lease with a quickly depreciating type of automobile.) A lessee can drive a nicer car for a smaller monthly payment than purchasing, although they have nothing at the end of the lease term. Despite leasing company hype, tax savings are about the same for leasing or buying. The person has the option of buying the car at the end of the lease for the residual (remaining) value If that is what they want to do, but simply buying the car from the beginning is less expensive. Dentists should buy or lease through the practice. (See Chapter 17 for a discussion.)

There really are two situations in which a practitioner should consider a lease. If they get a new car every two or three years, then it is financially better to lease. This way, they always have an automobile under warranty and do not have to worry about buying and selling used cars. If they plan to own the car for many years (or even run it until the "wheels fall off"), it is financially advantageous to buy. The other time when leasing may be an advantage is when they cannot afford the down payment or regular payments required of an automobile purchase. Here, they can lease a better car for a lower monthly payment. However, at the end of the lease, they do not have any equity and have to start over with a new lease or purchase. They never get to the point where they do not have an automobile loan payment. They should consider driving a less expensive type of car as an alternative.

OFFICE SPACE

Many dentists lease office space. In this arrangement, the person or company that owns the property (lessor, landlord) sells the right to use the property (lease) to the tenant (lessee). In return, the lessee pays rent to the landlord. Leases have a term or length associated with them, which may be one to many years. Although a short-term lease allows the lessee to move at the end of the term, most dentists have trouble simply picking up the office and moving it because of equipment, plumbing, and other office design needs and because patients get used to a particular location. So, most dentists negotiate longer-term leases (more years), often with options to renew. This also gives them a known future cash flow.

In theory, all lease arrangements are negotiable. Mostly, negotiating power is based on local market conditions. The lessee has more leverage if there are many empty commercial properties similar to the one being negotiated on. A tighter local market favors the landlords. With larger developments, landlords are often reluctant to allow an individual lessee privilege for fear that other lessees will ask for similar considerations. In an ideal world, a business owner will have two or more acceptable office spaces and be able to negotiate with each potential landlord over specific terms and items of the lease. In the real world,

the business owner must be prepared to walk away if the landlord does not meet their bottom-line terms.

There are several common types of commercial lease arrangements when leasing office space. These are named based on how the landlord charges tenants. A gross lease is a property lease in which the lessee pays the landlord rent. The landlord then pays all expenses associated with the property, such as utilities, repairs, insurance, and (often) taxes. A net lease requires the lessee to pay some costs associated with the property. (The landlord only receives, as rent, the portion of the payment that is net of expenses.) Several versions of net leases exist, the most common being the triple net lease. In a triple net lease, the lessee pays rent to the landlord, all taxes, insurance, and maintenance expenses associated with using the property. The landlord then passes all ownership expenses on to the lessees, protecting themselves (in part) from losses. Where there are several tenants in a property (such as an office building), the costs are usually pro-rated among the tenants based on the square footage leased. In this type of lease, the rent amount will change as the landlord's taxes, insurance, and maintenance costs change (usually increase). One contentious issue is often heating and air-conditioning repair or replacement. These can be large-ticket items that landlords typically assign to tenants in net leases.

The dentist should check out the local market to negotiate the lease amount effectively. Most leases are quoted on a dollar amount per square foot leased per year. For example, a landlord may quote a 2000 sq. ft. office at $15.00 per sq. ft. This means that the lessee will pay $30 000 per year (2000 sq. ft. × $15.00) or $2500 per month ($30 000/12 months) in rent. Most landlords want to include an annual price increase in the lease. If so, the lessee should insist on the increase being capped so that they will know how much they will have to pay in the future.

Tenant improvements are a large expense with most dental office leases. These include interior walls, cabinets and counters, special plumbing (e.g. vacuum, compressed air, nitrous oxide, oxygen, etc.), bracing for wall-mounted equipment, routine carpet, paint, and lighting. The cost of these improvements, even in a modest office, can easily run into hundreds of thousands of dollars. As a rule, the tenant pays for these "leasehold improvements." Often landlords will offer a modest amount of leasehold improvement cost within the lease terms, not realizing the extent of the improvements needed to establish a dental office. (If a dentist is looking at a site that was previously a dental office, many of these improvements may have already been made.) A negotiating point may be to have the landlord provide some or all of these improvements, writing their cost into the price of the lease. This saves the lessor from borrowing money for improvements, taking their costs from their capital and putting those costs instead into operating costs (the lease). This also allows the lessee to expense the costs over the term of the lease (say, 5 years) instead of depreciating them over 15 years if they pay them upfront. Dentists should note that if the lease is extended beyond the initial term, they have the cost of these improvements negotiated out of the cost of the ongoing lease.

It is important to try to get the right to sublease the space written into the lease. If the lessee wants to leave, they can then lease the space to someone else for the duration of the contract. (This gives them more flexibility, but is not a required lease term.) A potential lessee should be sure to check their ability to put up visible signs that identify their office. Many developments restrict the size or types of signs permitted for lessees. A lessee may negotiate other terms, such as being the only dentist in the development, if that is an advantage to them.

An obvious financial issue for a dentist is when they should lease office space and when they should buy or build it. There are both financial and non-financial issues at work here. From a financial perspective, purchasing is usually better than leasing, if the person is to stay in the same location for many (10 or more) years. Mortgage payments are usually fixed over time, unlike lease payments. The owner can depreciate the cost of the building and contents (but not land) over 39 years and deduct the cost of interest associated with office real estate. Although the entire cost of the lease is deductible, it may be more than the total cost of purchase. At the end of the time, with the purchase option, the dentist will have an asset (the real estate) that they can sell, hopefully at a profit.

Other considerations relate less to financial trade-offs. One is a personal choice. Many dentists do not want the headaches of property ownership. Others want the control and independence associated with ownership. Young dentists especially may not have the financial resources needed to buy commercial real estate. Most banks will lend 75–90% of the appraised value of a property. The borrower must then come up with 10–25% as a down payment. If they cannot, purchasing is simply not an option. Availability is always a question too. There may not be acceptable properties for either rent or purchase when and where the dentist is looking, although with the purchase option they may be able to find the right place and make changes to turn it into exactly what they want. Particularly with stand-alone dental offices, the eventual sale of the building and practice can be a problem. Because of the extensive remodeling, the building can only be used as a dental practice without a large expense. Selling a dental practice without its location lowers the value of the practice considerably. If the dentist cannot find a qualified buyer, they may be in the landlord business for a long while.

OFFICE EQUIPMENT

Most equipment leases in dental practices are operating leases for specific pieces of equipment. Dental suppliers often have purchase or lease "deals" for their clients. They may offer no down payments, favorable interest rates, or other inducements to purchase or lease the equipment. Practitioners should look at the terms and conditions of any purchase or lease deal carefully and consult their accountant.

A dentist should consider leasing equipment if they are already deeply in debt and banks are unwilling to lend them more money. Leasing companies often offer more flexible terms (e.g. graduated payments) than banks. Although lease contracts are more flexible, they are also more complex, so there can be more hidden pitfalls. Another reason to lease is that the practitioner may not have money for a down payment (often 20% or more of the price) required by a bank. Or they may have the money but want to hold it as a cushion in case they need it in the future. A lease does not appear on a credit report or balance sheet like a loan does. The payment is taken from operating capital, so a lease may be a good option if the dentist is profitable but greatly in debt. Finally, some aggressive tax strategies involve putting business property (real estate or equipment) in family partnerships and then leasing it back to shift income into family members' lower taxes.

Business Taxes and Tax Planning

Over and over again courts have said that there is nothing sinister in so arranging one's affairs so as to keep taxes as low as possible. Everybody does it, rich or poor, and all do right, for nobody owes any public duty to pay more than the law demands; taxes are enforced exactions, not voluntary contributions. To demand more in the name of morals is mere cant.

Justice Learned Hand, US Supreme Court, 1947

GOAL

This chapter will cover the tax obligations of the business owner. The methods and timing of tax compliance will be discussed, as well as various methods that the business owner can use to minimize the tax burden and potential problems with taxing agencies.

LEARNING OBJECTIVES

At the completion of this chapter, the student will be able to:

- Differentiate between a tax deduction and a tax credit.

- Describe depreciation as applied to a dental practice.

- Differentiate between deductible and non-deductible expenses for operating a dental practice.

- Discuss business taxes that impact a dental practice.

- Apply the basic principles of tax planning to a dental practice.

- Discuss the effect of the business entity on tax obligations.

KEY TERMS

179 election	business income tax formula	checkbook
accounts receivable	business loan payment	commission
ad valorem taxes	capital asset	constructive receipt
amortization	capital gain	cost of goods sold
audit	capital loss	cost of operations
automobile expenses	cash basis accounting	deduction

Business Basics for Dentists, Second Edition. James L. Harrison, David O. Willis, and Charles K. Thieman.
© 2024 John Wiley & Sons, Inc. Published 2024 by John Wiley & Sons, Inc.

depletion
depreciation
employee benefit plans
employee taxes
Employer Identification
Number (EIN)
FICA
Form W-2
gross income
gross receipts

income
Kiddie Tax
mandates
marginal tax rates
pass-through entity
profit
recapture
relicensure fee
returns and allowances
sales and usage taxes

Schedule C
state income taxes
tax credit
tax withholding
taxable income
temporary services
unemployment insurance
unwithheld expenses
workers' compensation
insurance

This chapter presents the common taxes that businesses pay. It only discusses federal taxes. Many states and municipalities have similar, additional taxes if the practitioner is practicing in their authority. These taxes also follow the same principles outlined here, but the specific implementation of those principles and rules may differ. An accountant will help compute and report these taxes.

Tax laws and rates change frequently depending on governmental priorities and values. Taxes are not solely a revenue generator but also serve politicians to make a political statement. When politicians say "Big companies need to pay their fair share" or "We want to help small businesses," they are making political, not governmental, financial statements. Tax laws, then, change for reasons other than purely revenue generation.

This chapter does not give specific tax advice or rates. Instead, it gives an overview of business taxes. Depending on the type of business entity, business owners will report these taxes to the government differently. The basic tax principles remain the same, though, regardless of the entity. Business owners report income and deductions, depreciate equipment, and pay employer-related taxes. An accountant will complete forms and do other paperwork for the business owner. However, the business owner needs to understand the principles to communicate effectively with their accountant and other advisors.

THE BASIC BUSINESS INCOME TAX FORMULA

The general business formula for determining profit or loss is the basis for Schedule C, partnership, or corporate income tax returns (Box 17.1). The prototype, Schedule C, is the tax form that an individual proprietor uses to report profit or loss from operating a business, such as a dental practice. If someone practices as a partnership or a corporation, they report this information in a different form,

| **BOX 17.1** | **BUSINESS TAXES – GENERAL FORMULA** |

Gross receipts
 – Returns and allowances
 – Cost of goods sold and/or operations

 = Gross income
 – Deductions

 = Profit or (Loss)

This chart gives the general formula for determining profit or loss from operating a business.

but it contains similar information. Only income and expenses relating to this business should appear on this schedule. If someone has more than one business, they will file a different form for each of them. (Multiple dental office locations are generally considered to be one business.)

- **Gross receipts**

 Gross receipts are the actual amount of money the practice collects, because most dentists use a cash basis for accounting. (If a practice owner uses an accrual basis, they must adjust this number.) This is not how much dentistry someone produced, but how much they collected in cash, patient checks, insurance checks, and capitation payments.

- **Returns and allowances**

 If a dentist refunds money to an individual or third-party payer (for an overpayment), they need to record it as a "return." They have already received this money and accounted for it as a gross receipt. In this section of the form, they take it back off gross receipts if the situation warrants it.

- **Cost of goods sold and/or operations**
  This metric is different for businesses that produce or sell a product (such as a dress shop) and businesses that provide a service (like dentistry). Product-based businesses have a cost of goods sold (COGS), while service businesses use a cost of operations (COO). Generally, both show how much a company spends on producing or providing its primary product or service. This does not include general business costs such as rent, front-office employees, or utilities. So, a product-based company would include the cost of raw materials, inventory costs, and labor for production. A service company would include direct labor for providing a service (e.g. the assistant or hygienist), dental supplies and materials, lab costs, and operatory equipment costs.

- **Gross income**
  Gross income is gross receipts reduced by any returns and the COO.

- **Deductions**
  Deductions are the costs of doing business that are not a direct cost of goods or operations. They include office rent, advertising, accounting, legal fees, and management salaries. All non-operating costs, such as interest and capital expenditures, are not costs of providing the services and so are included here. If an item is a capital expense (it lasts longer than a year), the business depreciates it, and that depreciation expense for the year is a deduction.

- **Profit or loss**
  The profit or loss is how much money is left after a practice collects fees and pays the costs of running the business for the year. If collections are greater than expenses, the result is a profit. If expenses are greater than collections, then the result is a loss.

PRINCIPLES OF BUSINESS TAXATION

The principles of business tax planning remain the same from year to year. Specific rules, amounts, and thresholds change constantly, however. Congress ties some to the inflation rate. It changes others as it attempts to affect social policy and the economy. If someone understands the principles, specific changes will make more sense and be easier to implement.

INCOME

The Internal Revenue Service (IRS) has a simple rule concerning whether money made is "income" or not for tax purposes. It considers any money made to be taxable unless it has made a waiver for that specific type of income in the tax codes. By this definition, almost any income gained by the dental practice is taxable. This includes collections from patient payments, money paid by insurance companies, capitation payments, interest or dividends earned, the gain from the sale of assets owned by the practice, the value of trade or barter, and rebates. (This does not include money that the practice borrows.) Some business entities (C corporations) pay income tax on any profits in the business at the end of the tax year. Others (proprietorships, partnerships, S Corps, and limited liability companies [LLCs]) do not pay income tax, but let income and deductions flow through to the individual owners. The tax forms from these flow-through entities tell the IRS who received money for the year. The IRS then checks to be sure that the individual has claimed the right amount of income on their individual tax return.

After the practice pays for the costs of doing business, the profit goes to the owner or employee of the business. The owner or employee then pays individual income tax on it. This includes profit from a proprietorship or partnership (self-employment income), wages paid from an employer (proprietor or corporation), bonuses paid, profit-sharing, and sometimes excessive employee benefits. The taxpayer must report the type of income because the IRS taxes it all differently. Ordinary income is the same as earned income. This money is from working. Individuals pay income taxes and Federal Insurance Contributions Act (FICA) or Self-Employment Contributions Act (SECA) taxes on earned income. Investment income (e.g. capital gains, interest, or dividends) is unearned income. The IRS taxes it at a lower rate. Because it was not earned, individuals do not pay FICA or SECA taxes on this type of income. Tax laws and rates frequently change at the whim of Congress. So this text does not include specific rates or amounts. Practice owners should check with their accountants for the current tax rates.

Most dental practices fall under the cash basis accounting rules. This means that someone realizes income when they take constructive receipt of it. Therefore, they only pay taxes when they have control of the income and can use it for whatever purpose they desire. For example, assume a patient has a bill for $1200. They pay $800 on December 31 of year X1 and the remainder ($400) on January 2 of the year X2. The practice owner pays income tax on $800 of income in year X1 and pays tax on $400 in year X2, the year they constructively received it. By this definition, the practice owner pays no income taxes on accounts receivable because they are not income until patients pay them. (It is not income until the check crosses the receptionist's desk.) Some large practices use accrual-based accounting rules. These are accounting rules that most large corporations follow. Accrual-based accounting causes income and expense recognition problems that do not favor the practice, so most use the cash basis rules.

If the practice owner sells a practice or a component of the practice (such as dental operatory equipment), they receive money for the asset(s). The IRS calls this money either a capital gain or ordinary income, depending on the circumstances. The difference is important, because a different tax rate applies to the two types of income. This leads to some obvious tax-planning issues, which are discussed later in this chapter.

BUSINESS DEDUCTIONS

Definition

A deduction is an expense that is a cost of operating or maintaining the practice. The dentist may need to prove the amount and necessity of this business expense to the IRS, so they need to keep a receipt and canceled check for the item. They must be sure to keep excellent records. Canceled checks, by themselves, are not enough documentation.

The IRS considers no expense to be deductible unless it has specifically granted deductibility in the tax codes. Common dental office deductions are listed in Box 17.2. For a business expense to be deductible, it must meet *all* the following criteria:

- It must be "ordinary," which means that it is common to other taxpayers in similar situations.

- It must be "necessary," which means that it is helpful in the conduct of a trade or business.

- It must be "reasonable in amount," which means that any other taxpayer would pay a similar amount for a similar good or service.

- It is *not* a personal expense (separate business from personal expenses).

- It is *not* a capital expenditure (accounted for as depreciation).

- It does *not* relate to tax-exempt income.

The IRS expects everyone to follow these rules for deductions when they file their income tax for the year. However, the only way the IRS knows for sure that someone has followed the rules is if it audits that person and finds a problem. Therefore, many taxpayers take a risk, get away with breaking the tax rules, and do not get caught. This is a risky

practice. If the IRS catches that person, there are substantial fines, penalties, and interest payments. They might even receive a prison sentence for gross or willful tax cheating. The IRS recently increased the audit rate on high-income individuals (such as dentists), decreasing the chances of getting away with breaking the law. Accountants are very reluctant to advocate any tax reporting that does not strictly follow the tax laws. Their accounting licenses could easily be in jeopardy.

APPLICATION

There are several common issues to consider about deductions:

- Expenses in getting to be a practicing dentist (or any other *new* occupation) are not deductible. Therefore, expenses for dental education and the first state board exam are not deductible. The IRS considers a specialty to be a new occupation, so those expenses are not deductible. (Dentists frequently challenge this point in the tax courts.) The costs associated with setting up a practice are deductible.

- Expenses incurred for maintaining an occupation or profession are a required expense of doing business and are, therefore, deductible. Relicensure fees, continuing education expenses, dues, professional books, and publications are all deductible once someone is a practicing dentist. They may deduct the costs of taking another licensing exam after they earn an initial license.

- Business loan payments are not directly deductible. The interest paid on a business loan is a cost of business and is therefore deductible. The principal portion of the loan payment represents a long-term asset. The value of the asset itself is deducted indirectly through depreciation.

- It never pays to incur an expense to "get a deduction." If it is an expense someone would take anyway, then that expense ought to be structured so that it is deductible. The deductibility of an expense only lowers the cost to the taxpayer, it does not eliminate it.

- The first step in maximizing deductions is to learn which items are deductible, so as not to miss one or more authorized deductions. Examples of deductible and non-deductible expenses for the dental office are in Box 17.2.

- The marginal tax rate influences the value of a deduction. (Chapter 10 describes the marginal tax rate.) A $1000 deduction in the 15% marginal tax bracket translates into a $150 tax saving. Conversely, the expense only "costs" someone $850 ($1000 − $150) instead of the full $1000. That same deduction in a 28% marginal tax bracket translates into a $280 saving.

BOX 17.2	COMMON DEDUCTIBLE AND NON-DEDUCTIBLE EXPENSES

Deductible expenses	Non-deductible expenses
Lease payments	Loan payments
Professional supplies	Mileage to office from home
Office supplies	Cost of land
Stamps	Disability insurance premiums paid
Stationery	Amounts uncollected from patients
Printing costs	Personal draw
Advertising	
Phone bills (utilities)	
Lab bills	
Malpractice Insurance	
Employee wages, taxes, worker's compensation, unemployment insurance	
Office insurance policies	
Continuing education	
Office taxes	
Mileage from office to lab, post office, etc.	
Interest on office loans	
Depreciation	
Collection costs	
Relicensure fees	
Magazine subscriptions	

- When establishing a checkbook register, the practice owner should be sure to establish categories that are the same as appear on Schedule C (business tax form). This makes tax time much easier in that they do not need to go back over all receipts and categorize them for tax purposes. They have already been allocated to proper categories. The owner uses the year-end totals. This also makes practice cost analysis much easier and more effective.

CAPITAL ASSETS AND DEPRECIATION

Definition

Some business purchases are assets that last for several years. These are "capital" assets of the business. For example, a dental chair will last for several years and a building for many years. Tax law says that because those capital assets have a lifetime greater than one year, the taxpayer must spread out the deduction for the expense of that item over the estimated "useful lifetime" of the asset. (The IRS has a list of asset categories that tells the useful lifetime of most assets.) If the IRS says that a dental chair ought to last

seven years, then the taxpayer can logically deduct one-seventh of the value of the dental chair each year. Another way to think of depreciation is wear and tear on long-term assets. By this definition, the dental chair "wears out" over its useful lifetime of seven years. The taxpayer writes off the cost of the chair over the same period.

- **Depreciation** is the term used for hard, tangible assets.

- **Amortization** refers to the depreciation of intangible assets. Intangible assets may also have a useful lifetime or wear out over time. For example, a restrictive covenant that lasts for three years has a three-year lifetime.

- **Depletion** similarly refers to natural resources, such as timber or coal deposits, that decrease in value as they are "used up."

Application

Depreciation is a complex tax subject that the practice owner's accountant will compute. The business owner ought to understand depreciation to plan appropriate financial strategies with their accountant. Some points they need to consider about depreciation are the following:

- The depreciation deduction starts the tax year the taxpayer places the asset into business service and occurs each year after that according to the depreciation law in effect in the first year. The IRS allows several accounting methods to set an asset's depreciation (wear and tear). These depreciation methods include:
  1. Straight line.
  2. Double (200%) declining balance.
  3. Modified accelerated cost recovery system (MACRS).

- As a rule, the alternative methods (2 and 3) speed up the deduction for depreciation over the straight-line method (1). A person gets a larger portion of the depreciation in the early years and less in later years with these accelerated methods. They do not need to know how to calculate these amounts, just that several methods exist that generally speed up the deduction.

- The business owner should discuss with their accountant whether to speed up depreciation deductions. The MACRS method loads the deductions much more heavily on the front end. That is fine if someone estimates that their income will be steady over the next several years. They will gain more of a tax saving immediately. However, if their income will be significantly higher in the future (as, for example, with practice growth), they may want to defer those depreciation deductions until they are in a higher tax bracket, thereby getting more "bang" for the depreciation expense. In the straight-line method, the person trades off the certainty of an immediate deduction for the possible higher value of a future deduction. They might find that later in the asset's life they have a cash-flow problem, in that they are still paying the loan for the asset (primarily principal) although they have used all the depreciation deduction for it.

- When someone puts an asset into service during the year affects how much depreciation they can deduct in the first year. If they buy an asset in January, they get to claim much more of a full deduction than if they buy it in December. The IRS also has several methods for calculating this amount. An accountant will do that. A business owner needs to know that they may not receive the entire deduction the first year when buying a large asset.

- Disposable assets (those used up within one year, such as dental supplies) are a deduction in the year purchased. They are not depreciated.

- Land does not "wear out" over time, so taxpayers do not depreciate it. Buildings do wear out over time. If someone buys a building and land, the appropriate percentages of the cost of each must be allocated, depreciating the building but not the land.

- A business may depreciate any piece of equipment that they purchase, even if it is used and someone else has already depreciated it. It is essentially "new" to the business for which it has a new useful lifetime. An asset may be depreciated as many times as it is bought. The sale price determines how much depreciation someone claims. The previous owner is subject to a capital gain or loss and recapture.

- If someone sells an asset that they have previously depreciated, they might be subject to "recapture" rules, meaning that the business must recapture any previously reported depreciation as income. For example, if a dentist bought a dental chair for $7000, then depreciated it (straight line) for three years of its seven-year life, they are telling the IRS that the chair is now worth $4000 ($7000 − 3 years × 1/7 × $7000). If that person sells that same chair for $5000, they have made a book profit or "capital gain" of $1000 ($5000 − $4000). The person must "recapture" this depreciation expense and claim the gain on this capital investment as ordinary income, which is a higher tax rate than a capital gain. This frequently happens in practice sales, where the seller has fully depreciated the assets of the practice.

- As a rule, any "high-tech" equipment for the dental office (computers, lasers, etc.) is a five-year property. Other dental equipment (chair, compressor, etc.) is a seven-year property. There is some capital equipment that does not fall neatly into these categories. Remember, these are IRS rules for depreciation. They do not mean that the actual "useful lifetime" is the same as the IRS lifetime. A business can use the equipment for as long as it meets its needs.

- Congress periodically enacts special tax rules to encourage businesses to purchase assets. One of these rules allows a business to immediately expense (take the value in year 1) the value of assets instead of claiming the value over several years through normal depreciation. (This is the "179 Election" because it refers to that tax code section.) According to these rules, someone may elect to expense (take in year 1) the deduction for many depreciable assets. This election can be an advantage for small business owners if they want to increase current deductions at the expense of future ones. That person may elect to deduct 0–100% of the allowable amount in year 1 of the asset and depreciate the balance. However, the problems are the same in choosing a depreciation method. Early in a practice's life, the owner may find it more advantageous to push those depreciation deductions into later years, when they can claim a larger dollar deduction. Congress frequently changes the rules on this deduction (including the maximum amount and the size of qualifying business).

- Depreciation is a "non-cash" write-off. This does not mean that a person writes a check that lists "depreciation" as the payee, but that they claim the expense for depreciation on their income statement. The person has taken the expensing write-off but has not paid any cash. This leads to differences between the income statement and cash-flow statement.

- If someone uses an asset for personal and business use (such as an automobile), they must allocate the proportion for each use. They then take as depreciation the portion they use for business.

TAX CREDITS

Tax credits are like deductions, but they are even more valuable. A deduction lowers income, and by that lowers tax. A tax credit is a dollar-for-dollar reduction in tax.

Congress often uses tax credits to encourage individuals and businesses to do certain things. For example, the government has had tax credits to encourage employee retention, remodel buildings for disabled accessibility, encourage paid family leave, and promote health insurance premiums. The list of credits changes frequently. Many apply to specific industries (e.g. electric cars, or railroads). Many are designed for small businesses, including dentistry. The practice's accountant will be aware of the list of credits. They can help decide if the credit is appropriate and useful for a particular situation.

NON-INCOME TAXES (MANDATES)

Governmental agencies also require business owners to comply with regulations written and enforced by the governing body. These mandates result in a hidden tax to which a business person must respond. A common current example is the Occupational Safety and Health Administration (OSHA), which requires that dentists (and other businesses) meet certain safety standards regarding the operation of the workplace. The business owner must finance the cost of these mandates, although no true "tax" is levied or paid. Other examples include the Health Insurance Portability and Accountability Act (HIPAA), family leave, and vaccination mandates.

EMPLOYER TAXES

A business owner will probably hire employees (98% of practicing dentists have one or more employees). If someone hires employees, they have another area of tax to be concerned about: employer taxes. An employer must withhold tax from each employee's paycheck, report the amount to the employee, and then send this withheld amount to the appropriate government agency. Chapter 27 details these taxes. The responsibilities of an employer are listed here. As before, an accountant or bookkeeper will help a business owner establish systems to pay and account for these taxes.

BUSINESS OWNER RESPONSIBILITIES

Any business that has employees must follow several rules enacted by the federal government. Some states and local authorities have additional requirements.

Obtain and Use an Employer Identification Number

If a business has employees, it must obtain, by application, an Employer Identification Number (EIN). There is one for federal and others for state and local tax reporting. (A federal number is often used for all; check the rules in each locality.) Once a business has an EIN, the taxing agency will automatically send it yearly instructions, rates, forms, and tables. The business owner uses this number when paying and reporting employer taxes.

Verify Employee Eligibility to Work

A US employer cannot hire individuals who are not authorized to work in the United States. So, they must verify an employee's immigration status. An IRS form (I-9) that the employer and the employee complete verifies the employee's status. The employer must do this after the person is employed, not before.

Withhold Income Taxes from Employees' Paychecks

A business owner must withhold a certain portion of the income from each employee's check. They then send this money to the government monthly. At the end of the year, each employee computes their actual tax liability and compares it to the amount withheld along the way. If an employer withholds too much, the employee gets a refund. If an employer does not withhold enough, the employee pays the difference. The IRS has tables to use when calculating withholdings. If state or local governments impose income taxes, they also provide tables and forms. Payroll software is updated annually to reflect changing tax withholding requirements.

Withhold FICA Tax from Employees' Paychecks

FICA includes the old-age, survivors', and disability insurance taxes, also known as Social Security taxes, and the hospital insurance tax, also known as Medicare taxes. These are employment taxes (tax on earned income) that fund these federal programs. Employers withhold this tax from employees' pay, similarly to income tax. Presently, the combined Social Security/Medicare tax is a flat amount (7.65%). There are upper limits on the Social Security tax portion.

Match FICA Taxes

An employer must match the FICA tax withheld with an equal amount from the practice. Presently, the total tax is about 15.3% (7.65% from the employee and 7.65% from the employer) for most employees. Again, there are upper limits on the matching Social Security tax portion.

Report Wage and Withholding Information to the Employee

Employers must report earnings and the amount of tax they withheld to each employee (or former employee) by February 1 of the following year. This report (Form W-2) details the employee's earnings and the amounts withheld for the previous year so that the employee can accurately complete their personal tax returns. The employer sends a copy to the government so that the government can check that the employee claims the proper amount. State and local taxing agencies have similar forms.

Report and Pay Withheld Amounts to Government Agencies

The employer pays the federal government the income taxes it withheld from employees' paychecks. The payment frequency depends on the size of the withholding (federal + FICA). Most practice owners make these payments monthly online at a special federal tax payment website. The IRS electronically debits (takes) this money from a business checking account. The IRS levies significant penalties if an employer misses a payment or filing date, even by one day. State and local governments have their own procedures for reporting and paying employee withholdings, so check with an accountant about setting up these payment mechanisms.

UNWITHHELD EXPENSES FOR THE EMPLOYER

Three items cost the employer money beyond wages for each employee. Legally, an employer may not withhold money from employees' checks to pay for these costs. Therefore, they are called "unwithheld" expenses.

Workers' Compensation Insurance

An employer must have this insurance before it hires any employees. The employer gets the insurance policy from a private carrier, paying an annual premium. These insurers must register with the state. The insurance covers job-related accidents and illnesses.

Unemployment Insurance

The state unemployment insurance program (SUTA) and the federal unemployment insurance program (FUTA) have coordinated state and federal unemployment insurance programs. This is really a tax, although it also has some characteristics of insurance. The state portion of the program requires quarterly reporting and payment. Typical total rates are around 2–3% of gross wages (on the first $8000 per employee), although this varies by state. The employer pays taxes separately to the state and federal governments.

Matching Portion of Social Security and Medicare Tax

As described previously, an employer withholds a portion (currently 7.65%) of employees' pay for Social Security and Medicare tax. An employer must also match that with an equal amount. The matching portion is unwithheld.

MISCELLANEOUS EMPLOYEE TAX ISSUES

There are several miscellaneous issues regarding employee taxes.

Commission

An employer may use a commission as a basis for pay, but only for dentists and hygienists (professional staff). If an associate dentist is an independent contractor, then the owner reports to the IRS income paid by the employer to the associate. The payee must file a Schedule C or otherwise account for income and self-employment taxes. If the associate has "employee" status, the practice owner withholds and reports commission employees as other payment methods. Depending upon the state employment law, a practice owner might pay a hygienist a commission.

Temporary Services

Businesses often contract temporary services through a temporary placement agency. The temporary worker is under contract with the temporary agency, not the employer. As such, the employer does not have to withhold taxes, match FICA, participate in a retirement plan, or be responsible for any of the other unwithheld expenses normally associated with employees. The temporary service agency is responsible, and it passes those costs on to a business when it uses temporary staff. If an employer uses someone long term (i.e. staff leasing), the IRS views that person as a bona fide employee, and the rules change.

Hiring a Spouse or Child

An employer can hire a spouse or child to work in the office. The employer gains certain tax advantages by doing this. The rules are different for spouses and children. To deduct the expenses for hiring a close relative (spouse or child), the employer must meet the following four tests:

- The service must be ordinary and necessary for the business operation.

- The fee charged must be reasonable or similar to what other dentists would pay for comparable services.

- The payment must be for a service actually performed. If the service was not done or was done by someone else, the employer may not deduct the payment.

- The money must change hands. That means the employer must write a check (or use another payment mechanism) and the relative must cash it.

If an employer hires a spouse, they can deduct the full cost of reasonable wages. These wages are subject to FICA taxes (if the employer is a corporation or partnership), which makes the spouse eligible for Social Security benefits for which they might otherwise not qualify. (Unincorporated doctors currently do not pay FICA taxes on their spouses or children.) The spouse is also eligible for employee benefit plans offered through the office. This way, an employer may take the full deduction for medical insurance premiums paid for the family. These wages are subject to all applicable income taxes, so the employer must do full withholding, just as if the relative were a normal employee. Tax rules in this area are complex, so the business owner needs to work with the accountant to ensure compliance.

If an employer hires one of their children, the employer gains some tax advantage for the family. (This must be a job for which the child is reasonably qualified.) A limited amount of the salary is taxed at the child's low rate. However, most are taxed at the parent owner's higher rate. The same goes for assets transferred to children (the "Kiddie Tax"). This is an area that the IRS looks at closely. The business owner needs to work carefully with an accountant to ensure compliance.

OTHER BUSINESS TAXES

Some areas have other business taxes.

STATE SALES AND USAGE TAX (SALES TAX)

Some states require vendors to charge sales tax on all services (including dentistry). Others require that a business owner pay this type of tax on items purchased from out-of-state vendors. Because in-state purchases already have paid sales taxes, this includes only purchases from out-of-state vendors. Examples of taxable items if purchased from an out-of-state vendor might include dental supplies, lab bills (materials only), printing services, and magazine subscriptions.

AD VALOREM TAXES

Ad valorem taxes are property taxes on the assets of the business. Generally, local taxing agencies levy them. As a rule, practice owners pay these yearly. Depending on the particular jurisdiction, assets may include financial items such as accounts receivable and "hard" assets of the practice, such as dental equipment.

EFFECT OF BUSINESS ENTITY

Depending on the business entity, an employer will pay and account for taxes differently. The total tax liability is generally the same. The difference is in whose name they are paid.

PROPRIETORSHIP

If someone is a proprietor, they are the business. They pay all employee taxes under their name and EIN. They pay any property or other taxes under their name as well. Because the employer is not an employee, the proprietorship does not withhold income taxes. Instead, the owner estimates their tax liability and prepays it quarterly to the IRS. They file a Schedule C along with personal Form 1040 to report profit from the practice as income. They pay SETA on earned income. Losses pass down to the owner personally and offset other forms of income.

PARTNERSHIP

If the owner is a partner, they report and pay employee taxes under the partnership's EIN. Like a proprietorship, the person estimates and prepays personal income taxes. The partnership will provide an information return to the IRS that details how much each partner reports for income and expenses related to the business. The owner pays SETA on earned income, and losses flow through to their personal return, according to the partnership agreement.

CORPORATION

A corporation is a separate tax entity. The corporation reports and pays employment taxes under the corporation's EIN. The dentist is an employee of the corporation. Therefore, the corporation withholds tax from the dentist's paycheck, similarly to all other practice employees. The corporation withholds FICA taxes and matches them, like other employees. The corporation then issues a W-2 at the end of the year that details how much the employee earned. If the dentist is an owner of the corporation, they may also receive dividends from the profit of the corporation. This is unearned income (not subject to Social Security and Medicare taxes), but the C corporation pays it from the after-tax profit of the corporation. If the C corporation has a loss or tax credit, it does not pass down to shareholders. Instead, it stays at the corporation level.

PASS-THROUGH ENTITY (S *CORPORATION*, LIMITED LIABILITY COMPANY)

S corporations and limited liability companies (LLCs) are separate entities that have elected to be taxed as a partnership. Pass-through entities do not pay income taxes. Instead, they divide profit or loss among the shareholders (members) who report these on their individual tax returns. (The term pass-through refers to the portion of the corporation's income, losses, deductions, or credits that passes through to the shareholder.) If income is a wage, then the corporation withholds and matches FICA taxes. If income is a dividend, it is unearned and not subject to FICA. (The IRS requires that someone take a "reasonable" salary for work done.) Single-owner LLCs are usually "disregarded entities" for tax purposes and report taxes as proprietorships (on Schedule C). Multiple-member LLCs report income as a partnership.

BUSINESS TAX PLANNING

RECORD-KEEPING

An employer must keep excellent financial records for many reasons. Tax compliance is one. Others include:

- To identify sources of income.
- To track deductible expenses.
- To determine depreciation expenses.
- To determine proof of payment.
- To support items on the tax return.
- To aid in the tax planning process.
- To minimize the possibility of embezzlement.

Employers can (and should) keep records themselves. They can train a receptionist or business office manager to take care of most financial issues in the office. The employer can (and should) verify those records. (Chapter 27 discusses specific procedures.) If someone has good financial records, accounting fees will be much less and they can use an accountant's knowledge to their best advantage.

TIMING ISSUES: RECOGNIZING INCOME AND EXPENSES

Most dental practices use the cash basis of accounting. This means that they recognize income when they receive it (the check or cash is in hand, or the credit/debit card transaction has cleared) and expenses when they pay them (write the check or sign the credit card slip). An employer can accelerate some deductions by paying or prepaying before the end of the year. For example, if a dentist receives their dental association dues statement at the end of December, they can pay them on December 31 (receiving the deduction this year) or on January 1 (receiving the deduction next year). As a rule, the employer should speed up deductions as much as possible. The owner must count any money as income that is in hand this year. If they or an employee do not go to the office and process the mail, any checks in the mail will not be income until the following year. As a rule, the practice owner should slow the recognition of income as much as possible.

SPECIFIC TECHNIQUES FOR OWNER–DENTISTS

There are several specific techniques that dental practitioners who own their own practices might use to take the best advantage of tax laws.

Using a Professional Corporation to Advantage

The biggest advantage of incorporation (from a tax perspective) is the tax deductibility of employee benefits. A dentist is an employee of the practice corporation. Medical insurance premiums are completely deductible for themselves and their family and tax deductible to the corporation.

As an employee of the corporation, the owner can use a medical reimbursement plan. This can be set up so that an insured medical reimbursement plan can be deductible to the corporation but not income to the owner.

Any business can establish a cafeteria benefit plan. In a C corporation, the owner–dentist is an employee, not just the owner. As an employee, they can participate in the cafeteria plan. In these plans, the doctor and employees carefully choose among various benefit options. Money that goes into the plan comes from the individual, not the practice. Employees buy $1 of benefits for 60–65% of the after-tax cost. The business withholds no payroll or income taxes.

Employees can do business with a separate entity, such as a corporation. They might own their office building in a separate entity, then pay the highest reasonable rent for the space. This makes the rental expense unearned income not subject to FICA or SETA.

There are monetary costs associated with a corporation. An accountant or advisor will "run the numbers" both ways to decide if incorporating is worthwhile. From a tax perspective, tax law changes are making it less advantageous to incorporate the practice.

Maximizing Business Write-Offs

A practice owner should take all deductions that are legitimate business expenses through the practice. In that way, they are fully deductible. (In the past, employees who itemized deductions could include business-related expenses. That is not currently allowed.) The following are expenses that practice owners should be sure to pay through the practice:

- Work-related travel and meal expenses.
- Depreciation on a computer or cell phone needed for work.
- Dues to professional societies.
- Professional continuing education.
- Home office expenses for part of the home used regularly and exclusively for work.
- Subscriptions to professional journals.
- Work clothes and uniforms.
- Business liability insurance premiums.
- Personal tax preparation expenses.

Using a Tax-Sheltered Retirement Plan

This technique works for most dental practitioners. Practice owners should have the right type of plan to reduce staff contributions and administrative costs, establish the plan as early in their career as possible, and fund the plan as early in the year as possible.

Maximizing Business Automobile Expenses

Typical dental practitioners take about 60% of their automobile costs as tax-deductible business expenses. A business owner should write off their most expensive car. If a dental practice is incorporated, the corporation should own the car. If unincorporated, the dentist should leave it in the practice's name. To maximize the deduction, the dentist should pay for all operating costs out of the practice. Record-keeping is critical. The dentist should prove business usage for one month of the year and then annualize this amount for the year.

Using 179 Election as Appropriate

Congress intended this deduction primarily for small business owners. The rules change frequently, but business owners should investigate with their accountants if this election saves money. If a business owner expects their income and tax bracket to increase significantly soon, they should put off depreciation expenses into the future using a slower depreciation method. On the other hand, if they expect their income and tax rates to decrease in the future, they should use 179 election to speed up depreciation expenses.

Putting Family Members on the Payroll

If a practice owner hires their spouse, the spouse qualifies for Social Security benefits, child-care credit, deductibility of travel expenses, and retirement plan income sheltering as well. An accountant will know the latest rules for hiring a spouse or family member.

SPECIFIC TECHNIQUES FOR EMPLOYEE DENTISTS

If a dentist is an employee of a practice (rather than the owner), they have special problems regarding tax savings. These stem from the fact that they do not make decisions concerning the practice; the dentist loses several advantages written into the tax laws that are an advantage to owners, and they file different returns than owners. However, dental practitioners who are employees might take advantage of tax laws by using several techniques.

Taking Advantage of Employee Status

If a dentist is an employee, they should participate in employee benefit plans and retirement plans. These are valuable benefits; they need to be maximized. If the owner has a cafeteria-style benefits plan, the employee should use it.

Having the Employer Pay for Professional Expenses

A dentist should have the employer pay the professional expense for the employee dentist. The employer then reduces compensation by an equal amount. This makes the expense deductible for the employee. For the employer, it is the same if they wrote a check to the employee or an organization for the employee. As a bonus, the employer saves the cost of FICA and Medicare taxes on the difference.

Establishing a Schedule C

As an alternative, a dentist can do some consulting or outside independent contract dentistry. This way, they can develop a Schedule C and deduct all business-related expenses on that schedule. The IRS requires that someone have a valid business to use this technique. Otherwise, it might declare it a hobby (not a business enterprise) and deny the deductions. The dentist needs to set the proprietorship up as a true company, have a separate checkbook, register with the state, and possibly have a website.

Maximizing Retirement Plan Contributions

Depending on whether an employee–dentist participates in the employer's retirement plan, they can establish an Individual Retirement Account. If an employee does participate in a plan, they should maximize the contribution.

Looking at the Home Office Deduction

Tax laws allow dentists to deduct part of their home as a "principal place of business" to include situations in which the home office is used for administrative or management activities if there is no other fixed location where they can conduct these activities. Although this will not affect most dental practitioners, a few can take advantage of the provision. If, for example, a dentist consults with an insurance company or does other non-practice professional activities, they can probably use this provision. It is important to consult an accountant about the home office deduction rules, because the deduction frequently triggers an audit.

Management Principles

CHAPTER 18

Lots of people confuse bad management with destiny.

Kin Hubbard

GOAL

This chapter acquaints the student with the meaning and importance of the concepts of practice management and the roles that the dentist plays as a professional and a business person.

LEARNING OBJECTIVES

At the completion of this chapter, the student will be able to:

- Define the functions involved in managing a dental practice.

- Describe the common types of decisions.

- Describe the roles that the dentist–manager plays.

- Differentiate between a business and a profession, and describe how a dental practice incorporates elements of both.

- Differentiate between an entrepreneur and a small business owner.

- Define the management competencies required by practicing dentists and describe why each is needed.

- Describe the types of behaviors commonly found in small groups.

- Describe assets and liabilities in group problem-solving.

KEY TERMS

controlling
dental practice management
entrepreneur
financial resources
human resources

leading information resources
organizing
physical resources
planning
practice philosophy

preferred future
profession
small business owner
roles of an owner–dentist

Most people who choose dentistry have weighed up their perceptions of various careers. The length of time in preparation, cost of training, qualifications for entrance, expected income, and expected lifestyle all contribute to their career choice. Most applicants to dental school understand that dentistry involves caring for people, technical and artistic expertise, and scientific and technical knowledge. Most profess loyalty to the notions of

Business Basics for Dentists, Second Edition. James L. Harrison, David O. Willis, and Charles K. Thieman.
© 2024 John Wiley & Sons, Inc. Published 2024 by John Wiley & Sons, Inc.

being independent (their own boss) and a member of a learned profession. However, few applicants pause to consider that they will be operating a small business. If they consider it, they probably do not understand all it entails. Most have the belief on entering dental school that they will have friendly patients, work on some teeth, make good money, and play golf or go fishing on Wednesdays. That vision is only partly accurate. They have loans to secure, taxes to pay, payrolls to meet, meetings with suppliers, staff disagreements, and patients who have unreasonable expectations. Dentistry becomes a richly rewarding career and a satisfying daily experience if they handle these business problems properly.

Success in dental practice comes from a combination of clinical, behavioral, and managerial skills. Each domain has a rich history and a large body of knowledge. Each can be taught and learned. Learning business principles is no different from learning the principles of operative dentistry. Once a dentist understands the fundamental concepts, they can apply them to each particular circumstance. Lacking the concepts, a practitioner will search for a new solution to every problem. If they understand business management principles and use them to develop a modern business model, then the dentist can run a practice that fulfills all their personal expectations. If they do not understand and practice sound business management, the practice runs the dentist, leaving them a victim of the practice's needs.

CHARACTERISTICS OF DENTAL PRACTICE

DENTAL PRACTICE AS A BUSINESS AND A PROFESSION

The dental practice has many characteristics of both a profession and a business, although dentistry and business management come from entirely different mindsets (Box 18.1). Dentistry (and therefore dental education) is scientific, procedural, and dogmatic. Most procedures have a right and wrong way to do them. Management is much less dogmatic. In fact, management teachers praise students and practitioners who do things differently than everyone else as innovators. They encourage students to try something different, even if it does not work. (Imagine the opinion of dentists to another practitioner who tries a new way of cutting an alloy cavity preparation!) Dentistry teaches us to conform; business management teaches us to be different. Dentistry teaches safe, proven, tried, and true methods; management teaches innovation and experimentation.

BOX 18.1	CHARACTERISTICS OF BUSINESSES AND PROFESSIONS

Characteristics of a business
  Provides an economic good or service
  Distributes goods or services at a profit
  Treats customers fairly and honestly

Characteristics of a profession
  Members possess special knowledge
  Long training requirements
  Necessary for society
  Self-regulation
  Members place the good of society above self-interest
  Members do what is best for patients

A dental practice is a business. A business is an individual or group effort to distribute goods or services for a profit. This is done by providing an economic good or service the public wants and needs. A business tries to make a profit. In fact, this profit motive separates businesses from public organizations, which are often held only to standards of accountability and not losing money. Society expects business owners to treat customers fairly and honestly, but not necessarily to look out for the customer's best interest. In fact, there is always some tension between the business and the customer as each tries to gain in a transaction. Dental practices are businesses in that society expects them to generate income, pay bills, and follow regulations like any other business.

Dental practitioners are also professionals. Society has created the professions and granted them certain privileges. To be considered a profession, members must possess special knowledge that the public does not have. Gaining this knowledge often involves long training requirements that are unnecessary for other vocations. Because the professions hold this advanced knowledge, society allows them to regulate themselves through licensure, education standards, and disciplinary actions. They are then relatively free from lay control. The knowledge that professionals hold and apply is necessary for the ongoing functioning of society, not something from which only a few benefit. Because society grants so much authority to the professions, it also expects members to place the good of society above personal interest. That is not to say that society expects a vow of poverty from the members of professions, but it does expect professionals to do what is best for patients, not just for their own pocketbooks. If professionals abuse this power, society can unilaterally change the rules through legislative actions.

Dental practitioners can satisfy both views in their practices when they understand these differences. In interactions with patients, concern for the patient must drive suggestions for treatment, and the treatment itself must be given by a professional. Business interests must not dictate or even influence patient interactions and care delivery. The structure within which a professional delivers the service *is* the business of dentistry. Here, systems and methods are established that allow a dental practitioner to profit from dental care. The hazy line that separates the two often leads to tension for the practitioner. Which side "wins" if a given insurance plan's reimbursement for a procedure is too low to allow for adequate profit but it is in the patient's best interest? Such problems lead professionals to rebalance business and professional interactions continually.

To add to the problem, the dentistry that is done in the practice is technically based. That is to say, dentists need to know the science and have the technical ability to do excellent dentistry. However, this is only a starting point for a successful practitioner. When this technical discipline is applied, it is done to people who bring their own set of wants, needs, preferences, and desires to the practice. These behaviorally based factors form the basis of doctor–patient and business–customer relationships. Dentists want to be the most proficient technical dentist with hand skills that amaze colleagues, but without a behavioral skill set that allows them to apply those technical skills, they cannot be successful.

To accomplish all of this, dentists must not only practice the art and science of dentistry properly, they must also practice the art and science of management. Practice management is based on a huge body of science and history in the business world. Its basis includes mathematics, psychology, sociology, and logic. Each manager applies management information differently, depending on their situation, needs, personal style, and frame of reference. Although management has a large scientific basis, its application, like dentistry, is more of an art applied to the science on an individual, day-to-day basis. As a practice owner and manager, a dentist's job is to learn and understand the basic principles of management and then apply them to best meet a practice's needs.

DENTISTS AS ENTREPRENEURS OR SMALL BUSINESS OWNERS

Many people believe that entrepreneurs and small business people are one and the same. In fact, studies have shown that the two types of people (and their resulting businesses) have different sets of goals, strategies, and needs from the business. Neither is right nor wrong. There are many obvious examples of dentists who fit into either type. People's view of themselves, the dental profession, and the practice's objectives will help them understand where they "fit in."

Entrepreneurs are builders. They try to gain market share and to make the business grow rapidly. Their purpose is to take over or acquire other businesses or sell the existing business to someone else. This means that the entrepreneur must use aggressive business practices, both externally and inside the business, to gain the speed of growth required by outside venture investors and initial public offerings. They may "mortgage the farm" or family fortune to finance the start-up phase of the business. They have a riverboat gambler's sense of calculated risk: they do not play the game without knowing the rules, the odds, and how to use them to their advantage. They investigate possibilities, estimate the chances of success and failure, and calculate the expected return from each possibility. Only then do they decide if a venture has an adequate financial return to pursue. They are maximizers. Adequate is not enough. If they can make $1 million this year, they will try for $2 million next year. Every city has dental entrepreneurs who accumulate offices, grow and sell practices, or build networks. Their vision is different from the individual lifetime practitioner's.

However, most dental practitioners approach their practice like a small business owner (Box 18.2). Few dental

BOX 18.2	CHARACTERISTICS OF A SMALL BUSINESS OWNER VERSUS AN ENTREPRENEUR

Small business owner	Entrepreneur
Low risk, low return	High risk, high return
Personal profit	Growth of business value
Informal systems	Formal systems
Social orientation	Commercial orientation
Personal (family) staff	Impersonal staff relations
Personal satisfaction	Financial return

practices fail as business ventures. People enter dentistry to be safe, not to take risks. Dentists understand that their income is limited by their personal skill and ability and by how much time they devote to their practice. Many could make more money if they worked longer hours, but they choose family and personal time instead. Most aspiring dentists do not plan to be rich, but they do plan never to worry about money. Because most dental services require that the practitioner personally deliver the service, the size of most practices is limited. Growth involves adding highly trained (and compensated) professionals. Most dentists want to satisfy themselves and others they are in contact with. Once they have established an adequate income, they may take Wednesdays off and play golf. Although they take some financial risk when establishing a practice, most dentists do not continue to grow the practice once it reaches a certain size and style.

CHARACTERISTICS OF SUCCESSFUL BUSINESS OWNERS

Successful small business owners has several important characteristics (Box 18.3). First, they have a vision of what they want the business to be. This type of dream is not a nebulous notion or a conglomeration of possibilities. Instead, it is a specific and concrete idea of what the business owner wants this specific business to be. This vision of a preferred future looks five hours, five days, five months, and five years into the future at once. Every action then supports the achievement of the preferred vision. Secondly, successful business owners show persistence. Nearly all businesses have difficult periods because of excessive growth, lack of business, staffing problems, or hundreds of other business problems. Successful business people take setbacks in their stride. They retain their preferred vision and continue to work toward its achievement. Finally, successful business people are willing to manage. Management is not pie-in-the-sky dreaming, it is "roll up your shirt sleeves," day-to-day work. Good management means that the business owner is involved in every aspect of the

business daily. Successful business people do not leave the details to others. Instead, they dig into the details of the business to make it run most efficiently.

For most of this book, it will be assumed that the reader aspires to be a dental practice owner, manager, and producer. That owner may have partners or associates in the office, but the essence of the ownership issue is that the owner is responsible for more than just doing dentistry. They are responsible for seeing that the office runs smoothly as a business, that it is compliant with all laws regarding businesses, that the staff (and owner) feel that each is a fairly rewarded and productive member of the practice, that the owner presents the proper professional image that they want to promote to the public, and that they are involved in professional activities to improve the profession and the community's access to healthcare services. It sounds like a huge task, and it is.

DEFINITION OF DENTAL PRACTICE MANAGEMENT

The definition of dental practice management is "to plan, organize, lead, and control the human, physical, financial, and information resources of the business of delivering dental care." Notice that this definition is composed of four functions and four resource areas. If this is considered a matrix, there are 16 different functional problems to manage in the practice. The dentist–manager must plan, organize, lead, and control each practice resource area (human, physical, financial, and information).

FUNCTIONS OF THE DENTIST–MANAGER

There are several business functions that dental practice owners routinely perform. These include the following.

Function 1: Planning

Planning is the process of determining courses of action, direction, goals, and objectives for the practice. Plans may cover long periods or be much more immediate (days or weeks). Plans start with the practice philosophy, which is the overall guiding vision of what the dentist wants the practice to be. They are supported by goals, which define an expected outcome or desired future situation. Once the dentist knows where they want the practice to be, they develop strategies for getting there. The owner should also identify likely barriers to overcome and a time for completion. Finally, objectives give concreteness to the planning process. Objectives define what the expected outcomes are. They should be measurable and specific to decide whether the practice has met them.

BOX 18.3	**CHARACTERISTICS OF SUCCESSFUL SMALL BUSINESS OWNERS**

A vision of a preferred future
Persistence
Willingness to manage

When a dentist decides to expand the office or move to a new location, they are planning. For major initiatives such as these, the dentist will probably use advisors, such as accountants, equipment representatives, and bankers. For many smaller initiatives, such as hiring an additional staff member or changing recall systems, the dentist will plan what to do with little outside help. In all these planning instances, a preferred future is desired, and changes are made to try to reach that goal.

Function 2: Organizing

Organizing means coordinating resources and activities by designing the physical facility and by structuring tasks and authority. The organizing function involves setting up the physical space and systems in the office, deciding information needs and solutions, deciding what types and numbers of staff to hire, and how the office will operate daily.

Many dental practitioners develop office manuals that contain policies, rules, procedures, and standard operational methods. They find instrument set-ups and sterilization methods that work effectively. They develop equipment maintenance and repair schedules, supplies vendors, office cleaning and redecorating schedules, and hundreds of other routine organizational policies that allow the office to function smoothly.

Function 3: Leading

Leading is selecting, motivating, and directing staff members to work at the peak of their abilities. Most dental offices have employees. As discussed previously, the planning and organizing functions describe the types and numbers of staff members that will be needed. Many new dentists believe that all a dentist needs to do is to plug people into the various slots. In fact, at this point the dentist must engage in what many people believe is the most difficult piece of the management puzzle: leading and motivating those employees.

Each employee brings their own set of wants, needs, family histories, backgrounds, and personalities to the workplace. The astute manager works to understand people so they can stimulate high performance from them, both as individuals and as groups. As the owner of the practice, the dentist sets the office environment. That environment consists of the compensation package (pay and benefits), the communication process, group interactions, and job duties. How the office environment is set up can either support or discourage motivated workers from doing their best at work.

Function 4: Controlling

Controlling means monitoring and evaluating activities to ensure that the operational and performance outcomes happen as planned. The owner must monitor the practice's progress as it moves toward its goals. If the practice is not acting in a way that will allow it to reach its "target," then the owner needs either to change processes or change the target.

In fact, controlling is an ongoing function in the office. At the end of each day, the dentist examines the office's daily production and collection numbers, looking for problems. They give immediate and constructive feedback to members of the dental team so that they know what they are doing correctly and incorrectly. The dentist examines previously done work and changes materials or procedures if problems are found. These are included in office control. Some are more formal than others, but all this feedback (and more) helps the dentist make better practice decisions.

RESOURCES OF THE PRACTICE

The definition of practice management is to plan, organize, lead, and control the practice's resources. But what are the major resource groups of the practice?

Resource 1: Human Resources

Most dentists in practice in the United States employ staff. Yet staffing the practice continues to be one of the practitioner's greatest problems. Staff typically is the greatest expense for a practitioner and the most important limit to practice growth. Dentists want long-term, committed individuals to be employees, yet generally do not know how to establish pay, compensation, and reward systems that optimize staff performance. Dentists and staff members work closely together in a physically confined space. They often become genuine friends, making employee discipline and rewards difficult to administer fairly. The variety of staff job duties and legal requirements of job classifications can lead to petty jealousies and interpersonal conflicts that the manager–dentist must arbitrate on.

Resource 2: Physical Resources

The physical resources include the office space and the equipment and supplies required for dentistry. Dentists typically rent office space, although many own their own buildings and space. Maintenance, upkeep, and decoration all add to the expense of the basic office cost. New equipment, especially high-technology equipment, has a short useful lifetime. (Most computers are obsolete within a few years of purchase.) Yet new techniques and materials are coming to the dental marketplace continually. This means that a dentist must plan for continual change and upgrades in the physical plant and equipment of the office.

Resource 3: Financial Resources

Dentists must properly manage the finances of the office to be profitable. Initial (start-up or buy-in) loans significantly affect cash flow. The dentist's plans and decisions regarding payment plan and credit policies, personal financial planning, retirement plans for themselves and staff, staff pay schedules, and even bill-paying schedules affect the practice's profitability.

Resource 4: Information Resources

Dentistry is currently becoming more of an information service and less of a product or personal service-based industry. Patients want information on their dental and general health conditions. Insurance carriers and third parties want information on services provided and their associated costs. Dentists need patient information for legal and ethical reasons and for mailing and other appropriate marketing services. Dentists need information about the profession, evaluations of new materials, descriptions of new techniques, and responses from third-party carriers. Information drives the practice. Modern dentists understand and manage the information that the practice needs.

ROLES OF THE OWNER–DENTIST

Private dental practice is both the long-term goal and result for most graduating dental students. The vast majority of these are in solo practices. Most of the rest are in two-practitioner offices. Because there are few practitioners in most offices, most dentists must play many different managerial roles. In larger organizations, one person can be responsible for staffing, another for supplies, and yet another for accounting. The small dental office is different because the owner–dentist must wear many different hats during the day (Box 18.4). The dentist must produce dentistry. Legally, the dentist is the only person in the office who can do many daily dental procedures. As the owner, the dentist must be a decision-maker. These decisions deal

---

BOX 18.4	ROLES OF AN OWNER–DENTIST

- Producer
- Decision-maker
- Information provider
- Mentor
- Teacher
- Technical expert
- Interpersonal facilitator
- Figurehead
- Accounting and operations manager

---

with the dentistry produced and the management in the office. The dentist possesses the primary storehouse of information for patients and staff. They are the technical expert in dentistry, the chief of accounting for the office, the personnel manager, the production supervisor, the vice president for marketing, and the ceremonial head of the practice. Add to this the many roles played outside the office (e.g. parent, spouse, church member, little league coach) and it is little wonder that some dentists are victims of personal and professional burnout.

The dentist who is a management student is better able to control the daily problems in the practice. In that sense, to do management properly in the office means that the study of management is an ongoing concern, just like the study of dental techniques and materials. It is not an end in and of itself but a road, path, or Tao. If someone understands basic management principles and applies them appropriately, they will take the first steps toward a lifelong career that is satisfying and rewarding in both a personal and financial context.

Planning the Dental Practice

It was the best of times, it was the worst of times, it was the age of wisdom, it was the age of foolishness, it was the epoch of belief, it was the epoch of incredulity, it was the season of Light, it was the season of Darkness, it was the spring of hope, it was the winter of despair, we had everything before us, we had nothing before us, we were all going direct to heaven, we were all going direct the other way—in short, the period was so far like the present period, that some of its noisiest authorities insisted on its being received, for good or for evil, in the superlative degree of comparison only.

Charles Dickens, *A Tale of Two Cities*

GOAL

This chapter aims to acquaint the student with the internal and external factors that affect the planning and operation of a dental practice.

LEARNING OBJECTIVES

At the completion of this chapter, the student will be able to:

- Describe external environmental factors that affect dental practices.

- Describe internal environmental factors that affect dental practices.

- Describe the amount of control the practitioner has over the various factors.

- Describe an environmental analysis.

- Describe how a SWOT analysis can be applied to a dental practice.

- Describe several environmental trends that are important for planning in dentistry.

Business Basics for Dentists, Second Edition. James L. Harrison, David O. Willis, and Charles K. Thieman.
© 2024 John Wiley & Sons, Inc. Published 2024 by John Wiley & Sons, Inc.

Starting a practice is much like having a child. A practice must be birthed, allowed to grow, and helped through problems before it becomes a fully functioning mature practice. The problems and opportunities faced by a child are different from those faced by an adolescent. Similarly, a start-up practice faces different challenges from a mature practice. With both children and dental practices, a well-articulated plan must be in place to move to the next level of development. In both instances, change happens regardless of whether there is a plan. Nevertheless, having a plan helps to guide the process and maximize opportunities that occur.

PRACTICE STAGES

Dental practices typically develop through several stages. Depending on where a dentist is in the practice development stage, planning needs and practice profiles will be different.

Four stages in a practice's growth are shown in Box 19.1. During the first stage (establishment), the practitioner is concerned with getting warm bodies in through the door. Marketing efforts are critical. Practitioners often use managed care, welfare patients, emergency call, or other methods to increase the number of patient visits. Efficiency is not as much of a problem as in later stages because there is often slack time. The second, growth stage sees an acceleration in patient visits. Schedules begin to fill, and the practitioner begins to "weed out" managed care and other less profitable patients. The third, maturity stage sees practitioners concerned with making the practice efficient on production, cost, and revenue bases. Finally, during the redevelopment stage of practice, the dentist readjusts the practice to meet their long-term personal and professional life goals. The practice is concerned with different problems in each phase of its development. Different problems and solutions will also be more important at different stages.

STAGE 1: PRACTICE ESTABLISHMENT

This initial stage begins with the practice's set-up, buy-out, or buy-in. The practitioner's main concern is to increase the patient base and to acquaint those patients with the style and personality of the practice. To this end, they will see virtually anybody, any time. Marketing and advertising are important to attract people into the practice so that they may be won over as regular patients. Profits are low or non-existent because revenue is slow to collect, whereas debts and start-up costs are high. Operational efficiency is not a big problem because extra appointments are often available, and the practitioner is increasing their clinical and management skills. During this time, the practitioner develops operational systems and management skills that will be the basis of later practice efficiencies.

STAGE 2: PRACTICE GROWTH

The growth stage occurs when the practitioner continues to acquaint the patient base with their individual practice style. Because of the unique style, patients begin to self-select for or against the practice. This leads to patients leaving the practice to find a dentist who is more compatible with their needs and wants, or patients who enjoy the style of practice will refer other patients with similar wants and desires. This internal referral process allows the practice to

BOX 19.1	STAGES OF A DENTAL PRACTICE

Stage	Major concern
Establishment	Warm bodies
Growth	The right warm bodies
Maturity	Becoming efficient
Redevelopment	Goal attainment

approach a "critical mass" of patients that will help it sustain itself from internal referrals.

Many marketing efforts begin to pay off as well. There is often so much new and previously deferred work that the practice begins to run the practitioner rather than vice versa. This can leave the practitioner with little time for personal growth or family interests. Although a large amount of money comes into the practice, there is low profit because the overhead is still high due to loan pay-offs and personal debt associated with typical family start-up expenses. This often leads to a "cash crunch" in which the practitioner has trouble paying the bills each month, though production reaches an all-time high. Operational efficiency becomes a large problem as the number of patients increases. The practitioner needs to assess carefully when to add staff, change hours, or make other critical operational management decisions.

STAGE 3: PRACTICE MATURITY (REALIZATION)

The practitioner reaches their intended level of practice busyness during the maturity stage. Referrals increase as the dentist concentrates on the types of work that are of greater interest to them for personal, professional, or financial reasons. The dentist takes control of the time spent with the practice and balances this commitment with personal and family time uses. Involvement with professional societies and organizations increases as the practitioner gains in professional and personal stature. Profits increase as fixed costs decrease from loan pay-offs. Production peaks and fees increase so that this stage becomes the most profitable. The dentist's time is the limiting factor to production, so office operational efficiency is vital to maximum profitability. Many dentists' goal is to maintain a mature type of practice for many years.

STAGE 4: PRACTICE REDEVELOPMENT

This stage of practice can take two different paths. One group of practitioners is content to continue the existing practice pattern. The patient pool begins to contract as patients move away, die, or have decreased need for dental care. If the practitioner has not encouraged children into the practice, the patients age along with the practitioner as the patients' families grow and move away. Often the treatment scope is fairly limited, especially if the practitioner has not incorporated the newer techniques, methods, and materials. The practitioner takes more time off for outside pursuits. Profits remain high because the overhead is low, although profits and revenues are decreasing due to the shrinking patient pool. Operational efficiency is not important if the practitioner is satisfied with the profit and workload of the practice.

The second group of practitioners wants to maximize the value of the practice. To do this, they take in associate dentists, sell a part to a new partner, or merge their practice with another. They find ways to continue to develop and grow the business so that the practice becomes more of the focal point instead of them. As the practice grows, they often require additional, specialized staff to run it. Office managers, sterilization clerks, and insurance management staff members do tasks that are shared in smaller practices. Operational efficiency is paramount to these larger practices maintaining profitability in the face of this increased bureaucracy needed to run the practice.

THE ENVIRONMENT OF DENTAL PRACTICE

A dental practice does not exist in a vacuum. It exists in an environment that affects the practice either directly or by influencing the climate in which it operates. These environmental forces may be external to the practice or may exist internally as management-related concerns or as personal positions taken by the owner–dentist. But each of these factors may profoundly affect how a dentist structures the practice. The individual practitioner should identify these forces, anticipate their effects, and use this information to plan practice growth in the most advantageous manner. An "environmental analysis" assesses the practice's environment so that the dentist can anticipate problems and make changes in its direction to increase their chance of success. This becomes the framework for planning a successful practice.

EXTERNAL ENVIRONMENT

The external environment, by definition, lies outside the practice itself and is composed of specific individuals and general groups. It includes those people who influence the practice and those whom its actions affect. This is obviously a large, diverse, and complex group of factors. Therefore, external environmental factors generally fall into two categories: general environment and operating environment.

General Environment

The general environment includes the business, regulatory, legal, technological, cultural, and social factors that affect the climate in which dental practices operate. It includes factors that affect the number and types of patients and the number and types of inputs into the practice (labor, supplies, etc.). The general environment is divided into several domains.

Sociocultural Domain The sociocultural domain consists of the demographics (e.g. age, education level, income level, etc.), values, customs, and historical interests of the people within the society the practice serves. Because dental practices exist to serve the needs of the population base, it is no wonder that these cultural factors should influence the organization and operation of the dental practice. The people the practice employs bring many of those cultural factors with them as background knowledge on the job. Social and cultural roots, for example, may in part determine an individual's "work ethic" or affect their personal interactions with the practice's clients.

Dental practices face a host of sociocultural influences. Demographic changes in the population will affect the practice's future productivity. The US population overall is aging, as well as becoming more affluent and better educated. Some 20% of the population move home in any given year. People value preventive healthcare and practice more "self-help" than ever before. The ethnic and racial composition of communities and the population at large is rapidly changing. The myriad positive and negative ways these factors might affect the dental profession overall (and a specific dental practice in particular) are considered the sociocultural factors of the external environment.

Economic Domain The application of sociocultural factors requires an exchange between the dentist and the population. This process results in the economic domain. On a macro level, general economic conditions such as inflation, unemployment levels, and benefits packages negotiated by workers affect the number and types of dental services patients demand. Interest rates, resource prices (e.g. gold, silver, computers, and dental instruments), and alternative employment possibilities all affect the general atmosphere that determines practice costs. Although the individual practitioner has little control over economic environmental factors, understanding how these factors can affect the practice is still important. In this way, a dentist may anticipate future effects and react appropriately to developing trends by anticipating the outcome and planning accordingly.

Technological Domain Technology is the third major general external environmental domain that affects dentistry. Technology is the means, knowledge, training, and systems used to deliver dental services. Just as robotics has revolutionized the manufacturing sector, research and technological changes have dramatically influenced dental practice. A few of the new dental technologies from the past 25 years include community water supply fluoridation, the high-speed handpiece, four-handed auxiliary skills, fiberoptics, lingual braces, castable ceramics, desktop computers and supporting software, light-cured composite restorations, spherical cut alloys, implant materials and techniques, computer-aided design and manufacturing (CAD/CAM) restoration formation, laser cutting, electronic insurance filing, improved non-surgical and pharmacological periodontal treatments, and newer filling and cementing agents. The rate of change in technology is accelerating rapidly. Future dental practices will be vastly different from today's in materials, techniques, and information processing. This will affect the nature and character of dental practice. A dental practitioner must constantly monitor the technological domain of the external environment for developments. They then decide how those developments might affect their own practice and incorporate them into the growth plan when appropriate.

Legal and Regulatory Domain The sociocultural environment strongly influences the legal and regulatory domain. In a sense, this is an outgrowth of our cultural norms. It defines what is acceptable and unacceptable behavior by members of society and translates that into laws and regulations aimed at controlling it. In this country, laws are formed by the legislature, enforced by the executive, and interpreted and judged by the judicial branch. As such, they are closely tied to the will of society.

The legal and regulatory environment has an obvious and profound impact on dental practices. Every dentist remembers the state board ("trial by fire") clinical exam required for licensure. State Dental Practice Acts define limits of auxiliary duty delegation and practice ownership. Through legislation and regulation, Congress affects how much money is spent on indigent care, workers' health benefits (and the tax deductibility of those benefits), and the inclusion or exclusion of dental care in health policies. The Occupational Safety and Health Administration (OSHA) and the courts are presently redefining the dentist's responsibilities to employees and patients when handling potentially infectious materials. The litigious nature of today's US society has caused many dentists to change how they practice dentistry. The individual practitioner should closely monitor the political and regulatory system to anticipate shifts in ideology and priorities among regulators.

Ethical and Professional Domain The profession of dentistry is relatively autonomous in that dentists decide the prevailing entrance and educational requirements of its members, set the practice and technological norms, define behavioral expectations, and discipline members who do not adhere to their norms. Society grants the profession this autonomy with the understanding that the professional will not abuse these powers and that they look out for the best interests of the public and individual patients under their control. So individual practitioners must respond to and follow a set of socially and professionally determined ethical norms. These ethical expectations change slowly over time as new influences in other environments change public and professional expectations and opinions.

Operating Environment

The operating environment is the direct influence that the general environment has on the dental practice. It is the environment in which the dental practice actually operates. In a sense, it is the concrete embodiment of the abstract general environment. The practitioner is in contact with and can exert some influence over its factors. For example, the general demographic trend is that, because of fluoridation and the end of the "baby boom," there are fewer young people with significant dental caries. The periodontist may feel the direct influence of this trend in the changing character of the service mix of the practice. Conversely, the local environment may not mirror the overall trend. Several new subdivisions in an area may bring an influx of new families, lowering the age of the patient base. Focusing efforts to cope with changes in the operating environment (e.g. the inclusion of orthodontics or adolescent marketing) is more productive than trying to fight or influence the underlying general trend. The operating environment is divided into several components.

Suppliers Suppliers provide the resources needed for the dental practice to operate and consist of much more than simply dental supplies. They also include personnel or labor (assistants and hygienists), financial capital (banker), subcontracted work (laboratory), and information (accountants, lawyers, continuing education courses, practice consultants). A dentist, for example, competes for labor with other local businesses that offer alternative forms of employment, such as grocery stores and manufacturing plants. If local employers are offering high wage and benefit packages, the dentist must compete for suppliers of labor by offering comparable compensation packages for comparable-level jobs.

Patients Patients (customers) are the second major component of the operating environment. Every dental practice serves a defined and segmented portion of the population. Marketing attempts to match the service provided to the wants and needs of a larger population segment. Producing profiles of those who actively use the practice's services is the first step toward developing a plan to increase the number of patients who would be patients. Customers have different amounts of bargaining power with the service provider. Preferred provider organizations (PPOs) are an example of the power a group may exert when bargaining for services. Plant openings or closings in the geographic area will increase or decrease the buying power and number of potential customers, and therefore enable them to exert indirect bargaining power with local dentists and other business people.

Influence Groups Influence groups become a real part of the operational environment every time a regulation is enforced. Zoning commissions can profoundly influence the growth plans for a dental practice by allowing or not allowing a favorable zoning change. Professional associations and organizations such as the American Dental Association (ADA) or the various specialty groups act as information exchange centers and may propose policies or laws that affect the general environment of the practice. Interest groups (such as parent–teacher organizations) may influence the immediate environment through concerted efforts (e.g. boycotts) or via informing and influencing their members and the public about their position.

Competitors Competitors influence the operating environment of the practice. If a patient is not satisfied with the service provided, they may find another practice that does satisfy their wants and needs. Desired growth opportunities may be shut off because of existing competition in the area. New forms of dental service payment plans (e.g. capitation plans) may alter the traditional competitive environment and cause patients to choose dental practices based on reasons an individual dentist cannot control.

Allies Allies are groups or individuals who develop an interdependent relationship with the practice. In this function, they share resources or information for the mutual benefit of both parties. Individual dentists may have well-established referral patterns, study clubs, group purchase plans, or kindred spirits with whom they share a special bond. More formal groups of allies may also develop, such as independent practice associations (IPAs), that seek to influence the marketplace through group action.

Internal Environment

The internal environment consists of the elements of the practice when viewed as a business. Personnel, marketing, financial, organizational, and production-related functions all fall within the practice's internal environment. The owner–dentist can control the quality and quantity of internal factors more easily compared with external factors. In fact, until and unless the practice is operating with excellent efficiency and effectiveness, it probably cannot take advantage of external environmental opportunities.

Internal Management Internal management issues are the focus of many practice management texts, lectures, continuing education courses, and consultants. Internal management includes marketing, staffing, the efficient provision of services, and office financial management. The dental practitioner has almost unlimited control over the internal manner in which their office will operate. It is important that the practitioner adapt their internal management philosophy and techniques to fit other internal and external environmental considerations.

Personal Style of the Dentist

Practice growth is a notion similar to "motherhood" or "the American way." People profess to believe in it, but each person would come up with a different definition and method of carrying out their plan for achieving it. This is because everyone approaches personal and professional decisions with a unique history, set of values, abilities, and beliefs.

The first step in analyzing the internal environment is to appraise individual circumstances regarding wants, needs, desires, and abilities. The result is that appropriate and realistic strategies will be formulated that fit a unique style. The four primary areas of self-appraisal are views of the profession of dentistry, personal risk aversion or attraction, personal position, and professional strengths and weaknesses.

Dentist's Views of Dentistry Some dentists believe that dentistry is a cottage industry; others believe that it is a multibillion-dollar-a-year service industry. Every dentist has a different view of dentistry and the dental profession. Many aggressive growth strategies (such as opening a satellite location or participating in a managed care program) require that the participants have a business-oriented view of the profession that would be anathema to a cottage-industry dentist. Conversely, a conservative strategy of internal referrals and community education may appear stifling and unimaginative to a dentist with a true entrepreneurial spirit.

Risk Aversion Everyone has a unique tolerance for and aversion to both risk and debt. The US hero is a swashbuckling daredevil entrepreneur who risks the family savings and mortgages the ranch on a new idea and wins. Few people truly have the riverboat gambler's tolerance for risk, however. In fact, most people avoid risk whenever they can, especially as they progress through their professional lives and accumulate assets representing goal attainment or making their lives more comfortable. People must decide how much risk and uncertainty they can tolerate.

Any growth action involves taking some risk. That may take the form of placing personal or professional assets at risk as collateral (financial risk) or may take the form of possible loss of professional standing, bearing, or reputation (professional risk). Including an associate dentist may decrease income due to increased expenses or a decrease in professional bearing in the community if the associate is not carefully chosen or acts unprofessionally. Using novel treatment approaches may lead to either new opportunities for patient satisfaction, poor clinical results, or the gain or loss of professional reputation. The success of a satellite office may paradoxically risk a decrease in personal and family time that the practitioner cherishes.

Every growth strategy or action has some attendant risk. The higher the risk associated with a growth strategy, the higher the pay-off should be. Otherwise, the dentist would choose a strategy with the same potential pay-off but less risk. The pay-off may be in financial or entirely non-financial currency. A feeling of success, service to people in need, religious goodwill, and other "good feelings" are adequate pay for many dentists in certain situations. Depending on how much risk aversion is identified through self-assessment, the dentist will pick a growth strategy that adequately compensates them for the associated risk. If the dentist is only willing to accept limited risk despite the potential returns, the acceptable strategies may similarly be limited to those with a limited return.

Personal Position Each dentist has a set of personal issues that act as profound factors in the growth decision. Families grow accustomed to certain income levels and time commitments from family members. Individuals need different amounts of personal time for such activities as hobbies, outside interests, and personal development efforts. Most professionals require time for personal health-related activities and spiritual and religious devotional efforts. Many require time and effort for political, environmental, community, or social causes. It is essential that each dentist continually explores and recognizes those personal factors that are critical for their spiritual, mental, and social well-being. Practice growth cannot occur until the personal position is identified, developed, and reconciled with professional opportunities.

Professional Strengths and Weaknesses A critical self-appraisal is also necessary for the professional arena. Every clinical dentist has areas of technical, behavioral, and managerial strengths and weaknesses. Dentists are often unaware of these, either through a lack of introspection or through the inability or unwillingness to gain an honest appraisal from themselves, patients, staff, or peers. An honest appraisal is difficult because it involves personal risk. They might find out something they do not want to know, or they might gain confirmation of something they suspected but wished were not so. Yet an appraisal is critical to successful growth.

A successful growth strategy uses an individual's strengths and reduces their weaknesses. The dentist cannot intelligently choose an appropriate and successful growth strategy without an honest appraisal of their professional strengths and weaknesses. For example, suppose someone identifies the need for a periodontal maintenance program for a particular patient. If the dentist does not have adequate skills or knowledge in this area, it would be foolish, destructive, and unethical to pursue this strategy without continuing education in the field. Or if staff members report that the dentist is particularly adept at interpersonal communication with apprehensive patients, the dentist could initiate a "Dental Phobic" program and expand office revenues by referral and program development in this area. Without an honest appraisal, the dentist might have been unaware of this staff-perceived strength and lost the opportunity for practice growth and patient service.

THE BUSINESS PLAN

Starting and running a successful dental practice has never been easy. This task has become even more difficult in the volatile and competitive marketplace that the profession now faces. One common trait of all successful dentists (and small business people generally) is that they have a solid plan for what they want to do with the business. A dentist's financial, personal, and emotional energies will be tied to the success or failure of their practice. They will invest a lot of their soul into a dental practice. Sadly, some dental practices never succeed or only barely "scrape by." Many of these unsuccessful dental practitioners are there by their own devices; they have failed to plan the small business adequately. Particularly during these competitive economic times, trying to start a business without a plan is akin to going to sea without a chart or a compass. Rational people would want to know where they are going, whether sailing the ocean or the financial seas. A business plan is a chart of someone's practice voyage. It is a plan for where they want to go or what they hope to accomplish with the business.

Most new dental practitioners will need to secure financing from a bank or lending institution. Bankers are in the business of lending money to people who will repay them. One of the best ways to help convince a loan officer that a person is a good business risk is to present a business plan with the loan application. Much of the information that is required in the loan application is also included in the business plan, so the additional work is not as formidable as it first appears.

Strictly speaking, a business plan is a document that someone uses to project the practice's future performance. It begins with general statements and conditions and moves through a more detailed explanation, ending with numbers that the dentist projects to represent the financial outcomes of the practice, based on previous conditions. The process of developing the business plan is important for more than just the pieces of paper that result. The dentist learns about their business through the process of writing the plan. This is where they write down concisely what they expect their financial health to be in a year and why. Developing a business plan forces the new practitioner to decide in an organized way rather than just letting things happen and responding to them in a crisis fashion. The banker or loan officer will be interested to see that they have thought through these problems, determined solutions, and committed them to paper.

Bankers may have specific forms that they need to be completed to process the loan application. Once the business plan is completed, the borrower will generally only need to shift information from one form to the other. The additional work is worth the effort when the bank approves the loan!

Many loan officers, especially in rural areas, may never have processed a dental practice loan. Often the borrower's job, as the applicant, will be to educate the banker on the special business needs that the dentist, as a practice owner, will have. The banker, or loan officer, usually cannot make the final decision on a loan. Instead, they must take the information that has been developed to the bank's loan committee, composed of senior bank officers, owners, or board members. They are the ones who make the final decision on a loan. The loan officer is the borrower's spokesperson in this process. The chances of a dentist gaining a loan under favorable terms will obviously increase if the loan officer is in their corner. The best way they can do that is by showing the loan officer that they have done background work, are well prepared, and have provided all of the information needed to represent them in front of the loan committee.

FORMAT OF THE BUSINESS PLAN

The specific requirements and format of the business plan are different for each bank. Some banks require formal written plans. Others may only require some background information and simple financial projections. The important common theme is the information that each contains. The topics that most business plans include are as follows.

Mission Statement

In this section, the applicant describes their practice philosophy, specifically:

- The type of services the applicant will offer.
- The planned relationship with the community, such as local organization membership.
- Any innovative technology, equipment, or services that they will offer.

Target Market

In this section, the applicant describes the expected patients of the practice, including:

- The number of potential patients in the area.
- Commercial or residential development in the area.
- Specific groups that may be underserved or other opportunities for patient generation.

Competition

In this section, the applicant describes the expected competition in the area, including:

- The number of currently active dentists in the area.
- Expected retirements or new dentists in the area.
- Breakdown of general and specialty care and referral patterns.
- How the applicant will fill an unmet need in the area.

Projections

In this section, the applicant provides financial projections for the practice, including:

- Expected income, based on patient visits.
- Expected expenses, based on industry averages and practice-specific plans.
- Expected cash needs, based on a cash-flow projection.

Capital Requirements

In this section, the applicant details how much money they need to borrow, specifically:

- Equipment and supplies that the applicant will purchase.
- Any tenant or other facility improvements planned.
- The amount of working capital or operating funds needed, and their purpose.

Marketing Plan

In this section, the applicant details how they will generate patients for the practice, specifically:

- The type and frequency of marketing efforts.
- Special marketing offers or promotions.
- Plans to use the current customer base to generate patient visits.
- Other relationships or tactics to use to generate additional patients.

SPECIFIC NUMBERS NEEDED

As part of this planning process, most bankers will require (at a minimum) several numbers. Some describe the community and patient pool the dentist will serve. Others describe the needs of the practice itself. The numbers that bankers commonly require include the following.

Community Description

- **Area population**
  To decide the area population, the practitioner first needs to know the service area; that is to say, where most of the patients will come from. It is less definite in urban and suburban areas but often centered on neighborhoods or sections of the city. Some practices (especially in urban areas) may be located downtown, where most patients come from nearby employers. Suburban practices often find the bulk of their patients from nearby neighborhoods. In rural areas, the service area is often the county. Often shopping (or buying) patterns help define the service area. Areas with significant retail growth (especially national chains or franchises) usually show where they think the population growth will be.

- **Number of dentists in the area**
  The number of active dentists in the area is another key number for planning a practice. Many dentists may be semi-retired or practice part-time in this area and

part-time in another practice. Adjust this statistic for full-time equivalent (FTE) dentists. If one dentist in an area is retired, another practices half-time, and a third practices full-time, then there are 1.5 FTE dentists in the area. Specialty dentists (except for pediatric dentists) are usually excluded from this statistic.

- **Dentist-to-population ratio (competition)**
  As a rule, a general dentist needs approximately 2000 active patients for a viable practice (1:2000 dentist-to-population ratio). (The military uses 1200 patients per dentist, but these patients must visit the dentist regularly.) Remember, only about half to two-thirds of the population visit a dentist in a year. Rural areas and lower economic areas have lower utilization rates and therefore need a higher population for each dentist.

Practice Description

- **Cost of Building or Renovation**
  If the dentist builds a new practice, they will work with a builder and designer from a dental supply house. They will help develop a complete listing of the cost to build out the facility and the cost to buy and install specific dental equipment (such as x-ray units and evacuation systems). The dentist who is buying an existing practice may also have significant renovation and improvement costs if the facility is old or in need of repairs.

- **Cost of equipment and supplies**
  If the dentist establishes a new (start-up) practice, they must develop a comprehensive list of supplies and equipment. The dentist buying an ongoing business will not have as large a list of equipment and supplies to update, although the amount can still be significant.

- **Financial projections**
  Most lenders ask for two types of financial projections – profit and cash flow. (These are detailed in Chapter 15.) The profit projection is often a three-year estimate of the expected profit of the practice. Most lenders ask for representative or average practice cost numbers and specific expected revenues. Cash-flow projections often cover the first year of business, when collections lag behind the practice's payments, leading to a cash-flow problem. The answer is to determine the amount of working capital needed to cover the shortfall.

SOURCES OF INFORMATION

There is no single source of information for potential dental practice owners to use in planning their practice. Instead, they will use various sources, depending on the information they need. These include the following.

Accountant or Management Consultant

If the new practitioner has an accountant or consultant, that person may have information that can be used in the business plan.

Practice Broker

If the new dentist is buying an existing practice, the selling dentist probably used a broker to help sell their practice. These brokers often have specific numbers for the area or dental practices they will provide. The new dentist must remember that the broker works for the seller, not the buyer.

Chambers of Commerce

The local chamber of commerce aims to help and promote businesses in the area. They have many statistics on the population of the area, and some have industry-specific information, such as the number of dental practitioners.

Organized Dentistry

At the local, state, and national levels, organized dentistry has information for its members. This is especially useful for specific practice numbers or averages when developing financial projections.

Dental Office Success Factors

SECTION 4

Successful dental practices do not just happen. They are managed by an owner who has a clearly defined vision of where they want the practice to be and works each day to guide the practice to that vision. That is the same as all good managers, from CEOs of Fortune 500 companies to start-up entrepreneurs, do every day. For people who have no training or background in business management that can seem like an overwhelming task. However, the philosophies, methods, and techniques that successful business managers use in other large and small companies can be learned by dental practice owners. If they apply those techniques to the business operation of a dental practice, the dental practice can prosper like any other well-run business.

The first step is to examine the business and decide what factors lead to its success or failure. Then try to measure (using some key performance indicators) whether those factors are being met, and if not what can be done to improve operations to be more successful. Financial ratio analysis is a common business tool that shows areas to be improved.

CONCERNS OF THE DENTAL OFFICE SUCCESS FACTORS SECTION

A successful dental practice is run in a business-like manner. That means that the owner understands the foundational principles of business management and applies them to the operation of the practice. These business foundations relate to three major goals:

- **Understand what makes a practice profitable**
  Several factors lead to the success of a dental practice. Financial ratio analysis is a technique that business

managers use to gauge the financial health of their firm. Just as someone's blood pressure is an indicator of their cardiac health, financial measures can show the financial health of a practice. When someone looks at the "numbers" of the practice, they are measuring whether they are meeting those success factors.

- **Understand how to manage an efficient and effective operation**
  Dental office owners must manage the daily operations of the business to develop a successful practice.

- **Know and manage the sources of risk in the dental office**
  Every business faces risk. Some of this is common to all businesses. Some risk is specific to the industry or individual firm. Regardless, a dentist needs to understand the risk so that they can reduce its effect on practice profitability and protect the practice from risk-related losses.

OBJECTIVES OF THE DENTAL OFFICE SUCCESS FACTORS SECTION

Given these three main goals, it is possible to define the factors that make the operation of a dental practice successful. These success factors become the indicators of a well-run dental business. The first chapter in this section describes the factors and how to measure them using key performance indicators (KPIs). The subsequent chapters then describe each factor and how someone can affect them.

- **Chapter 20: Financial Analysis and Control in the Dental Office**
  Dentists need to know the factors that lead to business success in a dental practice. They then need to know how they can measure whether they are achieving those factors. Key performance indicators assess each success factor. The rest of Section 4 gives more detail on each of

Business Basics for Dentists, Second Edition. James L. Harrison, David O. Willis, and Charles K. Thieman.
© 2024 John Wiley & Sons, Inc. Published 2024 by John Wiley & Sons, Inc.

these items, discussing how dentists can change their practice to improve these indicators and, therefore, the underlying factors.

- **Chapter 21: Maintaining Production**
  Production is the key to a practice's health. Unless a dentist is generating adequate production (and therefore dollars), then no amount of management skill can gain profitability.
  - **Part 1: Duty Delegation**
    If dentists can legally have staff members do tasks in the office that they themselves would have done, then the dentist has time to do other, more profitable procedures. This improves production.
  - **Part 2: Scheduling Patients**
    Dental offices need to keep an orderly flow of patients to use the practice resources effectively. This keeps patient visits, and therefore production, at a healthy level.
  - **Part 3: Dental Fee Policy**
    The fees that dentists charge, along with the number of patient visits, are the basis of office production.

- **Chapter 22: Maintaining Collections**
  Once dentists have done the dentistry, they must collect fees from patients and insurance companies.
  - **Part 1: Patient Financial Policies**
    Dental offices need to establish payment policies that encourage patients to have the needed work done and to pay for it.
  - **Part 2: Office Collection Policies**
    If patients do not pay for services as they had agreed, dental offices need to have methods that encourage patients to fulfill their financial obligation.

- **Chapter 23: Generating Patients for the Practice**
  Patient visits are the basis of all income generated in the practice. Dentists need to be sure that they generate enough patients to meet their financial goals.
  - **Part 1: Generating New Patients**
    New patients increase how much work dentists do in the practice. They often result in large, expensive cases that directly improve the profitability of the practice.
  - **Part 2: Managing Continuing Care**
    Existing patients of the practice have improved oral health outcomes when dental offices see them regularly for periodic maintenance of dental conditions. They also improve the financial outcome of the practice.

- **Chapter 24: Gaining Case Acceptance**
  Any patient who comes to the office may have additional dental work to be done. However, a patient does not automatically accept treatment recommendations. Dentists must properly communicate patients' needs to them and help patients to understand how the treatment will improve their health and life.
  - **Part 1: Communication in the Office**
    All human interactions involve some form of communication. If dentists understand how they transfer information, they can improve communication in the office.
  - **Part 2: Case Presentation and Acceptance**
    Dentists must turn a patient who has dental needs into a patient who wants treatment for those needs by using proper case presentation techniques.

- **Chapter 25: Controlling Costs in the Practice**
  Profit happens when someone keeps their costs less than their revenue. Dentists cannot eliminate costs in the dental office, but they can manage and control those costs. Understanding the nature of the various office costs helps dental office owners to manage costs in the most effective way.

- **Chapter 26: Promoting Staff Effectiveness**
  Successful practices have effective staff members. Effective staff does not just happen. The owner–dentist creates them by hiring the right people, compensating them well, and motivating them to high levels of performance.
  - **Part 1: Selecting and Hiring Employees**
    Dentists need to find people with the right skills to do tasks and the right attitude to fit into the staff team in the office.
  - **Part 2: Compensating Employees**
    Everyone works, to some degree, for compensation. Dental office owners need to develop a competitive pay and benefits package to attract and retain the best employees.
  - **Part 3: Motivating Employees to Perform Well**
    People work, to some degree, for reasons other than pay. If dentists understand what motivates people in the workplace, they can develop a system and atmosphere that promote employee performance.
  - **Part 4: Assessing Employee Performance**
    Employees want to perform well on the job. As employers, dental office owners need to communicate what they expect of employees, reward them when they do well, and discourage inappropriate behaviors.

- **Chapter 27: Maintaining Daily Operations**

  Dentists need to manage daily work in the office. They must ensure that supplies are ordered, laboratory cases are completed, instruments are sterilized, and payments are properly accounted.

  - **Part 1: Office Operations**

    The most profitable practices are those that use their resources effectively and efficiently.

  - **Part 2: Office Accounting Systems**

    Dentists need to establish proper accounting systems to use in the office.

  - **Part 3: Instrument Management Procedures**

    Each dental office needs to establish methods to clean, disinfect, or sterilize instruments and equipment used.

  - **Part 4: Office Supply and Lab Management**

    Each dental office needs to establish methods to ensure that there are enough supplies for procedures and that lab work is properly prepared and returned in time for delivery to the patient.

  - **Part 5: Dental Insurance Management**

    Dental insurance is a reality for most practitioners. They need to understand how dental insurance programs work so that they can manage the programs in the office.

- **Chapter 28: Managing Risk in the Office**

  Practices face many types of risk. Dentists need to identify and manage those risks so that they do not face a financially devastating incident.

  - **Part 1: Office Risk Management**

    Risk management identifies and decreases the sources of risk in the office. Risk may develop from the dentist's role as a practicing dentist or that as the owner of the business.

  - **Part 2: Regulatory Compliance**

    Dental offices must comply with regulatory agencies' requirements.

  - **Part 3: Quality Assurance**

    Many third-party providers require quality assurance through various assessment activities.

Financial Analysis and Control in the Dental Office

CHAPTER 20

Put all your eggs in one basket and WATCH THAT BASKET!

Mark Twain

GOAL

This chapter aims to examine the financial control process for use in dental practices. It discusses the factors that lead to dental office success and gives common financial ratios that assess the attainment of those success factors.

LEARNING OBJECTIVES

At the completion of this chapter, the student will be able to:

- Discuss the steps in the financial control process.

- Describe the common stages in the practice development cycle.

- Describe the six critical factors that lead to dental practice success.

- Compute typical office analysis in the areas of:
  o Office production
  o Office collections
  o Practice costs
  o Patient generation
  o Case acceptance
  o Staff effectiveness.

- Discuss the importance of and give common normal values for the following dental office financial ratios:
  o Overhead ratio
  o Office monthly production
  o Service mix
  o AR amount
  o Collection ratio
  o AR over 60 days
  o Managed care percentage
  o Managed care efficiency
  o Total staff percentage
  o Variable cost ratio
  o New patients per month
  o Recall effectiveness
  o Marketing dollars per new patient
  o Case acceptance ratio

Business Basics for Dentists, Second Edition. James L. Harrison, David O. Willis, and Charles K. Thieman.
© 2024 John Wiley & Sons, Inc. Published 2024 by John Wiley & Sons, Inc.

KEY TERMS

AR amount over 60 days
basic profitability formula
collection ratio
fee profile
key performance indicator

lab-to-labor ratio
managed care percentage
mix of devices
overhead ratios
staff efficiency ratio

standards
success factor
variable cost ratio

Financial control looks at the "numbers" of the practice to maximize its profit. Dentists can make the financial control process as simple or as complex as they want. The possibilities for gathering data are endless. The problem is often deciding which of the many reports and analyses they truly need. Practice owners should not inundate themselves with information and should look for major problem areas first. They should start with basic ratios (production, profitability, and collection ratios) and look for problems in these areas. If the owner finds no major problems, they probably do not need to do any in-depth analysis. Conversely, a practice may have problems in one area that needs additional attention. Other areas may be functioning well and only require periodic monitoring.

Most people think only of costs when they look at financial control. The revenue side is equally important. For example, costs may be under control, but low production leads to low profitability. Many also think business owners should reduce overhead wherever possible; however, there is "good" overhead and "bad" overhead. Good overhead is money that dentists spend that makes them more money. Bad overhead does not contribute to making more money; it is therefore wasted. For example, suppose a practice owner hires a new staff member with pay of $15 an hour. That staff member allows the dentist to produce an additional $50 per hour. That is money well spent (a good piece of overhead). However, if the office does not increase production enough to make up for the additional costs, the additional money spent on the staff member would be bad overhead. The problem is deciding which costs cause waste and which contribute to the practice's profitability. That is what financial analysis is about.

Many practice owners want to leave the numbers to an accountant. Such a policy is OK if the accountant is familiar with dental practices and understands the dentist's personal philosophy, goals, and where the practice owner wants the office to be financially. The problem is that most accountants do not know these things. They are more interested in tax numbers. If an owner finds an accountant who is knowledgeable about dental practice numbers, they should use that accountant to their advantage. If not, then they will need to be their own financial analyst.

THE FINANCIAL CONTROL PROCESS

Understanding the financial control process is important. Otherwise, someone might apply a simple rule that is not appropriate for the given situation. Chapter 16 presents the fundamental information on finances in the office. This chapter continues the analysis by examining how the dentist should interpret and apply those concepts.

STEP 1: DECIDE WHAT YOU WANT TO MEASURE (SET STANDARDS)

The first step is for the practitioner to decide what to measure. Office computer systems provide unlimited data to analyze. The practice owner needs to know what factors lead to the business's success ("success factors") and set standards to measure those factors. Otherwise, they may be overwhelmed by data that is not important for their purpose. (The next section of this chapter gives a set of basic success factors and their measurement that all dental offices follow.)

A standard serves as a mechanism to monitor practice performance and should meet the needs of a particular practice. Practitioners often use national or regional averages to set a standard. For example, the average overhead ratio is 65%. Does that mean that the practice *should* have a 65% overhead ratio? Not necessarily. A practice may be a start-up business in which the dentist is not fully scheduled. So, any time a practitioner compares their practice to others as a standard, they must adjust the analysis appropriately. The key is to decide the appropriate standard – what is it that the practice owner wants to measure? They should look for measures that relate to the changes made or suspected problems rather than trying to measure everything. In this way, they can make a higher impact by concentrating on specific target areas rather than trying a "shotgun" approach to measuring their practice.

STEP 2: DECIDE HOW TO MEASURE IT (MEASURE PERFORMANCE)

Although standards set forth "what should be," measuring performance examines what has happened in a practice. This reality measure is crucial to successful and effective practice management control.

After a practice owner decides what to measure, they need to find a number that gives good information about the standard. These are known as key performance indicators (KPIs). A KPI should be easy to access from the office computer system, schedule, or other common sources. Depending on the variable, the owner may make these KPI measurements daily, monthly, or annually. For example, they should assess collections monthly. If they look at collections daily, then the natural ebb and flow of the payments may produce an alarming (and wrong) analysis.

Practice owners should be sure to pick an appropriate period for their analysis. Many numbers and ratios may fluctuate widely over a given time range. If so, the owner would want to lengthen the period that they review. Practice owners might track some numbers daily. Some offices set daily production goals. Other offices feel that daily production is too unsteady and prefer to use monthly numbers instead. If someone examines a month in which they took two weeks of vacation, unrepresentative numbers may give skewed results. A quarterly analysis might be more appropriate. Most practitioners look at their numbers monthly. Others look quarterly, believing that this smooths out the monthly variations. Still other practitioners only look at numbers when accountants prepare their taxes. The final group never looks at them. They simply believe that things are going OK and they are making an adequate living, so why bother? All are perfectly acceptable.

Whatever system a practice owner uses, the KPI must relate directly to the standard to measure. It should also represent the entire dental practice and be reliable (consistent) and valid (measure what it is intended to measure). Reliable measures require, for example, that a dentist use the same survey questionnaire to interview patients who have completed treatment. Practice owners cannot expect to gain useful information if they ask different questions each time they give out a questionnaire. Valid standards measure what they are intended to measure. "Percent of recall patients seen by the hygienist" might be a measure of scheduling rather than hygienist performance, for instance.

STEP 3: MEASURE IT (COMPARE PERFORMANCE TO STANDARDS)

In this step, owners compare actual performance with what should have happened to decide if the office met the standard. The actual results and the desired outcomes for the KPI will rarely match exactly. A dental practice owner should set acceptable ranges for performance, evaluate the performance outcomes within these ranges, and then look for exceptions. Management by exception permits someone to concentrate on the significant problems that may arise in the practice without becoming overburdened with the minutiae of all the standards. For example, if someone has a standard of seeing 200 recall patients per month but only see 180 in a month and 197 the next month, they may not be too concerned about the two-month average of 188 recalls a month. However, if they saw only 55 recalls one month and 127 the next month, they would want to explore more fully the reasons for much lower than expected recall patient visits.

STEP 4: DECIDE WHAT TO DO ABOUT THE FINDINGS (CORRECT DEVIATIONS)

This is the essence of control. During this step, the practice owner takes action to adjust the plan or operation of the dental practice. There are four possible courses of action:

- **Do nothing**
  The office met the standard, so no corrective action is required. The office may set a new standard for upcoming measurements to improve office performance.

- **Address an immediate concern**
  The office may find a one-time fix for a given problem.

- **Reset office policies, procedures, and systems**
  The office may need to set or change an office policy or system to solve an ongoing problem or to encourage certain behavior.

- **Dig deeper**
  The office may need to find a more specific measure to analyze the problem further. For example, if the office does not meet the standard for office production, the practitioner needs to know if it is a scheduling problem, a lack of patients, or an issue of the mix of insurance patients.

Correcting deviations from planned standards requires astute problem-solving skills. Knowledge of dental practice management helps someone decide when to modify standards, replace personnel, restructure office policies, set up new staff development programs, and so forth. The key to setting up an effective control system is taking corrective action. Failure to act when someone detects a substantial deviation in a planned standard undermines the purpose of this evaluation system.

The plans that a practitioner started may be inappropriate for the actual conditions that develop. If so, they need to correct the plan itself. If they assume a steady economic climate and plan to expand the dental practice by finding additional office space, equipment, or staff and the general economy declines instead, they will need to alter the plan. If they only find slight deviations, they may decide to monitor the changes and act when these reach a certain point. For example, if a patient satisfaction survey reveals slight displeasure with the receptionist from one or two patients, the owner would probably choose to monitor this situation rather than discuss it with the receptionist. If other patients also reported dissatisfaction over a period, the owner may decide to speak to the receptionist.

STEP 5: FOLLOW-UP (MONITOR)

The office needs to follow up with any changes to be sure that the changes result in an improved outcome. This might be during regular monitoring activities or as a special follow-up review.

PROFITABILITY ANALYSIS

The basic statement that shows profitability is the profit-and-loss formula (Box 20.1). (This is also the profit-and-loss or P&L statement.) Practice owners want to maximize the "bottom line" and make the practice as profitable

as possible, given certain constraints. (Dentists could increase income by working 80 hours per week, but most are unwilling to do that.) There is no magic formula. To increase profit, practice owners can only increase revenues, decrease costs, or combine the two. So, they need to examine the components of the income formula (both revenues and costs) when planning an office analysis.

DENTAL PRACTICE REVENUES

Total collections (gross practice revenues) result from the number and type of procedures that dentists do, the fee that they charge for each of those procedures, any adjustments granted from the full fee, and the collection ratio shown by the office. Any of the four factors may be at fault if collections are low. The following formulas describe these relationships:

$$\text{Gross Production} = \text{Number of Procedures} \times \text{Fee}$$

$$\text{Gross Production} - \text{Adjustments} = \text{Net Production}$$

$$\text{Net Production} \times \text{Collection Ratio} = \text{Revenues}$$

- **Gross production** is the total amount of dentistry produced by the office for the period before any discounts or adjustments. Production levels vary with the number and types of procedures done and the fee charged for those procedures. Gross production is the combination of all individual procedures and fees. Production is obviously the cornerstone of practice profitability in dental practices because, without production, no money flows through the office.

- **Adjustments** are the amounts of money that the office "wrote off" for discounts because of payment plan (such as Medicaid) requirements, marketing efforts, or professional courtesies. Practice owners may decide to track types of adjustments to detect the plan's impact on the office finances. For example, someone may wish to track how much Medicaid plan payment the office adjusts each month or find the adjustment percentage of each plan to know which plans are more profitable.

- **Net production**, mathematically, is gross production minus adjustments. It is the amount of money that a practice owner wants to collect. Because dentists do not expect to collect the money they have adjusted, they should exclude those amounts from many analyses.

- The **collection ratio** is the percentage of net production the office collects from patients and insurance companies.

| BOX 20.1 | PROFIT-AND-LOSS STATEMENT |

Gross Production
  - Adjustments

Net Production
  - Uncollectibles
} **Revenues**

Revenues (Collections)
  - Fixed Expenses
  - Step-Fixed Expenses
  - Variable Expenses
  - Professional Services
} **Costs**

Net Practice Income
  - Owner's Expenses
} **Profit (Loss)**

Gross Personal Income

- **Uncollectibles** are the monies the dental office has given up trying to collect.
- **Revenues (collections)** are the amounts of money (i.e. cash, checks, and credit cards) that crossed the receptionist's desk for the period. Some of this may be from production this month, whereas the rest may be for dentistry done several months ago but now being paid for. Individuals, insurance companies, or government programs may make payments.

DENTAL PRACTICE COSTS

Dental practice costs fall into three conceptual categories: fixed, step-fixed, and variable:

- **Fixed costs** do not change with production. Rent, for example, remains the same regardless of whether the office sees 10 or 100 patients in a month.
- **Step-fixed costs** change with production, but only in discrete steps. These are employee costs. They are the largest single item of expense for a dental practice.
- **Variable** *costs* change directly with the level of gross production. These are supplies and laboratory charges. If someone produces twice as much dentistry in a month, they would logically expect to have twice the lab and supply bill from the increased amount of work.

The **cost of professional services** is the variable cost of hiring a dentist to provide dental services. This is a large expense item in a large group or dental management service organization (DMSO) practice. In a solo practice, it becomes part of the owner's compensation. It is only important because it helps calculate how much "entrepreneurial profit" the practice produces. This is a key metric if

someone wants to sell their practice, bring in a partner, or distribute profits to practice owners.

PROFIT

Profit is the money available for the practice owner to take from the practice accounts and use for personal benefit and enjoyment.

- **Net practice income (entrepreneurial profit)** is the amount that is available to the owner as profit from operating the practice. This shows the business's efficiency if the owner hires someone to do the dentistry. In a small or solo practice, the cost of professional services is usually included in this category.
- **Owner's expenses** are expenses that an owner has chosen to take from the practice that they could have taken as profit. Examples include personal automobile expenses, personal retirement plan contributions, and many continuing education expenses. Because taking these costs is discretionary, they are included in the practice profit. In a DMSO-type practice, these expenses are included in the cost of professional services.
- **Gross personal income** is the amount the solo practice owner claims for initial personal tax computations.

CRITICAL SUCCESS FACTORS

Seven factors lead to the business success of the dental practice. To keep the process simple, the practice owner only needs to look at a set of seven KPIs each of which measures one of these factors. If that KPI is acceptable, they do not need to do any additional analysis. If it is not acceptable, then the owner needs to dig deeper with other indicators for the factor to find the problem. Box 20.2 lists

BOX 20.2	KEY PERFORMANCE INDICATORS FOR BUSINESS SUCCESS
Success factor	Key performance indicator
Maintaining production	Monthly production
Maintaining collections	Accounts receivable amount
Controlling insurance adjustments	Insurance adjustment percentage
Generating patients for the practice	New patients per dentist
Staff effectiveness	Compensation system
Gaining high case acceptance	Case acceptance rate
Cost control	Overhead percentage

these success factors and the primary (KPI) that assesses office performance on meeting that factor. We then develop additional indicators to examine each of these critical success factors in more depth.

These factors form the basis of routine office financial analysis in the monthly (quarterly) review of KPIs. If a particular KPI has not been met, then go deeper.

FACTOR 1: MAINTAINING PRODUCTION

Production is the key to a practice's financial health. Unless dentists are generating adequate production (and therefore revenue), no amount of management skill can gain profitability. Production results from the number of procedures done and the fee charged for each procedure. The number of procedures completed is the result of all the management functions in the office. The front office influences this through scheduling. A dentist's abilities, wants, and the efficiency of the clinical personnel also affect production.

Primary KPI #1: Office Production per Month

This KPI tracks the total amount of dentistry (production) done by the entire office for the month (Box 20.3). Assuming an individual practitioner, production should remain steady or rise each month. (Obviously, if a dentist takes a week off, production may be down for that month.) Others may set daily production goals. The actual number for production varies by region. The fee for a service in a large east-coast metropolitan area is much greater than that in a small mid-western farming community. (Wages are also different.)

Some practitioners like to track gross production, others net production. Gross production describes how

---

BOX 20.3   KPIs FOR OFFICE PRODUCTION

Primary KPI #1: Office production per month
  No decrease

1a. Capacity utilized
  >90% utilized

1b. Mix of services
  One-third hygiene
  One-third non-lab-related
  One-third lab-related

1c. Fee profile
  50th–75th percentile

---

hard a dentist is working because it is before any insurance adjustments. It is a gauge of patient visits. Net production (after adjustments) shows how much money the office generates. It is a more accurate gauge of practice finances and insurance plan participation. Net production defines income, whereas gross production determines costs. Either is an appropriate indicator, depending on what someone wants to measure.

If the owner finds a problem in the KPI office production per month, they can use the following indicators to help identify the problem:

- **KPI #1a. Capacity utilized** assesses how well the facility is used. It is the percentage of potential patient visits (appointments available) that are filled by a patient. This measure includes capacity, the number of patients, and scheduling effectiveness. An office, regardless of size, should fill a minimum of 90% of the available appointments. Less than this, the office has slack (and unneeded) resources that drain profitability. This metric accounts for cancelations and no-shows. More importantly, it examines scheduling and the size of the patient pool. This measure can also help determine when an office needs to expand or add additional employees.

- **KPI #1b. Mix of services (procedure mix)** examines the types of services done in the office. To do production, the office must adequately schedule patients. "Adequately scheduled" does not just mean being busy. Instead, someone needs a good mix of highly productive procedures (such as crown and bridge) and preparatory procedures (such as restorations). As a rule, a general dental practice should have about one-third of the revenue generated from hygiene procedures, one-third from non-lab production, and the final one-third from high-margin lab-related procedures. This shows enough patients in the pipeline for diagnostic, basic, and complex procedures. If the practice mix is significantly different from this, then the dentist might look at new scheduling priorities.

- **KPI #1c. Fee profile** compares the practice's fees to the average fees in an area. Most practice owners want to position themselves so that they are in the upper half of fees in the area. More aggressive practitioners prefer to be above the upper 75th percentile. Owners must be sure to keep fees current for the area in which they practice. Even a small increase can have a dramatic influence on production numbers. Monitor fees regularly. Depending on the insurance plan, the dental office may not have the power or discretion to set fees for those patients.

FACTOR 2: MAINTAINING COLLECTIONS

Once the dentistry is done, the dental office needs to be sure to collect from patients and insurance companies for the work done (Box 20.4).

Primary KPI #2: Accounts Receivable Amount

This KPI assesses the office collection efficiency. It shows the proportion of production that dental offices are not collecting. A raw amount for accounts receivable (AR; e.g. $30 000) is meaningless. Was that from a practice that grosses $25 000 per month or one that grosses $90 000 per month? (AR will be larger for larger practices, all other things being equal.) This indicator says that for any practice, about 0.5–1 times the average month's net production is acceptable as an AR amount. Credit and collection policies will have an obvious impact on the indicator. Easy credit policies will generate higher AR; stricter policies lower. Practices that process a large amount of insurance (more than 60–70% of patients) will also have a larger AR as they wait for insurance companies to process forms and send checks. Immediate fee-for-service practices are on the low end of this range. This also assumes that the office processes insurance electronically rather than through paper and mail. These latter practices will have higher AR (up to 1–1.5 months' production) because of the slower insurance processing.

If the owner finds a problem in the KPI accounts receivable amount, they can use the following indicators to help identify the problem:

- **KPI #2a: Collection ratio** looks at the office collection effectiveness. It should be at or more than 98% of net production. Ideally, everyone should pay their bill. Most dental offices collect between 95% and 99% of net production. (Because dentists do not really expect to collect adjustments, those are not included in this ratio.)

BOX 20.4	KPIs FOR MAINTAINING COLLECTIONS

Primary KPI 2: Accounts receivable amount

    0.5–1 month's net production

KPI 2a: Collection ratio

    >98% of net production

    One-third counter, one-third insurance, one-third billed

KPI 2b: Accounts receivable amount over 60 days

    One-fourth to one-third of a month's net production

A lower collection ratio may suggest problems with collection procedures or a temporary surge in production, resulting in an increase in AR and potential cash-flow problems. A high collection ratio may suggest a credit policy that is too strict, discouraging patients from accepting large treatment plans. This may be a particular problem in younger, growing practices. Established practices with an excess patient base have more freedom to set stricter financial policies.

- **KPI #2b: Accounts receivable amount over 60 days** assesses the timeliness of the office collections. It tells a practice owner how well the front office collects the money from patients that the office has billed. a 60-day-old account is becoming a problem account. Any insurance payments should have cleared on these accounts. These amounts are becoming difficult to collect, and the practice owner has lost the use of the money for that time. Dental practices should see, at most, one-fourth to one-third of one month's production in this number. If this number is high, then either credit policies are too loose, or collection efforts are not strong enough.

FACTOR 3: CONTROLLING INSURANCE ADJUSTMENTS

Managed care programs (preferred provider organizations, dental maintenance organizations, etc.) significantly affect the financial analysis of a dental practice. For example, using gross production will give an unrealistic result in determining collection ratios. If the dental practice discounts 20% of the work done for insurance adjustments, then the highest that it can expect to collect is 80% of gross production. This is a seemingly abysmal amount that may be excellent for the circumstances. Using net production as a basis finds a more accurate collection efficiency. Few dentists in the United States want to deal with any managed care plans. However, most do. If someone does, they need to track how well they control managed care in the office.

Primary KPI #3: Managed Care Percentage

This assesses the amount of the office's insurance adjustments. It looks at the portion of a practice's gross production represented by managed care insurance plans (Box 20.5). (Here, a managed care plan is any dental insurance plan that requires less than full-fee reimbursement to the dentist.) This measure has two options. First, if total managed care production exceeds 50% of total gross practice production, then managed care is simply too great a part of the practice. Not only is the office losing a lot of

BOX 20.5	KPIs FOR INSURANCE ADJUSTMENTS

Primary KPI #3: Managed care percentage

Total managed care production <50% of total production *or*

Managed care adjustments <20% of gross production

KPI #3a: Largest insurance plan

<25% of gross production in any one plan

KPI #3b: Insurance plan efficiency

Total plan collections/full fee value of plan services

money, it is also losing control of the schedule, because managed care patients replace full fee-for-service patients. The practice may be in a "risky" position if the programs change reimbursement schedules or cancel provider contracts. A second measure is to look at managed care adjustments. These adjustments should represent no more than 20% of the total office production. This considers the efficiency of all the plans (in total) that a dental practice is working with, but does not assess an individual plan. Both measures give similar results. The first is a bit easier; the second is more accurate.

If the owner finds a problem in the KPI managed care percentage, they can use the following indicators to help identify it:

- **KPI #3a: Largest insurance plan** examines if a single insurance plan dominates the practice. No single plan should account for more than 25% of gross production. In this way, if that employer changes insurance plans, closes temporarily, or goes bankrupt, the change does not devastate the practice. This may be difficult to accomplish in areas with only one major employer, and the practice depends on that employer for a large portion of the patient pool. It also encourages locating a practice in an economically diverse area.

- **KPI #3b: Insurance plan efficiency** assesses how well each plan reimburses the practice. This indicator looks at each individual plan and asks what percentage it returned compared to a similar, full-fee patient. This way, practice owners know how much discount each plan requires. To calculate this measure, take the total collections from each plan (including any capitation payments) and divide them by the full-fee value. The full-fee value is the amount the dental practice would have charged if this were a private pay patient. Dental

offices need to track this regularly, because plan administrators often change their reimbursements and rules without telling providers. This is discussed in Chapter 27.

FACTOR 4: GENERATING PATIENTS FOR THE PRACTICE

Without patients, dentists have no practice. Patients are either existing (recall) patients of the practice or new to the practice, generated either from internal referrals or outside marketing efforts (Box 20.6). Patient satisfaction with a dentist's care leads to internal referrals. The money that dental practices spend on marketing programs leads to outside new patient generation. All are important sources of patients. Practice owners should monitor them regularly. Established practitioners can often live off internal referrals without the need or expense for external marketing programs. New and growing practitioners often need a planned marketing effort to generate the patient pool needed for success.

Primary KPI #4: New Patients per Month

This KPI assesses new patient generation. Because new patients present with most of the large cases in an office, it tracks this statistic. Each practitioner should see at least 20 new patients per month (or about one per day) to keep the practice adequately busy. "New" patients imply comprehensive care patients, not emergent or episodic care patients.

If the owner finds a problem in the KPI new patients per month, they can use the following indicators to help identify the problem:

- **KPI #4a: Recall effectiveness** examines recall scheduling. It measures the percentage of patients due for

BOX 20.6	KPIs FOR GENERATING PATIENTS

Primary KPI #4: New patients per month

20 per practitioner per month

KPI #4a: Recall effectiveness

>90% of recalls due

KPI #4b: Total active patients

1500–2000

KPI #4c: Marketing dollars per new patient

Treatment = 5 × marketing dollars

recall each year that the dental office saw for recall visits. This ratio examines how effectively the practice encourages patients to return for periodic maintenance visits. In established urban practices, production resulting from the recall visit and subsequent findings accounts for 60–75% of the total production. Managing the recall program is obviously an important component of overall practice management. Dental practices should expect some patient attrition as people move from the area, switch dentists, or forgo dental treatment. However, practitioners should try to reduce these two latter reasons through effective recall planning. Dental practices should strive to see 90–95% of the patients who are due for the month. If they fall short, the front-office person or hygienist (whoever is responsible for recall management) should begin procedures to increase recall acceptance. (This is also, in part, a scheduling issue.) Normal monthly variations suggest that an annual recall effectiveness ratio is better than the shorter, more volatile monthly analysis.

- **KPI #4b: Total active patients** looks at the adequacy of the patient pool or the number of active patients per doctor. Active patients are those who come regularly to the office for both periodic and treatment care. This does not include episodic patients or those who have not been seen for more than a year. There should be 1500–2000 active patients per full-time doctor.

- **KPI #4c: Marketing dollars per new patient** looks at the cost of generating a new patient with the production each new patient represents. If a dental practice is spending $10 to generate a patient who has a treatment plan of $800, the marketing program is obviously effective. Most office accounting software will track patient referral sources and dollars generated from the referral source. This is particularly important in assessing the cost–benefit ratio of specific marketing plans. Dentists should generate at least $5 of production for every $1 spent on marketing. Less than that may still be profitable, but only marginally. Another measure is that dental practices should not spend more than $100 to generate each patient unless the patients are highly profitable.

FACTOR 5: PROMOTING STAFF EFFECTIVENESS

Successful practices have effective staff members (Box 20.7). The owner–dentist creates one by hiring the right people, compensating them well, and motivating them to high performance levels. Analysis items that examine staff effectiveness do not have standard numbers

BOX 20.7	KPIs FOR STAFF EFFECTIVENESS

Primary KPI #5: Compensation system

    Compared to published averages

KPI #5a: Staff configuration

Clerical efficiency	7–9% office production
Clinical staff efficiency	10–12% doctor production
Hygiene efficiency	33–42% hygiene production

associated with them. They are specific to individual practices. However, some general guidelines are provided here.

Primary KPI #5: Compensation System

This examines the staff pay rates relative to others in the community. It helps reward individuals and the team for high performance. Compensation includes both wages and benefits. Staff members compare these with other similar jobs in the area. They then decide if they believe they are fairly compensated for their work. Practice owners should compare their compensation to published averages for the area. The total compensation package should be at or above average for the area. Although simply paying a high wage will not guarantee loyal, hardworking employees, paying an inadequate wage will almost guarantee an unmotivated workforce.

People work for many reasons besides pay. Social interactions found on the job, personal growth, and a belief they are contributing to improving people's lives all play a part. As the practice leader, it is the owner's job to tap into all these emotional reasons for working and to use them to build a cohesive and productive team that meets the philosophy and goals of the practice. That is the essence of motivation and team-building. Practice owners should check how well they are doing through their staff performance appraisals. In turn, staff members should be meeting or exceeding the practice owner's expectations.

If the owner finds a problem in the KPI compensation system, they can use the following indicator to help identify the problem:

- **KPI #5a: Staffing configuration**. Because staff costs are such an important part of the cost equation for dental practitioners, a series of ratios has been developed to assess whether the office is properly staffed. These are "negative" ratios. That means the lower the percentage, the better the ratio. These ratios are given as a range. A ratio above the range may show overstaffing in an area, but too low a ratio may indicate understaffing in that area. Remember to include all employment costs (e.g. wages, benefits, insurance, FICA, retirement plans, etc.) when calculating total compensation. Total employee costs are included in the cost control KPI.

○ **Clerical efficiency**

Clerical efficiency looks at total clerical compensation as a percentage of office collections. Typical practices run at 8–10% for this number. Higher than that, either the office is overstaffed, or its production or fees are too low. Less than that, the office may be understaffed, or the existing staff may be underpaid. If it is understaffed, front-office personnel probably cannot do billing, make appointments, or make collection calls in a timely manner. Problems with general office productivity may result.

○ **Clinical staff efficiency**

This ratio compares non-hygiene clinical labor costs and revenues. Ideally, clinical labor should run at 7–10% of the doctor's collections. (Hygiene labor and collections are excluded and calculated later.) The doctor's productive capacity and the state's expanded function laws will obviously influence this number.

○ **Hygiene efficiency**

Hygiene efficiency examines the relationship between the hygienists' total compensation (including taxes and benefits) and the hygiene area's production. The "exam" portion of the periodic visit is generally included in the doctor's production because that is the person who does that service. This is probably a better ratio than production per hour for looking at hygiene productivity, because areas with higher fees also usually have higher salary levels. (They balance each other out.) Hygienists should be producing 2.5–3 times their compensation. That is to say, compensation should be 33–42% of hygiene revenue (not production).

FACTOR 6: GAINING HIGH CASE ACCEPTANCE

Generating patients for the practice is only one step in generating income. Someone who comes to a dentist for an examination is only a potential patient (source of revenue). The dentist must turn each of those potential patients into patients who accept recommended treatment, becoming comprehensive patients of the practice (Box 20.8). How many accept the recommended treatment is determined largely by how the dentist presents the case and how the office completes the "sales" of dental services. The case

BOX 20.8	KPI FOR CASE ACCEPTANCE

Primary KPI #6: Proper case presentation
Case acceptance ratio >90%

acceptance ratios judge how well the dental office convinces patients to complete the recommended treatment.

Primary KPI #6: Proper Case Presentation

A dentist's case presentation technique is what turns a prospective patient into a comprehensive patient. It involves patient psychology, patient education, selling techniques, and ethical behavior. During the presentation, the dentist should establish what the patient wants and provide solutions to those wants. Everyone will have objections to the treatment proposed. This is a healthy skepticism that, if properly answered, leads to a commitment to act. Despite presentation techniques, not everyone will immediately accept the total proposed treatment. However, dentists should aim for at least 90% acceptance of complete treatment plans.

The appropriate sales technique involves all the office systems that help a potential patient commit to a dentist's treatment recommendations. These include a flexible payment plan, proper collection techniques, appointment availability, follow-up of missed or broken appointments, and reminders of upcoming appointments. If any of these fail, the patient may not initiate or complete the proposed treatment. The case completion ratio compares all the cases completed with those initiated (accepted). Dentists should complete at least 95% of the cases to which patients commit.

FACTOR 7: CONTROLLING COSTS

Because both output (revenues) and input (costs) contribute to productivity, dental practitioners obviously must control both to be productive. There is a cost of doing business. For example, dentists cannot practice without spending money on space or supplies. Any cost that adds to profitability is a "good" cost; any cost that decreases profitability is a "bad" cost. The key is to decide which is which. To accomplish this, most management experts compare a dental practice to norms or "average" practices of a similar type. Every dentist has a cost associated with renting (or purchasing) office space. If the "average" dental practice pays 9% of their production for rent and another dental practice pays 12%, then the rent may decrease the profit of the latter's practice.

Primary KPI #7: Overhead Ratio

This assesses the practice's profitability by rearranging the income statement's information (Box 20.9). Rather than showing how much profit the practice made, the overhead ratio shows how much it costs for a given amount of work. The profitability formula answers the question: "What percentage of production went to pay the bills?" (It also answers the converse: "What percentage of production was left as profit?") The traditional overhead percentage is the total cost of doing business divided by the total collections. This shows, in a rough way, the percentage of every dollar generated that pays the costs of the practice. The inverse (1 – overhead percentage) represents the practice's profitability. (If the overhead is 70%, the practice's profitability is 30%.) The profitability formula often uses total or net production instead of collections. This gives a more accurate picture of costs, especially in practices that participate in highly discounted insurance plans. However, most national reference numbers still use collections as the base. This can lead to confusing practice comparisons.

In general dental practices, overhead (and the overhead ratio) falls into ranges: more than 65% is high; less than 55% is good, and 55–65% is about average. This ratio balances out for different parts of the country. High-fee areas are also generally high-cost areas. If overhead falls into the "good" range, the practice owner may be satisfied, realizing that the trouble of additional analysis and control may not produce enough return to worry about. Conversely, someone may want to maximize the potential profit from the practice and continue the analysis to investigate areas further to increase profitability. If the overhead percentage is out of line compared with other practices, the practice owner needs to look at their numbers more carefully. Generally, the problem is that the overhead ratio is too high, but the overhead ratio may also be too low. This happens when dentists staff the office unrealistically, do not account for all costs (such as working spouses), collections surge because of anomalies in the collection pattern,

or they do not purchase adequate supplies, equipment, and material to keep up to date. Specialty practices have different acceptable ranges because of the different characteristics of those practices. This also assumes that the practice owner is not doing any fancy tax avoidance strategies (e.g. renting space from themselves or hiring family members at an unusually high price) that can skew the results.

When a dentist looks at their overhead ratio compared with others, they compare their practice with other dental practices. When making this comparison, they make two implicit assumptions: that the dental practice is like other practices and that practice owners are rational business people making similar, rational business decisions. These assumptions can be challenged; however, given a broad mix of practice types and styles, a practice owner can use these comparisons as a beginning point in understanding their financial structure.

The overhead ratio depends on a dentist's point in the practice cycle. If someone is in a start-up phase, with few patients and high debts and expenses, the overhead will obviously be very high. New practitioners are often paying off the buy-out or start-up loans. The interest and depreciation expenses represented by this outlay are additional costs that established practitioners generally do not have. New practitioners in a buy-out situation often must replace or update equipment, supplies, and materials at an additional cost. Finally, many new practitioners cannot do the volume of dentistry that established practitioners do. This may be from the need to increase the patient pool or the new practitioner's clinical inexperience. Regardless, if production is less than that for a comparable established practitioner, then the overhead, and most other ratios, will appear to be out of line. New practitioners can expect an additional 5% overhead for debt service while paying off loans. They may even run at a loss (more than 100% overhead) while building a patient pool.

Dentists' personal and professional wants, needs, and desires will modify what they consider to be an acceptable range in all these analyzes. For example, a dentist may be considering two practice options. Practice one produces $600 000 with a 70% overhead on five days per week ($180 000 net). Practice two produces $400 000 with a 60% overhead on four days per week ($160 000 net). They must decide whether the added management problems and time commitments are worth the additional net income.

If the owner finds a problem in office overhead, they can use the following indicators to help identify it:

- **KPI 7a: Specific cost ratios**
  This KPI looks at the same things as the overhead percentage, but begins to break them into specific units,

---

BOX 20.9	KPIs FOR CONTROLLING COSTS

Primary KPI #7: Overhead ratio

  55–65%

KPI #7a: Specific cost ratios

Staff ratio	22–30%
Variable cost ratio	13–20%
Office space ratio	8–10%

using typical ranges of costs for each area of cost allocation. These standards attach values to various components of the expenses of operating a dental practice. Most are related to a percentage of collections. (Some, such as variable costs, may more logically relate to gross production, but industry norms use collections as the basis of comparison.) When using these numbers, someone compares their practice to the "norm" or other similar practices. They can compare every cost if they want, but that is not a good use of time. They should concentrate on the areas where a change can have the most impact.

o **Total staff costs** involve all the expenses of hiring and retaining staff members. This includes gross wages (including withholdings), FICA matching, unemployment and workers' compensation insurance, retirement plan contributions, and any other benefits (such as health insurance) paid by the practice. The acceptable number is a range. $P = A$ practice without a hygienist should be at the low end of the range. Practices that employ a hygienist (or multiple hygienists) should expect to be at the upper end of the range. Staff is the single largest area of cost in the dental office. Little savings here can make a large difference in the bottom line. (Detailed staff ratios are in the staff KPI section.)

o **Variable cost ratio**. Variable costs change directly with production. The more dentistry is produced, the greater these costs should be. Variable cost ratios run at 13–20% for most general dental practices. Breaking these costs down further, dental supplies run from 7% to 10%, office supplies from 1% to 3%, and dental lab costs from 6% to 12%.

o **Office space ratio**. Practice owners should hold the total cost for office space (facilities) within the range of 5–10% of collections. (The average is about 7%.) This is true whether they own or rent space or whether the facility is freestanding or part of a larger situation.

The KPIs for the dental practice are summarized in Box 20.10.

Staff Accountability

Many business owners (including dental practice owners) assign areas of responsibility to a particular person in the office. For example, the hygienist may be responsible for scheduling their own patients. The practice owner may set a standard that the office should see 95% of available recall patients. The hygienist is then accountable for this metric. The person who is accountable needs to have the authority to ensure that they can affect the outcome. For example, if a front-office employee is responsible for hygiene scheduling, they, not the hygienist, should be accountable for the metric.

STAFF MEMBERS AND KEY PERFORMANCE INDICATORS

All dental team members are accountable for the dental practice's success, enabling it to continue to exist and provide for future growth. For an office to be successful, the team members must understand how they contribute to its overall success. Box 20.11 outlines the roles and responsibilities of each staff member and the KPIs they contribute to. Helping the dental staff understand how they contribute to the success of the overall practice is an important role the dentist plays in fostering practice success.

BOX 20.10	SUMMARY OF KEY PERFORMANCE INDICATORS FOR THE DENTAL PRACTICE

Key performance indicator (KPI)	Measures	Value
Factor 1: Maintaining production		
Primary KPI #1: Office production per month	Gross production	Increase
KPI #1a: Capacity utilized	Facilities use	>90%
KPI #1b: Mix of services	Types of services	1/3, 1/3, 1/3
KPI #1c: Fee profile	Fee relative to the area	50th–90th percentile
Factor 2: Maintaining Collections		
Primary KPI #2: Accounts receivable amount	Collection efficiency	0.5–1 month's net production
KPI #2a: Collection ratio	Collection effectiveness	>98% of net production
KPI #2b: Accounts receivable over 60 days	Collection timeliness	<33% of 1 month's net production
Factor 3: Controlling insurance adjustments		
Primary KPI #3: Managed care percentage	Insurance adjustments	<20% of gross production
KPI #3a: Largest insurance plan	Single plan dominance	<25% of gross production
KPI #3b: Insurance plan efficiency	Efficiency of each plan	
Factor 4: Generating patients for the practice		
Primary KPI #4: New patients per month	New patient generation	1/Dr./day
KPI #4a: Recall effectiveness	Recall scheduling	>90%
KPI #4b: Total active patients	Adequate patient pool	1500–2000
KPI #4c: Marketing dollars per new patient	New patient cost	Treatment = 5 × marketing dollars
Factor 5: Promoting staff effectiveness		
Primary KPI #5: Compensation system	Relative staff pay rates	
KPI #5a: Staff configuration	Total number of staff	22–30% of gross production
Clerical efficiency	Front-office staffing level	<9% of office gross production
Clinical staff efficiency	Clinical staffing level	<12% of doctor gross production
Hygiene efficiency	Hygiene staffing level	33–42% of hygiene gross production
Factor 6: Gaining high case acceptance		
Primary KPI #6: Proper case presentation	Case acceptance rate	>90%
Factor 7: Controlling costs		
Primary KPI #7: Overhead ratio	Overall costs	60–70% of gross production
KPI #7a: Specific cost ratios		
Staff cost ratio	Total staff cost	22–30% of gross production
Variable cost ratio	Total variable cost	15–25% of gross production
Office space ratio	Total facility cost	8–10% of gross production

BOX 20.11   ROLES AND RESPONSIBILITIES FOR KEY PERFORMANCE INDICATORS (KPIs) BY DENTAL POSITION

Dentist

Roles and responsibilities	KPIs	
Coach, measure, connect	Production	Average treatment presented
Patient experience	Production per hour	Production per visit
Clinical care	Treatment acceptance %	Supply/lab cost as %
Diagnosis and treatment planning	Average accepted per revenue/patient	of revenue

Dental hygienist

Roles and responsibilities	KPIs	
Periodontal therapist	Production	Fluoride acceptance %
Preventive specialist	Production per visit	# of sealants
Treatment advocate	Reappointment %	Treatment acceptance %
	Perio %	

Dental assistant

Roles and responsibilities	KPIs
Treatment advocate	New patient reappointment
Safe and efficient set-up and sterilization	Treatment or case acceptance %
Operatory organizer	Alignment with dentist goals

Office manager

Roles and responsibilities	KPIs	
Dental staff organizer/manager	Production	% of team members hitting
Practice performance optimization	Collections	performance targets
Process and system implementation	Collections %	Profitability
	Scheduling efficiency	Pre-appointment %
	Cancelations/no-shows %	
	Human resource cost as % of revenue	

Insurance coordinator

Roles and responsibilities	KPIs
Insurance processing	Accounts receivable days
Posting	% of claims <30 days
Denials/appeals	Collections %
Verification	
Statements	

Treatment coordinator

Roles and responsibilities	KPIs
Financial arrangements	Patient acceptance %
Scheduling treatment	Treatment acceptance %
Follow-up on unscheduled treatments	Follow-ups %

Front office team

Roles and responsibilities	KPIs
Answering phones	Call conversion %
Building and maintaining schedule	Cancelation/no-shows %
Over-the-counter collections	Over-the-counter collections %
Data entry	Scheduling efficiency

Maintaining Production

CHAPTER 21

Part 1: Duty Delegation

When a man tells you that he got rich through hard work, ask him: "Whose?"

Don Marquis

GOAL

This part aims to make students aware of the principles of delegating tasks to dental auxiliaries.

LEARNING OBJECTIVES

At the completion of this part, the student will be able to:

- Describe the types of dental staff and their duties.

- Differentiate between the types of supervision in the dental office.

- Describe the methods of labor substitution.

- Describe how state Dental Practice Acts affect duty delegation in the dental office.

- Describe typical extraoral tasks that dentists delegate.

- Describe typical intraoral tasks that dentists delegate.

- Describe the principles of duty delegation.

- Describe the steps in proper duty delegation.

- Describe the benefits of cross-training.

- Describe arguments for and against using expanded-function auxiliaries.

KEY TERMS

bookkeeper
chairside assistant
cross-training
dental hygienist
differential pay rate
direct supervision
doctor time
effectiveness
efficiency

expanded-duty dental assistant (EDDA)
expanded-function dental assistant (EFDA)
flexible staff time
general supervision
indirect supervision
insurance clerk
job sharing

labor substitution
laboratory technician
mid-level practitioners
office manager
outsourcing
receptionist
responsibility

Business Basics for Dentists, Second Edition. James L. Harrison, David O. Willis, and Charles K. Thieman.
© 2024 John Wiley & Sons, Inc. Published 2024 by John Wiley & Sons, Inc.

To schedule patient visits in the office effectively, dentists must decide which procedures various staff members in the office will do. They must schedule each staff member's time and their own time. Each staff member has a cost and allowable duties associated with their position. Duty delegation means time management. It fits procedures to the appropriate staff position. Dentists are trying to maximize their time by having other people in the office do some procedures or tasks that the dentist could do. They choose to delegate these tasks for any of several reasons, including:

- The dentist has other, more profitable tasks that they could be doing.

- The dentist does not enjoy the tasks and wants someone else to do them.

- A staff member is better at the task or procedure than the dentist.

Everyone in the office (including the dentist) should be busy throughout the day. If not, the office is probably overstaffed, incurring an additional, unneeded expense that decreases profit. To be efficient, dentists need to manage their own time in the office and their staff members' time. The principles of duty delegation are based on the idea that dentists have additional patients to see or additional work to do in the office. If not, the critical problem is to increase patient visits and decrease costs. Principles of duty delegation therefore become important for the cost-effective operation of a dental practice.

TYPES OF DENTAL STAFF MEMBERS

Dentists traditionally delegate many tasks in the dental office. They often think only of intraoral tasks when they think about duty delegation. Dentists can direct staff to a broad range of duties that frees their time for other, more lucrative procedures (Box 21.1). They must be sure that the staff member knows how to accomplish their duty and that they are given proper support.

Several types of dental staff members work in a dental practice (Box 21.2). The use of these auxiliary personnel depends mainly on the individual state's laws regarding what dentists can and cannot delegate to non-dentist personnel. Their pay rate depends on local market factors (supply and demand of workers), the skills and training necessary for the job, and the certification the job may require. Often one person may serve several functions in the office. Their overlapping roles typically evolve as the practice grows and hires additional staff members. Larger offices usually have more personnel doing more specialized tasks.

BOX 21.1 TASKS DENTISTS CAN DELEGATE

- Front-office tasks
- Bookkeeping
- Office cleaning
- Equipment maintenance
- Dental laboratory work
- Instrument management (sterilization)
- Supply management
- Chairside assisting
- Some intraoral procedures

BOX 21.2 TYPES OF DENTAL OFFICE EMPLOYEES

Clinical staff
Mid-level practitioner
Dental hygienist
Expanded-duty dental assistant (EDDA)
Expanded-function dental assistant (EFDA)
Dental assistant (certification)
Sterilization clerk

Clerical staff
Receptionist
Office manager
Insurance clerk
Bookkeeper

Other staff
Laboratory technician

CLINICAL STAFF

Mid-level practitioners have the highest independence. They function between a licensed dentist and a hygienist or other auxiliary who is present in the office. These people may operate independently (without a dentist present). They may do restorative work, prophylaxis, basic extractions, and other common dental procedures. Training requirements and allowed procedures are not standard but are evolving. Often a dentist must be available for consultation or follow-up care if needed. Some dentists may use these staff members in the office, freeing the dentist to do more complex restorative procedures. Proponents tout them as a solution to the problem of a lack of dentists in underserved areas, mainly rural and impoverished areas. State laws do not commonly allow this type of dental auxiliary, but they are becoming more frequent. This is currently a hot political issue in the dental profession.

State dental law usually allows **dental hygienists** to do prophylaxis, polishing, and deep scaling on patients, besides taking radiographs. Many states allow hygienists to administer local anesthetic or nitrous oxide conscious sedation if the hygienists have adequate prescribed training and certification. State law describes whether a dental hygienist is subject to general or direct supervision. Most states do not allow hygienists to diagnose intraoral disease, so they generally require some supervision. (A few states allow independent practice for dental hygienists.) They then refer to a licensed dentist for evaluation and treatment of any dental needs that are beyond the scope of their treatment.

Expanded-duty dental assistants (EDDAs) are the same as **expanded-function dental assistants (EFDAs)**. Each state is specific regarding what intraoral functions dentists may delegate to EDDAs. EDDAs generally can expose and process radiographs, place amalgam and composite restorations, fabricate temporary crown or bridge restorations, take preliminary or final impressions, and cement restorations. Although some states allow auxiliaries to perform all these tasks, others allow them to do few or none. Some states require formal training and certification for EDDAs, whereas others do not. Depending on the state where a dentist practices, they might delegate a significant part of many routine procedures to these trained auxiliary staff.

Traditional **chairside assistants** operate chairside, mixing materials and medicaments, passing instruments, and keeping the operating area clean and dry through rinsing and suction. Most states allow chairside assistants to expose and process radiographs if they have had formal training and certification. Formal programs often offer a certificate as a Certified Dental Assistant (CDA) through the Dental Assistants National Board (DNAB). The Commission on Dental Accreditation of the American Dental Association (ADA) accredits dental assisting programs. This shows a higher level of formal training for those who have passed knowledge examinations, and there is an annual continuing education requirement for recertification. Some states require certification, but others do not require this certification to act as a traditional dental assistant.

Many larger dental offices hire someone as a **sterilization clerk**. Their job is to clean, package, and process instruments for the rest of the team to use while seeing patients. Smaller offices require the dental assistant and often the hygienist to process instruments between patients and during designated times during the day. Although this job is critical to office functioning, it is a low-skill, low-training, entry-level job.

BUSINESS OFFICE STAFF

The number and type of business office staff members depend on the size of the office. As the office sees more patients, it needs more front-office (business) staff members (Box 21.3). In some offices, these additional staff members share all duties among themselves. More commonly, they specialize and are responsible for specific duties, such as insurance management, account collections, or patient scheduling. This allows staff members more skilled at specific functions to do those functions and decreases those people's training needs because their jobs become narrower but deeper.

A true **office manager** runs the business office. One to several business office staff members report to the office manager. The office manager can hire and fire staff, make office policies, and develop operational procedures. There is a continuum of responsibility from an office receptionist to a true office manager.

The office **receptionist** is responsible for running the business office in smaller dental practices. In larger offices they are often only responsible for patient interactions, telephone communications, scheduling, and computer entry.

Managing patient insurance has become one of the most significant jobs in many dental offices. Even

---

BOX 21.3	**BUSINESS OFFICE FUNCTIONS**

- Initial patient contact

- Meeting, greeting, and dismissing patients

- Answering and routing telephone calls

- Entering information into the computer system

- Developing financial plans for patients

- Collecting insurance information

- Collecting payments

- Sending statements

- Writing and sending checks as payments

- Processing office payroll

medium-sized offices will typically assign one person to be an **insurance clerk**. This person verifies eligibility and finds benefits schedules and benefits used for the year. Although it may not be the dental office's job, it is often in their best interest to maximize a patient's insurance benefits.

A **bookkeeper** is responsible for paying bills and verifying income from the office computer system.

OTHER STAFF

Dental lab technicians fabricate crowns, bridges, removable appliances, and other complex appliances that the dentist cannot easily delegate to clinical staff members. Most dentists have found it easier and more cost-effective to outsource this function to external laboratories.

LEVELS OF SUPERVISION

Each state has laws that govern the procedures that a staff member may do while in the dental office. Additionally, some states require specific education or certification of different classes of employees. Dentists must know the dental laws of the specific state they practice in, because some states even interpret the definitions of staff differently. (Most state dental boards have a website describing these duties.) However, some general concepts can be applied throughout the nation.

Levels of supervision are critical because they define how much work dentists can have staff members do, freeing the dentists to do other high-skill duties in the office. For example, dentists can delegate placing and carving restorations and many other procedures if a state allows expanded functions. A dentist with an adequate patient base can have more operatories and staff than in a more restrictive state. Hygienists can give anesthesia in many states, freeing dentists from this task. Some states permit hygienists to operate under general supervision, allowing them to see patients while the dentist is not in the office. Many states are now considering allowing some form of mid-level practitioner or dental therapist. Depending on the laws regarding the supervision of these paraprofessionals, the dental practice may take different sizes and forms:

- **Direct supervision** means that the dentist takes full responsibility for the work done. The dentist in the dental office personally diagnoses the condition, authorizes the procedure, and remains in the dental office. At the same time, the staff member completes the procedure and examines the patient before their dismissal. Direct supervision is the most common form of supervision in dental offices in the United States. Many states allow EFDAs to place and carve restorations if the dentist exercises direct supervision. The dentist may inject anesthesia and cut a cavity preparation. The assistant then would place the restoration while the dentist does other procedures in the office. When the EFDA is finished, the dentist evaluates the final product.

- **Indirect supervision** means the dentist is in the dental office, personally diagnoses the condition, personally authorizes the procedures, and remains in the dental office while the dental auxiliary does the procedure, although the dentist may not evaluate the final product or procedure. As an example, the dentist may authorize a prophylaxis by a hygienist or a lab procedure by a technician. The dentist may remain in the office for the procedure, although they do not evaluate the final product or service.

- **General supervision** means the dentist has authorized the procedures (often in writing), and the dental auxiliary carries them out according to the dentist's diagnosis and treatment plan. The dentist does not have to be physically present for the staff member to do the work assigned. For example, in some states a dentist may make rounds at a nursing home and write a prescription that certain patients should have their teeth cleaned by a licensed hygienist. The hygienist may then come to the facility later to do the prophylaxis. Some states allow a hygienist to see patients in the office without the dentist being present. Often this also requires a written prescription. States' requirements for general supervision vary considerably.

LABOR SUBSTITUTION

In dental practice, the labor cost (i.e. wages and benefits paid to employees) is the largest single expense item. Typically, an individual practicing dentist spends from 25% to 30% of collections to pay staff members. If dentists can decrease this cost, they will see the difference (after substitution expenses) as profit. Two major ways to decrease those costs are to control the number of staff members and the wage rate paid and to substitute other methods for labor. The cost of replacing the labor (over time) must be less than the cost of the labor itself. This results in either decreasing costs or allowing an employee to become more efficient (doing more work), thereby decreasing the cost of hiring an additional employee. Businesses use several common methods to substitute for expensive labor, as listed in Box 21.4 and detailed in this section.

CAPITAL (MACHINERY, COMPUTERS)

Industry commonly uses this method of labor substitution in large manufacturing plants, where machines and robotics have replaced many workers. This involves a higher initial cost but a lower long-term expense. It is also common

BOX 21.4	METHODS OF LABOR SUBSTITUTION

Capital (machinery, computers)
Outsourcing
Eliminating marginal jobs
Using lower-paid employees
Flexible staff time
    Part-time employees
        Time
        Duties
    Job sharing

in dental practices. For example, buying digital radiographic equipment involves a significant initial cost, but saves staff costs in processing and maintaining radiographic facilities. A new office management computer system (or software upgrade) may allow the existing person to do additional work rather than hiring an additional front-office person. Other dental examples include purchasing instrument cleaning systems, voice-activated charting systems, or computer-aided design and manufacturing (CAD/CAM) restorations.

OUTSOURCING

Outsourcing means that instead of hiring an employee, dentists pay another company to do the work the employee would have done. This is especially effective if the work is not full-time for someone in a highly skilled position. For example, dentists may hire a laboratory technician to make crowns and bridges in the office. Still, if the dentist does not do enough crown and bridge cases to keep the person fully employed, it is more efficient and effective to outsource the laboratory work by sending it to an outside lab. Similarly, the payroll and bookkeeping functions in large offices are often outsourced.

ELIMINATING MARGINAL JOBS (REDUCTION IN WORKFORCE)

A common method of labor substitution is to eliminate a staff line (through firings or attrition). The dentist then assigns that person's job duties to other people in the office. The work continues to be done but at no additional cost. The downside of this method is that the remaining employees may resent having to do additional work. If the remaining employees were fully busy before, some parts of their job will not be done. So, this becomes an appropriate efficiency method if the remaining employees are not fully busy.

USING LOWER-PAID EMPLOYEES

A related technique is to use lower-skilled, lower-paid employees to do the job that higher-paid employees do. This frees the higher-paid (more skilled) employee to do higher-margin, more profitable procedures. This is the basis of substituting for dentist time, but it also applies to other dental office staff. If two different people in the office can do a job, the lower-paid employee should generally do the job, if the higher-paid employee has other duties that they can be doing during the substituted time. Dentists may need to hire a lower-paid employee to do the job. For example, a hygienist can clean instruments and trays. However, if there are enough patients, they should see an additional patient, and a lower-paid employee (such as a sterilization clerk) should clean the trays. If there are not enough patients for the hygienist to see an additional patient, then a dentist should not hire a sterilization clerk but should have the hygienist clean trays instead of doing nothing. Likewise, dentists should not employ a hygienist if they are routinely sitting in their office working the crossword puzzle while the hygienist does the prophylaxis. Many dentists employ high-school workers part-time to file charts and do other routine, low-skill jobs, freeing the receptionist or office manager to call insurance companies, make collection calls, or arrange patient financing options. Box 21.5 shows an estimate of the percentage of the dentist's time that a trained and competent staff member could substitute for those procedures in which they are involved.

FLEXIBLE STAFF TIME

Using flexible staff time also controls staff costs. Hiring part-time employees instead of full-time employees saves in several ways. Part-time employees may not qualify for employee benefits. Dentists can have them work only peak hours so that the part-time employees are not "sitting around doing nothing" when the office is not busy. These

BOX 21.5	LABOR SUBSTITUTION IN THE DENTAL OFFICE	

Type	Hourly wage	Substitution
Dentist	$100	100%
Hygienist	$40	90%
Expanded-duty dental assistant	$30	65%
Assistant	$20	30%
Sterilization	$15	10%

peak times may occur during the week (Tuesday evenings) or at special times during the year (school holidays or local plant shutdowns). Part-time employees can be hired based on time (e.g. Monday mornings) or job duties (e.g. collecting accounts). If more than one employee wants to work part-time, dentists can often allow them to share a job. Job sharing allows the individuals flexibility in taking time off for vacations and family issues such as daycare. If one employee is present when dentists need them, job sharing can keep excellent employees engaged while meeting their individual time needs.

PRINCIPLES OF DUTY DELEGATION

Before delegating duties and procedures to staff members, dentists need to understand the principles of delegation.

KNOW WHAT THE EXPECTED RESULTS ARE

Both dentists and their subordinates should have a clear understanding of the expected outcome. This may involve a technical procedure, self-assessment, or interpersonal skills of the auxiliary. There is a line to walk between being a "control freak" who manages every decision and a pushover who does not care about the outcome of the decision. With proper training, dentists can let go of the authority to act and follow up where needed.

DELEGATE THE AUTHORITY TO ACT

Dentists must allow the subordinate to act independently. That implies that the subordinate can decide and act on decisions without asking the dentist. The dentist sets the boundaries within which the subordinate can act. However, the dentist must allow and encourage the subordinate to act independently within those boundaries, or the delegation will be worthless. For example, assume that a dentist wants to delegate responsibility to the receptionist for scheduling emergency patients. First, the dentist must decide what constitutes an "emergency" patient (e.g. pain, swelling, hemorrhage). Developing a script for the receptionist to determine if a patient is a true emergency helps in this. Then the dentist defines rules for how and when to appoint these patients. The dentist must also decide what the receptionist should do when a case does not fit the rules. Finally, the dentist should follow up with the receptionist to ensure they act appropriately within the established boundaries. If the dentist does not let the receptionist act independently in this area, they should schedule all emergency patients themselves.

DENTISTS RETAIN RESPONSIBILITY

Delegating does not mean that dentists are free from responsibility or that the auxiliary has all (or no) responsibility for a bad outcome. Both the dentist and the auxiliary share that responsibility. However, because the dentist is the employer and directs the employee to do the task, the dentist is ultimately responsible for the actions or (inactions) of the employee. Therefore, dentists must delegate appropriately to the right person (who has training, abilities, certification, etc.). Dentists must ensure that the work is done correctly. This means both from a technical standpoint (the procedure is clinically acceptable) and a behavioral standpoint (the auxiliary behaved appropriately while doing the procedure). Whether a dentist delegates oral prophylaxis on a nursing home patient to a hygienist under general supervision or delegates preliminary impressions to the chairside dental assistant, they retain responsibility for the correctness of the subordinate's actions.

USE DIFFERENTIAL PAY RATES

Different classes of employees earn different rates of pay in the office. This is based on the supply-and-demand considerations of how difficult replacing someone is. This, in turn, is based on the employee's abilities, training, and certification. Hygienists earn more than assistants because hygienists have additional training and licenses that assistants do not have. This allows the hygienists to do certain functions in the office (dental prophylaxis) that assistants cannot. The hygienist carries a higher financial value. Likewise, an EDDA demands a higher wage in the marketplace than a traditional assistant because they can perform more functions. As a rule, dentists should hire at the lowest pay level first, then hire higher pay-level employees as the demand for their service increases.

DELEGATE TO THE LOWEST PAY LEVEL

For maximum efficiency, dentists should delegate tasks to the lowest level possible. Three factors dictate this. The state Dental Practice Act defines what is legally permissible. For example, dentists may only delegate deep scaling to someone with a dental hygienist license. Dentists must delegate commensurately with the abilities of the staff member. Although delegating placing a composite restoration to an assistant may be legal, if no one has trained the assistant or they cannot do the restoration, the dentist should not delegate the procedure. Finally, dentists must keep the higher-paid employee busy doing higher-level tasks. Dentists should not delegate dental prophylaxis to a dental hygienist if the dentist does not have other (more lucrative) procedures that can be done simultaneously. For example, assume that a dentist's staff members consist of a hygienist (paid $50 per hour), an EDDA (paid $30 per hour), and a chairside assistant (paid $18 per hour). The dentist needs instruments sterilized. Legally, any of the staff can do the procedure. Why pay the hygienist or EDDA to do the procedure when the assistant can do it less expensively? (This assumes that the other staff members are doing other, more lucrative procedures.) If a patient needs a scaling procedure, then the dentist can do it, or they can legally delegate it to the hygienist. It is more efficient to delegate if the dentist has other, higher-value procedures to do while the hygienist is doing the scaling.

CROSS-TRAIN WHEN POSSIBLE

Cross-training means that a dentist trains someone who holds one job to do the tasks normally done by someone in another position (Box 21.6). Often the replacement will not do as good a job as the original person (because of lack of experience), but they can substitute for a short time. This is especially useful if a staff member becomes ill or must leave work for other reasons. (If the dental assistant can process instruments and the sterilization clerk must leave early, the assistant may fill in.) This helps to avoid paying overtime or using temporary employees, adding to office costs. This also promotes teamwork in the office because each employee understands and appreciates other employees' jobs. A dentist might also find an employee who has hidden talents. For example, the dental assistant may have excellent telephone skills and be interested in expanding their duties to confirm and schedule patients.

BOX 21.6 BENEFITS OF CROSS-TRAINING

- Avoids overtime and temporary employees
- Avoids being "held hostage" by key employees
- Promotes teamwork
- Handles peak demand more easily
- Uncovers hidden talent
- Helps prevent embezzlement

STEPS IN DELEGATING IN THE DENTAL OFFICE

Dentists should use the following steps to delegate procedures in the dental office:

- **Determine the state law**
  Each state has a Dental Practice Act that details which procedures dentists can delegate to auxiliaries and which they cannot. It also describes the training and certification requirements for each type of employee. Some laws are negative; that is to say, they describe the procedures that dentists may not delegate to a particular type of employee. Other states have positive laws, which describe the procedures that dentists may delegate to staff. Both types of laws describe the level of supervision dentists must exercise for the procedure. (Some states have different definitions for the levels of supervision from those given here. Each dentist should be sure to read their state's laws carefully.)

- **Decide which procedures to delegate**
  Depending on state law, dentists should decide which procedures they want to delegate to staff. Dentists may need to hire or train staff before legally delegating those procedures. Most extraoral and management procedures (except laboratory work) have few training requirements. Most intraoral procedures have significant rules to follow. Dentists should remember the delegation rules and determine the lowest level to which they can delegate. Box 21.7 gives several intraoral and extraoral tasks that dentists might delegate, depending on state laws.

- **Break procedures into steps**
  Each procedure is a combination of many procedural steps. Dentists can delegate some procedures entirely to staff members. For other procedures, dentists may delegate some steps but not others.

- **Determine which steps dentists can delegate and to whom**
  After dentists have decided what the steps are, they should decide which steps they can delegate and to whom.

- **Estimate the time needed**
  Each step requires a certain amount of time. Although each procedure is unique, dentists can begin to estimate the time required for each step of a "generic" procedure of that type. Box 21.8 shows the time breakdown for a hypothetical two-surface composite restoration. The state l allows trained staff to place and carve restorations

BOX 21.7   PATIENT TASKS TO DELEGATE

Extraoral procedures
Patient education
Oral hygiene instruction
Patient financial counseling
Medical history
Chairside assisting
Passing instruments
Mixing materials
Workspace management
   Evacuation, etc.
   Operatory set-up and breakdown

Intraoral procedures
Scaling
Prophy/polish
Examination
   Existing conditions – charting
   Periodontal charting
   Radiographs/photographs
Placing and carving restorations
Diagnostic impressions
Fabricating temporary restorations

but not to inject anesthesia. These are done under direct supervision. Each office will certainly be different as they estimate the time for procedures and the subtasks to delegate.

The steps in the procedure are in the first column. Steps 4, 6, and 13 are those that the dentist must *personally* do (they may not delegate them, as shown in column 2). The time estimate is for a generic two-surface restoration (personal times may vary). From this breakdown, the total *chair time* for the procedure is 61 minutes (13 + 15 + 33). Of that, the dentist is needed for 18 of those minutes, and they can delegate the rest. The first and last times for the dentist are so small (one or two minutes) that they are impractical to schedule. The only block of *dentist time* that needs to be scheduled is the 15-minute block for cavity preparation. The dentist will need to find time, among other activities, to inject anesthesia and evaluate the completed restoration.

- **Plan appointments**

When the dentist has decided who will do each step and how much time they need for that step, the dentist can plan the appointment, scheduling the patient for the correct amount of time. (The next part of this chapter

BOX 21.8   TIME ESTIMATION

Procedural step	Delegate?	Time (min)	
1. Seat patient	Yes	3	
2. Review medical history	Yes	3	
3. Apply topical anesthetic	Yes	2	13 minutes
4. Anesthetize (inject)	No	2	
5. Apply rubber dam	Yes	3	
6. Cut cavity preparation	No	15	15 minutes
7. Apply bases and lines	Yes	5	
8. Apply matrix band	Yes	3	
9. Place restoration	Yes	5	
10. Contour and finish	Yes	5	
11. Remove rubber dam	Yes	2	
12. Check occlusion	Yes	1	
13. Evaluate restoration	No	1	33 minutes
14. Postoperative instructions	Yes	2	
15. Complete record	Yes	3	
16. Dismiss patient	Yes	1	
17. Disinfect operatory	Yes	5	

describes how to use this information to construct daily patient schedules.)

- **Schedule Appropriately**

  The next part on patient scheduling describes how to use these planned appointments in a comprehensive office scheduling system.

USING DELEGATION IN THE DENTAL PRACTICE

Every office delegates some procedures to auxiliary personnel. The question usually focuses on the delegation of intraoral procedures, using expanded-function auxiliaries.

ADVANTAGES OF USING EXPANDED-FUNCTION AUXILIARIES

Using expanded functions develops a more efficient practice. This allows the dentist to see more patients in a given time. The office can participate in more insurance plans because dentists require a lower income to be profitable in the additional chair. This provides more care to people at a lower (insurance-mandated) fee. Although advocates have claimed that this would lead to lower fees, most dentists keep their fees and the resulting higher income. Patients benefit from more appointment availability and expanded insurance plan participation. Staff members have higher job satisfaction because of the increased responsibility and job enrichment accompanying expanded functions.

DISADVANTAGES OF USING EXPANDED-FUNCTION AUXILIARIES

The biggest downside to using expanded functions is the additional management required. Dentists have more staff members to manage, which leads to more interpersonal interactions that can sour. Preplanning the appointments takes additional time. A larger operation is riskier and more expensive. If a dentist is away from the office, the higher costs of a larger office continue in their absence. Some patients do not want auxiliaries to do technical intraoral procedures. (Studies have shown that dentists can decrease, but not eliminate, this with proper patient education.) Finding certified, competent staff members may be difficult, depending on state laws. In these cases, the certified staff members generally demand a premium wage. This concerns some practitioners, who worry that auxiliaries may "take over" the profession or demand independent practices.

Part 2: Scheduling Patients

This is the earliest I've ever been late.

Yogi Berra

GOAL

This part aims to demonstrate an appointment control system for the office.

LEARNING OBJECTIVES

At the completion of this part, the student will be able to:

- Define the prerequisites for proper appointment control.
- Differentiate between a treatment plan and an appointment plan.
- Describe an appointment plan, its use, and its construction.
- Describe the proper use of the appointment book.
- Describe treatment time codes and how they are used to plan dental appointments.
- Make appointments in a multioperatory office.

KEY TERMS

"outlining" the appointment book
appointment book
appointment control
appointment plan
confirming appointments
delegation of duties
direct supervision
emergency patients

indirect supervision
new patient appointments
primetime appointments
quick call list
series appointments
time units
treatment plan
treatment time codes

Traditionally, dentists have approached appointment control in a dental practice simply. They schedule patients one after another, usually for a standard amount of time such as one half-hour. The appointment may specify the type of treatment to be done, for example alloys. When a staff member seats a patient, the dentist will quickly review the patient's record and select the teeth they will try to restore in that half-hour appointment. With the constant pressure to "produce," the dentist often works over the half-hour, rather than select an amount of work they may finish early. Thus, what occurs is that the dentist gets off schedule with the first patient. They either must do little work on patients at the end of the day or work over at lunch and closing. This results in a practice where everyone rushes all day. Overtime is common. Everyone is nervous. There is low work satisfaction and high auxiliary turnover.

PURPOSES

Appointment control is a system carried out for the convenience of the dental office. A treatment plan is a listing of the procedures that will be done for a given patient. The appointment plan organizes those procedures so the office staff can schedule more efficiently and prepare for and execute those treatment procedures. Appointment control systems are valuable for several reasons.

An effective appointment scheduling system helps promote the office's smooth operation. It does this first by ensuring that dentists and staff members use their time efficiently and effectively. Second, it encourages dentists to see patients on time for their dental procedures. Finally, an effective appointment system helps to balance the patient treatment load and service procedure mix. Simply stated, a properly operated appointment system increases patient satisfaction and staff productivity.

A proper appointment control system is versatile. The dentist and staff should continually observe and receive responses from the practice. Dentists can adjust the appointment control system to meet the changing needs of the practice quickly. This system is for small or large offices. The appointment system described here works in large, expanded-function practices or small, individual practices. The important principles that underlie the system are that dentists do the following:

- Schedule the appointment for the time needed, not for a standard amount of time for all visits. All appointments do not take one hour. Some take considerably less, others more.

- Schedule procedures with the appropriate staff person. Dentists should schedule dental prophylaxes with the hygienist and basic restorative procedures with the EDDA, as permitted by law.

- Schedule dentist time separately from chair time. A patient's total visit may take an hour. Of that, the dentist may only spend 30 minutes with the patient. If dentists schedule correctly, the dentist can see another patient while the staff complete procedures on the first patient.

PREREQUISITES

Before starting an effective scheduling system, the office (dentist and staff) must meet several prerequisites.

WRITTEN TREATMENT PLAN

The first requirement of any effective appointment control system is a formally written treatment plan. This treatment plan is the basis for the entire scheduling system. The office schedule will reflect the accuracy of the treatment plan. Without a formal treatment plan, the practitioner must rediagnose each time the patient is seen.

PROPER DELEGATION OF RESPONSIBILITY AND AUTHORITY

In any practice, the keys to appointment schedule control are duty delegation and preplanning. To delegate effectively, the dentist must know the laws in the state they practice in regarding the delegation of duties to auxiliaries. As described in the previous part on duty delegation, dentists want to delegate any procedure to the lowest level legally possible.

For effective schedule delegation, dentists must give the receptionist enough information to schedule patients efficiently. Only the dentist can provide this information. If a dentist supplies this information each time they appoint the patient, they should make the appointments themselves because it is time-consuming. What the dentist needs are means of preplanning for each patient visit. That is called *process appointment planning* (and it will be discussed later).

The practitioner must delegate to a staff member the authority to keep the appointment book. In the traditional system, the dentist essentially does the scheduling, either by escorting the patient to the front office and telling the receptionist how long and when the next appointment should be, or by giving the receptionist standard appointment lengths (such as 30 minutes for a restorative visit) without regard for the actual time anticipated for the procedure. Either of these approaches is inefficient and inappropriate because the dentist, and a staff member, is doing the clerical duties of scheduling patient appointments.

APPROPRIATE APPOINTMENT BOOK

The third requirement of the system is that the appointment book accurately represents the scheduling needs of the office. If a dentist is using a computer system, they should be sure that the system adapts to the office's needs rather than requiring that the office adapt to the needs of the computer system. Before dentists can use the scheduling module of a computer system, they must set the preferences to meet their office needs. Setting up the computer program includes these steps:

- The dentist should "outline" the appointment book before making any appointments. Outlining sets up the appointment book "matrix" so that staff know what times are available for appointments. The dentist should mark off the times the office is closed; mark off holidays and note when the office is closed for staff meetings and other administrative functions; and show "buffer periods" if the practice uses them (e.g. for emergency patients, new patients). Professional meetings and other professional obligations should also be noted. The dentist should note local school holidays, because many teachers and parents want to find appointments on those days.

- There should be one (and only one) column for each operatory. (There can only be one patient in the chair at a time.) It is assumed that the auxiliary stays with the chair. So, if there is an EDDA chair, the EDDA stays in that operatory.

- Proper time increments should be set. Dentists should be sure that the time increments in the schedule are the same as in the appointment planning process. These must reflect the smallest increments of time for which a dentist is comfortable scheduling patient visits. Initially, a dentist will probably use a 15-minute interval. As they become more familiar with how long it takes to do the various steps of the procedures, it may be shortened to 10-minute intervals to schedule more efficiently. Some experienced offices use 5-minute intervals.

- The dentist should schedule dentist time separately from patient chair time. Dentists must schedule both the time the patient is in the chair and the time that the dentist is captive with that patient.

APPOINTMENT PLAN

The last prerequisite is that the dentist takes a few extra minutes at the time of preparing the treatment plan to organize and sequence the treatment procedures into a plan for the appointments. This requirement is fulfilled by using a worksheet called an appointment plan. The appointment plan is completed just after the dentist formalizes the treatment plan. This plan is how dentists preplan the treatment to be done at each visit, duty delegation (if appropriate), and the length of time required to complete each appointment. Using this method, dentists indirectly control the receptionist's appointment choice.

Appointment plans are helpful for grouping procedures together. Dentists can combine several different procedures or parts of procedures to reduce the number of patient appointments. Quadrant dentistry is much more efficient than single-tooth operations. The appointment book should reflect this.

Dentists can schedule appointments for the time needed. A simple occlusal alloy and a difficult pin-retained build-up obviously will take different amounts of time. The appointment plan allows the receptionist to schedule appropriately for those procedures.

Appointment plans help to organize multiple visit procedures into discrete units. This helps staff to have proper instrumentation, materials, and other needed items ready for the procedure. Staff members can schedule specific patients or procedures for specific operatories. If, for example, radiologic facilities are only available in one operatory, the receptionist can, through proper appointment control systems, ensure that they schedule procedures involving radiographs for that particular chair.

TREATMENT TIME CODES

A time code is always written as three digits separated by two dashes (e.g. 1-1-1). This is a three-digit time code. In any time code, both the first- and third-digit positions refer to an auxiliary. The time code designates:

- Who the primary operators are.

- Their sequence of operation.

- How much time each operator needs.

- Total chair time.

The middle or second digit always refers to the dentist. Thus, in a three-digit time code containing no zeros, the auxiliary operates first, the dentist second, and the auxiliary again operates at the end.

Set Time Increments

Dentists must have a consistent increment of time. It is recommended that one increment or unit is equal to 10 minutes for the experienced practitioner, and one unit is equal to 15 minutes for the less experienced practitioner. In this discussion and example, one unit is equal to 15 minutes. Thus, the digit "2" equals 30 minutes. Consequently, the time code 1-2-3 would mean the following:

- The first operator is an auxiliary needing 15 minutes (one 15-minute time unit).

- The second operator is the dentist needing 30 minutes (two 15-minute time units).

- The third operator is the auxiliary needing 45 minutes (three 15-minute time units).

- Total chair time is 90 minutes.

When the first operator is the dentist, use a zero in the first digit position (e.g. 0-1-2). A single 10-minute block is required for operatory set-up, breakdown, and disinfection, even if the designated auxiliary is not required during the visit.

Develop Standard Time Codes

To schedule dentist, assistant, and total chair time, a dentist must have a notion of how long the typical procedure will take to complete. A copy of this should be given to the receptionist. Unless the receptionist is instructed otherwise for a particular procedure, they should use these time codes to schedule appointments. For example, if Mrs. Jones has a particularly difficult alloy or a quadrant of composites to complete, note the three-digit time code needed for this appointment on the appointment plan.

Box 21.9 should be completed with numbers from a particular practice. Box 21.10 is given as an example only. A dentist's frequent procedures and time requirements for each procedure will differ from this example. These time codes will also change over the practice life as skills, abilities, staff, and the physical office change.

- **Code** is an abbreviation for the step in the procedure. For example, "E2M" means "Endo, 2nd visit, Molar." A dentist can decide which procedures the office commonly uses and an appropriate abbreviation for each. If the dentist generally takes 12 visits to complete a denture, then develop 12 procedure steps for dentures. If the office commonly does other procedures, add them to the list.

- **Treatment** is a description in words of the step code.

- **Delay** is the number of days between the previous visit and this visit. If, for example, the office routinely needs 10 days to get lab work back on crowns, a "10" is put in this column for the second crown visit.

CONSTRUCTING APPOINTMENT PLANS

The appointment plan has columns containing the procedures, time code, and date completed. The first step is to make a diagnosis and construct a treatment plan as usual. Then complete the appointment plan.

Decide Appropriate Operatory (Staff Person)

The dentist needs to decide which operatory the procedure will be done in. This is an indication of which auxiliary type will see the patient. If, for example, the office employs an EDDA who is trained and capable, then dentists schedule the patient in the EDDA chairs, freeing themselves of the time required to place and carve the restoration.

The dentist should estimate how long each standard procedure takes to complete, filling in a time code for each type of staff and each procedure. Each time unit should be the same as the appointment book (5-, 10-, and 15-minute intervals). The three-digit time code reflects how long:

- The staff member has to set up the operatory, meet, greet, and seat the patient, and begin initial treatment procedures, such as removing temporaries.

- The dentist will have with the patient.

- The staff member has alone with the patient for completing work, patient dismissal, and operatory breakdown and clean-up.

The three-digit time code also defines who the treating auxiliary is:

- **Units (traditional)** is the three-digit time code the office uses for this procedure if it is done with a traditional chairside dental assistant.

- **Units (EFDA)** is the three-digit time code the office uses for this procedure if it is done with an EFDA. Dentists should not bother with this column if the state Dental Practice Act does not allow these auxiliaries in the office.

- **Units (hygienist)** is the three-digit time code the office uses for this procedure if a dental hygienist does it.

BOX 21.9   TIME CODES

Code	Treatment	Delay (Days)	Units (Traditional)	Units (EFDA)	Units (Hygienist)
Initial exam					
IA	Adult		_____	_____	_____
IC	Child		_____	_____	_____
EM	Emergency		_____	_____	_____
Recare exam/prophy					
RA	Adult		_____	_____	_____
RC	Child		_____	_____	_____
Amalgam					
AM1	1 Surface		_____	_____	_____
AM2	2 Surface		_____	_____	_____
AM3	3 Surface		_____	_____	_____
AM4	4+ Surface		_____	_____	_____
Pol	Polishing		_____	_____	
Composites					
CM1	1 Surface		_____	_____	_____
CM2	2 Surface		_____	_____	
CM3	3+ Surface		_____	_____	
Complete denture construction					
CD1	Initial impression	_____	_____	_____	
CD2	Final impression	_____	_____	_____	
CD3	Jaw relations	_____	_____	_____	_____
CD4	Try-in/delivery	_____	_____	_____	
CD6	Adjustment	_____	_____	_____	_____
Endodontics					
E1	Initiate	_____	_____	_____	
E2M	File (molar)	_____	_____	_____	
E2A	File (anterior)	_____	_____	_____	_____
E3M	Fill (molar)	_____	_____	_____	
E3A	Fill (anterior)	_____	_____	_____	_____
Extractions					
EXT	Simple extraction		_____	_____	_____
EXTQ	Quadrant extract, alveoloplasty		_____	_____	
SUT	Suture removal	_____	_____	_____	
Crown and bridge					
CR1	Crown: prep, temp, imp		_____	_____	_____
CR2	Crown: seat	_____	_____	_____	
BR1	Bridge: prep, temp, imp		_____	_____	
BR2	Bridge: seat	_____	_____	_____	_____

This chart allows the dentist to fill in time codes for several common procedures. They can add or delete procedures as their practice dictates. The chart allows for time codes for three types of auxiliary employees.

BOX 21.10 EXAMPLE TIME CODES

Code	Treatment	Delay (Days)	Units (Traditional)	Units (EFDA)	Units (Hygienist)
Initial exam					
IA	Adult		2-3-1	2-3-1	2-1-3
IC	Child		2-1-1	2-1-1	2-1-1
EM	Emergency		1-2-1	2-1-1	2-1-1
Recare exam/prophy					
RA	Adult		1-3-1	1-3-1	2-1-2
RC	Child		1-1-1	1-1-1	2-1-0
Amalgam					
AM1	1 Surface		1-1-1	1-1-1	1-1-1
AM2	2 Surface		1-2-1	1-1-2	1-2-1
AM3	3 Surface		1-3-1	1-2-3	1-3-1
AM4	4+ Surface			1-3-1	1-2-3
Pol	Polishing		0-1-0	1-0-0	
Composites					
CM1	1 Surface		1-2-1	1-1-2	
CM2	2 Surface		1-3-1	1-1-3	
CM3	3+ Surface		1-3-1	1-2-3	
Complete denture construction					
CD1	Initial impression				
CD2	Final impression	3	1-3-1	4-0-0	
CD3	Jaw relations	5	1-2-1	3-0-0	
CD4	Try-in/delivery	5	1-2-1	3-0-0	
CD6	Adjustment		1-1-0	2-0-0	
Endodontics					
E1	Initiate		1-3-1	1-2-2	
E2M	File (molar)	3	1-4-1	1-3-2	
E2A	File (anterior)	3	1-3-1	1-2-2	
E3M	Fill (molar)	3	1-4-1	2-2-2	
E3A	Fill (anterior)	3	1-3-1	3-1-2	
Extractions					
EXT	Simple extraction	1-2-1	1-2-1	1-2-1	
EXTQ	Quadrant extraction, alveoloplasty	1-4-1	1-4-1	1-4-1	
SUT	Suture removal	0-1-0	1-0-0	0-1-0	
Crown and bridge					
CR1	Crown: prep, temp, imp		1-4-1	2-2-2	
CR2	Crown: seat	8	1-3-1	2-1-2	
BR1	Bridge: prep, temp, impression		1-6-1	3-2-3	
BR2	Bridge: seat	8	1-4-1	2-3-2	

This chart gives example time codes for several common procedures. Each office's codes will be different, depending on the speed and skill of the dentist and staff members.

Group or Split Procedure Steps into Appointment Blocks

The treatment plan lists all of the dental procedures that a dentist will do for a patient. Some of those procedures require several visits to complete. Dentists need to break them into their steps for treatment visits. Others are quickly accomplished and can be combined with other procedures in a single appointment. The appointment plan then groups those procedures with the procedural steps so that the dentist knows what will be done at each appointment.

In Box 21.11, the patient, Susan Smith, will have the procedures listed in the treatment plan done. The appointment plan shows that the treatment will be done in seven appointments. The first appointment, for 30 minutes, will be with the hygienist for scaling and root planing. The next appointment is to initiate endodontics on tooth 3 in the chairside assistant's chair. The next visit is also with the assistant for filling the endodontic preparation. The patient will then be in the EDDA chair to complete a core on tooth 3, then again with the EDDA for preparation, impression, and temporization of crowns on teeth numbers 7 and 3. The final visit is in the assistant's chair for the cementation of the crowns.

Group the treatment steps for each appointment based on efficient delivery. For example, if several teeth in a quadrant require restorations, restoring the entire quadrant at one visit is more efficient than restoring each tooth at a separate visit. (There is less operatory set-up and breakdown time, less time for anesthesia, etc.) In grouping procedures, there are no restrictions on grouping different types of treatment, such as preventive and restorative, at the same visit. Combining different types of treatment often results in better scheduling.

Notice several additional guidelines for allotting time. First, no time is allotted for an auxiliary to assist the dentist; the assistant is always at the chair. Secondly, no time is allotted for local anesthesia. Because this procedure generally takes such a small amount of time, it is not worth scheduling even the shortest appointment (e.g. 10 minutes) for that procedure. Thirdly, no time is allotted for evaluating procedures that have been delegated for the same reason. The quantity of time allotted in each digit is based on the number of procedures to be done, the difficulty of the procedure, the experience and speed of the operator, and individual patient management factors.

MAKING PATIENT APPOINTMENTS

Proper planning dramatically simplifies making appointments for the receptionist or other front-office person. Computer scheduling modules have evolved to become effective if the staff members set them up correctly. However, most programs still need effective appointment planning modules. A dentist may need to develop paper systems (like in this chapter) to communicate appointment planning needs. The process for making an appointment includes several steps:

- The scheduler uses the appointment plan for each patient to schedule the next visit. As the appointments are completed, the receptionist schedules the time code for the next appointment in the priority column. If the dentist has no appointment plan (e.g. for a new patient visit), the receptionist uses standard time codes to decide how much time to schedule.

- One person, usually the receptionist, should be in charge of making appointments. If a dentist finds problems or changes are required, they can deal with them

---

BOX 21.11	COMPARING A TREATMENT PLAN WITH AN APPOINTMENT PLAN

Treatment plan – Pt name: Susan Smith

Tooth #	Procedure
All	SRP&P
3	Endo
3	Core
3	FG crown
7	PM crown
19	MOD alloy
20	DO alloy

Appointment plan – Patient name: Susan Smith

Procedure	Time code	Chair
1. SRP&P	3-0-0	Hyg
2. E-1 #3	1-3-1	Asst
3. E-2 #3	1-3-2	Asst
4. Core #3	1-1-2	EDDA
5. R #19, #20	1-1-3	EDDA
6. CR1 #3, #7	1-4-2	EDDA
7. CR 2 #3, #7	2-2-2	Asst

This chart shows how a treatment plan relates to an appointment plan. The treatment plan lists the billable procedures by tooth number. The appointment plan shows which of those procedures (or parts of the procedures) will be done at each of the appointments.
Asst = assistant; EDDA = expanded duty dental assistant; hyg = hygienist. See the text for a description of the procedures.

by involving only one person. (Obviously, other office staff members should know how to make appointments if the primary person is out of the office.) If the hygienist is in charge of preappointing periodic (recall) visits, then they are in charge of that component of scheduling.

- The computer scheduling program should enforce the following guidelines when making appointments:
  - Do not overlap patients in a chair. (Only one patient can be in a chair at a time.)
  - Show dentist time and chair time.
  - Do not overlap dentist time horizontally across chairs. (The dentist can only be in one operatory at a time.)
  - Include the patient's name, phone number, and abbreviated procedural listing for the appointment.
  - Schedule appointments as determined on the appointment plan or with standard time codes.

EXAMPLE SCHEDULE

An example daily schedule is given in Figure 21.1. This conceptual appointment calendar shows the principles of proper patient scheduling. This conceptual schedule uses an arrow to represent the time the operatory is dedicated to the patient, either direct patient time or breakdown and set-up time. The barbells represent doctor time when the doctor is directly tending to the patient. Office management software systems use color codes that replace the arrows and barbells, hot links that show patient contact information and alerts, and other features that enhance the scheduling function. Nevertheless, the software *must* support the basic idea of scheduling chair time and dentist time as separate functions.

It is assumed that an auxiliary is associated with each chair. The first two chairs are dedicated to traditional dental assistants, the third to an EDDA, and the fourth to a hygienist. (In the example, state law allows an EDDA to place and carve final restorative materials.)

The dentist had previously determined the appointment increments when they developed the appointment plan and associated time codes for each visit. An example of determining these delegated time increments is given in Figure 21.1 (15-minute increments for both schedule and time codes are used in this example). In the schedule, Pat Greene has an appointment in chair 2 at 9:00 for the second visit for a crown on tooth 4 (Cr 2 #4). The dentist set a

↕ = Chair Time		⦚ = Doctor Time		Date: _____

	Chair #1 – Assistant	Chair #2 – Assistant	Chair #3 – EDDA	Chair #4 -Hygienist
Time	**Patient and Service**	**Patient and Service**	**Patient and Service**	**Patient and Service**
8:00				
8:15		Anne Woods	Mary Adams	Connie Judd
8:30		E-1 #9	New Patient	Adult Recall
8:45	Eva Sands	Confirmed		Left Message
9:00	Ext 1, 32		John Smith	Bobby Franklin
9:15	Confirmed	Pat Greene	Comp # 3, 4	Child Recall Confirmed
9:30		Cr-2 #4	Text	
9:45		Text		Mary Worth
10:00			Ted Ford	Quad Scale UR
10:15	Joe Morgan		Comp #14	Text
10:30	Br-1 4 X 6	Kevin Ross	Text	
10:45	Left Message	Suture Rem -Confirmed		Hank Studer
11:00			Amy Hand	Adult Recall
11:15		Bob Hoffman	Am # 19,20,21	Text
11:30		CD-3	Left Message	Jenny Combs
11:45		Left Message		Child Recall Confirmed
12:00	Lunch	Lunch	Lunch	Lunch
12:15	Lunch	Lunch	Lunch	Lunch
12:30	Lunch	Lunch	Lunch	Lunch
12:45	Lunch	Lunch	Lunch	Lunch
1:00				

This chart shows an example of a morning schedule for a hypothetical dental office. The arrows show chair time and must not overlap vertically. The barbells show dentist time and must not overlap horizontally.

FIGURE 21.1 Example schedule.

time code of 2-2-1 for this visit. This means that the patient is with the auxiliary for 30 minutes (i.e. operatory set-up, anesthesia, and temporary removal), with the doctor for 30 minutes (i.e. try-in, adjustment, and cementation), followed by 15 minutes with the auxiliary (i.e. clean-up, patient dismissal, operatory breakdown, and disinfection). Remember, no time block is assigned for anesthesia or checking completed work.

In the schedule, the lines with arrows (patient appointment time) cannot be overlapped vertically, or two patients would be in the chair simultaneously. Anne Woods will occupy chair 2 from 8:00 until 9:00, Pat Greene from 9:00 until 10:15, Kevin Ross from 10:30 until 11:00, and Bob Hoffman from 11:15 until 12:00. There are two 15-minute intervals when chair 2 is not scheduled this morning.

The barbells show the dentist's time with the patient in the indicated chair. Dentist time cannot be overlapped horizontally, or the dentist would need to be in two places simultaneously. The dentist is with the patient in chair 3 at 8:00 for 15 minutes, then in chair 2 to initiate endodontics on tooth 9 for 30 minutes. They then move to chair 1 for 30 minutes for extractions and then to chair 3 to prepare amalgam restorations on teeth 3 and 4. (The EDDA will fill these latter preparations.) The dentist moves to chair 2, chair 3, and so forth throughout the morning. As previously mentioned, no dentist time is scheduled for anesthesia or final evaluations. At some point during the first 15 minutes, the dentist will stop by chair 1 to administer anesthesia, and during the first hour they will attend to chair 4 (the hygiene chair) to check the adult recall on Connie Judd.

APPOINTMENT ISSUES

Several additional notes follow about appointments.

- **Patient communication**
  The receptionist should offer the patient appointment options. They should not simply ask: "When do you want to come in again?" (The patient may not want to come again!) They should offer the patient "Tuesday at 10:00 or 1:30." This allows the receptionist to fill one day before moving to another. The receptionist should also avoid the mind trap of just "filling holes" in the schedule. Instead, they should consider the procedure, the patient, and other procedures scheduled near and opposite this procedure.

- **Series appointments**
  Many patients prefer a series of appointments (e.g. every Tuesday morning at 8:30). For patients with long treatment plans, the advantage is that they provide a consistent time for the patient. However, patients may feel freer to cancel a series of appointments, knowing

that they have another already scheduled. Dentists should be sure that they allow time between appointments for lab turnaround, and that treatment does not go too far ahead of a patient's payment plan.

- **Vary the day**
  A variety of procedures should be scheduled during a typical day. Long, productive appointments should be scheduled during the dentist's best time (some dentists are morning people, and some are afternoon people). At least one "big-ticket" item (bridge, partial, or other large-fee procedure) should be scheduled for every morning or afternoon session.

- **"Primetime" appointments**
  Evening hours and Saturdays are high-demand times. Many dentists restrict these appointments to private pay or traditional indemnity plan patients. Others charge an additional fee for evening hours, not so much for the income as to make patients aware of how valuable those time slots are. Many dentists have especially strict cancelation and "no-show" policies for these prime hours.

- **"Look-sees"**
  A look-see is a quick evaluation of a small problem. The dentist does not plan to do anything, just to look at the problem and see what should be done about it. These visits may be for follow-up of previous treatment or as a triage method for emergent problems. The minimum time allotment should be used for these quick appointments. Some dentists have an extra operatory for such use.

- **New patient appointments**
  New patients should be scheduled as soon as possible. A maximum wait of 2–3 days is suggested. New patients are the lifeblood of a practice. They may have waited for months, building their courage to call. They may have just won the lottery. Whatever the reason, they are ready now. Dentists should get new patients an appointment quickly. They may schedule "buffer time," which is an hour allotted for new patients and is kept open for only new patients until the day before the appointment. The new patient should be told of the fee required and the need for insurance forms and plan information (if any).

- **Children**
  Children should be scheduled in the morning if possible. They are less tired and, therefore, better acting that way. Their parent may want the appointment after school, but the scheduler does not have to schedule it at that time.

- **Elderly patients**
  Many elderly patients do best in the mid to late morning slots. They can get up and dress, take their daily medicine, and get out before lunch or before they get tired in the afternoon.

- **Emergency patients**
  The dentist should have a standard list of questions for the receptionist to determine if the caller has a true dental emergency (Box 21.12). Depending on the availability of time and the practice philosophy, the dentist can set parameters for whom they should see and how quickly. As with all transactions in the office, the dentist should have a written script for the receptionist to follow in assessing and appointing emergency patients.

- **Confirming appointments**
  The dental office should confirm appointments daily for the following day. If the staff member cannot talk with the person at home, they should leave a message. The patient should be asked before they are called at work. Many people (and their employers) do not want to be bothered while working. Most dental office computer systems have automatic call or texting appointment reminders incorporated into the system.

- **Problem patients**
  All offices have "problem" patients. These patients are habitually late, consistently break appointments, or fail to show up for scheduled appointments. What a dentist does with these people is a matter of personal preference and where they are in the practice cycle. If a dentist has a young practice they are trying to build, they will tolerate more of this behavior than if they have a well-established, "full" practice. Some practitioners charge patients for broken appointments. The purpose is to try to instill the importance of the visit rather than try to generate any income. If the purpose is to anger people who break appointments and drive them away, then the dentist should use this technique also. It works well for that.

- **"Quick call" list**
  Most dentists maintain a "quick call" list. These patients live or work nearby and can come in at short notice to have work done. Most computer management programs have these lists built into the program. (A 3×5 in. file card box or a simple list on a legal pad is sufficient.) If a patient expresses a desire to be seen sooner than the office schedule otherwise permits, write their name, phone number, procedure, time code, and present appointment on the list. Whenever a cancelation occurs, the receptionist checks the list for an appointment code that will fit into the newly vacated time slot. The receptionist can easily update the code for the next visit when the dentist completes a patient's appointment plan.

  Quick call lists have several uses. The most obvious is filling a time slot when a patient cancels their appointment. This lets the office use their valuable (and expensive) time the best. It is also used when confirming appointments (usually 1–2 days ahead). If a patient cannot keep their scheduled date, staff members can fill it with the quick call list. Finally, many practitioners keep new patient slots open until the day before the appointment slot. (This allows the office to see valuable new patients quickly.) If the dentist has scheduled no new patients for the day, the receptionist can also use the quick call list to fill those time slots.

- **"Tickler" list**
  Dentists should keep a list of patients who have missed appointments and need to be rescheduled. Some patients will miss an appointment and forget to call back for another appointment. Others do not have their schedule with them or need to check conflicting appointments. Whatever the reason, keep a list of those missed appointments and call the patients back to make the appointment.

- **Production goals**
  Some offices set daily production goals for the scheduler. This can work if there are adequate patients to pick the procedures. (Other offices are more concerned with filling the appointments for the rest of the week.) As a rule, these scheduling philosophies stress scheduling high-margin (i.e. lab-related visits) first, then filling around these more profitable procedures with the other, less profitable procedures (i.e. restorations). The idea is that this keeps a steady flow of the more profitable procedures. If a potential appointment is lost, losing a lower-margin procedure is better than the more profitable ones.

BOX 21.12	QUESTIONS TO ASK AN EMERGENCY PATIENT

- Where is the pain?

- When did it begin?

- Is it constant or intermittent?

- Is there fever or swelling?

- Does anything trigger the pain (e.g. hot, cold, sweets, chewing)?

- Is there any recent treatment or injury to the area?

Part 3: Dental Fee Policy

It is a socialist idea that making profits is a vice; I consider the real vice is making losses.

Winston Churchill

GOAL

This part aims to present the basis of fee determination for the dental practitioner. The nature of dental fees and the behavior of the buying public regarding dental fees will be explored.

LEARNING OBJECTIVES

At the completion of this part, the student will be able to:

- Describe fee-setting objectives, giving an example from both general business and dental practice environments:
  - Market skimming
  - Satisfying
  - Market penetration.

- Describe fee-setting methods, giving an example of each from both general business and dental practice environments:
  - Cost based
  - Demand based
  - Competition based.

- Discuss the effect that managed care programs have on dental fees.

- Discuss consumer or patient sensitivity to fees.

- Describe how to raise fees.

- Discuss the effect of fees on practice profitability.

- Define "elasticity of demand" and relate it to dental fees.

- Calculate a procedure's cost-based fee.

- Describe the Consumer Price Index and its use in dental fee determination.

KEY TERMS

apparent fee
competition-based fee setting
consumer/patient fee sensitivity
Consumer Price Index (CPI)
cost-based fee setting
cost shifting
demand-based fee setting
elasticity of demand
fee objectives
market penetration
market skimming
practice profitability
satisfying

Fees dramatically affect practice profitability and patient perception. A profitable practice can only be attained by careful attention to the financial details of income generation and practice cost management. A dentist's self-esteem is closely tied to fees, both as a cause of low fees (the dentist must believe that the fee is fair and valuable) and in the resulting practice profitability. The fees that the practice sets have obvious and important implications for income generation. Principles from marketing and economics can help the dentist in setting practice fees.

PROFESSIONAL FEE OBJECTIVES

As a practitioner, a dentist should initially determine what they expect to accomplish with practice fees. Those objectives may include, depending on the type and style of the practice, market skimming, satisfying, and market penetration. Various strategies accomplish these alternative profit objectives.

MARKET SKIMMING

Skim pricing occurs when a business prices goods or services so high that only a few consumers can afford them. In the automotive world, Porsche and Bentley automobiles are sold on this basis. Dental practices that profit significantly from a few patients by charging high fees employ skim pricing.

A paradoxical value of high fees is that consumers may use them as an indicator of quality. A patient who perceives the quality of dental care as high is not as concerned about the cost of that care. Treatments for these patients are based on non-fee considerations, such as esthetics, image, treatment outcome, or personal interaction with the dentist and office staff. Often then, high fees may lead to higher patient satisfaction.

Market skimming also has limitations for use in a dental practice. The number of patients who will buy dental services without regard to the price is not large. So only a few practices in an area can use this skim pricing. Each of those practices must offer something unique for which the patient is willing to pay a premium price. Practitioners must be sure to differentiate themselves from other dentists in the area. In that way, a patient dissatisfied with the fee will be less likely to leave because they have no (or few) other substitutes or comparable providers. Patients with dental insurance may question a procedure fee when their insurance carrier notifies them that the charged fee exceeds the carrier's usual, customary, and reasonable (UCR) fee schedule. When other practices in the area discover these higher fees, they may provide similar services, market the service similarly, and charge fees similar to the practice that initially adopted a market skimming strategy.

SATISFYING

Many dental practices may not emphasize extreme profitability in the short or long run. These practitioners may exhibit behavior that produces satisfactory, rather than maximum, profit. Satisfying behavior is an economic notion that emphasizes attaining the desired level of something without maximizing anything. Ford Motor Company "satisfies" in its mid-sized line of automobiles. It produces adequate numbers of automobiles, charges a reasonable price, pays its workers a satisfactory wage, and earns a satisfactory profit. It could maximize profits in the short run by charging more, but might lose satisfied customers or workers. A dental practice that uses the satisfying strategy structures its fees so that everyone is "fairly happy." The practice meets current expenses and allows the dentist to live comfortably and to reward the staff adequately (*comfortable* and *adequate* have different meanings for different people).

Creating this perception of satisfying behavior helps the practitioner to earn a reputation for being fair and equitable. Studies on dental consumer satisfaction suggest that the attributes of professionalism, quality, and reputation are significant determinants of consumer selection and retention of a dentist. Patients who perceive their dentist is satisfying rather than maximizing may assume a higher level of satisfaction in the dentist–patient relationship. The cost of care alone does not lead to satisfaction but can significantly exacerbate patient dissatisfaction. (Patients will not become more satisfied if they believe the fee is fair but will become dissatisfied if they believe the fee is too high.) Therefore, a satisfying fee strategy is a practical component in developing patient satisfaction.

MARKET PENETRATION

Fees may be set at a low level to attract new customers or "penetrate" a new market. Many stores have grand opening sales to develop markets for new outlets. Ford Motor Company also uses this strategy in pricing its entry-level line of automobiles. The hope is that the low price will lure initial Ford buyers who will later upgrade to larger, more expensive (and more profitable) automobiles in the line. In dentistry, the price or fee may be set below that of similar services offered by other dental practices to attract potential patients based on lower fees and, hopefully, keep them in the practice. It is often used for services such as initial exams, cleanings, economy dentures, or even orthodontics.

Many high-volume retail dental operations use this pricing objective. They aim to attract patients based on a lower price for a common service, such as an initial exam. By doing this, they hope to attract enough patients to penetrate the market. Once they establish a patient load, the retailer may adjust fees upward to approximate those of other dentists in the area.

Advertising dentists who offer initial price reductions in their advertisements or coupons use a similar strategy. A free or reduced-price examination, prophylaxis, or radiograph attempts to penetrate a market and generate new patients for the practice. This strategy is especially effective for cost-conscious dental consumers. It is much less effective for consumers for whom cost is not a significant deciding factor. These groups include families with higher discretionary income and managed care participants.

Managed care dental plans often use a similar strategy to become established in the dental benefits market. Their goal is to price the managed care plan at a low entry-level price compared with conventional dental reimbursement plans. By doing this, the dental plans hope to rapidly attract companies or organizations as clients and build a market share. Once they build this share, they may eliminate the introductory offer, and prices may rise. Profitability to the participating dentist under this objective is small or may not exist during the plan's growth phase.

Using a low-price market penetration strategy is only advisable under certain circumstances. The markets in which this strategy is most effectively used include markets highly sensitive to fee levels (demand for a service increases as the fee declines), in which a lower fee would discourage competition, and those in which a lower fee does not equate with poor quality. Whether the traditional dental practice marketplace meets any of these criteria is debatable. Many patients may use price as an indicator of quality, particularly for intangible services like healthcare. Dentists must also inform potential patients of the price, which means that they may incur expensive advertising costs to inform the potential patients. However, advertisements rank low as an important dental consumer decision factor. Therefore, undue emphasis on advertising dental services may be counterproductive to the effective marketing of dental services. A market penetration strategy may be used by independent practice associations (IPAs), preferred provider organizations (PPOs), or other groups competing based on price and willing to accept low profits to build a presence in a particular market.

FEE-SETTING METHODS

Once a dentist has established an objective and strategy for setting fees, they should select a method to determine them. Setting professional fees can include casual conversation at a professional meeting, "gut-level" estimates, or analytical business techniques. These fee-setting methods can be grouped into three broad categories: cost-based, demand-based, and competition-based methods.

COST-BASED METHOD

One standard method that dentists use to set fees (price) is based on the practice's cost structure. The dentist determines the total office cost per hour and the time required to do each procedure, then computes the required fee based on the time needed to complete the procedure and any additional costs (e.g. lab). A regular or desired profit (personal income) can be added to the overhead cost to decide the fee. For example, assume that a dentist knows that the practice must generate an average of $200 per hour to meet the operating costs, and they want $100 per hour in profit. If the dentist also knows how long it takes, on average, to do a given procedure, then they can calculate the amount required to "break even" on that procedure. If they can do the "average" two-surface alloy in 20 minutes, they should charge $100 ($200 per hour overhead + $100 profit divided by three procedures per hour) to meet this projection. These numbers are given as examples only. Individual practice numbers will, of course, vary.

This fee planning is essential if a dentist participates in managed care or contract dental plans. In this instance, dentists must know how much a given procedure will "cost" the practice to produce. Because the practice receives a predetermined fee for any procedure, dentists must know the cost structure of the practice to determine if they will be making or losing money by participating in the program. A capitation plan may decrease the fixed costs of a practice (by supplying a monthly fixed revenue amount) but not pay a high enough fee to recover variable practice expenses. If the managed care plan fee will not cover at least variable expenses, it will cost the dentist money to participate in the plan and treat patients covered by it. There may be reasons other than simple profit for participating in a plan. The marketing and practice growth implications of gaining additional patients for the practice may outweigh the strict financial justifications.

Cost-based fee determination has its shortcomings. It leads to a satisfying fee strategy. Its intent is to be "fair" to all parties involved and accomplishes that end. However, it is not an aggressive fee strategy and does not lead to the maximum profit or income for the practitioner. Most practitioners want to be viewed as fair and not overly concerned with money. This strategy reduces the dissatisfaction of all parties. It involves considerable calculation work, however. Dentists must have excellent time records, which involve considerable time with a stopwatch, consistent schedule records, or a good guess. This can also lead to the clinically faster dentist being compensated less than the slower dentist.

DEMAND-BASED METHOD

A second method used to set a fee is based on consumer demand for a service or product. This method is represented by the adage "charge what the market will bear." This infers that the firm or dentist will charge the highest fee at which enough people will buy the product or service. It is important to note that there is no price at which everyone will buy dental services, nor is there a price at which no one will buy services. Demand-based pricing says that some people will be dissatisfied with the price or fee and go elsewhere to purchase the service or not purchase the service at all. However, demand-based pricing also says that other people who value the good or service will pay the price. Demand-based pricing is a technique used for specialty and image-based goods and services. Luxury automobiles, designer clothing, and gourmet restaurants set prices on a demand basis. The business could sell more products or services at a lower price, but not enough to make up for the income lost from lowering the price. Thus, these firms optimize profit rather than the number of goods or services produced.

For example, assume that a dentist could "sell" 30 gold crowns monthly at a fee of $900 each. If the fee for a gold crown were raised to $1200, some people would not buy a gold crown that would have previously been purchased at $900. Assume that the dentist could sell only 20 crowns at this higher fee. Which fee would result in a higher income for the dentist? If one assumes a

$150 laboratory fee for each crown, then selling 30 crowns at $900 results in an income of $22 500 per month ($30 \times [\$900 - \$150]$). Selling fewer crowns at a higher price results in a higher income of $26 250 ($20 \times [\$1200 - \$150]$). Here, the dentist has increased income by selling fewer crowns at a higher price.

The obvious problem is figuring out how many people will purchase various services at various prices. Economists determine this by estimating the elasticity of demand for a product or service. *Elasticity* is a term that describes how much "give" or "flex" will occur in purchase amounts because of a price change. Demand is elastic if a large change (either increase or decrease) in the amount purchased results from a price change. An example is the purchase of soda drinks. If someone's favorite cola brand raises its price, many consumers will switch to a competitor's brand. Demand is inelastic if there is no significant change in the amount purchased because of a price change. An example of inelastic demand is the purchase of pharmaceuticals. If a particular drug gives relief of symptoms, a person will purchase the drug at virtually any price. Dental services appear to fall in a mid-range of elasticity. That is, patients are not sensitive to changes in price (fee). Increasing dental fees causes some (but not all) potential patients not to purchase the service. The elasticity of demand for dental services varies considerably with socioeconomic and demographic factors. People with higher disposable incomes are less sensitive to price changes or economic conditions.

Dentists can use the Consumer Price Index (CPI) and disposable income estimates as indicators of how much change in demand there may be in response to dental fee adjustments. If the CPI increases, the public is generally aware of higher prices and will accept increases in dental fees as a matter of course. If, on the other hand, prices (i.e. the CPI) are stable, then the public will expect a smaller increase in dental fees. Whether or not people can pay these higher fees will be influenced more by their disposable incomes than by the CPI. If income goes up faster than prices, people will have more money to spend on discretionary or optional services, such as routine dental care. They will be less sensitive to increases in fees. If the price index rises faster than income, people will have less money to spend on such services and will be much more sensitive to increases in dental fees.

Traditional dental indemnity insurance plans tacitly encourage demand-based fee determination. The insurance portion of the total fee will essentially absorb any fee increase. Capitation dental plans, on the other hand, virtually eliminate demand-based pricing because the fee is contractually determined. Interestingly, the sponsoring organization then uses demand-based pricing (in reverse) to set fee reimbursement levels. If enough dentists are willing to provide the needed quantity of services at the given contract price, the price will hold. However, if the market of dental providers is unwilling or unable to provide the services at the prescribed fee level, the contract plan would have to raise the reimbursement level until enough dentists would be willing to participate to provide the required number of services.

Demand-based fee determination is an aggressive strategy. It leads to maximum profit for the practitioner, although many patients may be dissatisfied with the high fees and leave the practice. This is acceptable if a practice is mature and has a backlog of patient demand. If one patient becomes dissatisfied, another will take their place. New practitioners growing their practice and practitioners in competitive markets find it difficult to use this aggressive strategy. Managed-care plans are irrelevant to the demand-based fee practice. Because fees are high, managed care is not involved.

COMPETITION-BASED METHOD

The third major method that dentists can use to set dental fees is based on what the competition charges. This is the method that dentists traditionally use when they "casually discuss" fees. With the addition of third-party payers, competition-based pricing becomes more complex. The basic problem with this fee determination system is verifying the source of information about other dentists' fees.

The most common information source is asking other dentists in a geographic area what their fees are for given procedures. This method has several shortcomings. Besides being possibly illegal (because of price-fixing), the other dentist may need to accurately represent their fees. The inquiring dentist often asks friends and contemporaries about dental fees and only gets a partial cross-sectional sample of the dental community.

A second and more accurate source of information concerning competing dentists' fees is the data published regularly in the dental literature. This data is often broken down by region of the country, city size, and dental specialty to make the comparisons more meaningful.

The third source is for the dentist to establish a system in the office to track insurance and other third-party reimbursements. Dental insurance carriers will generally keep fees for a specific area or region, often to the point of establishing UCR fees for part of a metropolitan area or even an individual zip code. By gradually raising fees, the dental office can determine when the "cut-off" occurs for a particular plan. For example, if a plan will pay the UCR fee up to the 80th percentile, a dentist can learn that when

Table 21.1 The effect of fees on practice profitability.

	Dr. Red	Dr. White	Dr. Blue
Fee level	10% below = $90	Average = $100	10% above = $110
Gross collections	$450 000	$500 000	$550 000
Practice costs	$300 000	$300 000	$300 000
Practice profits	$150 000	$200 000	$250 000
Profit difference	25% below	Average	25% above
Overhead ratio	67%	60%	55%

their fee for that procedure reaches the 80th percentile for the area, the insurance carrier will no longer reimburse the full amount. Because most offices see different plans with different payment schedules, a dentist can develop an accurate notion of prevailing fee levels through this method. To make this system work, the dentist must have a detailed knowledge of each plan's limitations and do constant monitoring.

Once a dentist has a range of fees for their geographic area and type of practice, they must decide how to position fees compared with other practitioners in their reference group. Many practitioners want to establish fees at the mean or average level. Others are more aggressive and prefer the 75th or even 90th percentile. (That is, their fees are higher than 75% or 90% of the practitioners in the area.) If a dentist's fees are too high, patients will quickly notice it. If a dentist takes this approach, they should have a "name" in the community. Also, if the dentist's fees exceed the 80th percentile, third-party carriers may not reimburse the total amount. Patients may require extra education to understand their relationship with the third-party carrier in this case.

IMPLICATIONS FOR DENTAL PRACTICE

Price is a factor in almost every purchase decision that consumers make, although it is only one decision factor. Everyone has some price that will cause them to switch to a different brand, style, or model, or healthcare provider. For dental consumers, switching behavior results from the practice's uniqueness, consumer discretionary income, third-party involvement, and consumer attitudes to dental healthcare.

EFFECTS ON PRACTICE PROFITABILITY

Dentists' fees affect practice profitability tremendously because the most significant part of a dental practice's costs is fixed. Once this fixed cost component has been met, additional revenue becomes almost pure profit. (For more

explanation, see Chapter 25.) Table 21.1 illustrates this point. Assume that there are three equal dental practices, Drs. Red, White, and Blue. Their practices are in the same building, employ similar staff members, and have the same exact cost structures. In this example, Dr. White charges the average fee for the area, $100 for a procedure. Dr. Red's fees are 10% below the average for the area ($90); Dr. Blue's are 10% above ($110). They all do identical numbers and types of procedures for the year. Table 21.1 shows the financial results from this scenario.

Dr. Red made 25% less than Dr. White and 40% less than Dr. Blue, although they had identical practices. The actual difference in fees for a given procedure was small (in the example, $90, $100, and $110), but the outcome was quite dramatic. The overhead ratio changes considerably as well. Because costs are the same among the three practices, increased revenues affect the overhead ratio. Because fee level impacts productivity, it seems that all dentists could raise fees and become more profitable. Several constraints keep dentists from charging whatever fee they want to charge. The most significant constraints are patients' sensitivity to fees and the effect of insurance plans.

CONSUMER OR PATIENT FEE SENSITIVITY

Most people shop for certain goods based solely on price. This is the basis of selling many commodity-type goods, such as generic soap, paper products, or canned tomatoes. Some people also buy dental services solely based on the professional fee. The patient who calls the dental office and asks about the price of an extraction or denture is "shopping" for services and will buy primarily based on price. Some dentists are concerned about attracting these people and desire to use a low-fee or penetration-fee strategy to make them "regular customers." Dentists should be aware that people who shop on price often look for specific, not comprehensive, dental care. Therefore, these patients may not represent a significant potential source of income. Because the patient was initially won on price, the dentist can just as quickly lose them because of price. If they find a dentist who will do dental services more cheaply, the patient might leave the practice and patronize the new dentist. Therefore, using a low-fee strategy often does not result in establishing a stable patient pool for the dental practice. It may, however, generate an initial patient pool that can be a referral base. Additionally, dentists can convert some of those who initially won on price to buy dental services based on factors other than price. These patients may become loyal patients. However, many dentists are too sensitive to these "price shoppers."

Dental consumers are concerned with a service's apparent or out-of-pocket cost. The third-party payer decreases out-of-pocket expenses. If a patient has dental insurance that reimburses 50% of a procedure that costs $800, the apparent cost to the patient is $400. Patients are not particularly sensitive to the price of dental services, but they are sensitive to payment options and other forms of credit (see Chapter 22). A patient will balk at an $8000 treatment plan the same as at a $9000 treatment plan. Using the same principle as automobile leasing, if someone can make the monthly payments affordable, the cash-flow price for the consumer becomes tolerable. Dental consumers are also more concerned with and knowledgeable about frequently "bought" procedures. Many patients know when a dentist raises the price of a "recall" exam by $1, but are oblivious to a $25 increase in the price of a crown because they have never bought a crown.

EFFECTS OF DENTAL INSURANCE PLANS

Managed care is any plan in which the dentist provides services for a contractually reduced fee. Managed care plans change the traditional relationships between the dentist and the patient. They do this by upsetting the usual methods of reimbursement for services. Managed care plans take much of the power to influence the purchase behavior of clients away from the dentist. It is now vested in the payment plan administrators through their choice of participating dental offices. This changes the "rules" that have governed competition between dentists. Non-participating dentists find competing based on demand or price criteria difficult or impossible. Participating dentists find their traditional cost structures changed and their traditional pricing decisions eliminated. The public find their dental shopping choices severely limited. (Judging from the continuing growth of these plans, this may not be as significant an issue to the public as dental practitioners hope it would be.)

Closed panels, capitation, and PPO plans remove the elasticity of demand as a criterion from the dental purchase decision. Fees become irrelevant to the consumer except in a yes–no participation criterion. If a dentist is a plan participant, their fees (and, therefore, the patient's monetary costs) are fixed and inelastic. The non-participating dentist's fees are prohibitively high by comparison. The purchase decision is then governed by elasticity. Patients will purchase a few services at this higher (non-participant) price. This also negates the possibility of competition-based pricing by non-participants because the fees that the competition sets are irrelevant to the demand for the service.

Managed care plans severely limit the dentist's ability to raise fees. If the patient participates in the plan, then the dentist has signed a contract that stipulates what the fee for the procedure will be. It does not matter what the office charges enrolled patients for the service. The dentist will only collect what the plan allows. The plan may raise or lower the fee schedule. The dentist then must decide whether to continue to participate in the plan. Practitioners can negotiate fee schedules with insurance plans. Individual practices or practice networks that see many plan patients have more negotiating leverage than a smaller plan participant. Chapter 27 discusses these issues more thoroughly.

Managed care plans also affect the participating dentists' cost structure and cost-based pricing. If a PPO or capitation plan reimburses at a 65% level and the office cost or overhead is 65%, then the dentist or participant barely covers costs. (For a more detailed explanation, see Chapter 20.) The practice's full-pay patients provide the profit. Here, the dentist must either accept a lower income or charge the full-pay patients more to make up the difference. This is called price differential "cost shifting." It occurs when the practice shifts the profit lost on the managed care patient to the traditional insurance and private payment patients in a hidden way. Using different prices for different patients may seem unethical or at least unsavory to many healthcare providers. However, this is a common practice in the business world. Hotels charge different rates depending on a particular convention or group. Senior citizen discounts, volume discounts, buying cooperatives, and preferred customer plans are all examples of charging different customers different prices for identical goods or services.

RAISING FEES

Most management experts agree that dentists should adjust dental fees, at a minimum, annually. January 1 and July 1 are the most common dates, with the first of the calendar year being the most prevalent. Many practitioners time staff members' raises to follow fee increases closely. This has several advantages. It helps staff members remember that practice revenues dictate their pay. If patients question fees, the staff member will be more interested in justifying the fee. Staff members will look forward to fee increases because they know their salaries will soon increase.

Many dentists use the CPI to set changes in their practice fees. The CPI is an index that measures the price change of a hypothetical "basket" of goods and services that the "average" consumer might purchase. It is a statistical index computed by the US government based on selected urban standard metropolitan statistical areas and a few sample cities. The CPI includes payments made for housing, food, transportation, and healthcare costs. Dentists assume that their cost of doing business will generally rise in proportion to the CPI. When dental practice costs rise, it is logical to assume that dental fees should rise with that change in cost. Dentists have a much better measure of their practice costs than the CPI: they have the actual costs. The CPI is valuable in determining changes in compensation levels for employees because their cost of living is reflected in the index's basket of goods and services. The CPI is not as useful for cost-based pricing decisions. It is, however, more useful in assessing the public's demand for services.

Some fees, such as the fee for a routine periodic oral exam or prophylaxis, are visible to the dental consumer. Because these services are the most commonly performed, many patients can use them as benchmarks or comparison figures, either between practitioners or over time. One strategy to cope with this problem is to list every procedure done on the maintenance visit. Rather than list "Recall exam, Prophy" on the patient's statement, a dentist should list everything to be done. This should include a medical history update, oral cancer exam, blood pressure check, home care instructions, radiographs, toothbrush, floss, hard and soft tissue exams, and any other education or services routinely provided during a maintenance visit.

Other procedures, such as cast posts and periodontal surgeries, are less frequent. Patients have a much more difficult time comparing the costs of these procedures. Dentists may thus have more discretion when setting fees for these procedures. Routine patients become accustomed to fees for routine procedures. Often problems arise when dentists confront patients with procedures that are uncommon or that they have not seen in many years. A form of "sticker shock" sets in. Like an automobile consumer who has not priced cars for several years, these patients are amazed (and appalled) at the total price for the package of services. ("The last crown I got in 1948 cost me $30, and it was all gold!") A dentist's patient education skills become essential at this point.

Maintaining Collections

CHAPTER 22

Part 1: Patient Financial Policies

Every tooth in a man's head is more valuable than a diamond.

Miguel de Cervantes, *Don Quixote*, 1605

GOAL

This part aims to present guidelines for formulating credit and collection policies.

LEARNING OBJECTIVES

At the completion of this part, the student will be able to:

- Define the elements of a patient financial policy.

- Describe the common methods of payment in a dental office.

- Establish a credit policy for a dental practice.

- Establish payment plan alternatives for patients.

- Describe typical methods for presenting financial plans to patients.

- Describe the effects of financial policies on office operations.

KEY TERMS

account aging	credit	personal checks
account guarantor	credit bureau	professional courtesies
accounts receivable management	credit cards	recourse
cash	credit check	returned checks
cash discounts	financial policies	statements
collection agency	in-house collections	third-party payers
collection calls	interest on unpaid amounts	truth-in-lending laws
collection policy	payment plan	
collection techniques	payment plan policy	

Business Basics for Dentists, Second Edition. James L. Harrison, David O. Willis, and Charles K. Thieman.
© 2024 John Wiley & Sons, Inc. Published 2024 by John Wiley & Sons, Inc.

Every dental office and every business has a financial policy, whether they know it or not. The consumer is aware of the policy. When someone goes to a fast-food restaurant, they know their credit policy: cash at the time of purchase. Yet many patients continue to believe that they can (and should) get a bill from the dental office at the end of the month, let it sit for another 20 days, then write a check for the part they owe without worrying about late charges or accrued interest. The office's job is to inform the patient if this is not the case.

There is a high cost to the business owner who does not collect the accounts promptly. Figure 22.1 shows the decrease in an account's value as it ages. This is due to many factors. The older an account is, the less likely it is that the business will ever collect it. Collecting accounts has an associated cost, including office personnel cost, postage, and time taken from other essential tasks. The dentist loses the use of the money until they collect it. If they use an outside collection agency, then that agent also costs the business money. Finally, the dental practice may lose the patronage and goodwill of the patient, their family, and friends over misunderstood collection issues.

Practice owners must decide before the fact what their policy is regarding payment for services. Patients need to have this information to make informed treatment acceptance decisions. They will also become angry if a dentist springs a financial surprise on them without informing them ahead of time. Having a written policy improves patient compliance, increases collections, decreases uncollectible accounts, improves scheduling (by reducing broken appointments), and leads to more appreciative patients. Although they may not like the policy, at least they know and understand it.

ELEMENTS OF A FINANCIAL POLICY

Dental office financial policies commonly contain several elements (Box 22.1).

WHAT PATIENT INFORMATION TO COLLECT

Every person that a dental practice agrees to allow to pay them over time is essentially applying for an interest-free loan. If the practice offers extended payment plans, they want to have some indicators of the creditworthiness of the account guarantor or applicant for the loan. If a patient does not pass the test, the practice does not have to offer them credit. That patient must pay for services as the dentist provides them, or the office does not offer the patient another appointment.

The dentist (or office staff) needs to gather certain information to ensure payment for services from patients who do not pay in full at the time of service. The account guarantor is the person who is responsible for paying the bills. They "guarantee" the patient's account. The guarantor may be the person themselves, a spouse, or the parent of a minor child. An adult child may be a guarantor for a marginally capable elderly adult. A divorced parent who lives in another city may be the guarantor for a child who comes to the dentist with their custodial parent. A trustee or guardian may have financial control over an incapable adult. The account guarantor may or may not be a patient of the practice. Regardless, the office's job is to ensure that they know who the guarantor is and to let the guarantor know the practice's financial policies. (The guarantor, not the custodial parent or anyone else who does not have payment responsibility, should sign financial agreements.) Offices also must send any bills to the guarantor, so offices need to keep a current address and telephone number for the guarantor. A Social Security number is important to

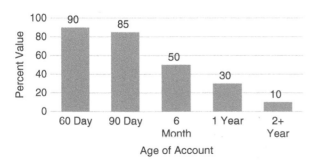

FIGURE 22.1 Losses from slow accounts.

BOX 22.1	ELEMENTS OF A FINANCIAL POLICY

Patient information collected
Qualifications for credit
Payment conditions accepted
Payment methods accepted
Charges for late payments
Rules regarding dental insurance plans
Marketing incentives in place

track people down or check on credit histories, but they are becoming more difficult to obtain. Driver license numbers are also valuable for tracking people down.

Offices can legally make a credit check (order a credit report) on any patient who makes a financial commitment to them. In practice, dental offices will use this only for large amounts. What is a "large" amount? That is up to the practice owner to decide. A $1000 treatment for one dentist may be appropriate; another will not bother getting a credit report for amounts less than $10 000. Dental practices can join a credit bureau. The cost is several hundred dollars per year. Personal credit histories may still cost an additional fee. The report does not give the practice a yes–no reply, but instead describes the person's history of payments on credit cards, loans, and mortgages. It is up to the practice owner to interpret that information and decide if they want to extend credit. The office must have the patient's Social Security number to run a credit check on them. The office can refuse to offer credit if the patient does not provide that.

WHO QUALIFIES FOR CREDIT

Credit occurs when someone buys a good or service but does not entirely pay for it until some time in the future. The office credit policy dictates the conditions under which patrons are allowed to pay in the future for dentistry done today. It describes to whom the office is willing to extend credit. The practice lends patients money when it agrees to send a bill at the end of the month. Practice owners should qualify ahead of time to whom they are willing to lend, to whom they are not, and under what terms they will lend to patients.

Dentists do not have to extend credit to anyone. They may require a full cash payment when they provide service, with no exceptions. The problem is that a credit policy that is too strict may discourage people from proceeding with treatment plans (i.e. "buying the dentistry") who might otherwise go on with treatment. Patients are not particularly sensitive to fees, but they are sensitive to credit and collection policies. Think about a patient who has $8000 of dentistry to be done. They are interested in having the work done. They cannot discriminate between a total price tag of $8000 and one of $9000. One price over the other will not make their decision. However, the difference between 100% immediate payment and a payment plan of $1000 per month can help them decide whether to have the treatment. The real issue becomes how they fit the payment into their monthly family budget rather than the simple cost.

Not everyone that a dental practitioner treats deserves credit. Dentists may consider the public's creditworthiness a continuum, from very creditworthy (will always pay as agreed) to not creditworthy (will never pay) and everything in between. Their job is to decide how far they will go on the continuum to generate the desired production. Dentists should be aware that only 30% of Americans qualify for a VISA or MasterCard with more than a $1000 limit. If these companies do not extend credit to someone, the dentist should seriously consider if they will.

WHAT PAYMENT CONDITIONS TO ACCEPT

If a dentist decides to extend credit to patients by sending a bill, they must decide the repayment conditions in their financial policy. Will the dental practice allow people to send $50 per month to pay off a $5000 treatment plan? Will the practice require 50% down before starting any treatment or a specific procedure (e.g. a bridge)? Does the practice's payment plan policy differentiate between cash (fee-for-service accounts), traditional insurance accounts, and managed care accounts? Some of these payment conditions include the following.

Written Plan

Dental practices should have a definite repayment plan for every patient to whom they extend credit. This arrangement should be written, not verbal, and require the account guarantor to sign it. This does not make the debt more legally binding. (The patient owes the dentist for the service whether they signed a piece of paper or not.) What it does do is place in the patient's mind the idea that they have signed an agreement to pay the dentist for the service. The patient thinks that it is more binding to see it in black and white. Practices should develop a payment plan for a complete treatment plan. If they create separate requirements for individual procedures, the patient may become confused.

Down Payment

The size of the required down payment affects treatment acceptance. A lower down payment means easing the dental practice's credit policy. A requirement for a higher down payment tightens the practice's credit policy. The dental practice should get an initial payment large enough to cover lab bills. That way, at the least the dentist will not lose money if someone does not pay their bill. Many dental practices require half the fee for the procedure as a down payment to begin treatment. Require a down payment of 33–50%, even if there is no lab work.

Length of Payment

Dental offices should only extend billing up to three months after they have completed treatment. If the payment period extends further out than this, patients often "forget" to complete their scheduled payments.

Amount of Plan

The total amount of the payment affects the options the office offers. For example, an office might set a financial policy that patients must pay all amounts less than $200 at the time of service. Amounts more than $200 but less than $1000 may be paid in three monthly installments (with an acceptable credit check). For amounts more than $1000, the patients must gain financing through a health credit card.

WHAT PAYMENT METHODS TO ACCEPT

Dental offices may or may not accept any of several methods of payment for their services. Each has advantages and disadvantages and may be part of a financial policy.

Cash

A patient may make a payment in cash. If offices often have patients who pay with cash, they must have extra cash to make change for large-denomination bills. Dentists know that cash will not "bounce" as a personal check might, but offices also must be careful to account for all cash accurately. Cash can be a problem in the office. It is difficult to track and, therefore, easy to steal. In the unlikely event of a robbery, cash is easily spent, while checks and credit card slips are not.

Personal Checks

Dental practices may refuse to take a personal check at any time. From their perspective, they want to ensure that someone's check is "good." In other words, the practitioner wants to ensure that the patient has enough money in their account to cover the check. From the consumer's perspective, they must ensure that offices protect their personal information. If offices put personal information on a check, that information is open to their office staff and throughout the paper trail through which the check travels. As a result, states have passed laws governing what offices can and cannot do regarding check verification. Each state is different, but the general rules are:

- Dental practices cannot require a consumer to show a credit card as a condition of accepting a check.

- Dental practices cannot condition accepting a check on a consumer's authorizing charges to a credit card if the bank returns the check (i.e. it bounces).

- Dental practices can require and record someone's name, address, and phone number on a check.

- Dental practices can require a driver's license or another form of photo identification.

If the bank returns a check, the practice owner has a problem. The first thing to do is for the office to call the patient and determine the problem. The office may and should charge the consumer a "reasonable" fee for reprocessing the check. (Often the bank charges the office to reprocess the check.) The office should add this fee as a separate code to the patient's ledger. (This is a charge adjustment but not part of the production numbers.)

When the bank returns a check from a patient, they will stamp it with one of four reasons:

- **Insufficient funds** means the patient does not have enough money in the account; the check bounced. This is the most common reason for returned checks. It might not be a big problem. The receptionist should call the patient when they discover it. The patient may have a reasonable explanation for the problem ("My paycheck was late"). In this case, the office should tell the patient they will process the check a second time. If it clears, then the office has payment. If it bounces again, the practice owner must take legal action. They should give the check to a lawyer or collection agency for immediate action.

- **Payment stopped** means that the patient has stopped payment on a check. The office should call the patient immediately to find out the problem. Often, it is because the patient is dissatisfied with the work the dentist has done. (Hopefully, the practitioner will know about this before the bank returns the check.) The dentist should discuss with the patient how they can correct the problem.

- **Closed account** means that the patient has closed the account. Sometimes this shows intentional fraud by the patient. At other times it may be an honest mistake if a patient closed an account and "forgot" that they wrote the check or their spouse wrote it. In these cases, the office may let the patient make payment immediately (generally in cash) rather than sending the check for prosecution.

- **No account** usually shows fraud because the bank has no record of any such account. The office should try to call the patient (but they may not find them). Unless the patient has some unusually inventive excuse, the practice owner will probably need to turn this type of check over to a lawyer or call the local sheriff or police department to prosecute the patient for intentionally writing a bad check.

Credit and Debit Cards

Most practitioners accept bank cards (e.g. VISA, Master-Card) for payment of dental services. Practice owners will have their bank establish a deposit account in their name, often the bank in which they have their office checking account. The bank then deposits any charges that patients make to that account. The owner can withdraw money from that account whenever they choose. The upside of this process is to speed up cash flow through the practice and encourage patient payment. The downside is that the issuing bank retains approximately 2–4% of the amount charged as its fee for processing the account. The bank calls this a "discount." This probably saves the dentist money if they send these people bills at the end of the month. If the practice collects in the office at the time of service, it is more costly.

Electronic Fund Transfers

An Automated Clearing House (ACH) network transfer is the movement of money electronically between banks. Many insurance companies use ACH to transfer payments to practitioners. Personal fund transfer companies (e.g. Venmo, CashApp, PayPal) use the ACH structure to transfer money between individuals.

Most dental offices accept electronic fund transfers (mobile bill pay). The dental office should use a business account to receive payments, not a personal account. The fund transfer companies report all annual transfers of more than $600 to the Internal Revenue Service (IRS). The IRS then checks (via a computer program) to be sure that the receiving business has reported the income on its annual tax return. Be sure to report all money received in this fashion to avoid compliance problems.

Online Bill Payment

Online bill payment has become a standard method. Currently, more than two out of every three bills are paid in electronic form in the United States.

Bank Plan or Health Card

Another common payment mechanism is a bank line of credit for the patient. In rural areas, banks offer these more often. In urban areas, finance companies offer them more frequently. Either way, the method is the same. In this arrangement, the office tells the bank the estimated amount for treatment. The bank then qualifies the patient (checks their credit history) and lends the patient the amount of the service. The bank pays the office for dental services. The patient then pays the bank over time as an installment loan. These arrangements have the advantage of keeping the dentist out of the money-lending business, speeding up payment, and decreasing billing costs. The bank generally charges the patient the costs of originating the loans.

Several national companies offer this service calling themselves "health credit cards" or other similar names. They often have websites and can qualify a patient for payment for services while in the office. The practitioner will need to sign up for these services (generally at a small charge). The patient then pays the finance company over time, with interest included for the finance company. (Depending on the size of the case and the payment history, the loan may be interest free to the patient.) The finance company pays the dental practice as the work is completed or sometimes when the work is scheduled. Each has different rules, so the practitioner should check them out to find the one that best suits their needs. These plans take the dentist out of the finance business. They do not approve everyone for credit. (Currently, they approve about 60% of applicants.) If an independent credit agency refuses to extend credit to someone, the dentist should consider whether they can offer that person credit.

Special Cards

Patients may have flexible spending accounts (FSAs) or other employer-sponsored payment methods. The tax advantage of these plans encourages many people to participate. This becomes a significant stimulus for demand. The plan may require patients to bring a receipt for reimbursement of services, or the sponsoring organization may issue a special debit card for the person to use in healthcare offices. Dental practices process these cards like any other.

CHARGES FOR LATE PAYMENT

Dentists may charge interest on any unpaid amounts. If an office does charge interest, they must be sure to meet the truth-in-lending laws. These laws state that the dentist must make a complete disclosure of all financing costs to the borrower, the dentist must calculate the annual percentage rate, and the borrower must sign a statement containing this information. Dental offices need a computer system and software designed for this task. (Most of the major dental management software contains this option.) If they want to charge interest, the dentist must know and abide by all the laws. Many offices find it easier to charge a nominal "billing charge" (such as $5 per month) to all accounts that have aged more than 60 or 90 days. No one intends this monthly charge to make money, but rather to induce patients to pay. Because they do not charge interest, they are free of the requirements of truth-in-lending laws. Good dental office management software allows dental practices to set up various patient payment plans. Most will also print out payment coupons for the office to remind the patient of the payment due. The software may also have truth-in-lending forms, interest calculators, and other requirements if the dentist charges interest.

RULES REGARDING DENTAL INSURANCE PLANS

Third-party payers are insurance companies, managed care companies, and others who write a check to reimburse the cost of care for a patient. A traditional indemnity dental insurance plan is a contract between the patient and the insurer. The dentist has no legal responsibility in the contract. However, most practitioners help patients by completing insurance forms, often allowing the benefits (payments) to be assigned or paid directly to the dentist. Managed care contracts are different in that the contract does involve the dentist, who has legal obligations to fulfill. This topic is covered in more detail in other chapters of this book.

Whether or not a dentist accepts the assignment of benefits for insurance payments is an integral part of their payment policy. If they do not accept the assignment of benefits, patients must pay the full amount and then receive reimbursement from their insurer. This means the patient must come up with more money up front, resulting in a stricter credit policy. Patients have been known to take their insurance reimbursement check and buy other desired goods or services, putting off payments to the dentist. If the dentist accepts the benefits assignment, they should have the front office estimate the patient portion of the bill, then charge them for their portion when they complete the service. When the insurance "clears," the office reconciles any difference and charges or refunds the patient the difference between the estimated and actual amounts. This speeds up cash flow through the office. If the office keeps accurate computerized insurance information and uses pretreatment estimates appropriately, there will be few differences. If the office waits for the insurance to clear, cash flow slows considerably. Offices must wait several weeks for the insurance process to complete and then send a statement of the remainder to the patient. This may be at the next billing cycle, which may be several weeks. If the patient is late or makes a partial payment, many weeks may elapse before the office records complete payment.

MARKETING INCENTIVES

Many practitioners offer cash discounts, either as part of a marketing plan or as a payment incentive. If patients make a cash payment ahead of service, some practitioners offer a 3–10% discount (5% is probably the norm). This speeds up collections and cash flowing through the practice. It also saves the dentist money through decreased billing costs. Marketing discounts are those that dental practices offer to encourage patients to come to their offices. They might offer a 10% senior citizen discount to those seniors who pay cash (or check) at the time service is initiated for a patient portion of more than $500. (Practice owners may offer similar discounts to members of their church, temple, mosque, or employees at a spouse's place of employment.) Other practitioners offer professional courtesies or discounts to other professionals, such as physicians and optometrists, and they return services similarly. Managed care plans may require dentists to offer discounts to their members as a condition of being a provider. If dental practices offer any of these discounts, it is a good idea to require payment in full at the time of service for the remaining portion. After all, the practice owner has already reduced their return by offering a discount. Requiring the patient to pay the remainder in full is reasonable and appropriate.

Offices may have different financial arrangements for the type of patient visit. Communication is crucial for patients who are making their initial office visits. This is a delicate balancing act. Dental practices must let patients know their financial obligations without appearing to be concerned only with money. It is a good idea to send a "welcome to the practice" letter that describes the financial policies. The receptionist should remind new patients on the phone to bring any insurance information and payment for the initial visit. Emergency patients require a similar type of arrangement. If the emergency patient is a regular patient of the practice, then they should be aware of the payment policy. Emergency patients who are not regular patients of the practice are another matter. Here, dentists want to be sure to collect the fee for any work they do, but they also (probably) want to encourage the patient to become a regular patient of the practice. Practice owners should be sure that the receptionist informs the patient professionally what the estimated fee is and that the office expects payment at the visit. Patients who are making routine office visits should know the policies. One type who may not be fully aware is the long-term patient without significant work. They have had routine prophylaxes, recalls, and occasional fillings completed. Then they break a tooth, requiring root canal therapy, core, and crown. The receptionist should be sure to review payment options with this patient rather than assuming that they know the policy.

PRESENTING FINANCIAL PLANS

Practice owners should be certain that their office presents financial plans when they outline a treatment plan. Then the patient will have an accurate estimate of costs and length of treatment. The practitioner will also have the patient's commitment to proceed with the treatment. Part of that commitment is understanding how the patient will handle the financial arrangements. Office personnel should make financial arrangements in a quiet area of the office that is away from other patients. Many people view financial discussions as a private issue and do not want other people listening to their private conversations. Other patients in the office do not need to overhear treatment plan amounts. The patients may worry that their treatment may be as costly.

Who presents the financial arrangements is a matter of personal preference. Some dentists make all the financial arrangements for their patients. They quote amounts based on treatment plans and know the financial policies thoroughly so that they can define payment amounts and conditions. These conditions may encourage patients to go on with their planned care.

Other practitioners gain treatment acceptance from the patient, with a general understanding of the cost. After that, they turn over the patient to the office financial coordinator (receptionist or business manager) to arrange payment amounts and conditions. Then, the financial coordinator provides truth-in-lending forms, payment coupons, contracts, or other financial forms. An advantage of this approach is that the dentist presents themselves as looking out for the patient's oral health interest. It is the financial coordinator who insists on payment conditions. Through this method, the office sets up a "good cop, bad cop" scenario in which the patient understands that the dentist is looking out for their needs rather than "selling" a service they may not believe they need.

EFFECT OF FINANCIAL POLICIES

The office's financial policies affect practice production and profitability. The policies are among the most important methods of increasing case acceptance, and therefore productivity. Obviously, dentists cannot please all patients (unless they give away the dentistry or allow people unlimited time to pay). Practice owners need to design their policies so that they get the best balance of money flowing through the practice and patient acceptance of treatment plans. To a degree, what is customary in the community in which they practice will dictate their financial policies. If the community norms are that patients pay the full amount at the time of service and the insurance company reimburses them, then develop a policy with similar parameters. That same policy would not be as effective at generating patients in an area where dental practices customarily accept the assignment of benefits and offer credit through extended payment plans. This does not mean that a dental practice must follow community dictates. However, the practice owner must be aware of community norms, especially as a beginning practitioner. The owner can tighten the credit and collection policy as they build the patient pool. Their financial policies will probably change over time as the character of the practice changes. A credit policy can be too strict, decreasing the proportion of patients who would have work done with a more generous policy. However, a plan can be too generous as well. If the dentist extends credit to everyone (even those who do not need credit), they hamper the practice's cash flow, resulting in large accounts receivable and uncollectible amounts.

Payment plans are important in stimulating demand for dental services. A patient generally will not know if a fee of $8000 for a set of procedures is too high. They often will not let that be the deciding factor in whether to have the procedures done. However, the patient will know if they can afford a monthly payment of $800 and will often make that a deciding factor in whether to have the work done. In this sense, payment options are more important than the actual fee in influencing patient acceptance of treatment recommendations.

Poorly designed financial policies cost dental practices money in several ways. They may lose the patronage and goodwill of a patient and all their future referrals to the office because of misunderstood financial policies. The patient may never pay the practice the amount that they owe. The longer a bill is outstanding, the less likely it is that the practice will collect it. The older a bill, the more it costs the office to collect. Dental offices pay billing expenses, postage, and staff time to prepare bills. The money that the practice receives becomes "less valuable" over time as inflation eats away at its value. Finally, they will have lost the interest they could have made on the money if they had it to invest instead of the patient having it.

Part 2: Office Collection Policies

It is the wise dentist who collects the fee while the tooth is still hurting.

Chinese proverb

GOAL

The aim of this part is to present guidelines for developing an office collection policy.

LEARNING OBJECTIVES

At the completion of this part, the student will be able to:

- Describe the elements of a collection policy.
- Determine accounts receivable and properly age patient accounts.
- Establish a collection policy for the dental office.
- Describe common office collection techniques.
- Describe common outside collection methods.

KEY TERMS

account aging	dunning messages
accounts receivable (AR)	factoring service
collection agency	in-house collections
collection calls	Small Claims Court
collection policy	statements
delinquent accounts	writing off accounts

A dental office's collection policies describe how it plans to collect payment from people who owe it money. These people represent failures of the office's financial policies, because if the financial policies qualified people properly and established timely payment procedures, nobody would fail to pay on time. This, of course, only happens in an ideal world. In the real world, people intentionally abuse kindness with no plan ever to pay their bills. Others may have life circumstances (a family death or job loss) that make it difficult to meet payments

BOX 22.2	PERCENTAGE OF DENTISTS COLLECTING PAYMENT

Net production collected	Dentists
99–100%	18%
97–98%	34%
95–96%	23%
93–94%	14%
92% and less	11%

as agreed. Still others may fully intend to pay what they owe but decide to use their currently limited financial resources elsewhere.

The office collection policies should integrate with patient financial policies. Patient financial policies describe how patients usually pay for services. The collection policy describes what happens when they do not (Box 22.2).

An issue that healthcare providers face that non-health business people do not is whether to continue treatment on patients who have not paid for past or current treatments. The dentist–patient relationship demands that a patient not be abandoned or harmed by failure to pay. This means that if a patient has treatment partially completed, the dentist should not stop in the middle of treatment because the patient might be harmed. So, if a patient has several teeth prepared for crowns, the practitioner must complete those treatments because the patient might be harmed by the dentist's failure to complete treatment. However, if a patient has had several quadrants of restorations and needs several more, the dentist could halt treatment until payment is up to date. Patients also have an obligation in the relationship to pay for the service. With large-ticket items, be sure that the financial policy calls for an adequate down payment and that the office staff follow the policy.

ACCOUNTS RECEIVABLE

Accounts receivable (AR) are the amounts that patients owe. This is a running tally. It changes when the office bills a procedure, opens the mail, and posts a payment. There is no absolute acceptable level for AR. That depends on the office production level, insurance amounts, practice philosophy, and even the time during the year. (Patients are notoriously slow paying just after the holidays.) As a rule, the practice is healthy if the AR value is about 0.5–1 month's net production. This amount may be higher in practices with significant (greater than 80%) numbers of insurance patients, especially with those insurance companies that do not process claims electronically. It may be lower in practices that accept no assignment of benefits and have other strict credit policies. AR will change over time. If the dentist has an excellent month (from a production standpoint), it may take several months to see all those payments across the receptionist's desk as payment.

BILLING SYSTEMS

Most dental offices with computer management systems process bills and send them to patients. The sequence of sending bills to patients is important. Most offices send bills once per month. The office should be sure to use a consistent date so that the patient remembers the bill. Larger offices may need to send bills several times per month. This helps smooth the workload and cash flowing through the office. For example, an office may send accounts with last names beginning with letters A–M on the first of the month and N–Z on the fifteenth. Other offices send a second bill two weeks after the primary bill with a special "dunning message" (see later in the chapter) to all accounts over 60 days old. This is an attempt to encourage the older accounts to pay.

     Billing is expensive. It involves staff time to process entries, staff time to review and print bills, mailing charges, costs of stationery and other paper products, and lost implied interest earned. Some estimates have put the total cost of sending a single bill at $16.00. If it requires two statements to collect, the cost rises to $32.00 for each patient, essentially eating away the profit on smaller cases. It obviously pays to collect fees as soon as possible. Box 22.3 shows that in a typical dental practice, offices collect about a third of the fees at the front desk. The collection ratio on these accounts is 100%. Offices send about a third of the fees to insurance carriers. The insurance also pays these at virtually 100%. The fees that offices send through statements (the last third) account for almost all the uncollectible amounts. If the total collection ratio is 97%, the actual collection ratio (on the billed amount) is much less, perhaps 91%. The uncollectible ratio is then in fact 9%. Few practice owners would be happy with a 91% collection ratio, although that number is a more accurate reflection of the actual collection percentage in this practice. The obvious solution is to move more collections to the front desk, leaving less in AR. Dental practices do this by asking for payment, making payments easy, and providing an accurate estimate of insurance payments.

BOX 22.3	TRUE COLLECTION RATIO
One-third front desk	100%
One-third insurance	100%
One-third statements	91%
Total	97%

3% uncollectible = 9% uncollectible ratio

33% billed

BOX 22.4	ELEMENTS OF A COLLECTION POLICY

Collection techniques
Delinquent accounts
Outside collection methods

COLLECTION POLICY

If the office financial (credit) policy has failed to screen bad credit risks adequately, the office will have a problem collecting money owed by patients. The collection policy determines the office's rules for collecting that money. It establishes collection techniques, defines a delinquent account, and decides on methods outside the office that the dental practice uses for collecting problem accounts (Box 22.4). Offices can use any or all of several different collection methods.

COLLECTION TECHNIQUES

Collection techniques describe the methods the dental office uses to collect money from patients.

IN-HOUSE COLLECTIONS

The best way to collect money that patients owe is to collect it at the time of service. By using this "in-house" method of collecting, dental practices do not need to worry about sending a bill, uncollectible amounts, or AR. Patients are free of worrying about paying later. However, many dentists are reluctant to have their staff members ask for payment. Staff members should remind every patient, as they leave the operatory and pass by the receptionist's desk, what their new current balance is and ask for payment. If a patient comes for treatment and owes money before receiving any treatment for the day, staff members should try to collect all they owe, not just the day's amount. Practice owners should develop scripts for staff members to use with patients who do not make a payment at this time. These might include patients who say "I forgot my checkbook" or "Just send me the bill."

STATEMENTS

A statement is a printed report sent to the patient that details the status of their financial account. Computerized accounting systems allow dental practices to customize the process, choosing whom to send statements to, when to send them, and to add special messages and account charges. Often the program will allow several types of statements, depending on how the practice wants the statement to look. The office should be sure that the statement contains a return envelope to make it easy for people to pay. Most offices set a minimum amount to bill. If a patient owes less than $5, sending the bill is probably not worth the trouble or expense. (This may also anger otherwise good patients over the trivial amount owed.)

Most offices place "dunning messages" on statements (Box 22.5). A "dun" is a repeated or insistent request for payment. Computer programs allow offices to place ever-more insistent messages on statements, depending on the age of the account. Accounts that are 30 days old receive a polite reminder for payment. Accounts that are 60 days

old receive a not-so-gentle reminder. These messages are marginally effective for people who have forgotten to pay their bills. They are not effective for people who have intentionally not paid.

LETTERS

Personalized letters are more effective than messages on monthly statements. Using an in-office computer, the receptionist can generate word-processed letters personalized with the individual patient's personal information and payment history.

TELEPHONE CALLS

A telephone call from the office staff is the most effective collection method. Unfortunately, it is also the least enjoyable and least liked by staff members. They will find all sorts of other tasks to do first and devise many valid excuses for not making collection calls.

There are several things to keep in mind when making collection calls (Box 22.6). Have the staff member find an area away from the patients to make collection calls. Patients in the reception area or those waiting to make an appointment do not need to hear a collection call in progress. Office personnel should ensure there are accurate records and review the chart and account before contacting the patient. A collection call is worthless and destructive if the patient has sent payment as required, but the caller discovers this fact too late. A caller should not say that they will do something if they will not. For example, if they say they will send an account to a collection agency if the payment is not received by this Friday, they should do it. Idle threats are illegal and unwise. The office personnel should show concern and understanding for the patient. Sometimes people lose their job or have an illness or other personal life difficulties. A new payment schedule can be arranged if the patient truly needs one. The office should

BOX 22.5	EXAMPLE DUNNING MESSAGES

Age	Message
30 days	We have not received your payment. Please send it as soon as possible. Thanks!
60 days	We have not received a payment from you in more than 60 days. Please pay your bill immediately to keep your account current.
90 days	Your account is seriously past due. Please send payment immediately to avoid collection action.
120 days	We have not received a payment from you in more than 120 days. If we do not receive payment in full within three working days, your account will be turned over to a collection agency for further action.

BOX 22.6	COLLECTION CALL BEHAVIORS

- Be accurate
- Be truthful
- Show concern and understanding
- Be persistent

be persistent, nevertheless. It is an unpleasant job, but they should keep it up. If patients know that the office will give up the collection effort, then they will expect that to happen and behave accordingly. Any required follow-up should be noted on the financial record. For example, if a patient has promised to make payment and has not done so, the office should call on the day the patient promised payment. The staff member should let the patient know that they have not forgotten. Finally, laws (such as the Fair Debt Collection Practices Act) govern how offices can conduct telephone collection calls.

When the staff member makes the collection call, most responses fall into one of four categories. The most common excuses patients give are:

- **It was an oversight**
  The most frequent response is "The check's in the mail." Often, the patient quickly writes a check, and the payment comes in the mail in several days. If it does not, follow up immediately.

- **The patient has a temporary financial problem**
  This results from seasonal jobs, illness, or other reasons that limit the patient's cash flow. People often will not call to tell the office they are not making payment. They just do not make it. A new payment schedule can be set up if required.

- **The patient wants their insurance to pay for the procedure**
  Patients often believe (erroneously) that their insurance will cover all, or most, of the cost of a procedure. They then want to put the dental office in the position of advocating with the insurer to get them a higher reimbursement. Dental practices should be sure that patients understand their portion of the fee before beginning treatment. Patients must also understand that they are responsible for the bill if the insurance changes or alters the reimbursement. As insurance contracts become more complex, more patients are confused by their contracts and need help understanding their benefits.

- **The patient is unwilling to pay**
  Generally this is because the patient is dissatisfied with the work they had done. At this point, the dentist should try to satisfy the patient by making the work right. They can then continue to press for payment or pursue payment less aggressively. The decision rests on how sure the practitioner is that the work is proper and how willing they are to face a potential malpractice suit. (The single largest cause of malpractice claims is continued collection effort.) Some states have a one-year statute of limitations. This means that the patient has one year from the date of discovery of a problem to initiate a lawsuit. If the office waits 366 days to initiate aggressive collection efforts in one of these states, it should be safe. Practice owners should check with a lawyer to find the statute of limitations in their practice state.

DELINQUENT ACCOUNTS

Delinquent accounts are the next level of the collection process. The first step at this point is to define a delinquent account. This means that the office must have a system to "age" the accounts. When accounts are aged, they are categorized by how long it has been since the office made the unpaid charge. (Some people use the time since the last payment on the account. Either system works.)

AGING ACCOUNTS RECEIVABLE

Keeping track of the age of accounts is important because the older the account, the less valuable it is to the dental office. The office may have already spent much money sending statements to collect the account. It has a lower chance of collecting the account, will have to allocate additional staff time and the cost of postage and supplies trying to collect it, and the dentist has gone longer without the money. Because of these problems, the account's value decreases significantly as it ages. Figure 22.1 shows the estimated value of an account as it gets older. As it demonstrates, an account that is six months old is only worth 50% of its original value.

An account that has a charge made less than 30 days previously is "current." Account aging classifications generally run in 30-day increments, up to 120- or 150-day-old accounts. A "30-day" account is one in which no payment has been made in at least 30 but not more than 60 days. A "60-day" account is one in which no payment has been made in at least 60 but not more than 90 days, and so forth. That means that the patient (or the account guarantor) has not made a payment in at least that time. The account will be older than the listed amount. If, for example, a patient made a payment on the first day of the month and the office aged the accounts on the last day of the month, that account would be current because the patient had made a payment within the 30-day window (even though there have been 29 days since the last payment).

The account aging report gives a listing of all the patient accounts that owe money, categorized by the time

BOX 22.7 EXAMPLE ACCOUNT AGING REPORT

Pt. No.	Account name	Balance	Current	30+ days	60+ days	90+ days	120+ days
12 568	Abel, John	235.50	0.00	0.00	135.00	100.00	0.00
	Last Pay: 50.00		Pay Date: 04-22-24		Phone: 123-562-9863		
9 522	Edgars, Ann	1675.00	0.00	0.00	1200.00	0.00	475.00
	Last Pay: 75.00		Pay Date: 04-22-24		Phone: 123-562-2593		
7 620	Hass, Timothy	855.00	0.00	855.00	0.00	0.00	0.00
	Last Pay: 100.00		Pay Date: 04-22-24		Phone: 123-638-5842		
5 131	Nante, George	190.00	0.00	0.00	190.00	0.00	0.00
	Last Pay: 50.00		Pay Date: 04-22-24		Phone: 123-562-7412		
8 569	Powell, Dawn	550.00	0.00	0.00	0.00	0.00	550.00
	Last Pay: 200.00		Pay Date: 04-22-24		Phone: 123-638-8790		
11 658	Smith, Roy	1650.00	0.00	0.00	0.00	1000.00	650.00
	Last Pay: 250.00		Pay Date: 04-22-24		Phone: 123-562-1436		

since the last payment (Box 22.7). A dental office management system will quickly generate this report. The front office staff should use it to make follow-up telephone calls and send letters to patients who are late in their payments. Often the 30-day accounts are waiting for insurance to clear before making the final payment. The 30–60-day accounts are the ones that staff should pursue aggressively so that they do not become older, harder-to-collect accounts. Any account more than 60 days old is becoming a problem account. The office should pursue these accounts more aggressively.

PURPOSES OF PURSUING DELINQUENT ACCOUNTS

Dental practices have two purposes in collecting delinquent accounts. First, they want to get the money owed. After all, they did the work; the patient should pay for it. If possible, the dentist also wants to retain the patronage and goodwill of the patient. That patient may have future work to do; they may refer patients to the practice, or they may have friends or family members who are patients of the practice. If the dentist or their staff are too aggressive, they risk angry or embarrassed patients, counter-claims, suits, malpractice suits, and adverse publicity. Again, dentists should be sure their work is above reproach before aggressively pursuing a delinquent account.

OUTSIDE COLLECTION METHODS

Since collection efforts represent failures of the office's patient financial policy, outside collection methods represent failures of their in-office collection policy. When the dentist has decided that an account is delinquent, they have several avenues to continue collection efforts. By this point, the dentist's costs will probably equal any money they gain from continued efforts. Often the dentist will pursue collection efforts just to feel vindicated.

COLLECTION AGENCY

The most common method dental practices use to collect delinquent accounts is a collection agency. A collection agency really cannot do anything to collect an account that the dentist cannot do in their office. The collection agency should not be a significant source of income if the dentist and staff are doing their jobs correctly. The collection agents know the system and can access credit reports that the office may not, however. Collection agencies take a percentage (generally from 33% to 50%) of the amount they collect from patients as their fee. (Some also have membership or retainer fees.) Therefore, it is worth little of their time to work a $50 account. The collection agent usually spends time with larger accounts to improve their return. The practice owner is satisfied knowing that the delinquent patient knows they are subject to collection action. The collection agency should put a notice in the delinquent patient's credit report so the next time they try to buy something on credit, they will at least have a problem.

In selecting a collection agency, the practice owner should be sure that the agency has the proper credentials and that the state has licensed and bonded the agency. The practice owner should ask for a list of dentists and other health professionals in the area who use the agency's service. They should contact several of them to see if they are satisfied with the results. The practice owner should have the agent explain the exact sequence of steps they use when attempting to collect and note what the agent does with accounts that are not paid. Poorly handled collection efforts reflect badly on the dentist's practice.

SMALL CLAIMS COURT

Every county in the United States has a Small Claims Court. The purpose of these courts is to settle civil claims of low value (generally $1500 or less). The court is informal, but there is some initial essential paperwork. Anyone can sue or defend themselves or bring an attorney. Small Claims Courts use no juries. A judge listens to both sides of the story, views evidence brought by the parties, and renders a decision.

Some dentists use the Small Claims Court to collect money that patients fail to pay. If the dentist has evidence that they rendered the service appropriately and the patient owes the bill, the dentist will probably receive a judgment in their favor. However, they may also not get paid even then. A judgment is a legally enforceable court order, but the dentist is still responsible for collecting the money (which is why they are there in the first place). The practice owner may need to return to court to get a garnishment of the patient's wages (if they are employed) or an attachment of personal property. Post-judgment collections can be difficult, time-consuming, and tricky. The dentist might even need an attorney to collect on their judgment.

Some dental practice owners are true advocates of using the Small Claims Court as a collection method. Others find that their time is better spent in the office doing dentistry or on the golf course relaxing. They can send staff in their place to present their case in court, but then the dentist has the added expense of the staff salary, with still no guarantee of collection.

LAWYERS

Another standard method of collecting overdue accounts is to have a lawyer write a letter to the non-paying patient. Letters from lawyers usually get action. The dentist must be willing to pay the lawyer to write the letter (usually a small fee) and then continue with the case if a patient refuses (potentially a hefty fee).

SELLING ACCOUNTS RECEIVABLE (FACTORING SERVICE)

Some offices sell their AR to a bank to collect. Such a service is also called factoring. Factors generally pay the practice owner about 80% of the face value of the accounts. The problem here is that they generally only buy accounts less than 90 days old, because the banks realize the problem in collecting older accounts. So essentially, they collect the easy-to-collect accounts, leaving the office with the difficult, older accounts. The primary use for these services is during practice sales or transfers when other arrangements do not work out.

WRITING OFF ACCOUNTS

Offices should write off uncollectible accounts regularly and periodically (usually annually). When it "writes off" an account, the office declares doubt that it will ever collect the money owed by that patient or guarantor. The office then removes it from their AR total, resets the account balance to zero, and removes the account from their files. If the patient ever returns and pays the account, the office reactivates the account and all unpaid balances. Offices should write off accounts when they turn them over to a collection agency or third-party collector. The office writes back any money the collector receives to a reactivated account.

Periodically writing off accounts lets the office keep an accurate running tally of the AR total. Without writing off uncollectible accounts, the AR total continues to rise. This is important so that the practice owner knows if there are problems with normal collection efforts. If dentists need to value their practice for any reason (e.g. bank requirements, practice sales), they also require an accurate AR figure.

KEYS FOR EFFECTIVE COLLECTIONS IN THE OFFICE

Offices should be honest and upfront about fees (Box 22.8). They should let patients know what the patient's estimated portion of the fee will be. Dentists should believe in what they are doing and in what they are charging. If they believe the service is overvalued, they cannot effectively convince patients that it is appropriately valued. New practitioners should practice telling

BOX 22.8	KEYS FOR EFFECTIVE COLLECTIONS

- Dentists should be honest about their fees.

- Dentists should believe in what they are doing and what they are charging.

- Dentists should practice telling people how much the service is going to cost.

- Dentists should never assume that a patient does not want or cannot afford the best dentistry that they can offer.

- Dentists should be sure that patients understand, upfront, what their portion of the fee will be.

- Dentists should have a written policy and should give it to all patients.

- Dentists should train staff and delegate to them.

people how much the service will cost. Some go as far as to practice in front of a mirror until they are comfortable with "selling" a service. Dentists should never assume that a patient does not want or cannot afford the best dentistry they can offer. They should be sure that patients understand, upfront, what their portion of the fee will be and what portion they can expect their third-party carrier to cover. Offices should always remind patients that the bill is the *patient's* obligation, no matter what a third-party carrier will pay. Offices should have a written policy and give it to all patients; they will appreciate that the office informs them before beginning treatment. Offices should have a definite plan for every patient. The dentist should train staff and delegate to them because they can arrange payment plans as easily as a dentist if given the proper direction.

Generating Patients for the Practice

CHAPTER 23

Part 1: Generating New Patients

So you think that advertising doesn't pay? We understand there are 25 mountains in Colorado higher than Pike's Peak. Can you name one of them?

The American Salesman

GOAL

The aim of this part is to present the basis of marketing professional services. It explores the nature of dental services and the behavior of the buying public.

LEARNING OBJECTIVES

At the completion of this part, the student will be able to:

- Describe the evolution of marketing of professional services.

- Discuss the relationship between professional ethics and marketing.

- Define what marketing is and is not.

- Compare the nature of services with that of products, and discuss how this affects their marketing.

- Describe the stages of the growth of a dental practice and its relation to the marketing effort.

- Define the "four Ps" of marketing and relate them to marketing dental services.

- Describe why people purchase dental services.

- Describe ways to segment the dental marketplace.

- Describe how common internal marketing efforts generate patients for the practice.

- Describe how common external marketing efforts generate patients for the practice.

- Describe the market planning process.

- Describe some common problems in marketing professional services.

Business Basics for Dentists, Second Edition. James L. Harrison, David O. Willis, and Charles K. Thieman.
© 2024 John Wiley & Sons, Inc. Published 2024 by John Wiley & Sons, Inc.

Dentists use many methods to help attract new patients to the practice, retain existing patients, and convince patients to purchase services. Every management decision that dentists make in the practice has implications for patient generation. These efforts are *marketing*. External marketing looks at generating new patients for the practice, whereas internal marketing aims to retain existing patients. Both are necessary for a successful practice. The hours that dentists keep, the fees they charge, insurance plan participation, and the types of services that dentists do all affect patient generation and retention. Together, these are marketing efforts.

Depending on the competitiveness of the practice area, dentists will need to put more effort into marketing. If the practice is as busy as it wants to be (or busier) with the right kind and mix of patients, there is less need for marketing expenditures. Even practices that have a full complement of patients and do not advertise continue to market the practice through their communications and management of the office.

DEFINING MARKETING

Marketing is a managerial process that focuses a practice's activities on the benefits sought by a target group of clients, thereby satisfying their needs and desires more effectively. Notice that marketing looks to satisfy the needs of a group of patients. The primary task is to learn clients' needs, wants, and preferences, and then to develop services and products that satisfy those needs. This affects how dentists deliver their services and even how they organize the practice. It means listening to people and providing goods and services that they demand (or want). Marketing means that dentists view the practice through the patients' eyes, thereby generating and retaining patients in the practice (at a profit).

It is as instructive to say what marketing is *not* as to start to define marketing. Marketing is not advertising, although advertising can be a part of marketing. Marketing is not the sales technique of a used car salesperson, although sales technique is a component of marketing. Marketing does not mean high-pressure techniques, convincing people to buy what they do not need, or slick four-color ads.

Marketing looks at dental consumers' desires (not dentists' professional assessment of their needs). Those desires fall into three broad categories:

- To avoid something, such as pain, disfigurement, noise, odors, x-rays, or cost.

- To gain something, such as health, a pretty smile, or relief from pain.

- To prevent something, such as pain, disfigurement, or embarrassment.

Consumers do not want amalgams, composite restorations, partial dentures, or bridges. Instead, from their perspective, they are avoiding, gaining, or preventing something from happening to them. Dentists can provide a service that helps a patient achieve their goals. That service may be a prophylaxis, tooth whitening, or orthodontics. If it solves the patient's wants, the dentist has acted with a marketing orientation. Part of the marketing orientation is to provide information to patients so that they know the available procedures and techniques. This education process makes consumers more aware of their needs, raising their level of wants and, therefore, their desire for dental services.

WHY DENTISTS MARKET

Dentists market to gain patients for the practice. Dentists have marketed their services since the first dental practice. In recent years, dental marketing has become much more sophisticated as dentists have brought business techniques to bear on professional practices. Several factors have fostered this.

The increased competition among dentists for the available patient pool has stimulated marketing. As described in Chapter 12, this is a question of the relative supply of practitioners and the relative demand for patients. Factors such as the number and age of dentists, auxiliary use patterns, technology, and practice patterns influence the supply of practitioners. The number of patients, usage patterns, disease patterns, third-party reimbursement, and efficiency of preventive measures influence the demand for services. When dentists see gaps in their appointment book, they first try to encourage more patients to come to the office. In other words, they market their services.

Dentists have two kinds of competition. The first is to gain the potential patient's attention and to have the patient patronize them instead of another nearby dentist. In this sense, dentists compete against each other for their share of the available patient pool. A dentist's internal operational policies (such as the hours the office is open) and external marketing strategies (such as advertising campaigns) help attract new patients. Once the patient comes to the office, then the dentist faces a second, equally important marketing problem. That is to educate and convince the patient that their dental needs are important enough to spend (often large amounts of) money to meet. Because most dental procedures are discretionary in nature, dentists compete against other forms of discretionary spending for the consumer's dollar. In this sense, dentists do not compete against other dentists but against travel agents, home remodelers, big-screen television sales agents, and fine-dining restaurants. Convincing the patient to come to a dentist involves external marketing plans. Once the patient is in the chair, internal marketing and sales techniques become more important.

The changing nature of third-party contracts has encouraged many dentists to market their services. Various contract organizations (capitation plans and referral plans) may limit where patients can go for reimbursed dental care. Deciding whether to participate in one of these plans is a marketing decision because it addresses the patients' desires for reimbursed dental care. Beyond that, a practitioner may see patients who sign up with a given plan leave the practice. The dentist then feels that they need to generate additional traditional fee-for-service patients to compensate for the managed care patients who have left.

A practice's insurance plan participation becomes one of its most critical marketing decisions.

The rise of consumerism and a revised legal and ethical climate in the profession have increased marketing in dentistry. In years past, the profession considered any advertising to be unethical. The American Dental Association (ADA) Code of Ethics and many state Dental Practice Acts described advertising as illegal. In 1977, a court decision (*Bates and O'Steen* v. *Arizona*) effectively ended professional prohibitions against advertising. This case stated that a professional must be allowed to advertise their services if the advertisements are not false or misleading. Simultaneously, consumerism was beginning to become an underlying trend in the United States. This trend advocates for more information for consumers to use while making informed decisions. According to this tenet, a consumer should differentiate among dentists. Dentists must tell the public how they are different from others. Some professionals have a problem with this notion. The public agrees with it.

Changing technologies have brought many new services to the arsenals of practicing dentists. These address consumer desires by fulfilling the benefits sought. Patients want to know about these services. Dentists who provide them want patients to know about them. Marketing answers both desires.

WHAT DENTISTS MARKET

Before a practice begins a marketing policy, the dentist needs to understand the characteristics of dental services to develop appropriate marketing strategies.

DENTISTS MARKET A SERVICE, NOT A PRODUCT

A product is a tangible object. Services, on the other hand, are intangible. Consumers can see the results of the service and feel or hear the service. However, they cannot pick it up and examine it. So services are, by nature, different from products. These differences also lead to a significant difference in how dentists market products and services.

Services Are Inseparable from the Provider of the Service

Retailers or other third parties can buy, repackage, and resell a product. They can put a different label on it and move it across the country or the world, but the product remains unchanged. On the other hand, services cannot be separated from the service provider. The delivery of service is the service. If someone else delivers the service, it becomes a new service.

Services Are Variable

Because services show low standardization, the providers of the service and the service itself are inseparable. Food preparation is a tremendously variable service. Virtually every restaurant prepares food differently. Fast-food franchises have decreased variability through strict standard operating procedures. Someone knows that a "quarter-pound burger" from a favorite fast-food franchise will be the same whether they buy it in New York, Atlanta, or San Francisco. This standardization essentially turns a service into a product.

Services Are Perishable

A service is perishable. The producer cannot put it into a warehouse or inventory as they can a product. This means that timing is critical. Because there are only a given number of hours in a day, one person can only provide a given amount of service. Once time is lost (through a "no show" or cancelation), it is lost for ever. Production cannot make up for the lost time.

Services Are Intangible

Services are intangible. A marketing maxim is to "tangibilize the intangible, and intangibilize the tangible." This means that dentists should try to provide an intangible service as a reminder of a tangible product and give a tangible reminder of an intangible service. Whether it is a little sign in a yard from the lawn service company, a mint on a motel bed pillow, or a toothbrush after a dental prophylaxis appointment, tangible gifts serve as reminders that someone provided an intangible service.

Services Are Intestable

Consumers are unable to test services before they purchase them. They cannot pick them up, examine them, take them for a test drive, or kick their tires to check for soundness. Instead, they use surrogates to test the service before they purchase it. Patients are similarly unable to test dental services before they purchase them. Instead, they use surrogate measures for testing the quality of the services. Those surrogates include reputation, recommendations from trusted others, cost (as a reverse measure), and familiarity. The inability to test the service beforehand leads to more post-purchase testing and dissonance.

DENTISTS MARKET BASED ON THE "FOUR Ps" OF MARKETING

Marketers often speak of the four Ps of marketing. Nearly all marketing efforts involve these four major concerns:

- **Product** is the good or service that the producer provides. It involves both the core product and all product extensions in the bundled services purchased.

- **Price** is the money that the consumer pays for the good or service. It includes not only the price for the core product but also all extensions. For example, the total price of a veneer includes the fee charged, how much work time the patient missed, the payment plan offered, and how much the insurance pays.

- **Place** is where the producer delivers the good or service. Generally, for dentists the core place is the dental office. The extended place includes parking and public transportation availability, disabled accessibility, office decor, and cleanliness.

- **Promotion** involves all the efforts someone makes to make people aware of their good or service. For the dentist, it includes the core advertising efforts and extended promotions such as signs, community service, and health promotion efforts by the dentist and office staff members.

WHY CONSUMERS BUY

The consumer buys to satisfy their wants and needs. People want their purchases to solve a problem for them. In that sense, they buy benefits, not features of the good or service. The expected outcome is generally not simply to own the good or service but instead to use it for some end. Consumers do not really purchase aspirin; they purchase relief from a headache. If another product (acetaminophen or ibuprofen) offers a better benefit at a reasonable cost, they will purchase the other product. They do not care about how the producer makes the product or delivers the service. Box 23.1 summarizes these differences for implant services.

DEFINITION OF FEATURES

A feature is a characteristic of the good or service that the producer sells. Patients do not need to know the features, such as the type of metal, the characteristics of the material, and the method of making the product. That is vitally important when fabricating a dental restoration or appliance. However, consumers do not care about the features of the product. In the example, an implant has the features

BOX 23.1	WHY A CONSUMER WOULD BUY IMPLANT SERVICES

Features

　Titanium
　Osseointegration

Advantages

　No clasps or wires
　Do not cut down adjacent teeth

Benefits

　Look great
　Function like natural teeth

BOX 23.2	BENEFITS OF DENTAL SERVICES

Gain

　Health, sex appeal, relief of pain, function

Improve

　Function, speech, chewing, appearance

Avoid

　Pain, disfigurement, cost

Prevent

　Pain, embarrassment, disfigurement, cost, inconvenience, disease

that it is made of titanium and osseointegrates with the bone, and a porcelain crown is placed on top of the implant.

DEFINITION OF ADVANTAGES

Advantages are the characteristics of one feature over another that make a product or service different. They help the consumer to differentiate among choices, but the advantages do not cause the consumer to buy. An implant has the advantage that there are no clasps or wires to look unnatural, and dentists do not have to cut on adjacent teeth to replace a missing tooth. Advantages compare the features of one solution with the features of another.

DEFINITION OF BENEFITS

A benefit is the expected outcome of a purchase. Consumers do not purchase a filling, a partial denture, or cosmetic bleaching. They purchase the benefit of a more attractive, youthful smile or the ability to chew food effectively. The more consumers see the benefit as solving their problem, the more they are willing to pay for the solution (Box 23.2).

Most dentists sell services based on the features of those services, not the benefits the consumer wants. When dentists talk "to" patients about their proposed treatment plan, they discuss the features of the bridge (what materials it contains, what steps the procedure requires) rather than the benefit that the patient can expect (a better smile and improved chewing). Any given patient will weigh the alternative solutions (partial vs. bridge vs. implant vs. no treatment) and determine, in their mind and their case, the best solution to their problem. Patient education is vital in helping people understand their dental problems and the benefits of the various treatment choices. In the end, it is the patient's perception of a solution to their problem that they buy.

PATIENTS BUY A "BUNDLE OF SERVICES"

People do not buy a simple good or service. Instead, they buy a bundle of goods and services combined to make the purchase decision. When someone buys a car, they buy the core product, which is the automobile. However, they also buy the reputation and location of the service facility, the car's delivery date, and financing options. These all make up the extended product that they purchase. Likewise, patients buy more than the core dental service. They purchase not only a veneer, but the time that the office is open, the date they can have the procedure completed, payment plans, and the dentist's reputation. The simple price of the service often will be one of many determining purchase factors.

MARKETING PLAN DEVELOPMENT

When dentists are ready to begin marketing their practice, they must develop a marketing plan. Developing this plan makes the dentist look at the people they will serve to meet their needs. It also makes the dentist consider what they are doing well, what they need to improve, what competitors are doing, and how they will tell their story. It should fit with the dentist's strategic plan and vision for the practice. The desired marketing outputs (e.g. additional new patients) are a function of these marketing inputs. The marketing plan consists of several discrete steps.

DEFINING THE MARKET

The first step is to define who the patient base will be. This defines the market. The location of a practice is one of the most important marketing decisions the dentist makes because it is crucial in defining their market. Most patients live within five miles of a dental practice (in urban areas).

If a dentist intends to develop an upper-class "white-collar" practice, but their practice is on a "blue-collar" side of town, they need to appraise their goals and possibilities honestly.

SEGMENTING AND TARGETING THE MARKET

Segmentation of the market refers to dividing the population into smaller groups of similar individuals. Dentists may assign these groups on several bases. Geographic segmentation groups people by where they live or work. People who use direct mail will probably look at zip codes to decide where to send mailings. Demographic segmentation groups people by some outward characteristic, such as age, gender, race, or income level. Many dentists aim marketing efforts at people who subscribe to a particular insurance plan. When someone advertises in a senior citizen's newsletter, they employ demographic segmentation in the marketing effort. Psychographic segmentation does not care about someone's outward characteristics. Instead, this form of segmentation groups people by how they think or feel about a particular issue. If someone develops a fear reduction program to attract fearful dental patients, they have used psychographic market segmentation. Behavioristic segmentation groups people by how they act. It is well known that people who display high general preventive health behaviors also have higher dental usage rates. When someone places flyers in the local fitness center or health foods store, they employ behavioristic market segmentation.

Market segmentation is the true art of successful marketing. Segmentation tries to group people so that the marketer can appeal to a particular group more effectively, with less wasted advertising effort and money. This is *target marketing* (as opposed to *mass marketing*). The target marketer is much more efficient because more of the marketing message reaches the person for whom they intend it. There are no fixed rules about market segmentation. A dentist can set and develop their own target groups (Box 23.3).

DEVELOPING THE MARKETING MIX

Dental office marketing consists of a mix of procedures and techniques for getting the word out about an office. The key is to decide who the target market is and then develop strategies that appeal to that target group. The office is likely to need several strategies to deliver the message. Even a well-defined target group uses several channels to find information.

BOX 23.3	EXAMPLE DENTAL MARKET SEGMENTS

- Fearful patients (dental phobics)
- Smile seekers (esthetic conscious)
- Status seekers (perfect smiles)
- Utilitarians (basic care that works)

This gives an example of marketing segments a dentist might develop. It is not intended to be an authoritative listing of segments, but rather to show how someone might group the potential patients in their area. They could then use different marketing and delivery strategies to appeal to each of these groups.

TRACKING THE EFFECTIVENESS OF MARKETING EFFORTS

Marketing efforts are expensive and time-consuming for the practice. Therefore, the dentist should track how many patients each marketing effort generates so that they can decide if the marketing has been worth the cost and time spent. The best way to establish how a patient found out about the office is obvious: ask. When the patient first calls the office, the receptionist who takes the call should ask "And how did you hear about our office?" The patient may respond with one specific method ("Doris Smith referred me") or may mention several methods ("A friend told me about you and looked up your web page online"). All modern dental management computer software has fields for entering this information. At the end of the month (or quarter), the practice then generates a report that lists all the patients who listed each marketing source (e.g. website) and the amount of dentistry treatment planned and completed for the source. By comparing the cost with the amount generated, the practice can decide if a particular marketing program is worth continuing.

When looking at this relationship in more depth, the cost to generate a patient needs to be allocated by type. For example, assume that the practice spent $1500 per month on Yellow Pages ads, generating three patients, each with $400 worth of dentistry. It also spent $3000 per month on a direct-mail program, generating 15 patients with an average of $400 per month. The Yellow Pages ad patients "cost" $500 each, losing $100 each. The direct mail patients cost $200 each, earning the dentist $200 each per patient. The direct-mail campaign, although more expensive, is more profitable given these numbers.

MARKETING STRATEGIES

Marketing strategies are the methods that dentists use to get their message to their target group. These efforts are grouped into two types, internal and external (Box 23.4). Internal efforts focus the attention on the existing patients of the practice, whereas external efforts focus on people who are not current patients.

INTERNAL MARKETING STRATEGIES

Internal marketing efforts are those that dentists have traditionally called "professionalism." These efforts cater to the existing patients, hoping they will stay with the practice and bring in additional new patients.

Branding

Branding is an internal function with enormous external implications. A dentist's brand is the image of their product in the marketplace. It is how consumers perceive the dentist to be different from similar providers in the area. A patient's information and expectations about their dental experience should be the same as their actual experience. If so, they will see a particular dentist as both relevant to solving their problem and unique in that ability. Branding involves all the intangibles that drive consumer perception of a business. These include logo, stationery, advertising, office decor and ambiance, staff training and attire, and website. These should all be consistent and offer the same messages about the value of the service provided. If the practice can establish a strong brand image, it will have more freedom in pricing and other management decisions, leading to increased profitability.

Performance

The most critical trait of a dentist (according to public opinion surveys) is the quality of care they deliver. Quality care is the basis of the "product" that a dentist provides. Quality dentistry is necessary for a successful practice. But quality dentistry alone is insufficient to guarantee a successful practice. A dentist's performance on the technical side of dentistry is an assumed trait by the public. If a dentist violates that assumption, the patient will be dissatisfied and probably leave the practice. It is not even the dentist's actual performance that the patient judges, but rather the patient's perception of the performance compared to the patient's expectation of the performance. The patient's expectations then become crucial to their satisfaction. If the dentist does not meet the patient's expectations, the patient will be dissatisfied with the service, even if their expectations were unrealistic in the first place. (To their mind, the expectations were realistic!) Even if a dentist does the most technically perfect procedure, the patient will be dissatisfied if they do not like it (or how it was delivered). If a dentist builds patients' expectations with slogans such as "special care," "painless," "low fees," or "cowards welcome," then they need to deliver what they promise. The worst thing a dentist can do is to gain someone's trust to come to the office and not deliver the promised services. Patients are concerned with the total time of treatment. From the dentist's perspective, time is the chair time in treatment. From the patient's perspective, time is the total time involved in the dental visit: travel time, waiting time, return-to-work time, and additional time to go to the babysitter, school, or other places. Other examples of influencing patients' expectations include promptness, pain control, availability, and the amount of health information provided.

Marketers have coined the "0-2-10 rule," which describes customers' expectations of their office experience compared with the actual experience. By this rule:

- If the customer had simply the experience they expected, they will tell no one.

- If the customer had a better experience than they expected, they will tell 2 people.

- If the customer had a worse experience than they expected, they will tell 10 people.

While this rule is an oversimplification, it points out how important it is to meet or exceed the client's expectations for service, not our expectations of the service we provide. By this rule, the worst thing we can do is underperform and not meet someone's expectations.

Insurance Plan Participation

Whether or not a practice participates in a particular insurance plan has an impact on how they generate

BOX 23.4	TYPES OF MARKETING STRATEGIES

Internal	External
Existing patients	New patients into the practice
Current patients of record	Target group
Traditional "professional"	Non-traditional methods
Existing resources within the office	External resources, media
Less costly	More costly

patients for the practice. People generally gain dental benefits through their work, often with little input into which plan to choose or the plan's specifics. The plan administrator then gives them a list of dentists who are providers for the plan, among which they patient chooses. The insurance carrier then steers hundreds or thousands of patients to participating providers. From a practitioner's perspective, they may gain many patients if they are a participating provider. (The dentist must also offer the patients substantial discounts from standard fees.) If the dentist is not a participating provider, they may lose patients whose insurance package at work changes. Because of this, the practice will need to compare insurance plans and decide with which, if any, it wishes to participate. This is currently one of the most significant marketing issues faced by dental practitioners.

Fees

Depending on its objectives, the practice will have different fee strategies. Those strategies and their uses are described in Chapter 21, and the various methods of determining fees (cost, demand, and competition based) are also in that chapter.

If a dentist wins a patient today based on price, the dentist can also lose them tomorrow based on price. When patients call asking about the fee for a particular service (e.g. a denture), try to deflect the answer (e.g. "the dentist will need to do a complete exam and determine the best course of treatment for your particular case"). However, the dentist should not worry about stating the fee because while they may have chased the patient away, was that patient going to be a valuable practice asset in the first place?

If a dental practice is different, the price is less important to patients. If it offers a unique service or offers a particular service uniquely, then the patient will find it more challenging to go to another dentist to have the service done. As patients bond with the dentist and the staff, the personal relationship also becomes unique. The value attached to a product or service is proportional to the ability to solve the problem for the consumer. The patient is seeking a benefit or solution to a problem. The better the service solves the patient's problem, the more they are willing to pay for the service.

Customers (patients) buy clusters of values for a multiplicity of reasons. Those reasons may not always be obvious to the dentist. Patients buy based on their values, not the dentist's. Dentists should be careful of *should* statements. (These statements imply the dentist's values, not the patient's.) The process of being sold (not just the product or service) sells the service. How the dentist delivers the

service is as important as the service itself. A dentist might make the most esthetic crowns in town, but if they cannot convince the patient of the value of those crowns, they will not make any of them.

Credit Policy

Every practice has credit and collection policies, whether they know it or not. (Chapter 22 discusses this in detail.) The public and all patients become aware of that policy every time they say "Just send me the bill." An easy credit policy encourages people to have work done and continue with treatment plans. A stricter plan requires patients to have more money upfront and discourages some from accepting planned treatment. Dentists want to establish a policy consistent with the clientele they serve in their practice. If the practice is too lenient when extending credit, its production will grow along with the accounts receivable and bad debts (uncollectibles) as people take advantage of the dentist's kind nature. On the other hand, accounts receivable may be too low, suggesting that the dentist may be losing some "sales" and production because of an excessively restrictive credit policy.

The credit policy interacts with fees to be a powerful marketing influence. Patients refer other patients based on how they perceive they were treated in the office, including payment plans. Patients look more at the monthly cost of a payment plan than the total cost of the procedure. The credit policy, therefore, greatly impacts how much dentistry the practice can "sell."

Facility

A facility is the "place" in marketing dentistry. The public expect cleanliness in a healthcare facility. (Cleanliness includes the degree of dust, cobwebs, and fingerprints.) Dentists should match the decor to the desired clientele. Decor includes color, lighting, furniture, and open or closed operatory arrangements. Accessibility for disabled and geriatric patients is important for those groups. Dentists should try to keep the reception area isolated from the noise and odors of the treatment area. Labs are usually messy. They should be hidden from view by either placing them in the back of the office or keeping the door closed. Most practitioners try to have diversions in the reception area, including reading material appropriate for their patients. Many others have an aquarium or a "kid's corner" to use as a diversion for patients.

A facility-related marketing strategy is the hours the practice keeps the office open to see patients. A dental practice is a business that "sells" dental services to the public. Successful practices make those services available at times that are convenient to the clients or patients. Many dentists aim to work only traditional hours during the day. However, new practitioners may find a wealth of patients by providing services during non-traditional hours. Changing demographics in the United States point to a continued decline in the "traditional" family unit (wage-earner father, non-working mother, and two school-aged children). Patients may be single parents or two-wage-earner couples who find it difficult to take off work for dental appointments. These people often have either dental insurance (or dual coverage) or discretionary money to spend on sophisticated dental care. As a result, many dentists find their non-traditional hours (evenings and Saturdays) to be the most productive. On the downside, neither the owner-dentist nor the employees may want to work during these hours. The providers want time with their own family or for outside personal interests. Depending on family situations, some people may not be able or willing to arrange schedules, daycare services, or other obligations to work these hours. Some dentists have hired part-time workers to fill times when other staff members cannot work.

Communication

Communication is the "advertising" of dental office internal marketing. The dental office communicates in several different ways. Verbal communication is the most apparent form. A dentist's (and staff's) choice of words is critical. A word with a common and innocuous meaning to the dentist may strike fear into the heart of an apprehensive patient. (Does *operatory* mean that the dentist will do an operation?)

Non-verbal communication is as important as the conversation itself. The tone of voice of the provider or person on the telephone tells more than the words themselves. Patients understand kinesics (body language) and proxemics (personal space) intuitively. Dentists should be aware of how they and their staff use these techniques.

Written communications should all convey the professionalism that the practice wants the office to project. It is a good idea to have a logo or other style of stationery used on all office communications. These include letters, brochures and information, postoperative instructions, and payment options and plans.

Recall (Recare) Systems

The practice's recall (recare) system is one of the most visible internal marketing efforts. (*Recall* implies defective care, as in a product recall. *Recare* or "periodic maintenance" implies ongoing care.) Dentists should aim all their efforts in this area to help patients achieve an optimum level of oral health. All communication should support this idea.

Information for Patients

Dental patients want information to make healthcare decisions. They want information about dental and general health, so many dentists provide brochures about these topics. (For example, "What is a root canal?" or "How can I stop smoking?") Many dentists also have video or DVD presentations about dental-care topics that they can show patients. This helps educate patients about complex procedures, assists in the informed consent conversation, and decreases the time the dentist spends in direct patient conversation.

People who use dental services preventively usually have a preventive health lifestyle that shows as other healthy lifestyle habits and procedures. They also exercise more, smoke less, eat healthier foods, and use seatbelts more than those who do not use dental services preventively. This preventive lifestyle group especially value health information. They appreciate and recommend the dentist because of it.

Asking for Referrals

One of the best ways to encourage patients to send additional patients to the dentist is simply to ask them. Often patients need to learn that dentists are looking for new and additional patients. Many dentists have developed reward systems for thanking patients for referring their friends or coworkers as patients of the practice. After a referral, the office may send a nice note of thanks. After several referrals, the office may send a note with a gift card or another more tangible method of thanking the referral source. Box 23.5 gives a simple formula method of verbally asking a patient for additional referrals.

BOX 23.5	HOW TO ASK A PATIENT FOR REFERRALS
Thank the patient by name	Mrs. Jones, thank you for coming to see us.
Say what you want	If you know anyone who is looking for dental care,
Ask them to send the referral	please have them call us.
Confirm your care	We would love to see them and will take excellent care of them.

EXTERNAL MARKETING STRATEGIES

External marketing efforts are those that dentists have not traditionally used. These efforts are to bring new patients into the practice. The hope is that those patients will stay with the practice and bring in even more new patients. Most external marketing involves advertising and promotional efforts because dentists are trying to reach a new group of patients.

Public Relations

This strategy often involves speaking to groups. Dentists must identify to whom they will speak and what they want as the outcome. Is the desired outcome a better-educated group? Or does the dentist want to generate three patient referrals from the presentation? Depending on the desired outcome, the talk will have a different orientation.

Public relations efforts frequently involve brochures or newsletters. Dentists may write these or purchase them already written (prefabricated or off the shelf). Writing a newsletter involves a significant amount of time that might be spent more productively doing other tasks. Practitioners can purchase prefabricated newsletters from many dental form and stationery companies. They can then have the dentist's name printed on them to customize the look.

Professional Relations

Interacting with other professionals is another essential part of the external marketing effort. Dentists need to let other professionals know where they are and what they can do for the other professionals regarding patient referrals. This usually includes announcements to physicians and other area dentists when a dentist opens a practice. Dentists should join local study clubs to learn and share special procedures and agree to take emergency calls for established local dentists, ensuring that their patients return to the dentist of record for follow-up treatment. Specialists appreciate referrals from generalists and often refer different patients to the generalist. A dentist should not be afraid to get on the phone and ask for help if they encounter a complex problem. If they refer regularly, the specialist will usually be glad to help. Many dentists give a bonus to their staff members who refer patients and send gifts to the staff of their referring dentists.

Signage

Office visibility is crucial for a dentist's success. The public need to know that they exist and where they practice. Where a dentist places the office is important in this regard. The most visible location is on a busy arterial feeder street through which thousands of cars pass daily. If the practice has a visible sign on such a busy road, thousands of people will see the location every day. Keep the sign simple. The "40–40 rule" says that someone should be able to read a sign from 40 yards away at 40 miles per hour as they drive past. This does not mean that they will all come to see that dentist, but when they do decide to see a dentist, this will be one of the dentists they consider. The dentist should "cut through the clutter" of other signs in the area. If all businesses have 20-foot-wide neon signs, the passersby will not see a 1-foot-wide black-and-white sign. Internal lighting makes it viewable at night. If the office is on a site that is not easily visible, then the dentist will need other forms of marketing to make up for the problem location.

Advertising and Promotions

Advertising and promotion bring a service to the attention of potential and current patients (customers) to increase patient visits. That media can be the Yellow Pages, direct mail, radio, or television advertising, a website, or social media. Advertising intends to inform the public of the services offered.

A promotion is an intentional effort to increase sales over a short period. Promotion adds something of value to the service offered. It helps to stimulate sales for reasons other than the face value of the service's benefit. For example, if a dentist sends a direct mailing to the households in the zip code surrounding their office, that dentist has engaged in advertising. If they include a coupon for a complimentary whitening tray, that dentist has included a promotion with the advertising. Promotions are effective in stimulating potential patients to action. The advertising informs them of the services offered, but the promotion gives them a reason to come and see that dentist.

Depending on the target market, a dentist will use different advertising and promotional efforts. Direct mail is more effective in blue-collar neighborhoods than in white-collar ones. Websites and social media are more important if the practice targets a younger, more affluent group. Senior citizen newsletters, high school sports brochures, and new mother publications are effective media for their target audiences. A dentist is only trying to get the potential patient to come in to see them, not to complete the treatment decision in the ad.

Network and franchise practices have an advantage over individual practitioners when conducting advertising and promotions in the mass media. Radio and television ads are effective, but also expensive. When someone places an ad in these venues, the ad goes to everyone. It is not targeted by geography or other demographic variables.

Most of the patients come from nearby practices. So using mass media wastes many contacts because it has too extensive a reach for the individual practice. If the franchise or network has practices throughout the media market, then each of those outlets shares in the benefits of the marketing effort, drastically reducing the cost of acquiring each patient. This means that an individual practitioner often takes a more focused marketing strategy that targets patients who are more likely to come to the practice.

Professional advertising differs from advertising many other goods and services. It must be more factual (office hours, services offered, location, etc.) with no "puffery" or other claims of superiority. What is customary in the area influences professional advertising. Using a radio ad in one area may be mainstream for the dental market but may label a dentist as a pariah in a more traditional marketplace. Although the dentist may legally use such advertising, the dental community may be small and close-knit. The dentist needs to interact with fellow practitioners to be aware of local customs in this area.

Good advertisements draw someone's **a**ttention, generate **i**nterest and **d**esire for the product, and result in an **a**ction by the person (called AIDA in marketing). Professionals often accomplish these goals by developing a list of potential problems that someone can identify with (e.g. dry mouth, floppy dentures). They may show examples of their work (such as before-and-after photos) or have people give testimonials of the excellent care they have received. Most have a call to action ("Good for the next week" or "for a limited time"). Incentives are often used to evoke action by the patient (Box 23.6).

Websites

Websites are becoming a critical source of information for consumers. This depends on the clientele the dentist seeks. For example, if a dentist has an orthodontic practice that seeks young, affluent families, then a web presence is essential. If they have a prosthetic practice that seeks elderly patients with prosthetic needs, then a website is less valuable as a marketing tool. Other forms of distributing a message (such as senior newsletters or Yellow Pages advertising) are more important for this group. A website can introduce services, introduce the dentist and staff members, inform prospective patients of hours and policies, and provide health information. The practice can also post forms (such as for a health history or the Health Insurance Portability and Accountability Act [HIPAA]) for patients to download and complete before they come to the office.

Social Media

It used to be that having a website was enough of an internet presence for a dental practice. Today, nearly 90% of practices use social media as part of their patient acquisition and retention strategy. Social media marketing has become the new standard for a presence on the Internet. Using social media helps a dental practice stop focusing on what they do (dentistry) and on what they make possible. An example might be "A confident smile boosts your health." It gives the practice a platform and stage to tell the story of the patients and the office. The practice's social media activity sets it apart from other practices, develops powerful one-to-one connections, and increases its perceived value.

The following are some must-have components for a social media marketing effort to be effective:

- **In-Practice Support**
  Team buy-in and participation are keys to having an effective social media presence. Team members have relationships with current patients and live in the community. They have extended family members, gym buddies, church congregations, and neighbors. A team that is solidly behind a social media program will help to grow its presence. The energy that comes from heightened friendships and engagement with patients is contagious.

- **Participation**
  Engaging patients to participate in social media accounts is critical. Dentistry is a relationship-based business. Connections occur as connective points are discovered between the patient, the doctor, and staff members. There are many strategies to get patients involved. Some offices have employed a "patient-of-the-month program." Others have people take a photo in the office and tag the practice on their social media pages as a way to get participation. When getting participation

BOX 23.6	EXAMPLE ADVERTISING INCENTIVES
Bonus	Call within 3 days and receive free x-rays.
Discount	Bring this coupon before September 1 and get 50% off a new patient exam.
Motivation	Come in today and begin your life with a beautiful new smile.
Consequences	Do not wait. Dental problems only get worse without treatment.

from patients, they must give express written permission. The patient must clearly understand how the information will be used and the purpose of sharing their details. A signed agreement with clear indications of how the information will be used must remain on file. This is essential to confirm the patient's willingness to participate. Verbal agreements are not sufficient permission. Lack of physical proof of permission may result in HIPAA violations.

- **Content**
  Great content engages, provides value, shares practice culture, demonstrates passion, and connects. Most savvy practitioners do not try to "sell" dentistry with their posts. While they publish content that informs people and supports excellent dental care, they rely on personal interaction to convince a patient of the care needed for their specific case. Besides dental content, practitioners should find at least three interesting and relevant non-dental topics that current and prospective patients will enjoy and find useful. An example might be "How does sugar affect your overall health?" Content needs to change over time to remain fresh and exciting.

- **Online tools**
  Various social media apps and tools are available. Many of these change or disappear over time, so a social media marketing strategy should not be dependent on any one account. The practitioner should think of these platforms as spokes on a wheel. The more spokes are present, the more likely it is that the social media presence will be felt and the less likely it is to suffer if one format goes away.

- **Consistency and patience**
  Like any marketing effort, consistency and patience are key. Putting together a social media calendar allows the practice to plan the posts and be consistent.

In the end, a practice's social media return on investment will be seen in four ways. The first is greater patient retention. Even if the practice only retains an additional 1% of patients through relationship-based marketing, this leads to saving thousands of dollars each year. It is much more profitable to retain a patient than to replace a patient with a new one. The second is through increased case acceptance. As mentioned earlier, social media helps to educate and tell stories of others who have experienced the same as your patients are looking for. This helps to "preheat" patients so that they enter the practice looking for a solution to their problem. Thirdly, social media marketing is primarily an internal way of getting new patients. Word of mouth increases referrals and generates top-of-mind

awareness. Fourthly, a digital marketing presence is more sustainable and effective than search engine optimization (SEO). This increase in the patient pool contributes to practice value.

MAILINGS

Direct mailings can inexpensively reach potential patients. These can target zip codes, areas near the office, or other target groups. Dentists can purchase brochures and mailing packages from marketing firms or develop their own. Direct mailings are especially effective for a working-class neighborhood, especially when they include a coupon or other saving enticement. The dentist should use such direct mailings for at least three to four months to imprint their name on the minds of those who receive them. Another form of direct mailing is to send current patients newsletters or other information about the practice. When a dentist purchases a practice, the outgoing practitioner often has a bank of patients that have not been active (seen in the practice) for one to several years. Sending a letter to these people is a cost-effective way to generate additional patients for the practice.

YELLOW PAGES

Many people still use the Yellow Pages (or another paper directory) to screen possible choices in dentists. They may use location in a large city or services offered as a screening criterion. (Dentists should include a map of the general location in their ad so that people can easily find the office.) A Yellow Pages ad can be expensive, especially as the size increases or the placement of the ad moves to be more noticeable. If it generates enough patients, though, it can more than pay for itself. As mentioned, older clients use Yellow Pages searches more than younger people. Dentists should identify and target the market to set the most effective use of their advertising budget.

FINANCIAL IMPACTS OF MARKETING

Given the high cost of marketing efforts, dentists need to understand how marketing and patient generation affect the practice's finances.

MARKETING IS NECESSARY FOR SUCCESS

Marketing brings both new and repeating patients to the practice for treatment. Without patients, there is no practice. Many dentists claim "I can't afford to spend money on marketing because of the office budget." This view assumes that marketing is an optional practice activity. The correct view should be "What do I need to spend on marketing to drive the number of patient visits I need to meet my financial projections?" This second view says that marketing is the engine of practice growth. If the dentist wants to grow the practice, they need additional patients. Marketing expenditures bring these patients to the practice. To the extent that a dentist limits marketing expenditures, they limit practice growth.

VALUE OF A NEW PATIENT

Each new patient is worth a specific dollar value to the practice. That value is the average amount of dentistry the practice does on new patients. Dentists can find it by adding the total collections for dentistry done on all new patients divided by the total number of new patients. Compare that dollar value to the average amount spent on marketing per new patient. On a basic level, if the dollar value of the patient is higher than the amount spent to generate the patient, the marketing program was worthwhile. If not, it was not.

MARGINAL COST OF PRODUCTION

Taking this analysis one step further, the cost of doing the dentistry should also be allocated to the new patient to decide profitability. The issue is whether the dentist has "slack resources" or empty chair time. If they have no slack resources (chairs are all completely booked), then all the office costs should be divided and allocated to all patients. If, on the other hand, they have empty chair time, then the cost of seeing an additional patient is only the variable costs associated with production (dental supplies, dental lab, and office supplies). The dentist has already paid the rent, the utilities, and the employees. The dentist's only costs for seeing another patient – the marginal costs of production – are small (the additional costs associated with lab and material for doing the dentistry).

REPETITION

Effective marketing means repetition. Dentists, who are used to the scientific method, believe that if something works once, it will always work for all similar circumstances. When sending a message to people, the dentist must tell them repeatedly. People hear a message when they are ready to listen, not simply when someone is ready to tell them. They may drive past the office every working day for five years, but it is only when they decide they need to find a dentist that they will notice the dentist's sign. For the same reason, Procter & Gamble constantly advertises Tide laundry soap so that when someone is ready to buy laundry soap, they will think "Tide." This "top-of-the-mind" awareness means that the dentist may not see an effect of their marketing efforts in the first week, month, or even several months. Repetition supports even a good marketing message. Although this appears to increase the cost of the marketing effort, it also increases its effectiveness and value.

Part 2: Managing Continuing Care

Remember that credit is money.

Benjamin Franklin

GOAL

The aim of this part is to present guidelines for developing the continuing care function in the dental office.

LEARNING OBJECTIVES

At the completion of this part, the student will be able to:

- Describe the patient care reasons to develop the continuing care function in the office.
- Describe the economic reasons to develop the continuing care function in the office.
- Describe common methods of setting continuing care appointments.
- Describe the effect of the retention rate on continuing care production.
- Compare the cost of acquiring a new patient with a continuing care patient.

check-up   preheating
periodic maintenance   recall
preappointing

Internal marketing aims to generate patients from within the practice and to encourage existing patients to remain with the practice for their continuing care. This is healthy from two perspectives. It improves patient care and oral health and makes good financial sense for the practice. Supporting continuing care is indeed a mutually beneficial situation.

Different offices have different names for the continuing care function. Although this seems a trivial exercise in semantics at first, how dentists convey to patients what they do has a tremendous impact on the patient's perception of them. Words do matter, and patients form opinions based on the words they hear. Although different patients may have wants and needs that a dentist cannot control, they can control how they communicate services to the patients.

The most common name is the recall system. This is an office-centric view of the function. Dentists recall the patient for their purpose and their procedures. In the patients' minds, this is like a defective product recall, where the manufacturer must repair or replace a defective part. (Is the gas tank going to explode? Did a filling go bad?) Because all dental services have a lifetime that is often dependent, in part, on the care taken by the owner, moving from dentist responsibility to partnered responsibility for long-term function seems appropriate. Some offices call the function *recare*. This moves the focus toward the patient's health and away from the office procedure. It helps the patient and staff members realize that the purpose is to care for the patient's oral health needs. Other offices call the process *periodic maintenance* or *continuing care* to emphasize the ongoing nature of the procedure and relationship. If the process is called maintenance, patients understand that they have a part in ensuring that their dental health remains good and their dental work remains defect free. Part of their responsibility is regularly returning for a follow-up evaluation and necessary treatments. Finally, some offices call the process a *check-up*. Although this infers the ongoing nature of the process, it also trivializes the vital function of the process in the individual's oral health.

VALUE OF PREVENTIVE SERVICES

PATIENT CARE PERSPECTIVE

Continuing care, adequately applied, prevents additional restorative work for the patient (Box 23.7). Through a personal preventive orientation, patients can avoid recurrent caries and the replacements that result. This also decreases the severity of future work, as each time dentists replace a restoration, it necessarily becomes larger and the tooth weaker. Regular prophylaxis and reinforcement improve periodontal health and decrease the severity of this disease. Other oral problems – caries, periodontal, or pathological – can be found and treated earlier. This improves the patient's oral health and decreases the total amount they spend on personalized dental care. Finally, ongoing care visits help the patient and doctor develop a more personal relationship instead of simply a client–provider relationship. This trusting relationship helps in communication, patient involvement in treatment decisions, and personal health awareness and ownership. All are important outcomes from both personal and public health perspectives.

FINANCIAL PERSPECTIVE

From a financial perspective, encouraging continuing care makes good sense for the practice (Box 23.8). Dentists charge for preventive services such as periodic exams, diagnostic radiographs, and prophylaxes. Although not enormously profitable, these services do generate revenue and profit when properly managed. At the periodic exam, dentists often identify dental problems that need treatment. This generates additional revenue and profit for the practice. Frequently this work is complex, generating higher-margin procedures and adding to the practice

---

BOX 23.7   VALUE OF PREVENTIVE SERVICES: PATIENT CARE PERSPECTIVE

- Prevents additional work
- Decreases severity of future work
- Improves periodontal health
- Develops relationships
- Improves oral health

BOX 23.8	VALUE OF PREVENTIVE SERVICES: FINANCIAL PERSPECTIVE

- Value of the work itself
- Additional work generated
- Higher-margin work generated
- Preparing patients for necessary work
- Improved treatment acceptance

profit. Routine visits help to "preheat" patients for future necessary work. When dentists remind a patient of a given problem ("That tooth needs a crown to avoid breaking"), they prepare the patient so that if the problem happens, the patient is ready for treatment. Dentists do not have to convince the patients of the need for the procedure. Finally, patients need to trust that the dentist is looking out for their best interest, not merely the dentist's pocketbook, before they commit to complex and expensive treatments. Periodic visits help build that rapport and resulting trust.

Economic Value of a Continuing Care Patient

The economic value of a continuing care patient comes from several sources: periodic work, additional work generated, and referrals from the patient.

The first source of revenue is from the periodic visit itself. Box 23.9 shows the revenue generated from hygiene visits over five years, given the assumptions shown. Over this time, hygiene production by itself rises to $285000 per year.

The second way in which continuing care patients add to the practice's financial health is through additional work generated. For example, assume that a single patient comes to the practice every six months for periodic maintenance visits and never has any other dental work done. The value of the visit is $100, inflation increases the price by 4% per year, and each patient makes two visits per year. As seen in Box 23.10 column 3, the pure cumulative financial value of the periodic visits for that patient after 10 years is more than $2400.

Now assume that, beyond the periodic visit procedures, the patient needs one additional restoration per year. That restoration has a value of $150, also compounded at 4% per year. Box 23.10 shows that the cumulative value of the restorations is approximately $1800. The total cumulative value of that patient over the 10-year example period rises to more than $4000 (Box 23.10 column 6). This is for a

BOX 23.9	HYGIENE VISIT PRODUCTION

Months	New patients	Recall patient visits	Total hygiene patient visits	Total hygiene production per month	Total hygiene production per year
1–6	20	0	20	$2500	
7–12	20	20	40	$5000	$45000
13–18	20	40	60	$7500	
19–24	20	60	80	$10000	$105000
25–30	20	80	100	$12500	
31–36	20	100	120	$15000	$165000
37–42	20	120	140	$17500	
43–48	20	140	160	$20000	$225000
49–54	20	160	180	$22500	
55–60	20	180	200	$25000	$285000

Assumptions:

Start at 0 patients; add 20 new patients per month (20 × 6 = 120/6 months; and keep 100% of patients for 6-month periodic visits).

Total hygiene patient visits = periodic patients + new patients

Average hygiene periodic production = Exam + Prophy + BWs/2 + Pan every 5 years = $105

BOX 23.10   ECONOMIC VALUE OF A CONTINUING CARE PATIENT

Year	Value of periodic visits	Cumulative value of periodic visits	Value of restoration	Cumulative value of restorations	Total cumulative value
1	$200	$200	$150	$150	$350
2	$208	$408	$156	$306	$714
3	$216	$624	$162	$468	$1093
4	$225	$849	$169	$637	$1486
5	$234	$1083	$175	$812	$1896
6	$243	$1327	$182	$995	$2322
7	$253	$1580	$190	$1185	$2764
8	$263	$1843	$197	$1382	$3225
9	$274	$2117	$205	$1587	$3704
10	$285	$2403	$213	$1801	$4202

This chart shows the economic value of a single continuing care patient over 10 years. The third column shows the value of just the periodic visits. The sixth column assumes that the patient has one restoration done from each periodic visit.

patient who has no complex or high-value procedures done. Higher-margin items (crowns or complex restorative services) increase the value. This example only shows 10 years. The value also increases quickly over a longer time as the fee compounds.

The third way continuing care patients contribute to practice finances is through referrals. If each continuing care patient refers one additional patient every year, Box 23.11 shows the total number of periodic visits that result. If each of those patients also refers an additional patient with similar habits and needs, the value compounds dramatically. This does not include any additional work that might be found on periodic visits.

The rate of retention of patients for periodic visits is also important. The previous analysis assumed that a practice retained 100% of the periodic patients. Box 23.12 shows the effect of lower retention rates. As dentists retain a smaller proportion of patients, the effect decreases hygiene production significantly. Every continuing care patient then is vital for the economic health of a practice. The loss of even a single patient, especially early in the practice cycle when the compounding effect is greatest, can significantly impact long-term office finances. The importance of actively managing the system should be obvious.

Cost of a Periodic Maintenance Patient

Marketing aims to generate patients for the practice through internal (existing patients) or external methods (new patients). Depending on the method used, a new patient may cost tens or hundreds of dollars to generate. Some of these new patients will come with significant, complex cases. The cost of retaining existing patients is much less than generating new patients for the practice. An existing patient costs the practice a postage stamp or a few minutes of staff time for a telephone call. Existing patients know the staff and doctor and have developed trust with the practice. They often participate in favored insurance plans, so the staff do not need to investigate their benefits or insurance plan requirements as often. These are higher-volume, lower-cost patients. Both contribute to practice profitability.

PERIODIC MAINTENANCE MANAGEMENT

Several issues are common in managing periodic maintenance systems.

COMPLETION OF TREATMENT

When the office completes a patient's active treatment and places them on maintenance status, staff members should show the date in the computer program. Dentists can also code special instructions (such as required premedication) in the appropriate area. They should set an exact date for the next visit. Many insurance companies pay for prophylaxis every six months (to the day) since the last one. If a patient returns for a periodic exam one day early, the insurance company may deny benefits.

BOX 23.11	PERIODIC VISITS GENERATED BY ONE PATIENT'S REFERRALS

Year	Number of periodic patient visits									
	Pt #1	Pt #2	Pt #3	Pt #4	Pt #5	Pt #6	Pt #7	Pt #8	Pt #9	Pt #10
1	2									
2	2	2								
3	2	2	2							
4	2	2	2	2						
5	2	2	2	2	2					
6	2	2	2	2	2	2				
7	2	2	2	2	2	2	2			
8	2	2	2	2	2	2	2	2		
9	2	2	2	2	2	2	2	2	2	
10	2	2	2	2	2	2	2	2	2	2
Total	20	18	16	14	12	10	8	6	4	2
Cumulative total visits	20	38	54	68	80	90	98	104	108	110

Assumptions:

Each patient has two periodic visits per year. If each of these visits is valued at $100, the total value is $110000.

Each year, the initial patient refers one patient who also has two periodic visits per year.

None of these patients leaves the practice.

This does not include any additional dental work required.

This chart shows the cumulative number of periodic maintenance visits generated by one patient (Pt #1) who refers one other patient per year (Pt #2–10) to the practice.

BOX 23.12	EFFECT OF RETENTION RATE

Retention rate	Hygiene production
100%	$285000
95%	$270750
90%	$256500
85%	$242250
80%	$228000
75%	$213750

SETTING APPOINTMENTS

There are two standard methods of setting appointments: pre-appointing and month of recall. Which method a dentist uses depends on trial and error and what is customary in the community where they practice. Depending on the patient's needs and wants, the practice may use a combination of the two.

Many offices make periodic appointments for patients as they leave the office, preappointing the patient's next periodic visit. This requires that the office has a defined schedule at least six months in advance. If patients are on a yearly frequency, office schedules must be determined at least that far ahead. This limits the patient's ability to take time off for continuing education courses or personal enjoyment without significant rescheduling problems. Offices using this method claim they are first on a patient's schedule. The patient then schedules other items around their dental appointment. The office can generally fill the appointment with anotherr patient if someone cancels. It also allows the practice to decide the appropriate level of future hygiene staffing. Many dentists who use this system leave blocks of time available for new patient prophylaxes or patients who must reschedule an appointment. Staff members should still call patients before the appointment for confirmation. Using this method works particularly well in offices with multiple practitioners because these offices can ensure that the office will be open and "covered" in the future.

The second method is to wait until the month before the maintenance visit to appoint. The office either sends a computer-generated card reminding patients to call to schedule a periodic visit, or computer generates a list of patients due and calls them to remind and appoint them. If a practice uses this method, they should send reminder cards at least two weeks before the month due so that they can schedule people appropriately early in the month. Otherwise, a six-month maintenance visit turns into a seven- or eight-month one, compromising both the patient's oral health and the office maintenance system. Offices that use this method claim that it gives more flexibility in scheduling vacations and other time off. They also claim that patients often change appointments when they make them six months ahead, so it is easier to schedule once rather than adjust appointment books. Some patients do not want to commit to a specific time that far in the future.

FOLLOW-UP

Contact patients who do not have an appointment during their scheduled month. Then appoint and place them on the appropriate monthly list or on inactive status. Follow-up and constant system monitoring are crucial to effective periodic system management.

RESPONSIBILITY

Responsibility for maintenance of the continuing care system varies from office to office. The receptionist or office manager often oversees maintaining and updating all periodic patient information, mailing reminder cards, and scheduling appointments. In offices where a hygienist earns a commission, they are usually responsible for maintaining the system because their productivity and income depend on the effectiveness of the continuing care program. One person, whether business office personnel, hygienist, or clinical assistant, should be responsible for the system. If problems occur, the dentist can identify the responsible person and take corrective action.

SCHEDULING PERIODIC VISITS

Dentists should set a standard time cod" for periodic visits. Hygienists on a salary generally want to see one patient per hour; those on a commission basis will schedule one patient every 30 minutes. Accurate scheduling differs from the practice philosophy and skills of the practitioners. Hygienists can generally complete children's visits in 30 minutes. They can usually complete adults with routine "prophy" needs in 45 minutes. Adults with significant calculus present or periodontal conditions may require reappointment for definitive periodontal scaling and root planing.

If dentists schedule the hygienist to do only hygiene procedures and an assistant to do non-hygiene procedures (such as history updates, charting, and radiographs), then the dentist can almost double hygiene production for each hygienist. This substitutes the ass'stant's time for the hyg'enist's time for those procedures the state law allows the dentist to delegate to the clinical assistants. It frees the hygienist to do hygiene-only procedures on a second patient while the assistant begins or completes the patient in the first chair. Some hygienists feel this becomes a "prophy mill" as they move from patient to patient without the personal interaction that many cherish.

Some offices have operatories expressly set up for hygienists, often using older or inferior equipment. Although older equipment saves money in the short run, it has negative consequences. Not only does it slow treatment, it also sends a subliminal message to the patient and the hygienist about the importance of the continuing care system. The additional cost of fully equipping an operatory over minimally equipping a "hygiene" operatory is small. Fully equipped operatories are more flexible and can be used for minor procedures on maintenance visits or when the hygienist is not working in them.

As the maintenance function becomes larger, some practices dedicate a day a week in which the entire office sees periodic maintenance patients (e.g. "hygiene Thursdays"). The office hires part-time hygienists to see patients in chairs they usually schedule for dentist visits. The dentist then spends the whole day assessing periodic maintenance patients and treatment. This allows the office to see many periodic patients without constantly interrupting dentist–patient procedures.

DENTURE PATIENT MAINTENANCE

Many successful practices insist that all complete denture patients return to the office once per year for a denture check-up. These visits consist of an oral cancer exam and a denture fit and function check. These practices generally find the time and effort well spent.

Gaining Case Acceptance

CHAPTER 24

Part 1: Communication in the Office

All great writers have a built-in, infallible crap detector.

Ernest Hemingway

GOAL

The aim of this part is to present guidelines for communicating with patients in the office.

LEARNING OBJECTIVES

At the completion of this part, the student will be able to:

- Describe the steps in the communication process.

- Describe the common methods of communication in the dental office.

- Describe the types of non-verbal communication.

- Describe how proxemics affects patient interactions.

- Describe how patient position affects patient interactions.

- Describe the oral communication process.

- Define common barriers to communication.

- Describe the types of listening.

- Describe how to deal with common "problem patient" communication issues in a dental practice.

KEY TERMS

active listening
body language
content listening
decoding
effective feedback
encoding
feedback
interpretive listening
intimate zone
medium

message
noise
oral communication
personal zone
proxemics
public zone
receiver
relationship listening
script
selective perception

self-disclosure
semantic problems
sender
social zone
therapeutic listening
value judgments
verbal/non-verbal incongruity
written communication

Business Basics for Dentists, Second Edition. James L. Harrison, David O. Willis, and Charles K. Thieman.
© 2024 John Wiley & Sons, Inc. Published 2024 by John Wiley & Sons, Inc.

Communication is key to successful dental practice. Dentists must communicate with staff members to ensure the office operates effectively. They must communicate with vendors and other professionals to ensure excellent patient treatment. And they must communicate with patients to inform them of their needs and to gain acceptance for treatment options. A successful practitioner must be a great communicator. This part discusses the communication process and how dentists can improve their patient communication process and abilities.

Communication, in its most basic form, is simply the transfer of information from one person to another. This seems simple on the surface. However, digging deeper into the process, communication involves speaking, writing, thinking, and a heavy dose of psychology. It involves transmitting not just facts but also ideas, opinions, emotions, and attitudes. It is the primary method of forming interpersonal relationships. For example, to formulate a treatment plan for a patient, the dentist needs to understand their frame of reference, wants, needs, and desires. The only way to find this out is through interpersonal communication. Although many forms of communication are used in the office, face-to-face communication is the most common. It is also the richest method for processing issues, especially those with high uncertainty or a large emotional component to the decision. Other communication channels, such as letters, email, or telephone calls, do not share the depth of understanding that someone gains from face-to-face communication.

THE COMMUNICATION PROCESS

The communication process is a shared experience between two or more people, with importance given to sending and receiving information. All interpersonal behavior involves communication, either intentional or not, because most actions convey some meaning. Communication involves eight key elements. All eight must work for there to be an effective sharing of ideas. The important point in understanding this process is that any of the eight steps may be the cause when communication fails. If someone understands the steps, they can decrease problems in the process.

- **Sender**
  The sender is the person who wants to transmit the idea or information to another person. A dentist may offer an idea, or the patient may want to express an emotion, fact, or concern to the dentist. The role of sender and receiver shifts back and forth as communication progresses.

- **Encoding**
  Encoding happens when the sender translates the communication into a language the receiver will (hopefully) understand. If practitioners use too much dental jargon that the patients cannot comprehend, their failure to properly encode may harm the communication process.

- **Message**
  The message is the result of the encoding process. It is the idea that the sender wants to send to the receiver. It may be information, a feeling, a value, a belief, or an attitude.

- **Medium**
  The medium is the process that carries the message. The most obvious is the meaning of the spoken words. Other examples include text messages, emails, tone of voice, or body language.

- **Receiver**
  The receiver is the recipient of the message. Receivers decode and interpret messages, developing their own meaning for the message. This may be different from the sender's meaning.

- **Decoding**
  Decoding happens when the receiver translates the message into their "language." They must interpret the direct words and any additional messages the medium carries. Because some media, such as face-to-face oral communication, are much richer (i.e. they contain more additional information), they also incorporate more room for misinterpretation and error. The receiver's perception of what was said is a reality for them. Therefore, their values, attitudes, beliefs, and concerns all influence the receiver's perception of the message.

- **Feedback**
  Feedback occurs when the receiver responds to the message. A direct response (verbal reply, facial expression) allows the sender to assess whether the receiver received the message and if it had the intended result.

- **Noise**
  Noise is a factor in the system that distorts the intended message. The receiver may not accurately interpret the message if there is too much distortion. Examples include physical noise in the conversational space, such as other people talking, and psychological noise, such as fear, different frames of reference, and preconceived notions by the communicators.

METHODS OF ORAL COMMUNICATION

People use several ways of communicating in face-to-face situations. Verbal communication (either written or oral) is the most obvious. However, how someone present verbal communication tells the receiver about their state of mind during the process. Perceptive people use these cues to come to a deeper understanding of what the sender meant to say, as opposed to what they actually said. This means that people have both intentional communication (e.g. the meaning of the words) and unintentional communication (e.g. the unease exhibited by nervous fidgeting during the conversation). The best communication occurs when these two match. Although this sounds simple, the process becomes muddied by people's perceptions, cultural and family histories, state of mind, and current conditions.

VERBAL COMMUNICATION

Verbal communication is the most common form of professional–patient communication in dental offices. Too often, dentists assume that when they say something, the other person understands what they said, why they said it, and the nuances of what they said. This involves the two sides of speaking and listening. People use verbal communication to transmit or obtain information, share experiences, or bring about change in another person. Depending on the purpose of the conversation, they rely on different elements. As noted, the dental practitioner needs to practice appropriate techniques for sending and receiving verbal communication. Sending involves speaking. Receiving involves the equally important listening function.

SPEAKING FUNCTION (SENDING INFORMATION)
Word Choice

The words that someone uses may have different meanings to someone else. This occurs especially when people discuss a topic that is familiar to them but unfamiliar to the other person, or if someone has preconceived ideas about the topic. For example, dentists are familiar and comfortable with endodontics, but many patients fear the dreaded "root canal." Patients may have heard stories or jokes that have given them preconceived ideas about how horrible the procedure is. So, a dentist using the more technical term *endodontic procedure* over the emotionally laden term *root canal* may avoid a negative reaction from a patient. Box 24.1 gives several other common dental office terms that may generate negative responses from non-dental people. The more non-dental terms dentists and their staff can use, the less likely it is that they will generate negative emotional responses from patients.

BOX 24.1	WORD CHOICE IN THE OFFICE
Dental term	**Non-dental term**
Waiting room	Reception area
Operatory	Treatment area
Price	Fee
Investing	Paying
Oral exam	Check-up
Recall	Routine visit

Effective Self-Disclosure

Self-disclosure occurs when a person intentionally gives information (verbally or non-verbally) to someone else about themselves. Self-disclosure is important because it conveys openness. Openness is one requirement for developing a trusting relationship. Trust is an element that is necessary for a patient to communicate effectively and accept proposed treatment.

People can see self-disclosure in the response statements "Really? I've had a similar experience" or "I've often felt the same way." When a practitioner shares that experience or feeling with the patient, the patient understands that the dentist's opinions may come from a similar reference and, therefore, be more valid.

Effective Feedback

The only way to know if the patient received and processed a dentist's message with the same meaning as was meant is for the dentist to ask. A simple question such as "Does that make sense?" or "Do you have any questions?" asks for a response that tells the practitioner if the patient understands what they said. Several other techniques also test for understanding. Parroting is a simple repetition of what the person said, and paraphrasing does the same thing, only rephrasing what the person said in the listener's own words. Both are good ways to encourage additional discussion of an issue.

Listening Function (Receiving Information)

As busy professionals, dentists become accustomed to talking but not listening to patients. However, listening is only half the communication process. To be an effective listener, a dentist must stop talking and listen. (This can be difficult for some people!) Dentists also must listen for more than facts by keenly observing the patient during the conversation.

Each person uses several levels or types of listening in their role as a practitioner. They shift between the types depending on the purpose of the conversation they are holding.

Listening for Content   The basic level of listening is to hear and comprehend the meaning of what the other person said. This requires that people have an appropriate vocabulary and understand the rules of grammar and syntax to understand what others are saying. Some words carry more importance than others. Understanding the content requires that people rank key facts from the long stream of words that make up many conversations. When a practitioner listens to a patient's medical history, they must initially listen for the simple, factual content of what the patient says. Once the dentist gathers this information, they can move to higher levels of evaluation and interpretation.

Listening for Interpretation   The next level of listening is where a person makes judgments about what the other person says. People listen to decide if the other person is telling the truth, how strongly they believe what they are saying, and if they have other hidden agendas. When people interpret what they hear, they must also listen visually. When someone notices the cues that body language provides, it helps them assess if what another said verbally is congruent with what they said through actions and mannerisms. This type of listening is important as dentists interview patients about their wants, needs, and desires in dental treatment. If dentists try to persuade a patient to change their health behaviors, that patient will use interpretive listening as they weigh the pros and cons of the dentist's position to decide if it makes sense for them.

Relationship Listening   Sometimes the reason that people listen is to develop or maintain a relationship. (Lovers talk for hours about things that would bore them when listening to someone else.) In relationship listening, a person tries to learn more about the other person, how they think, what they enjoy, and what motivates them. This type of listening is vital in developing both business and personal relationships. Before a patient commits to an extensive treatment plan, they must believe that the practitioner is looking out for their interests, not the dentist's. For a dentist to gain that level of trust takes time to build a relationship.

Therapeutic Listening   In therapeutic listening, people gain an understanding of how others are feeling. The purpose is to use this personal relationship to help the other change or develop. To get others to expose these deeper and more sensitive parts of themselves, people need to show understanding and empathy toward them, not just in words but in how they ask questions. Practitioners must be sensitive to the patient's unease in a way that encourages self-disclosure. A typical example in the dental office is discussing treatment history with a dental-phobic patient. These patients are often embarrassed about their dental condition and behavior in the dental setting. Through therapeutic listening, a dentist may find the root of the dental aversion and help the patient respond appropriately.

Active Listening

Active listening is a process that uses different types of listening. This process intends to improve understanding between speaker and listener. The listener frequently checks with the speaker to be sure that their interpretation of what the speaker said is what the speaker intended.

Active listening focuses attention on the speaker. The listener must be sure to listen fully, not think of other things, such as what they will ask next. The listener also observes the speaker's behavior and body language, incorporating those into the content and interpretation of the conversation. Having listened, the listener then paraphrases the speaker's words, not necessarily agreeing but simply checking what the speaker said. In emotionally charged conversations, the listener must recognize those emotional bases. The active listener often describes their observation of the underlying emotion ("You seem to feel angry" or "I sense that you feel frustrated. Why is that?"). This validates the speaker's emotional statement in a non-judgmental way. It allows and encourages the speaker to discuss their emotions in a positive fashion for the conversation and leads to effective therapy.

VERBAL COMMUNICATION BARRIERS

People have often heard someone say during an argument "What you heard is not what I said." This points to a breakdown in the communication process. Several common reasons that oral communications fail in the dental office (barriers to communication) include the following:

- Different frames of reference occur when people have different and valid views of similar issues. These come from different backgrounds, experiences, and values. For example, dentists value excellent oral health. Some of their patients may not share that view. If a dentist discusses treatment options based on their frame of reference, they may not "get through" to the patient because of this different frame of reference.

- Selective perception occurs when people hear what they want to hear, blocking out information that conflicts with their beliefs and values.

- Value judgments occur when the receiver decides the value of the message before they receive the entire message.

- Semantic problems occur when words and terms have one meaning to one person and a different (or no) meaning to the other. If practitioners use too much dental jargon or words too casually (root canals can have a negative meaning for many patients), they may impede communication.

- Poor listening skills can occur, especially under times of stress. Many patients find the dental office to be a stressful environment. Others may be in severe pain or worried about a diagnosis or the cost of a procedure. This can make effective listening difficult for them.

- Verbal–non-verbal incongruity occurs when the verbal message does not match the non-verbal message sent. If a practitioner shakes their head back and forth but verbally says "Yes," the patient will become confused. More subtle incongruities exist when a practitioner fidgets while trying to sound confident or grins when telling a patient bad news about the patient's dental condition.

IMPROVING VERBAL COMMUNICATION

Dentists can improve interpersonal oral communication in the dental office by using the following techniques:

- Follow up on messages to be sure the listener received them correctly. The simplest way is for the practitioner to ask the patient if they are clear about what is happening. This verbal feedback assures the dentist that the patient received and properly interpreted the message.

- Simplify language by not using too many professional terms. A dentist may find it helpful to make a list of dental terms and acceptable alternatives in daily communication.

- Watch body language. The dentist must be aware of the body language they project and take time to read the body language of patients. If a patient is sitting cross-armed with their lips pursed, they are probably not accepting the dentist's message, regardless of the verbal response. (There is more on body language in the next section of this chapter.)

- Work on effective listening skills. These are skills that people can learn and improve if they take the time and make an effort.

- Ensure that non-verbal messages support verbal messages. If these are not congruent, the listener will hear the worse one.

NON-VERBAL COMMUNICATION

Communication is the transfer of information from one person to another. This is usually thought of as simply the spoken word. However, face-to-face communication carries much more information than simply words. People can view the other's facial expression and hear their tone of voice or the emphasis they place on particular words or points in a way that is not possible if there is no personal encounter (e.g. think of an email message that is factual without any embellishment). Psychologists estimate that as much as 85% of the information conveyed in face-to-face communication is non-verbal. People use these non-verbal cues to learn additional meaning and emotional background. By examining the context of the communication, people validate or refute what was said verbally. They examine the other's body language, or what the person has said beyond the simple spoken word, to have a richer communication encounter. People do this continually and subconsciously. Even someone who is inactive or silent may be sending an intended or unintended message: that they are bored, depressed, or angry.

People must also remember that the other person is assessing them similarly. Therefore, the dentist must be careful of the non-verbal messages they send to others (patients and staff) and manage that part of the communication process.

Verbal and non-verbal information is related. Non-verbal information is usually the more powerful of the two. When they are congruent, the non-verbal message reinforces the verbal message. When they are not congruent, cognitive dissonance indicates that something is wrong. (Think of a person who has anger in their words and voice but is calm and smiling.) Cultural and gender differences play a role in non-verbal cues as well.

POSTURE

A person's posture clearly states how they feel about themselves. An upright but relaxed posture shows confidence and honesty. Slumping suggests lower self-esteem. Crossing arms may feel like a relaxed position, but to observers it can indicate that a person is shutting themselves out. Fidgeting (including twisting hair, drumming fingers, or examining fingernails) shows boredom or nervousness.

EYE CONTACT

Direct eye contact suggests honesty and openness, especially when speaking to someone else. A person looking down or away while speaking shows boredom. To be effective, people must try to make eye contact for the first and last 15 seconds of a conversation. This creates a feeling of concern and honesty that it is difficult to gain otherwise. However, eye contact should not be held for too long, because others will see that as hostile.

PHYSICAL CONTACT

People expect to be touched when they visit a dentist. However, they expect a "therapeutic" or "professional" touch, not an aggressive or sexual touch. Dentists still must respect a patient's personal zones, only entering the closer zone when they are invited. Hand-shaking is a ritualistic way to move from a social to a personal zone. (A person's emotional state is often shown by their hand. Are they cold and clammy? Warm? Sweaty?) A pat on the shoulder is a less ritualistic way of making a symbolic connection with someone.

FACIAL EXPRESSION

Facial expressions give away a person's emotions. People can read surprise, happiness, anger, or other emotions by carefully watching a patient's facial expression. Squinting can be read as aggression. Facial pallor or blushing can also share an emotional state.

TONE OF VOICE

The tone of someone's voice can be a giveaway to their emotional state. People can show (or see) anger, fear, boredom, or happiness depending on how they emphasize words and their tone. Practitioners see this when a patient talks with them or when a dentist or a staff member talks with patients. For example, consider the children's game where the speaker emphasizes a different word in the same sentence – entirely different meanings result:

I love my job.

I *love* my job.

I love *my* job.

I love my *job*.

Because no one knows how they sound to someone else, dentists should record themselves talking with a patient, then listen to the tape privately to evaluate their vocal delivery. That allows them to develop one or two specific things to work on. If they have difficulty speaking with patients, they should consider getting a voice coach, who will help them develop their tone and method of oral delivery.

PROXEMICS (PERSONAL SPACE)

Proxemics is the study of space and how people relate to space. Understanding people's comfort zones can help a dentist influence their communication and professional relationships with their patients.

Everyone has a personal space that surrounds them. The social relationship that someone has with another person defines this space. Psychologists have proposed that the reasons may lie in evolutionary behavior. When a person keeps another person at a distance, they cannot surprise with an attack. As people are invited closer, it becomes easier to talk with them. When people are brought even closer, intimacy or affection is being invited. Someone may deliberately threaten another by invading their space without invitation. Anytime someone enters a personal zone without invitation, it creates anxiety for the person whose space is invaded. This is seen as a threatening action. Some people do this intentionally to signal that they are more powerful.

Box 24.2 lists the comfort zones. The public zone is generally more than 12 ft. When people encounter each other in public, their tendency is to leave space between them. When adequate space cannot be left, people begin to feel uneasy. The social zone allows a connection with other people. People can talk with others but still keep them at a distance. Friendly people in a social setting adopt this distance. The personal zone is one in which people who know each other may directly converse. When each person is close enough to touch the other, they are in the intimate zone. They can harm or touch each other in intimate ways. There must be significant trust for the two to be comfortable in this area.

BOX 24.2   COMFORT ZONES

- Public zone – more than 12 ft
- Social zone – between 4 and 12 ft
- Personal zone – between 1.5 and 4 ft
- Intimate zone – less than 1.5 ft

The sizes of these zones vary by culture (people from Latin America and the Middle East have smaller personal spaces; those from Romania have larger personal space requirements), gender (women have smaller spaces), and personality. For example, males in some cultures find it unnerving to have a woman touch them or be proactive in invading their space.

In the dental office, practitioners see all of these spaces. Patients sit as far from each other as possible in the reception room. In the operatory, they are prepared for their intimate space to be invaded. Dentists then touch them and invade their bodies by putting their hands in the patients' mouths. This can be disconcerting, especially for someone who is not accustomed to dental visits or may be from a different culture. The practitioner should reduce space step by step by meeting the patient, shaking hands, and gradually decreasing space before the dental procedure. Patients who are supine in the dental chair are in an exposed and vulnerable position. (Think of dogs, who roll on their backs, exposing their bellies, to show submission.) When a practitioner discusses treatment options with a patient, they should do so with the patient upright with their eyes level or in a treatment conference room. This is a coequal position that promotes trust and open conversation.

SCRIPTS

Most communication in the office is repetitive for the dentist and dental staff members. Some staff members are more skilled at saying things in a way that elicits a positive response from the patient. Others have a difficult time talking spontaneously talking. Many offices have developed scripts for staff to use when talking with patients to solve this problem. For example, dental assistants may need to learn the words the receptionist uses when they answer the telephone. If the receptionist is sick or away from the desk, the fill-in may need to learn to answer the phone correctly. A script the replacement can read the first few times ensures that they answer the telephone correctly, gathering the correct information for patient care and scheduling.

A practitioner can write scripts for every typical interaction in the office. They can then use staff meetings to practice and refine the scripts. In that way, they can be sure that all staff members are saying what they want to be said in the way that the dentist wants it said.

WRITTEN COMMUNICATION

Written communication has become less common in professional settings. Because of this, its use can be more powerful as a tool. From a marketing perspective, the office owner should be sure that the stationery and other communication devices (websites, etc.) have a similar look and "feel," including logos, slogans, and other branding devices.

TREATMENT PLANS

Dentists often think of a treatment plan as a technical exercise in procedure sequencing. However, the treatment plan is also an excellent form of communication. It allows the patient to see the procedures the practitioner proposes and the cost associated with them, and for the dentist to gain consent for and acceptance of treatment. If a dentist provides different treatment options, then these can be the basis of a discussion about the advantages and disadvantages of each and open a discussion of patient wants and values. The patient's "chief complaint" is more than a line on a form. It is the reason the patient came to see the dentist. The plan must acknowledge and address this.

PAYMENT PLANS

As with a treatment plan, a payment plan is really a patient communication device. It allows the office personnel to discuss finance options and requirements with each patient. A verbal contract, such as a patient agreeing to pay, is legally binding. When a patient signs a payment plan, it becomes more binding in the patient's mind. It also removes any "he said . . ., she said . . ." discussions if the patient misses a payment.

TREATMENT LETTERS

Many offices follow up on treatment with a posttreatment letter. This letter will include before-and-after photos showing the improved esthetics. It will also thank the patient for their patronage and ask for referrals from friends or colleagues.

COMMUNICATION ISSUES IN THE DENTAL OFFICE

A dentist is the communication leader in the office. How they speak, act, respond, and relate sets the tone for everyone else in the office. Staff members will follow the dentist's lead, doing as they do. If a dentist finds someone with a different communication style, they should use that person's strengths to the office's advantage.

ADDRESS THE PATIENT IN THE WAY THEY WANT

Patients come to a dental office with different backgrounds and value systems. Some, especially elderly patients, are more formal than others. All office personnel must call the patient by title and last name – "Mr. Jones," "Mrs. Smith," "Dr. Brown" – until the patient invites them to do otherwise. ("Oh, honey, call me June.") Office personnel must not assume that someone wants to be called by their informal name (Steve instead of Steven, Kate instead of Katherine). The simple way to find out is to ask. People enjoy hearing their name, which says that the dentist recognizes them individually. Office personnel should use the patient's name often but correctly.

Pronouns are extensions of our human identities, just like our names are. It may be just as disrespectful and rude to use the wrong pronouns for someone as it is to call them by the wrong name. On the other hand, using someone's legal name and pronouns shows respect for their identity and welfare. For transgender, non-binary, gender-fluid, or non-conforming individuals, being referred to by the wrong name or pronouns can be an annoying or embarrassing experience.

The best way to learn someone's pronouns is to ask them! Their pronouns should not be assumed, may not match their gender expression, and may change over time. People may also choose to use a variety of pronouns. To learn someone's pronouns, lead by example and share your pronouns first during introductions. For example, "My name is James. I use he/him/his pronouns." This provides an invitation and creates space for others to share theirs. You can also simply ask "What are your pronouns?" or "What pronouns do you use?" With practice, this becomes routine. If you do not know someone's pronouns and would like to refer to them, it is best to call them by their name.

IDENTIFY PATIENT WANTS, NEEDS, AND DESIRES

Each patient comes to the office with a unique set of needs, wants, and desires regarding their dental condition and treatment. Not everyone feels free to discuss them with others, especially strangers. A dentist's job is to determine what the patient wants so they can respond effectively. The best way to do this is by using the following aids.

Using DISC Profiling When Speaking to Dental Patients

Building solid relationships is part of giving excellent dental care. Knowing how to speak to patients to help them understand their dental treatment and feel comfortable with moving forward with their treatment is one of the foundations of building successful personal relationships and gaining case acceptance.

The first step for the dentist is to know their own preferred communication style (their DISC profile – **d**ominance, **i**nfluence, **s**teadiness, **c**onscientiousness) and realize that all of their patients will not respond well to it. For example, the dentist may want to move quickly and get right to the facts. Some patients prefer to build personal relationships or understand complex treatment options before accepting treatment. The practice owner can be in a position or have enough influence to demand that their staff work with them in this manner, but they cannot hold all their patients to that standard. This is not to say that a dentist should be a chameleon and change their style for every patient. However, they can adapt their communication and presentation to better meet the patient's needs if they understand how they might be perceived.

The second stage is learning about other DISC profiles and how to spot them. The dentist can recognize each style using a quick list of behaviors. When the dentist shows patients that they appreciate what is important to them, they are more likely to consent to treatment. The following are things to look for in matching the dentist's presentation style with the patient's profile.

D Represents Dominance The D in DISC stands for dominance, and this kind of patient prioritizes achieving outcomes. These patients are not as concerned with details or personal relationships, and the dentist should get straight to the point and respect their time.

I Represents Influence The I in DISC represents influence. This individual values forming connections with others and enjoys socializing. They do not need to know every aspect of the treatment. This personality type will be more likely to consent to treatment if the dentist takes the time to engage in a conversation with them that interests them, addresses any shared problems, and then goes on to arrange treatment.

S Represents Steadiness The S in DISC stands for steadiness, and this calm personality type emphasizes collaboration and reliability. Most of these patients are silent and probably anxious, so gently explaining what to expect, even if they are not asking questions, is essential.

C Represents Conscientiousness The C in DISC stands for conscientiousness. This style might be challenging since such people have many questions. This patient prioritizes excellence, precision, knowledge, and competency. They are interested in specifics on the necessity for therapy and what to anticipate. They like it when the doctor or hygienist can explain everything in detail using a booklet, printout, or video. These patients require more time from dental experts, since they often ask several questions regarding the alternatives, materials, price, treatment process, and recovery.

Once the dentist understands these personality styles, they and their staff can talk to the patient in their preferred style to help them understand and accept the treatment.

Use Communication Aids

Adults learn best in many ways. Some use the spoken word, but most (about 80%) learn best visually, through pictures and videos. A practitioner must use all the patient education tools available to help inform the patient about their condition and treatment choices. This not only shows good sales skills, it is the ethical basis of valid informed consent. The dental office must have a variety of suitable educational materials available.

Speak the Patient's Language

A dentist must speak with the patient based on their level of understanding. The practitioner should avoid dental jargon or hot-button words. It is essential to find the line between talking down to a patient and talking over the patient's head.

Use Co-diagnosis

A practitioner should use a mouth mirror or intraoral camera to show patients problems that they find. When a dentist shows a patient a problem directly, the patient generally wants to know what to do to fix it. The patient will be actively involved in the diagnosis, asking for treatment options, rather than passively being told what they need.

Watch the Dentist's Body Language

Practitioners can easily send conflicting messages to a patient. They may discuss treatment options verbally. However, if a dentist does not maintain eye contact or if they slouch or fidget, the verbal message says that the dentist cares, but the more powerful non-verbal message says that they are distracted or uncertain. An upright posture conveys confidence.

Watch the Patient's Body Language

Patients will send clues to their emotional and physical state through their body language. A dentist must read the message a patient sends and respond appropriately. If the patient's hands are sweaty when shaking hands, they are probably nervous. A patient with crossed arms usually indicates they are shutting out the dentist's ideas. The more the dentist studies the subtle body signals patients give out, the better they will interpret the communication.

SPECIAL PATIENT PROBLEMS

Dental practitioners see several common "problem" patients in the office. These are often the result of a communication breakdown. Sometimes, the dentist (or the staff) can help resolve the problem.

Angry Patients

When a patient is angry, what is most important for office employees to do is to listen to the problem. Often the angry patient believes that the dentist or staff has ignored them or brushed them off. The dentist must not try to rationalize or counter every point the angry patient makes. They must give the patient time to talk and explain their side of the problem thoroughly. (They must allow the patient to "vent.") When the patient has finished, the dentist should use active listening methods and paraphrase one of the patient's points without being defensive or hostile. They should reflect on the issues the patient brought up. (Often, that is all that the patient needs. The patient just wanted a forum to explain their side!) The dentist should ask the patient what they want to happen to resolve the problem. Sometimes it is simple ("I need an extra month to pay off my bill"). Sometimes the patient will ask for another action the practitioner cannot do immediately. They need to tell the patient what they plan to do ("I will call Dr. Smith and discuss the problem with her"). They must tell the patient when they will be back in contact with them.

Non-compliant Patients

Patients who do not follow up with appointments, take medications as prescribed, or complete recommended home-care procedures risk developing additional problems. This can be both a treatment and a legal problem for the practitioner. Therefore, if a patient is routinely non-compliant, the dentist needs to address the non-compliance. The practitioner must note any compliance in the patient chart non-judgmentally. If a patient misses a follow-up visit, the practitioner should note the miss and any attempts to call or reschedule. The office needs to determine why the patient is non-compliant (misses appointments or does not follow through with recommendations) to address those concerns. The practitioner may need to write a stern and factual letter to the non-compliant patient that describes the additional problems the patient may face if they do not follow through with recommendations ("If you do not complete the root canal procedure that we started, the tooth might abscess and spread infection throughout your body. It also might break, resulting in significant pain, and require the surgical removal of the pieces at a specialist"). If the patient remains non-compliant, the practitioner should dismiss the patient from the practice, as described in Chapter 28.

Anxious Patients

Patients may be anxious in the dental office for many reasons. They may have experienced past pain or discomfort or fear upcoming procedures because of stories they have heard from friends, family, or acquaintances. They may worry about the cost of treatment or feel guilty for failing to seek care sooner. Some fear that they will receive bad news or that the doctor will find out they are afraid (the "he-man" syndrome). Regardless, the best solution is to deal with the issue directly. The dentist must acknowledge to the patient that it is normal to have such feelings. An open discussion using adequate disclosure and feedback will often help to find the "real" cause of the anxiety. The dentist can then try to address the cause of the anxiety instead of simply trying to reduce the anxiety itself.

Part 2: Case Presentation and Acceptance

I have never worked a day in my life without selling. If I believe in something, I sell it, and I sell it hard.

Estée Lauder

LEARNING OBJECTIVES

At the completion of this part, the student will be able to:

- Describe the common types of consumer purchases and relate them to dental office treatment.

- Define the common treatment acceptance decision points.

- Define the steps in presenting a case to a patient.

- Describe the common methods of gaining patient commitment.

A dentist's case presentation skills convert the patient's interest in dentistry into an action step: deciding to continue with treatment. Case presentation is analogous

KEY TERMS

adjournment close	problem-solving
concession close	purchases
direct close	routine purchases
extended cost of service	testimonial close
opportunity cost close	

to "selling" in the business world. In the professional practice, dentists look out for a patient's best interest, not to "oversell" what they can do or what the patient needs to have done. However, if dentists genuinely believe that a particular course of dental care is in the patient's best interest, it becomes their duty to fully inform the patient of the options, presenting the advantages and disadvantages of the options. In this way, practitioners develop valid informed consent before proceeding to treatment. The problem develops when practitioners take the information presentation step and turn it into a coercive or manipulative process, either stressing or withholding information to make their point, which does not involve a free decision by a fully informed patient. However, dentists want the patient to accept the treatment. First, they believe it may improve the patient's life, and secondly, it improves their bottom line. If patients do not accept treatment, practitioners have limited production, and therefore limited profit.

TYPES OF CONSUMER PURCHASES

Marketers say that consumers have two types of treatment decisions: routine and extended. Patients behave differently and use different purchase criteria for each type. A practitioner should appeal to patients differently in each type as well.

ROUTINE PURCHASE DECISIONS

Consumers buy many low-cost, frequently used goods and services. These are *low-involvement purchases* because they do not involve much thought or consideration by the consumer. These purchases do not involve much financial or psychological risk. (Examples include soap, fast food, and routine dental care.) The buyer often has a brand preference (or loyalty) that is strongly affected by "top-of-the-mind" awareness rather than conscious decision-making. When they go to the store to purchase bath soap, they generally do not agonize over the decision, weighing the merits of each type of soap and researching the values and other consumers' preferences for each. Instead, most shoppers pick up their usual brand without thinking much about it. (This is brand loyalty.) Advertising keeps the brand at the top of the consumer's mind so that when they are ready to make the purchase, they remember the brand.

In dentistry, regular dental patients make routine purchases every time they respond to a call for a "recall" or "periodic maintenance" visit. Most of the dental work at this visit is routine for most patients. (This includes cleanings, fillings, and often basic crowns.) Patients, as dental consumers, do not think about whether to purchase the service or not and from whom to purchase it. Like buying their usual deodorant at the store, they purchase based on familiarity and habit.

Routine purchase behavior works to a dentist's advantage when a patient returns for routine periodic maintenance without consideration of going to another dentist. It works to a dentist's disadvantage when consumers do not have brand loyalty to their office but instead go to an office on their insurance panel. In this sense, consumers view dental care as a commodity with no brand loyalty. They do not have much involvement in the purchase decision. They simply look for the most inexpensive care, which their insurance plan may dictate. In these cases, practitioners should try to develop "brand loyalty" for their practice. Nevertheless, they must realize that they may lose some consumers (patients) to other "brands" (dental offices) because of the insurance pricing inducements.

PROBLEM-SOLVING PURCHASES

These purchases involve the purchase of high-involvement, generally expensive items that have a long lifetime. (Examples include new cars, home entertainment systems, and reconstructive dental care.) The buyer must first learn the criteria for selection, then shop for the good or service based on those criteria. When buying a new car, many people research the various makes and models, check *Consumer Reports* or other online consumer guides, and agonize over the model, color, and options. This is all because automobiles are generally purchases that a person will live with for several (or many) years. They are expensive, so there is a high desire to be satisfied with the decision. (Many people even justify a poor purchase decision to reinforce their previous decision.) If someone finally admits that they made a poor choice, chances are that they will tell everyone about the shortcomings of the item they purchased.

In dentistry, dentists see problem-solving purchase decisions each time the patient worries about the treatment. This may be because of large costs, potential side effects, or excessive fear. (A simple alloy may be a significant life-altering event for a highly fearful patient.) Before a patient commits to spending many thousands of dollars for complex treatment, they may check with trusted friends or family members. The patient may research the expected treatment or get a second professional opinion. A dentist must not see these efforts as distrust, but instead as the consumer's search for information and an evaluation of alternatives before committing to treatment. In other words, this is healthy consumer behavior. Because patients evaluate the service after they complete it, dentists need to follow up with the patient, ensuring that they are satisfied with the work and trying to solve any problems identified. In this way, practitioners encourage a positive postpurchase evaluation by the patient. This encourages the patient to recommend the dentist to friends, family, and trusted others.

PATIENT TREATMENT ACCEPTANCE DECISION POINTS

Patients base whether to accept a dentist's treatment recommendation on four significant points. These are all patient perceptions, *not* facts. Patient perceptions are as real to the patient as concrete facts, so the practitioner must address them as such. A dentist must satisfy each of these points to gain treatment acceptance.

OFFICE ATMOSPHERE

Patients often make a conscious or subconscious decision about a dentist within the first minute after they arrive at the office. They make this based on their feelings about interpersonal relations and the office atmosphere. Patients who perceive a warm, trusting relationship between the dentist and the staff will assume that the same trusting relationship will develop with them. Likewise, they will perceive a rigid, formal, or controlling atmosphere as not leading to trust. Many patients view office cleanliness as a surrogate measure for the dentist's attention to detail.

TRUST

Patients must believe that a dentist is working in their best interest, not the dentist's own. This is especially true for extensive, complex treatments. Simply telling a patient "Trust me, I'm a dentist" is usually not enough. The practitioner must prove it through their actions and office personnel interactions. It may take a long time for some patients to develop that trust. That is why dentists may see patients for several years of routine maintenance visits before the patient feels comfortable enough to commit to a large, expensive treatment plan.

EXTENDED COST OF SERVICE

Money is always a consideration in the treatment decision. The absolute price is not as important as the conditions of payment. How long do patients have to pay, and how will the payment fit into their family budget? If payments are reasonable (a patient perception), most patients accept this decision.

PREVENTING DISCOMFORT

A dentist must not cause pain before, during, or after treatment. This means the dentist practices excellent injection techniques, using sedation (nitrous oxide/oxygen or chemotherapeutic agents) when indicated and halting treatment if the patient has pain. The practitioner can ease discomfort with a soothing atmosphere, music headsets, and other distractions. Nearly 15% of the US population are true dental phobics who need exceptional help (beyond that generally done for patients) to have a pain-free dental experience.

STEPS IN CASE PRESENTATION

The case presentation is a combination of patient education and sales techniques. There are several steps to follow in gaining patient case acceptance.

ESTABLISH A RELATIONSHIP

A dentist must establish a one-to-one personal relationship with the patient. Most people will only commit to large treatment plans once they establish that relationship.

Patients may make smaller, routine purchases (such as a "cleaning" or basic fillings) but generally will not commit to a large, high-involvement purchase (such as an oral reconstruction) without a relationship and the trust that is inherent in the relationship. Often, patients will not "buy" expensive treatment for months or years until they have developed the trust required for such a commitment. The patient comes to a dentist knowing that they are the expert. The patient must gain trust by discovering that the dentist is looking out for the patient's interests.

LEARN PATIENT WANTS

In this step, a dentist's listening skills become critical. They must ask probing questions and listen to the answers. This allows them to offer solutions that satisfy the patient's needs, not the dentist's technical solution to a dental problem. Understanding the patient's "why" is essential to understand what might motivate them to seek treatment. The practitioner should listen to the emotional side of the patient. (The previous part of this chapter on communication gives several techniques, including feedback and self-disclosure.) The patient may make an off-hand comment about how pretty someone's teeth look. They may be saying that they would like a mouth that looks as good and healthy.

DECIDE PATIENT NEEDS

Here, a dentist's professional skill, care, and expertise come into play. A dentist must decide the various treatment options based on their clinical and patient examinations. Helping the patient to understand their condition is also important. Patients who do not perceive a need are less likely to accept the recommendations. Part of a patient's understanding of their condition is to link the condition to the consequence. Using such phrases as "I'm concerned about. . ." or "Because that leads to. . ." will help patients connect their condition to the consequences, especially when no treatment is done. Many patients present routine, small-involvement needs that are easy to decide. Patients with complex treatment, psychological, and medical needs may require significant time from the practitioner to reach a decision.

TEST THE BUY-IN

It is important to test the buy-in to know if the patient understands the condition and its consequences. A simple question of "How concerned are you with. . .?" can help gauge if the patient fully understands their condition and its consequences. If they do not understand these two critical pieces, discussing solutions will only lead to them not accepting treatment. If the patient does not understand their condition and consequence, more time is needed to educate them on those factors.

OFFER SOLUTIONS

In this step, the dentist uses their diagnostic and planning skills to decide on the appropriate plan of treatment that addresses the patient's health or disease state and resolves the patient's treatment wants. Many adults learn best through methods other than oral communication (Box 24.3). Audiovisual aids, such as videos, pamphlets, or flip charts, can help show a patient the problems and solutions. The solution to a patient's need is the technical procedure that a dentist does, but the solution to the patient's wants is the benefit of treatment.

ANSWER OBJECTIONS

Many dentists are offended by patients who challenge or question their treatment recommendations. Really they should view this as a positive step because the patient has not discounted what the dentist has said and recommended. Instead, the patient is processing the information and trying to understand and internalize it. They must do this before they agree to treatment. They are interested, but have significant questions that the dentist must help them to resolve. What if this crown has bad esthetics? What happens if the implant does not integrate? Are there less expensive alternatives? The objections often involve the four decision points: discomfort, trust, time, and money. The practitioner should view each probing question as an opportunity to educate the patient about the proposed treatment and to educate themselves about how the patient perceives the dentist. Some people want technical information about the procedures. They decide logically, trying to exclude emotions. Others want more assurance that the dentist can solve their problem. They decide on a "gut" or emotional level. By finding the type of objections, a dentist

---

| BOX 24.3 | AIDS TO PROBLEM SOLUTIONS |

- Printed material
- In-office videos
- Intraoral camera
- Physical models
- Website/social media

---

can often respond in an appropriate way that satisfies the patient's reluctance to go on with the suggested treatment.

GAIN COMMITMENT

The final step is to have the patient commit to act. Several techniques from the sales world work well in the dental situation. The practitioner's technique may include combining several of these closing techniques based on the individual circumstances.

- **Direct close**

  The simplest way to do this is for a dentist to ask the patient if they are ready to go on with treatment. This is called a *direct close* in the business world. The salesperson asks the customer to purchase the good or service.

  "Mr. Jones, can I go ahead and schedule an appointment to start the reconstruction?"

- **Adjournment close**

  This technique does not ask for commitment now. Instead, it gives the patient time to think about it. This is especially useful when the dentist perceives that there are still unresolved objections that the patient needs to work through. It helps build trust and relationships because the dentist is not using a "hard sell" sales technique.

  "Mr. Jones, I can see that this is an important decision for you. Do you need additional time to consider all the implications? Should we discuss the details further at your next appointment?"

- **Concession close**

  When the patient offers an objection, the dentist can make a condition of resolving the patient's objection that they make the purchase. This is based on solving the patient's objections to satisfy their needs. Use an "If I . . . then will you. . .?" statement rather than an "If you. . . then I will. . ." statement. This focuses on the dentist trying to solve the patient's objection rather than the objection itself.

  "Mr. Jones, if we can work out the financing for you, are you ready to go with the treatment?"

- **Testimonial close**

  A dentist can use a satisfied patient to help convince this patient. Because a patient cannot prejudge services (until the dentist has delivered them), they may rely on others who have had similar services done. (Be sure that the testifying patient agrees or is anonymous.) In these cases, letters or before-and-after photos are valuable.

"This patient had a similar case to yours. I think you will agree from the photos and her letter that the treatment was very successful."

- **Opportunity cost close**
  This technique stresses the cost of not going on with treatment. It shows the patient that the apparent cost is lower than it appears compared with future costs. Costs involve more than price (money). The costs may include future inconvenience, pain, additional cost, or disfigurement.

"Mr. Jones, if we do not replace that tooth now, your teeth will drift, leading to gum problems, poor chewing, and a much more expensive solution in the future."

There is a big caveat to be born in mind regarding closing techniques. Patients who feel tricked or otherwise manipulated will not commit to treatment and may leave the practice. They may also tell friends and acquaintances, turning them against the dentist.

Controlling Costs in the Practice

CHAPTER 25

A penny saved is a penny earned.

Ben Franklin

GOAL

This chapter examines the nature of dental office costs. It divides costs into types and defines the amount of control the practitioner has over each of those types of costs. Finally, it examines representative data and measures for controlling costs in the dental office.

LEARNING OBJECTIVES

At the completion of this chapter, the student will be able to:

- Describe the elements of dental office costs.

- Allocate typical costs in the dental office into fixed, step-fixed, or variable categories.

- Perform a basic break-even analysis.

- Perform a basic "What if. . .?" analysis.

KEY TERMS

break-even analysis	fixed costs	total costs
break-even point	practice cost analysis	variable costs
cost allocation	step-fixed costs	"what if. . .?" analysis

Increasing income and controlling costs are the two methods to improve profitability in the dental office. Cost control is easier to understand because a dollar saved through reducing costs adds directly to the bottom line.

TYPES OF COSTS

Dental practice costs fall into three categories: fixed, variable, or step-fixed. These differing costs can be displayed graphically, where it becomes more apparent how each type of cost behaves as production changes.

FIXED COSTS

Fixed costs do not change with production (Figure 25.1). Whether someone produces $30 or $30000 per month, fixed costs are constant. For example, rent, dental association dues, malpractice insurance, and many other costs

Business Basics for Dentists, Second Edition. James L. Harrison, David O. Willis, and Charles K. Thieman.
© 2024 John Wiley & Sons, Inc. Published 2024 by John Wiley & Sons, Inc.

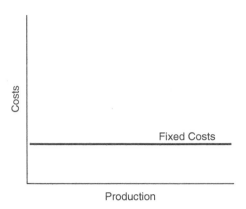

FIGURE 25.1 Fixed costs.

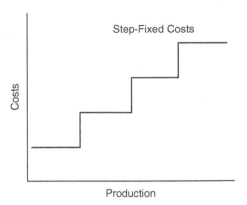

FIGURE 25.2 Step-fixed costs.

remain constant regardless of production. These may not be the same from month to month, but are generally consistent. Fixed costs consist of the following:

- **Office space and equipment** are the largest categories of fixed costs. They consist of all costs associated with operating the physical space and equipment of the practice, including rent, utility, tax, and other charges associated with the occupancy of the building. Dentists should also include an estimate of the depreciation expense for the office and equipment because this represents wear and tear on those assets, and any equipment replacement programs.

- **Other fixed costs** include bank charges, office insurance, advertising, and legal and professional expenses.

STEP-FIXED COSTS

Step-fixed costs vary with production but only in discrete steps (Figure 25.2). The existing staff will work harder as production increases. However, finally the load becomes too great, and dentists must hire an additional staff member to help the office function efficiently. Therefore, the cost jumps in a discrete step when the practice hires a new person. Dentists hire staff members as entire people (or increments of people). These costs are "fixed" over their range so that when the office owner hires a new person, this establishes a new set of fixed costs. Unless they hire an additional employee or lose one of the present staff members, these costs will be relatively constant or fixed in the range of the analysis. For that reason, dentists often include staff costs with fixed costs.

- **Staff costs** include direct wages, benefits, payroll taxes, retirement plan contributions, hiring and training expenses, and any other costs that are a direct result of

employing office staff members. Dentists can divide labor costs into clerical (front office), hygiene, and chairside-assisting personnel and should categorize them individually for detailed analysis:
- Clerical (front office) compensation.
- Chairside-assisting compensation.
- Hygiene compensation.

VARIABLE COSTS

Variable costs change directly with the production level (Figure 25.3). If someone produces $30000 of dentistry in one month, then their costs for dental supplies will be approximately 10 times more than a month in which they produce $3000. If the dentist has no production, theoretically they will have no variable costs. Variable costs change with production levels, not just collections. Dentists still must purchase supplies for procedures that they discounted or did not collect. In the dental office, variable costs consist of dental lab, dental supplies, and general office supplies. These costs often appear the month after the office purchases them because of typical

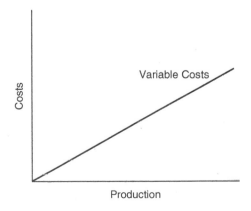

FIGURE 25.3 Variable costs.

billing and inventory cycles. Nevertheless, conceptually these costs are directly related to production. The following categories are tracked separately:

- **Dental lab costs** are associated with contract laboratory work. The costs of laboratory supplies in the office (stone, waxes, etc.) are dental supplies. If someone employs a laboratory technician in the office, they should include all costs associated with the laboratory operation (e.g. salary, benefits, supplies, and lab space rent) in this category.

- **Dental supplies** are the materials dentists use when doing dentistry. They include expendable supplies (e.g. cotton rolls, anesthetic, alloy, and composite material) and small-instrument replacement.

- **Office supplies** are the costs associated with materials for the front desk operation. This includes paper products, computer program fees, postage, magazine subscriptions, pencils, and other items used in processing patient visits.

- **Owner's expenses** are items that the dentist benefits from directly. The dentist could have taken them as profit from the practice, but instead they elected to pay for them, appearing to reduce the practice's profit. Common examples include self-employment taxes, automobile expenses, continuing education programs, travel, meals, entertainment, and retirement plan contributions for the dentist.

TOTAL COSTS

Total costs are the sum of fixed, step-fixed, and variable costs (Figure 25.4). (Step-fixed costs are fixed over their range.) Likewise, the diagram of the total cost is the combination of these various types of expenses. Total costs begin with fixed costs at a production of zero. As production increases for the period, total costs increase the same as variable costs.

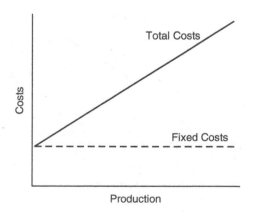

FIGURE 25.4   Total costs.

DENTAL OFFICE COST ALLOCATION

DEVELOPING CATEGORIES OF COST CONTROL

Cost control techniques can be grouped into general categories that are applied to specific practice areas.

Know the Costs

Dentists need to have an accurate and detailed compilation of office costs. This is an easy task if there is an accurate categorization in the office checkbook. The dentist should look at the numbers on an annual and quarterly basis. More frequently than that, they might identify false problems because of the usual ebb and flow of production, collections, and expenses over time.

Concentrate on Major Cost Items

Staff member costs typically are more than twice laboratory costs. Therefore, a 5% saving in staff leads to a larger return than 5% in the laboratory cost area. When the practice has the major costs under control, the dentist should work on smaller costs. Remember, a dollar saved still increases profit, regardless of the source of saving.

Look at the Income Too

Profit comes from both cost and production. If dentists increase collections more than they increase costs, income increases. They should negotiate reimbursement rates with insurers. Although the individual practitioner does not have as much leverage as a network of practices, they can often gain an increase. Most insurers will negotiate reimbursement rates. Dentists should eliminate less profitable (deeply discounted) insurance plans and keep fees up to date through regular comparisons and increases.

COMMON COST CATEGORIES

Dentists can develop a list of common dental practice costs for financial analysis. One place to begin is to examine the previous year's tax return. A Schedule C is a report of most dental office expenses. A complete checkbook register will also contain expenses grouped by category. The allocation of these costs into specific categories is somewhat arbitrary. Business office expenses, for example, vary slightly with an increase in patient visits through an increase in office supply usage and postage, although dentists may list them as fixed. Which specific category someone uses should result from the individual practice history.

Typical dental offices show the highest costs in the staff (step-fixed) category, typically about 25% of collections

BOX 25.1   BUSINESS OFFICE EXPENSES

Fixed costs	Variable costs	Step-fixed costs
Advertising	Supplies	Employee wages
Bank service charge	Dental laboratory	Employee benefits
Automobile expenses	Office supplies	
Dues and journals		
Insurance		
Equipment loans		
Legal and professional		
Rent or mortgage		
Repairs		
Travel or continuing education		
Utilities		

(Box 25.1). Variable costs of production generally run at about 15% of production, with fixed costs accounting for the rest, at 25% of collections. (This results in the average overhead ratio of 65% of collections.) That explains why small increases in production and collection lead to a large increase in profit. Dentists have already paid fixed and step-fixed costs. The only cost of seeing a few additional patients is the variable cost of production (about 15%), leaving the rest (85%) as profit.

BREAK-EVEN ANALYSIS

Proper allocation gives a more accurate understanding of practice costs than the simple traditional "percent overhead" figure. The break-even analysis technique is a valuable tool for using this information. This financial analysis technique relates the office's costs to the production and profit of the practice. Although, as its name implies, dentists can use it to detect the point of zero profit (the break-even point), it has a much wider use by providing insights into the cost behavior of the practice and the riskiness of many courses of action.

The basic equation used in the break-even technique is:

$$\text{Collections} - \text{Variable Expenses} - \text{Fixed Expenses}$$
$$= \text{Net Income}$$

This equation brings mathematical sense to an intuitive idea: that all the money someone collects, minus all expenses (fixed and variable), leaves a profit or loss. If three of the numbers of the equation are known, the fourth can be found through substitution.

The break-even analysis can be depicted graphically as in Figure 25.5. Essentially, this is the cost structure diagram superimposed on a production diagram. The point of intersection between the revenue (collection) line and the total cost line is the break-even point. Any production above this point results in a profit; any production below this point results in a loss. The production above the break-even point is "more profitable" because the fixed costs have been paid, and now only the lower variable costs must be paid. This also happens when someone takes an associate or offsets hours with another dentist. Only step-fixed and variable costs remain. Any additional dentistry produced is on a better margin for the owner–dentist. The incremental cost of producing more is small compared to the initial cost ratio. This is also critical to understanding capitation or other reduced-payment third-party plans. If there is slack chair time, then the only costs associated with the managed care production are the variable costs. However, if these patients replace traditional, fee-for-service patients, then the cost must also include the loss from the forgone production of those traditional patients.

For example, assume that a dentist, Dr. Sample, wants to understand his office finance better and has asked his accountant to prepare an income statement for the previous year to use the results for a more detailed analysis of the practice finances. From that statement, he allocated costs into various categories and arrived at the financial outcomes for the past year in his office shown in Box 25.2.

In the example, Dr. Sample produces $460\,000$ per year ($38\,333$ per month). He collects 97% of production.

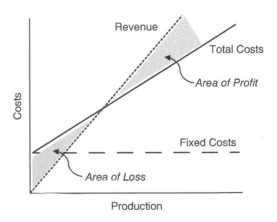

FIGURE 25.5   Break-even analysis.

BOX 25.2	INCOME STATEMENT FOR DR. SAMPLE

Category	Amount	
Production	$460 000	
Collections	$446 200	97% of production
Fixed costs	$107 088	24% of collections
Step-fixed costs	$116 012	26% of collections
Total variable costs	$75 854	17% of collections
Total costs	$298 954	67% of collections
Total profit	$147 246	33% of collections

Using the formula and previously given cost data, his income for the year would be:

$$\text{Collections} - \text{Variable Expenses} - \text{Fixed Expenses}$$
$$= \text{Net Income}$$

$$\left(0.97 \times \text{Production}\right) - \left(0.17\,\text{Production}\right)$$
$$- \left(\text{Step} - \text{fixed Costs} + \text{Fixed Costs}\right) = \text{Net Income}$$

$$\$446\,200 - \$75\,854 - \$223\,100 = \text{Net Income}$$

$$\$147\,246 = \text{Net Income}$$

Dr. Sample netted $147 246 by producing $460 000 of dentistry, collecting 97% of accounts, and paying all fixed and variable expenses. He calculates his actual production break-even point, where net income is $0:

$$\text{Collections} - \text{Variable Expenses} - \text{Fixed Expenses}$$
$$= \text{Net Income}$$

$$\left(0.97 \times \text{Production}\right) - \left(0.17\,\text{Production}\right)$$
$$- \left(\text{Step} - \text{fixed Costs} + \text{Fixed Costs}\right) = 0$$

$$\left(0.80 \times \text{Production}\right) = \$223\,100$$

$$\text{Production} = \$278\,875$$

This says that if Dr. Sample were to produce $278 875 of dentistry this year ($23 240 per month), he would barely pay all the bills but not make any profit, having a net income of $0.

WHAT IF. . .? ANALYSIS

What if. . .? analysis takes the basic formula for break-even analysis and uses it to answer practice finance questions. For example, assume the same numbers as in Dr. Sample's

break-even analysis. What if he wants a net income of $200 000 per year? He can use the same formula to calculate the production required to produce that income:

$$\text{Collections} - \text{Variable Expenses} - \text{Fixed Expenses}$$
$$= \text{Net Income}$$

$$\left(0.97 \times \text{Production}\right) - \left(0.17\,\text{Production}\right)$$
$$- \left(\text{Step} - \text{fixed Costs} + \text{Fixed Costs}\right) = \$200\,000$$

$$\left(0.80 \times \text{Production}\right) - \$223\,100 = \$200\,000$$

$$\left(0.80 \times \text{Production}\right) = \$423\,100$$

$$\text{Production} = \$528\,875$$

Dr. Sample would need to produce $528 875 to gain the desired income. If he cannot do this, given the present office configuration, then he would need to estimate new costs based on a different configuration, changing the values in the formula.

SPECIFIC COST-CONTROL TECHNIQUES

These cost-saving techniques are described in detail in other sections of this book and are briefly described by category here. No magic cost bullet suddenly makes the practice profitable. Instead, someone should keep an eye on small items that accumulate in large amounts. Some of these savings involve long-term costs, such as office rent. It may take years to see savings. Others are more immediate. Regardless, dentists should keep a constant eye on the costs of the business. Many do this through quarterly meetings with their accountant or practice financial advisors. The practice owner should annually appraise general office costs, such as insurance.

RENT

Office rent is not controllable in the short term. In the long term, a dentist can negotiate different terms before signing a lease. Property owners like professional tenants. They are stable, profitable, and have a positive clientele. This gives a dentist some bargaining leverage when it is time to negotiate or renegotiate a lease. They may gain a longer-term lease at a steady price or may negotiate lower-rent escalators in future years. They may push some expenses (e.g. snow removal) on to the owner. If they are making significant leasehold improvements, they might negotiate the cost of those into the lease payment (the owner initially pays for them). This decreases the practice owner's immediate out-of-pocket expense and time to claim depreciation expenses (though special tax rules apply here). The lease payment will be higher as a result. If the landlord refuses to negotiate terms, the practice owner should consider moving the office to a better location with better terms. If they own the space, they should look at leasing the space from a family partnership or other entity to recharacterize the rent as unearned income.

UPKEEP

Practice owners should know which upkeep costs the landlord pays and which the tenant pays. (These expenses often are exterior compared with interior expenses.) If, for example, the dental office shows water damage from a leaking gutter, the landlord (or owner or condominium association) may be responsible for repairing the problem and associated damages that have occurred in the dental office. The dentist should do upkeep and maintenance or hire a family member to do this. That not only keeps the payment within the family, but it also has a positive income tax effect and helps to teach teenagers a work ethic and the value of a dollar. Upkeep items may include mowing the grass, small repair or painting jobs, cleaning the office, or decorating the office with seasonal decorations.

EQUIPMENT

Routine maintenance is always less expensive than replacing expensive equipment. The dental office should have an equipment maintenance program for both large and small equipment. This includes the furnace and air conditioner, compressor and evacuation system, and processor and computer equipment. Follow manufacturers' recommendations for handpieces, curing lights, and other small equipment. When the dentist has paid off the start-up loan, they should redirect some of that payment into an equipment replacement fund so that funds are available to replace or upgrade equipment when required. The practice owner should consider tax savings by gifting equipment to a family partnership or other entity and leasing the equipment back, keeping the income in the family, and making those expenses unearned income.

TOTAL STAFF COMPENSATION RATE

The dentist should calculate the total compensation rate for staff members annually. This is the total cost of employment (which is also the total compensation for the employee). It includes direct pay, any benefits, and all unwithheld expenses. The practice owner needs to pay appropriate total compensation. External comparisons (such as surveys) and internal comparisons (for employee equity) should be used. Paying an excessive rate does not guarantee a better employee. However, paying a substandard rate will almost always guarantee an unsatisfied one. Start a cafeteria-type benefit plan. Each employee gets to choose the benefits that are most important for them and then pays for the benefit through salary reduction. The practice owner should check with an accountant or financial advisor about health savings accounts (HSAs) or other health insurance savings plans. Dentists should also require employees to take time off when they close the office for vacations or other reasons.

The dental practice should pay employees on a wage (hourly) basis. Paying a salary only ensures that employees make a minimum amount. It does not limit costs for overtime. Many offices now give an annual bonus instead of a raise. The bonus is a one-time amount. The raise goes onto the employee's base pay and carries forward for ever unless the employer cuts the employee's pay rate.

MOTIVATE STAFF MEMBERS WITH INCENTIVES OTHER THAN PAY

People work for many reasons. Only one of them is pay. The practice owner should pay attention to the social aspect of the job environment and promote employee skills development. This skill development encourages performance through social and personal growth rather than financial compensation.

HIRE THE RIGHT PEOPLE

Proper delegation of duties involves hiring lower-cost staff members and freeing higher-cost staff members to do more income-generating work. Dentists should use part-time employees as needed and base their pay on the time they work or the functions they do. Because employee turnover is so expensive, business owners should take time to hire the right employees. A practice owner can use computer lists to generate potential employees or hire a spouse or other family member. The tax savings may be significant. The dentist should train and cross-train employees. If an employee is sick, they may not need to hire an expensive temporary during that time.

SUPPLIES

Dentists should keep an accurate inventory control system to end excess inventory costs or stockouts. They should make staff part of the solution by encouraging them to shop wisely. Dentists should negotiate costs with suppliers.

If a supplier has a special offer on a needed product, another supplier will often meet the discounted price rather than lose the sale. Many offer convention specials, where the supplier discounts products bought on the convention vendor floor. The office owner also should investigate buying cooperatives. As corporate and chain practices increase, independent dentists are banding together to gain the economies of scale represented by the large networks.

DENTAL LAB

The greatest cost savings from the lab come from doing the procedure correctly the first time. Remakes cost chair time and materials that the practice cannot recover. The practitioner may use different labs for different procedures based on the quality and price of the specific procedures.

Promoting Staff Effectiveness

CHAPTER 26

Part 1: Selecting and Hiring Employees

You're only as good as the people you hire.

Ray Kroc, Founder of McDonald's

GOAL

This part aims to prepare new graduates to select and hire staff members for the dental office.

LEARNING OBJECTIVES

At the completion of this part, the student will be able to:

- Describe the employment process for finding dental office employees.

- Differentiate between a job description and a job specification.

- Define the purposes of conducting a job interview.

- Differentiate between legal and illegal job interview questions.

KEY TERMS

directive interview approach
employment application
employment interview
employment process
human resource management

job description
job-related behaviors
job specification
non-directive interview
observation of work

probationary period
references
résumé
temporary placement services
working interview

Properly trained and motivated staff are essential for survival in today's dental practice world. Although this at first appears to be a singular task, in fact dental practice owners must meet several steps or objectives along the way. These objectives include:

- To hire the best applicants possible.

- To compensate employees appropriately

- To motivate employees to perform well.

- To assess employee performance.

To accomplish these goals, practice owners must organize and manage the staffing part of the practice. Staffing is a critical resource area (along with financial, technical, and physical areas). It should be called "human resource management," to equate it in importance with the other management areas of the practice.

Business Basics for Dentists, Second Edition. James L. Harrison, David O. Willis, and Charles K. Thieman.
© 2024 John Wiley & Sons, Inc. Published 2024 by John Wiley & Sons, Inc.

Chapter 21 describes various types of dental staff members. Each practitioner will need to decide the type and number of each category of employee they require in their practice. Because dental staff is the single largest expense item in most practices, the practice owner should take care that each employee is fully used before deciding to hire another.

ATTRACTING THE BEST APPLICANTS

The obvious purpose of the employment process is to place the most appropriate person in a position so that the dental office can operate efficiently and effectively. This apparently simple process depends on several background facts. A dental practice owner must specify what the position entails and determine what characteristics and training they need in a person who would hold that position. The problem then becomes matching and finding the right person to fill the job.

JOB DESCRIPTION

The first step in the hiring process is to write a job description that explicitly lists the job holder's duties. The reason for doing this is to clarify the qualifications that are important for an applicant to possess. In addition, the practice owner can discuss in more detail with each interviewee the tasks that they will do based on the job description.

The practice owner must know what is needed to perform effectively in the given position. What are the duties of the person who will hold the job? Who will the person in this job interact with, and what are the responsibilities associated with the job? The job description defines the duties of the role. The dentist must write this description, so it is easy to understand, succinct, and yet detailed enough that a person who applies for or holds the position knows what they are expected to do. The description should consist of specific, observable, job-related behaviors rather than attitudinal or general characteristics that are immaterial to performance on the job. A useful offshoot of developing a job description is that this essentially becomes the performance appraisal instrument. Because it consists of what a person is supposed to do on the job, assessing performance on these specific behaviors is easy. If you have someone currently working in the role, the easiest way to write a job description is to have that person write down all the procedures they do during a typical day or week. If you are starting up a new practice, then developing a job description becomes more difficult. The list of what they do on the job must be the basis of the job description.

RECRUITING FOR AND ADVERTISING THE POSITION

Recruiting involves the development of a pool of potential employees. Advertising is one obvious method to gather these people, through either newspapers, internet bulletin boards, or through internal (staff) referral. Each approach has advantages and disadvantages.

Advertising is the most common form of identifying potential employees. Generally, the practice owner places an advertisement on internet lists or in the local newspaper (Sunday employment section). The ad should be specific for the job the dental office is filling, be positive in tone, and avoid misleading or discriminatory statements (Box 26.1). Several techniques can help an advertisement to stand out from the others. Simply making it more prominent, placing borders or white areas around it, or using bold or a different typeface can draw a prospect's eye to the advertisement. Unless the practice owner wants many calls or is looking for a fresh face, they should consider including the phrase *experienced* or the more restrictive *dental office experience required* in the advertisement. The practice owner may want to have the applicant phone or send a résumé to the office.

Internet bulletin boards and lists are rapidly replacing newspaper advertising for many dental offices seeking employees. They are inexpensive and common. Not everyone knows or uses these information sources, nevertheless. A dental office might miss many qualified potential employees, especially older workers, if it uses only internet advertising.

Another common form of recruiting is having existing practice employees identify friends or associates who may be searching for a change in employment. The

BOX 26.1	WHAT TO INCLUDE IN RECRUITMENT ADVERTISING

- Location of the practice

- Qualities the dentist is looking for

- Experience required

- Skills required

- Days and hours of the job

- Statement about the practice that generates enthusiasm

- Name of contact person, hours, and telephone number to call

practice owner can then contact them to determine their interest. A dentist must not "raid" neighboring dentists of their staff. Suppose the potential employee is presently working for another dental practice in the area. In that case, that person (employee) must initiate the contact and express an interest themselves before the hiring practice owner has any dealings with them. Although this may not eliminate ill will between the hiring dentist and the other practice owner, it should reduce it. Some practice owners offer a bonus or reward for an employee who identifies a new employee for the practice. If the present employees are happy and satisfied working there, they should be some of the best recruiters.

Some dental offices may keep a list of acceptable candidates from previous job opportunities in their practice. Others may use a private placement service or a university-based workforce service. The practice owner should know that private placement services charge a substantial fee for finding an employee that a dentist can find just as quickly.

If the dental office keeps a list, it can also use it for short-term and part-time employees. Or temporary placement services furnish employees on a daily basis. The dental office might use them as an opportunity to "try out" several people, looking for the person or the characteristics that are needed. Again, such services are expensive, but they do offer a solution to limited-time needs for the practitioner.

SELECTING THE BEST OF THE APPLICANTS

When a dentist has attracted several applicants, they must select the best one for their office.

THE APPLICATION

Unless an office owner wants the office staff to be unaware that they are hiring a new person, the potential applicants should phone the office. (The dental office should not use the primary patient lines in the advertisement and should have the applicants call a private number, if possible.) This allows the receptionist to assess the applicants' telephone communication skills. It also allows them to screen out unacceptable candidates by briefly describing the job and asking qualifying questions, such as salary requirements and experience. If the job has some undesirable component (e.g. evening hours two nights a week), the dental office should tell prospective applicants at this point rather than wasting everyone's time with an interview. If the prospect passes the primary screen, the practice owner should have them come to the office and pick up an application, complete it, and return it by mail to the receptionist, or send a résumé to the office instead of an application.

Some dentists prefer to use experienced employees only. They do not want to take the time to train a person who is new to the job. Others believe that dental offices must find a person with the personal characteristics they want; the dentist can then train the person to do the components of many dental office jobs. It is an individual choice. The dental practice will pay more for an experienced staff member, and that person can help the office learn additional ways of conducting the practice. However, that person may have previously learned undesirable habits and may be difficult to control, believing that they know more than the dentist about how the office should run.

As a rule, new practitioners should hire an experienced receptionist. An experienced person can help establish the business systems that every office requires. Otherwise, a new practitioner and a new receptionist will be searching for answers that may be common knowledge for a more experienced person. After several years, the established receptionist and the now more confident dental practitioner will often have control problems in the office (i.e. who is really the boss?). By then, the office should be running smoothly enough, and the dentist should be knowledgeable enough to hire another receptionist that fits the office's personality.

The application form should ask for information about the individual's qualifications and ability to do the job that the dentist has previously described. The practice owner can gather information about an applicant's credentials, background, and qualifications more efficiently through a written format than through interviews. They can also determine a basic level of written and expressive abilities by having an "essay" section on the application form. Applications are better than résumés because a practice owner can ask specific questions that may be important to them. The practice owner should also have the person fill the application out by hand to assess their handwriting skills and neatness.

However, many dentists prefer to have prospective employees send a résumé instead of filling out an application form. If a dentist requests résumés, they need to review them carefully. The person who wrote the résumé will try to place themselves in the best possible light. The practice owner should look for gaps in employment history or frequent jumps from one employer to another. They also need to examine the form and neatness of the résumé. References given on résumés are seldom helpful because people are obviously only going to give details of referees who support them. A practice owner may get more valuable and honest appraisals from former employers, although even this is doubtful in today's litigious society. A résumé may also not give the practice owner the specific information they need about a particular candidate (e.g. can the person use a computer?). Nevertheless, résumés are a good method for screening many potential applicants. Often business office applicants will have résumés prepared. Assistants or hygienists typically will not have a résumé prepared and might not apply if the office requires that. The practice owner may be missing a group of qualified candidates for these positions if they require a résumé from them.

THE EMPLOYMENT INTERVIEW

One means of gathering additional information is the employment interview, which is the final step in the employee selection process. The purpose of the interview is twofold: to aid the dentist in gathering information to select the best-qualified applicant, and to provide information so the applicant can decide whether they want to work for the practice. The practice owner, therefore, may use the interview to "sell" the prospective employee on the practice.

As mentioned previously, the dentist needs to know as much as possible about every applicant. If the applicant has filled out an application form, the practice owner should review it carefully before proceeding with the interview. They do not need to request any information they can obtain from the application form or résumé during the interview. However, if there are any questions about the information provided, the dentist needs to raise them. If, for example, the application shows a gap in recent work history, the interviewer should ask the interviewee to explain this unaccounted-for time. It may be as simple as time off for a family move, or it may show a problem, such as a job the interviewee was fired from that they did not include on the application.

Purpose of the Interview

The employment interview is a required step in the recruiting and hiring process. The interview serves several useful purposes, including the following:

- **To verify information on the application or résumé**
  Most people will not actively lie on an application or résumé (although one management study showed "inaccuracies" in nearly two-thirds of all applications examined). Nevertheless, everyone wants to put their best foot forward. A person may, for example, not include a specific part of their employment history because of a probable poor reference from the employer. Other people may embellish their duties, abilities, and responsibilities. The interview allows the practice owner to ask more in-depth questions of the applicant and to find information that is missing from the written application.

- **To find out additional information that is not on the application or résumé**
  Practice owners can assess many skills and attributes from a résumé. For example, does the person have the required years of experience, training, or background required of the job? However, they cannot glean other attributes simply from the application. How well does the applicant communicate? Are they able to think quickly on their feet? How do they react when put in a difficult situation? Practice owners can often deduce these and other traits and abilities during the employment interview when they are not evident from the application.

- **To let the applicant assess the dentist and the office**
  A prospective employee wants to know about the office for which they will be working. The interview gives that person the opportunity to meet the dentist and staff, and to see the physical and operational components of the dental practice.

- **To actively recruit the applicant**
  The marketplace for skilled dental auxiliaries is competitive. An excellent staff member may have several possibilities for employment. Therefore, the dentist may have to convince the prospective employee that their office is the one for which the applicant wants to work.

- **To assess personnel and compensation policies**
  It is challenging to learn what a fair wage and benefit package is, compared with what other dental offices and other forms of comparable employment are paying. During the interview, the office owner can find out if they are "in the ballpark" regarding their compensation package. Many employees are looking for a particular situation (hours, benefits, etc.) that is not apparent until they are asked. A practice owner might satisfy that person through a minor adjustment to personnel policies.

Findings from the Interview

The practice owner must try to answer three questions about each applicant.

- **Can the applicant do the job?**
  By reviewing an applicant's training and work experience, the practice owner ought to be able to answer this question with a high degree of certainty. The question relates to information that ought to be readily available. However, the practice owner must scrutinize these qualities closely to make an objective evaluation.

- **Will the applicant do the job?**

This question is more difficult to answer than the first one. Even if the applicant has the skills to do the job, a lack of motivation may impede job success. An objective evaluation may not be possible from the information obtained before selecting an applicant. For these reasons, practice owners ought to ask previous employers and educational personnel from whom the applicant received instruction how willing they are to do what they are asked.

- **How does the applicant get along with people?**

The practice owner wants to know how the applicant will respond to them as the employer, other personnel in the office, and patients. An organization such as a dental practice has many interpersonal relationships. An employee needs to relate effectively with other people. In the interview, the applicant should talk freely and easily. If the applicant has difficulty carrying out a conversation or dislikes working closely with others, the practice owner would suspect that the applicant might have difficulty working in a dental office.

Structure of the Interview

After reviewing the application form, the dentist is ready to talk with the applicant. An introduction is an easy way to begin an interview because it immediately lets the interviewee know that the practice owner is the person for whom they will be working. In addition, it avoids that awkward situation in which both the dentist and the applicant are at a loss in beginning a conversation.

At this point, the interview may continue in one of two ways. The practice owner may use a non-directive style, or find that a more structured approach is appropriate (Box 26.2).

Non-directive Approach In a non-directive (or non-structured) interview, the interviewer does not try to direct the applicant's conversation. The non-directive approach can be helpful when the interview is not yielding enough information. Business owners conduct this kind of interview in a conversational manner, with the chief difference being that the interviewer listens and occasionally comments in ways that encourage the applicant to talk freely about any subject of interest. For example, the candidate may wish to talk about their scholastic background, but the interviewer may be more concerned with work experience. At this point, some direction may be necessary to elicit the kind of information in which the practice owner is interested. Experience has shown that if dentists let applicants

BOX 26.2	SAMPLE INTERVIEW STRUCTURE

Introduction of participants
Description of practice
Job description
    Primary duties
    Secondary duties
    Wage (salary base)
    Benefits available
Office policies and procedures
Investigation of applicant
Discussion of qualifications and résumé
Self-description
Asking for further questions
Plan of future action

talk at length, they will likely discuss most of the topics in which the interviewee is interested, rather than what the interviewer needs to know.

The main advantage of non-directive interviews is that they put the applicant at ease and create an atmosphere in which they feel the interviewer is accepting and understanding. Such interviews are also excellent for assessing the employee's organizational, communication, and interpersonal abilities.

The primary disadvantage is that the interview may result in little exchange of information occurring between the interviewer and the applicant. If the practice owner does not elicit any information that helps them to choose among applicants, they have wasted the interview time. Veteran interviewers can use this technique productively, but a more direct approach is likely more productive for the novice.

Structured Approach In a structured (or directive) interview, the interviewer assumes a more active role than in an indirect interview. The topics discussed are those of interest to the interviewer. Rather than waiting for points to emerge during the interview, the interviewer usually gives information or asks questions about those points. Applicants for openings in a dental practice are usually interested in the following:

- Duties they will perform

- Types of personnel employed

- Working hours

- Scheduling of vacations

- Number of holidays
- Sick leave policy
- Professional development
- Insurance programs
- Dental care at a reduced cost
- Salary level

Covering these points directly is easier for the practice owner and less time-consuming than using the indirect approach and hoping that points that they want to discuss will arise. Therefore, the interviewer must control the discussion and mention those things that they feel are important rather than waiting for the interviewee to ask questions about them.

Interview Questions

As a rule, whether the practice owner uses a directive or non-directive approach, they should try to use open-ended questions whenever possible. Open-ended questions typically start with "How. . .?," "Why. . .?," "What. . .?," or "Tell me about. . ." Responses to these questions allow the dentist to assess the interviewee's communication skills and enables the applicant to explain their answers in much more detail than a closed-ended question. For example, the closed-ended question "Did you like your last job?" asks for a simple "Yes" or "No" response from the interviewee. However, the more open-ended "Tell me what you particularly liked about your last job" causes the respondent to give a discourse rather than a simple one-word answer. The interviewer will then be in a much better position to assess the person's communication skills. Box 26.3 gives several questions that an interviewer can ask during an interview. It is not the ultimate list of all possible interview questions; it is a list of suggestions for questions that a practice owner might ask to gain the most effect from an employment interview.

The interviewer must listen to the answers to the questions asked. Many people are so concerned with preparing to ask the next question that they fail to listen to what the interviewee says in answer to the previous one. Listen attentively. If something sounds strange or wrong, ask a follow-up question. If the person struggles with an answer, allow them to struggle for a moment. This way, the prospective employer can tell how the applicant may react under pressure.

Legal and Illegal Questions An employer may legally ask an applicant any question concerning the work or their ability to do it. It is illegal to ask any questions that are

| BOX 26.3 | SAMPLE INTERVIEW QUESTIONS |

Experience

What did you particularly like about your last job?
What did you particularly not like about your last job?
Who did you get along with the least at your former job?
What did you do about the problem?
Describe your previous employer's management style. How would you have liked to see it change?

Training

What educational experiences would you like to do over again? Why?
Describe your present job duties and responsibilities.
How has your education, training, and experience prepared you for this job?

Skills

Why should I hire you for this position?
What skills and abilities do you bring to this position that other people do not?
What is the best skill that you bring to this job? Give an example.
If you take this job, in what areas do you feel that you would need additional training?
What should the other staff members know about you to work effectively with you?

Interests

What do you want to be doing 10 years from now?
Why did you select a career in. . .?

Job attitudes

Describe the perfect boss.
Describe the perfect employee.
Why did you leave your previous employer?
What are you looking for in a job that you are not finding now?
What is your greatest disappointment regarding your career to this point?

discriminatory in nature, or that do not apply to the job. It is illegal, for example, to ask someone if they have any children. That has nothing to do with their ability to do the job. However, an applicant with children in daycare may be unable to work the extended hours required when an emergency patient calls. That affects job performance. Practice owners must be sure to ask work-related questions. While the question "Mary, do you have any children?" is illegal, instead practice owners can ask "Mary, due to the nature of dental services, we often must work late, often until 7:00 p.m. Is that a problem for you?" If Mary has daycare issues, that may be a problem. On the other hand, she may have a spouse or other family member who can pick the children up from daycare if necessary. Box 26.4 gives several examples of illegal questions.

Common Interview Pitfalls Several practices and habits may make an interview a frustrating experience for both the dentist and the applicant. To reduce these frustrations and make the interview more productive, the interviewer should follow these suggestions:

- **Do not allow interruptions during the interview**
  Staff members should hold calls and not interrupt the practice owner's time with the applicant. This is both efficient and courteous.

- **Beware of dangerous first impressions**
  People often intuitively judge a person in the first minute after meeting. A familiar style of dress, smile, or tone of voice can lull an interviewer into a false first impression that cannot be overcome throughout the interview.

- **Do not be too formal or too authoritative**
  It is important to exchange a few pleasantries and develop rapport to make it easier for the applicant to relax and talk freely.

- **Plan the questions**
  The practice owner should plan what they intend to ask of each applicant before the interview. Lack of planning may result in them not obtaining information that could aid them in selecting the best-qualified applicant.

- **Do not talk too much**
  One purpose of an interview is to determine whether applicants can express themselves verbally. If the dentist does most of the talking, it is unlikely they will be able to assess the applicant's verbal skills.

- **Do not mislead the applicant about the duties involved**
  An interviewer may inadvertently do this if a clear job description is not available. They need to be prepared to discuss duties and responsibilities in some detail. If a job turns out to be different from what the applicant expected, the new employee may quit within a short time.

- **Do not make the interview too short**
  This makes it difficult to obtain anything but the most superficial information about the applicant. Lack of information frequently leads to errors in selecting the best-qualified applicant.

BOX 26.4

ACCEPTABLE AND UNACCEPTABLE INTERVIEW QUESTIONS

Name
Acceptable:

- "Have you ever worked under another name?" if needed to verify information

Unacceptable:

- "What is your maiden name?" to a married woman

Residence and birthplace
Acceptable:

- "Can you furnish proof of citizenship?"

Unacceptable:

- "What is your citizenship?"

- "What is your birthplace/the birthplace of your parents?"

- "Do you own your home, rent, board, or lives with your parents?"

Religion
Acceptable:

- "The job requires you to work on [hours and days], is that OK for you?"

Unacceptable:

- "What is your religious affiliation?"

- "Are there any church, parish, or religious holidays that you observe?"

National origin
Acceptable: None

Unacceptable:

- "What is your lineage/ancestry/national origin/parentage?"

- "What is the nationality of your parents/spouse?"

References
Acceptable:

- "Can you give me the names and contact details of some character or professional references?"

Unacceptable:

- "What is the name of your pastor or religious leader?"

(Continued)

Gender or marital status

Acceptable: None

Unacceptable:

- "What is your gender orientation?"
- "What is your marital status?"
- "Are you pregnant or planning to become pregnant?"
- "How many children do you have?"
- "What is your spouse's occupation?"

Arrest and convictions

Acceptable:

- "Do you have any convictions that are relevant to the job?"

Unacceptable:

- "How many times have you been arrested and what for?"

Disabilities

Acceptable:

- "Do you have any disabilities that would prevent you from performing the job?"

Unacceptable:

- "Do you have any mental or physical disabilities?"

- **Keep the discussion focused**

  Discussions about mutual acquaintances or common interests may be entertaining, but they probably do not aid in judging the applicant's qualifications.

- **Do not be overly influenced by the applicant's physical appearance, dress, or grooming**

  Appearance only peripherally relates to the tasks customarily expected of a dental auxiliary.

- **Avoid making assumptions**

  Just because a previous employee with a particular background did good work, the practice owner must not assume that another person with a similar background would also be a satisfactory employee. Each person needs to be looked at individually.

- **Avoid biases**

  Age, education, and background are important only as they relate to job performance, so the dentist should avoid prejudging applicants on the basis of these qualities.

- **Use intuition carefully**

  The practice owner must not base a decision about a job applicant purely on intuition. Careful analysis and objective decisions need to be part of the selection process. The owner should only use intuition to complement these decision points.

Working Interviews

Many dentists have a potential employee work for a day in the office. This allows them to assess the applicant's knowledge, skills, and abilities and to observe their interpersonal relations with patients and other employees. It also allows the potential employee to assess the dentist's office as a workplace. The practice owner must pay applicants for these "working interviews." It may be difficult to arrange a suitable interview time if the employee is currently employed. The owner must also be sure that the employee understands that this is not regular employment but is only to assess their skills and compatibility for the prospect of employment. Given these caveats, working interviews can be a valuable final step in the selection process.

References

The practice owner should check references and former employers, if only as a formality. Few applicants will offer dissatisfied former employers as references. Equally, few businesses give honest references or appraisals of former workers (for fear of slander suits). As an example, suppose a potential employee worked at another dental office. The previous owner fired them because they caught the employee embezzling from the practice. However, the owner did not press charges because of the time and trouble involved in prosecuting the case. (They were happy to be rid of the employee.) The potential employee now has no criminal history. (They were not convicted of a crime.) When asked, the previous employer will not say that they caught the employee embezzling because there is no record or proof, and the previous owner fears a possible slander suit. The prospective employer thus has no way of knowing the potential employee's past.

It is still worth the small effort required for the practice owner to pick up the phone and ask. They may get lucky and find an honest evaluation. Many previous employers will only give the dates that the person worked there. Most others will not even give that information. The practice owner should still call any previous dental employers; they might give valid appraisals. The critical question is: "Is this person eligible for rehire?" If they are not eligible for rehire, there must have been a significant problem.

THE HIRING DECISION

The decision of which of the final applicants to hire should be based on all the information the practice owner gathers through the process. It includes the application form, the interview process, reference checks, work history, and staff information. Personality and skill tests are legal (if they test attributes essential to the job), but their high cost and low reliability make them impractical for the typical dental office.

Once the owner decides who to hire, they need to move quickly! Excellent employees seldom remain available for long. The new employee should be contacted (preferably by telephone) and offered the job. The practice owner should be prepared to negotiate with the potential employee. The top applicant may have several other possible employment opportunities. The practice owner must send a follow-up letter detailing the expectations of staff in the office, the duties of the person holding this job, the pay rate, and any benefits the person will receive.

Once the person accepts the job, the other final applicants need to be contacted immediately and informed of the decision so that they can continue with their job searches. If more than one applicant was acceptable, the owner should ask that person if they can keep their name as an applicant if another opening becomes available. This may shorten the recruiting process in the future if the owner needs to fill another position.

PROBATIONARY PERIOD

Many offices hire employees into a "probationary" status that typically lasts 30, 60, or 90 days. They can try out the employee, then terminate them if they cannot perform the job duties or do not fit in with the other personalities in the office, without fear of legal repercussions. The practice owner also does not pay employee-related benefits for the probationary period. If the employee passes the probationary period, they often are rewarded with a raise and qualifying for the employee-related benefit package.

Many large organizations have moved away from probationary periods. They believe that their time is better spent being sure that they select the right employee and training them appropriately. Most states support at-will employment, meaning dentists employ persons at their own will. They can also fire these persons at their own will. Paradoxically, a probationary appointment may imply that once an employee passes the probationary period, they can only be fired for cause, essentially nullifying the at-will employment idea.

If a practice owner wants to use a probationary period, they ought to call it a *waiting period*, which does not imply long-term employment and supports at-will employment. The office benefit policy can state when employees become eligible for various benefits, eliminating this justification for the initial period. A good hiring process does more to ensure excellent employees.

INTEGRATING THE NEW EMPLOYEE INTO THE OFFICE

The employment process does not stop with job acceptance. The practice owner must orient the new employee to the office procedures and possibly train or send them for education or certification. Taking time for orientation helps to encourage the employee's loyalty to the office, promote positive interpersonal relationships among staff members, and acquaints new personnel with all facets of the job. The following are tasks for new employee orientation activities:

- **Start a personnel file**
  This must include the person's résumé or application, W-4 and K-4 (state) withholding forms, Social Security number, and any other necessary tax-related information or work permits. Include a copy of the employee's application so that if it is found later that they misrepresented themselves or lied on their application, the employer can immediately fire them.

- **Have the new employee fill out any benefit or insurance forms**
  Give the employee pamphlets and policies describing those benefits (if applicable).

- **Verify and display their license or certification**
  Many states require the employer to post licenses or qualifying certifications for employees.

- **Require the employee to read the policy and procedures manual for the office**
  The dentist or office manager should review each section of the policy and procedures manual and the personnel manual with the new employee. The practice owner should have the employee sign that they have read and understand the manuals.

- **Explain opening, closing, and emergency procedures**
  The owner should have the employee sign for office keys, if applicable.

- **Give a detailed tour of the office**
  The practice owner should show the new employee where they store instruments and materials, and where to put personal effects during working hours.

- **Introduce the new employee to all existing employees**
  The practice owner should assign one employee who functions in a similar capacity to be the "information contact" so that the new employee knows whom to ask office procedural questions.

- **Arrange for OSHA and HIPAA compliance**
  The new hire must have hepatitis B vaccination within 10 days and must have the training required by the Occupational Safety and Health Administration (OSHA) and the Health Insurance Portability and Accountability Act (HIPAA) when feasible.

Part 2: Compensating Employees

It's not the employer who pays the wages – he only handles the money. It is the product that pays the wages.

Henry Ford

GOAL

This part aims to prepare new graduates to develop a compensation system for the dental office.

LEARNING OBJECTIVES

At the completion of this part, the student will be able to:

- Describe the basic principles of establishing a wage and benefit package for the dental office.

- Define when an employee may be paid a salary and when they are an "exempt" employee.

- Describe the benefits that employers must provide to employees.

- Describe a flexible benefits plan for the dental office.

- Describe an annual employee total compensation report.

- Describe how to process staff paychecks.

KEY TERMS

benefit	pay equity
flexible benefit plans	required benefits
jury duty	salaried employees
maternity leave	Section 125 plans
military leave	total compensation
non-exempt employees	unpaid leave
optional benefits	wage
overtime	

Dental practitioners compete with each other when recruiting staff for the office. Genuinely excellent dental office personnel will often have several offices to choose from when looking for a new employment opportunity. Why would they choose one office over another? One reason may be the pay and benefits package. A new practitioner probably cannot pay the top-dollar wage and benefit package that an established colleague or other business venture can. So a starting practitioner will face a dilemma: they do not have the immediate cash flow to pay for the best employees, yet they need the best employees to become profitable.

HOW TO SET STAFF COMPENSATION LEVELS

Usually, dental offices will pay the "going rate" for comparable employees in their area. The going rate is what most employers pay for similar positions with similar job requirements. This is determined by the technical skills or knowledge required, interpersonal abilities, and availability to work at certain times. There also may be legal or licensing requirements (such as a hygiene license or assisting certification) that limit the number of potential employees, driving up their cost to the practice owner. In the end, the supply and demand of the labor pool determine what practice owners pay employees. If hygienists in the area typically earn $45 per hour, then a practice owner will pay about $45 per hour for a hygienist. (There is a range around that average figure.) Various groups do periodic staff salary surveys, including the popular dental press and organized dental groups. These are good places for a practice owner to start when looking for comparable wage levels.

When thinking of "pay," the practice owner needs to consider the total compensation package, composed of the hourly wage, legally required benefits, and any optional benefits offered. Wages and benefits are, to a certain extent, interchangeable. A wage of $20 per hour with no benefits may be comparable to a wage of $17 per hour with a health insurance plan. Every employee is different. They will value the balance between pay and benefits differently, according to their own needs. Benefits hold tax advantages for employees over straight pay. Many dental office employees would prefer part of their total pay to be in the form of benefits. However, many others, especially low-paid employees, do not appreciate this and would rather have cash in hand. Benefits like salary help recruit, hire, and retain employees. However, some employees have a poor understanding of benefits. Often, they do not understand benefits' actual value and view them as employee "rights" rather than forms of additional compensation. Any paid time off (holidays, vacation) is additional compensation and comes from office profit. Unpaid time off decreases office production. To bring these confusing ideas together, many dentists compute the total compensation for employees each year at wage adjustment time. An example total compensation sheet is shown in Box 26.5. Adding a staff member is a significant investment, but if they increase office collections more than they cost, the addition is a good investment.

STAFF PAY

Equity means fairness in the reward system. There are many reasons for promoting equity besides the altruistic desire to treat employees fairly. As a business, a dental practice competes with other businesses for the pool of labor in the community. Dentists compete with other dentists for the services of assistants, hygienists, and receptionists, and with the local bank and grocery store for the general labor pool. Although people work for many different reasons, one reason certainly is pay and benefits. Therefore, dental practices must pay competitive wages and benefits to hire and retain excellent employees.

The Fair Labor Standards Act (FLSA) governs many pay issues in the dental office. This is a federal law that is carried out at the state level, so some state-to-state variation exists in its implementation. Practice owners must check with the state's Bureau of Labor Standards (or similar state organization) for the exact interpretation in their state.

HOURLY WAGE

Hourly employees earn an hourly wage. Their total pay is based on the number of hours they work multiplied by their hourly wage. Most dental office employees earn an hourly wage for their work.

To figure out total pay accurately, practice owners must have accurate information describing how many hours each employee worked for each day of the week. Either a written pay record (pay sheet) or a time clock accomplishes this legally. If a dental office uses a written record, the person needs to record "time in" and "time out" for each session (morning and afternoon). Simply recording eight hours is not adequate documentation. Also, many dental offices require each person to sign the timesheet or time card. This says that they agree it accurately describes the time they worked. Most office management computer systems have built-in time clocks to help in recording hours worked. This also makes it easier to process payroll.

SALARY

Salaried employees earn a fixed amount (salary) regardless of their work time (given some limitations). Some practice owners prefer paying a salary for several reasons. Accounting is easier to calculate. Each pay period, the owner calculates how much Social Security tax, federal, state, and local (if any) income taxes, and voluntary employee contributions to withhold from each employee's gross pay. Salaried employees make the same gross pay and therefore have the same amount withheld each pay period, making this function easier. Some practice owners erroneously believe that any salaried employee can work for an unlimited time. (In fact, only "exempt" employees can work overtime without additional pay.) On the downside, a salaried employee is paid for a whole week's work, even if they work fewer hours.

BOX 26.5	EXAMPLE ANNUAL EMPLOYEE COMPENSATION

Employee Name:

Direct compensation

Gross pay	$41 600	Assumptions
Overtime	$900	Employee's wage rate = $20.00/hour
Bonuses	$200	Employee works 40 hours/week
FICA (7.65%)	$3 182	Employee worked 30 hours overtime (30 × 30 = $900)
Unemployment insurance	$400	Employee receives 2 weeks of paid vacation
Retirement plan contribution	$2 080	Employee receives 6 paid holidays

Employee fringe benefits

		Employee receives 5 sick days and 2 continuing education days
Medical insurance	$4 800	Dentist makes 5% contribution to retirement plan
Dental care	$150	Dentist provides single health coverage ($400/month)
Group life insurance		Dentist provides a continuing education trip every year (value $500)
Dependent care allowance		Dentist gave employees a $200 holiday bonus
Gifts and awards		Dentist paid professional dues of $200

Career benefits

		DentiDenDentist provided routine dental care value $150
Continuing education payments	$500	
Tuition and travel reimbursement	$200	
Lodging and meals		
Professional dues/subscriptions		

Total compensation	$54 012
Total hours paid (52 × 40)	$2 080
Total hours not worked	$154
Total hours actually worked	$1 926
Nominal compensation/hour	$20.00
Actual compensation/hour	$28.04

This is an example of how benefits, time off, and unwithheld expenses add to an employee's total compensation.

COMMISSION

Dentists may pay specific staff a percentage of the work that they produce. This pay mechanism works for employees who control their own production, such as an associate dentist or hygienist. Most state labor laws require the business owner to pay non-professional staff (such as assistants or receptionists) on a salary or wage basis. The typical range dentists pay their hygienists is 30–35% of their production. The dentist is still responsible for ensuring the quality of work in the office. Associates are often paid based on a percentage of production (or collections). The specific percentage varies across the United States as supply and demand dictate.

Paying a commission to a hygienist has some inherent problems. One is to decide which procedures should be in the hygienist's base for commission. The periodic exam, for example, can only be done (in most states) by the dentist, so it should not be included. Radiographs, although taken by the hygienist (on the dentist's equipment), must be interpreted by the dentist. Eliminating these procedures for compensation significantly decreases the hygienist's compensation and can lead to dissatisfaction. Money may not motivate an employee to work harder. They may be working more for personal growth or social reasons. Tying their pay to production does not motivate these employees.

EXEMPT EMPLOYEES

Exempt employees are exempt from the wage and hour (overtime) laws. This means practice owners must pay non-exempt employees overtime (generally, at a rate equal to 1.5 times their wage for any time they work more than 40 hours per week). Dentists may pay an employee a salary with no overtime (i.e. they are *exempt* employees) if they meet all three of these criteria:

- They regularly supervise two or more 40-hour employees.

- Their salary is at least at a state-determined level.

- They spend less than 20% of their time doing the same duties as those they supervise.

Professional employees are exempt as well. An associate dentist (and, in some states, a dental hygienist) is a professional employee and therefore exempt from overtime laws.

Given these restrictions, the only people who genuinely qualify as exempt salaried employees in a dental office are a dentist associate, a true office manager, and, in some states, a dental hygienist. Dentists may pay dental auxiliaries on a salary basis. However, auxiliaries are still non-exempt employees. Because dentists must pay them overtime, putting them on a salary does not make much sense. (The dentist loses if they work more or fewer than 40 hours per week.) Wage and hour laws vary from state to state. They are also subject to change by regulators. Therefore, the practice owner should check with their state's labor cabinet before setting up a compensation system.

OVERTIME PAY

The FLSA requires business owners to pay overtime to employees who work more than 40 hours a week. (Four states base their overtime on 8 hours per day instead of 40 hours per week.) Overtime pay is a minimum of "time and a half," or 1.5 times each employee's regular hourly wage for those hours worked more than 40 per week. Each workweek stands alone regarding overtime. That says the employer cannot accumulate multiple pay periods (one week the employee worked 42 hours, the next week 38 hours) and not pay overtime. Business owners also may not legally substitute compensatory time (i.e. letting people take equivalent time off) for overtime pay, even if the employee agrees.

Determining the "base hourly wage rate" can be a bit tricky. What is (or is not) included in the regular wage is important because it determines overtime pay (Box 26.6).

| BOX 26.6 | DETERMINING OVERTIME PAY |

Problem: Mary, a dental assistant, earns $10 per hour. This week she works 45 hours. Determine her gross pay for tax determination.

Solution: Mary earns "time and a half" for any hours more than 40 per week. In this case, she earns $400 base pay (40 hours × $10/hour) plus $75 overtime pay (5 hours × $15/hour).

The regular pay includes all money received for employment, except reimbursed expenses, gifts, discretionary bonuses, and paid time off. A bonus is "discretionary" if it is not given in exchange for action by the employee. So, dentists should include a production bonus at the regular rate but not a Christmas bonus (unless it is based on production for the year). If a dentist has questions concerning overtime pay, they should check with their accountant about what they must include and exclude.

PAID TIME OFF

The FLSA does not require that employers pay for any time off for employees. This includes holidays, paid or unpaid vacation days, and sick or personal days. Some states do have this requirement, so the office owner ought to be sure to check with their local accountant or attorney. Most employers offer some time off to compete with similar businesses when hiring employees.

Office owners must decide their policy regarding staff working when they take time off from the office. In a solo office, when a dentist is not working in the office, the office generates no income, and most employees have little to do. If a dentist is gone for a day (e.g. to a continuing professional education course), they can usually find enough work to keep employees busy. This includes deep cleaning, checking inventories, maintaining equipment, updating periodic maintenance and other patient lists, contacting insurance carriers, making collection calls, and many other tasks the office is behind on. If the dentist is gone for a week, the issue is more of a problem. Some practice owners require staff members to take vacation days when the office is closed. In small offices, it is especially a problem to let an employee take time off when they choose because of the negative effect on daily operations. The employees are there when the practice owner needs them, and they are not there when the dentist does not need them. (One person may represent a fourth of the workforce.) Some have certain employees (e.g. the front-office staff) who work but not others (the clinical staff). Others who pay their employees a salary give employees the time off with pay.

BENEFITS

An employee benefit is something of value, besides cash, that an employer provides for their employees. Benefits are valuable for employees because they are generally tax free. They are also generally a tax deduction for the employer. The law requires employers to provide some benefits, but others are optional.

COST OF BENEFITS TO THE PRACTICE

Employers may pay for benefits to their employees beyond their hourly wage. Here, the benefit cost is tax deductible to the employer, and the benefit accrues to the employee without them having to pay income taxes on the value of that benefit. Tax deductibility helps to reduce the cost to the employer of providing the benefit, but it does not eliminate the cost. The employer still must pay for the benefit.

The benefits that practice owners provide will depend largely on what is customary in the economy of the local community. The practice owner will compete with other dentists and other forms of employment in the area for excellent staff members. Early in a dentist's career, the practice is not as profitable as later. When the patient pool is larger, the dentist's skills have increased and they have paid off the start-up loans. A new practitioner may have difficulty developing a compensation package that competes with other established practitioners in the area. Nevertheless, that is precisely what the new practitioner needs to do to compete effectively. The practice owner should try to make the workplace environment an advantage in these cases. They ought to sell the office as an excellent place to work. They probably cannot attract everyone as an employee, but neither do the established practices.

VALUE OF PAY AND BENEFITS TO EMPLOYEES

Staff members want both pay and benefits in varying amounts. Employee benefits can be powerful employment motivators. Many staff (or potential staff) members understand the value of employee benefits. Some (especially those with solid union family ties) believe that it is the practice owner's obligation as the owner (management) to provide a complete benefits package for employees. Others, especially low-paid employees, often struggle to make ends meet and would rather have as much compensation as cash as possible. Those who make a higher wage (such as

hygienists) may want more compensation in tax-advantaged benefits because their basic income needs are satisfied. Some may have family benefit plans through their spouse's employer. As a practice owner develops their compensation package for employees, they need to balance these competing desires. They cannot satisfy all employees and potential employees without overpaying. One solution is a flexible benefits plan, which is described later in this section. The workplace environment and employee motivation techniques (in the next section of the chapter) also affect employee job satisfaction.

REQUIRED BENEFITS

Federal or state laws require employers to provide certain employee benefits.

Required Insurances

The law requires the employer to carry (and pay for) specific insurance on their employees. The three required insurance benefits are as follows:

- Workers' compensation provides an income to workers who are temporarily unable to work because of an injury on the job. This is insurance that the owner must purchase and carry on their employees.

- Unemployment insurance provides income to employees who lose their job through no fault of their own (e.g. layoffs, plant closings). This is a federally mandated program administered through the state via unemployment taxes.

- Social Security provides income to retirees and people with disabilities. It is a federal program jointly funded by workers, employers, and self-employed people. Social Security provides income when a family's earnings are reduced or stopped because of disability, death (survivor protection), or retirement. The government requires employers to participate in the Social Security system by matching contributions from employee withholdings.

Time Off from Work

Federal, state, and local laws require an employer to offer several types of leave. Federal law does not require this leave to be paid, but individual state or local law may require the employer to pay all (or part) of the time off.

- **Jury duty** is a function of good citizenship. Employers must allow people time off if the courts have called them for this duty. The employer must hold a comparable job open for someone who does jury duty, but the employer does not generally have to pay the employee for the time on jury duty. (Some states require employers to pay employees for time served on juries.) The employer may also require employees to return to work if their jury duty ends before regular work hours.

- **Military duty** is also a function of good citizenship. Employers must allow people the time to fulfill their obligations if they are in the military reserves. The employer may fill the position permanently or temporarily, but they must have a comparable position available for the employee when they return from active duty to work.

- Employers must allow **maternity leave** of six weeks for women who are going to give birth to a child. If their doctor says they must have more time, the employer must grant it. Further, the employer must hold a comparable job for the woman to return to, although they can temporarily fill it in her absence. Other types of family leave vary by state.

- Many states believe that **time off to vote** in major elections is an act of good citizenship. This varies from state to state.

Contracts and Benefits

Laws or contracts may require certain other benefits. These include the following:

- Depending on the **retirement plan**, tax laws may require the employer to include employees in the plan. These plans may require the employer to provide all the funds for an employee's retirement account or match the amount the employee elects to save for retirement.

- Certain **group health plans** may require minimum group participation.

- **OSHA and HIPAA** have requirements that the employer must meet regarding worker safety. This includes a worker's protective gear and clothing, supplies, vaccinations, and medical tests related to their job.

- A **contract** between the employer and employee may require that the employer provide certain benefits, such as paid time off for continuing dental education.

Unwithheld Expenses

The cost of a worker's wage is one part of the total compensation package. The required benefits are an additional cost to the employer. These are called "unwithheld" expenses because they are additional expenses to the employer, but they may not be withheld from the employee's pay. For

BOX 26.7	"UNWITHHELD" EXPENSES

Type	Percentage
FICA (including Medicare)	7.65%
SUTA (state unemployment)	2.80%
FUTA (federal unemployment)	0.80%
Workers' compensation	0.50%
Total unwithheld expenses	11.75%

every dollar of payroll, these unwithheld expenses typically cost the owner approximately an additional 12 cents. Typical unwithheld expenses are listed in Box 26.7.

OPTIONAL BENEFITS

The employer may provide many benefits to workers. Generally, these are business expenses and are therefore tax deductions for the employer. Besides the legally required benefits, any paid holidays and vacation, sick, or personal days are costs to the employer above the pure cost of employment (plus the lost production and income). If the costs of retirement plan participation and even a modest benefits package are added, the total compensation package often runs 20–40% above an employee's pure salary cost. Many employers give employees a detailed description of the entire cost of employment (see Box 26.5). The purpose of this is not to defend the wage being paid. Instead, it is to make employees aware of how much they earn because such a large portion of their compensation may be in unseen benefits.

The employer may pay for benefits for employees besides their hourly wage. Here, the benefit cost is tax deductible to the employer, and the benefit accrues to the employee without them having to pay income taxes on the value of that benefit. Tax deductibility helps to reduce the cost to the employer of providing the benefit, but it does not eliminate the cost. The employer still must pay for the benefit. As an alternative, in a properly structured plan the employer can withhold from the employee's gross pay the money needed to pay for a given benefit. The employee then, through a salary reduction, pays for the cost of the benefit. This decreases the staff member's direct pay, which also decreases the unwithheld amounts that the employer contributes. So, every dollar an employer converts from salary to benefit saves them an additional 13–24%. As a final alternative, the employer may choose to share the cost of the benefit with the employee through a combination of salary reduction and an additional compensation plan.

The employer must pay for certain other costs associated with employees (besides the required benefits listed previously). If the employer requires staff to attend a specific continuing education course, they must not only pay for the course but also pay regular wage rates for the time that the employee attends. The employer must also reimburse meals, tuition, and travel expenses. If an employee voluntarily attends a course in non-work time, the employer does not have to pay or reimburse them, even if it is practice related.

There is a long list of benefits that an employer can offer to employees. These vary significantly across the United States and within regions. Benefits should be set based on what is common in the practice area so that practice owners can compete effectively for employees. A practice owner will not provide all the benefits detailed here – the cost would be too great – but it gives an idea of commonly provided benefits in dental offices.

- **Paid vacation days**
  Many US dental practices (about 90%) offer paid vacation days. Typically, employees may receive 1 week of paid vacation after a year of employment, 2 weeks after 5 years, and 3 weeks after 10 years of employment. Dental office owners often require that employees take these vacation days when the office is closed.

- **Paid sick or personal days**
  Many dental offices (about half) offer additional sick or personal days for staff members. Others require staff to use vacation days (or generic time off) for sickness or personal reasons.

- **Health insurance**
  About half of dental offices offer health insurance as an employee benefit. They often do this through sharing arrangements, such as a salary reduction or contributing up to a certain amount toward the health insurance premium. This is an expensive benefit that many employees require in the workplace.

- **Dental care**
  Almost all dental offices offer their employees dental care, free of charge or at a reduced rate. Some require that employees pay any direct costs, such as laboratory bills. Some offer the benefit to immediate family members as well.

- **Retirement plan contribution**
  About half of dental offices contribute to a retirement plan. There are many types of plans, and the contribution amount varies greatly. Generally, the rules for retirement plans state that if the office has a plan, all employees must participate.

- **Continuing education**
  More than half of dental practices pay for continuing education for their staff members. This improves the abilities of staff members and increases their sense of personal fulfillment on the job.

- **Bonus plan**
  About a quarter of dental practices offer a bonus plan, where staff can make additional income by meeting targeted goals. Some employees respond accordingly to the desire for additional income.

FLEXIBLE BENEFIT PLANS

Each staff person will have their own needs, wants, and desires regarding a benefit plan. For example, the worker whose spouse works at a Fortune 500 company and receives a complete benefits package will have a different set of benefit needs than the single parent. Many benefits, such as health insurance, are costly for employers. Others, such as paid time off (vacation or sick days), result in payments to the staff member and lost production from not having that person in the office. Giving all benefits to all employees would therefore be prohibitively expensive, even for a well-established practitioner. One solution is to develop a flexible benefit or "cafeteria" plan. In these plans, an employee who does not need health insurance could decide to have dependent care expenses withheld for their children who are in daycare. These plans consist of a group of benefit possibilities that employees may choose among, like choosing a meal at a food cafeteria. The employees probably cannot get all the benefits, but they can get the ones most important to them. An employee may choose health insurance, another dependent care allowance and life insurance. In contrast, a third employee may choose to take no benefits and receive the entire amount as taxable income. Tax laws are explicit on this topic but are subject to change. Practice owners must consult an accountant or tax planner regarding their current deductibility.

Benefits cost the employer less than paying an equivalent amount in wages. This is because the employer does not have to pay the unwithheld expenses. Benefits also hold a significant financial advantage for employees in that they do not have Social Security/Medicare taxes withheld and because they gain the full value of the benefit without having income taxes withheld. For example, assume an employee wants a health insurance package that costs $200

	No benefit plan	Flexible plan	Employer-paid plan
Gross pay	$20 000	$17 600	$20 000
Pretax insurance	$0	$2400	$2 400
Taxable income	$20 000	$17 600	$20 000
FICA taxes (@ 7.65%)	$1 530	$1346	$1 530
Retirement plan contribution (@ 5%)	$1 000	$880	$1 000
Net, pretax cost of employment	**$22 530**	**$22 226**	**$24 930**

BOX 26.8 — THREE TYPES OF BENEFIT PLANS AND TOTAL COST OF EMPLOYMENT

This chart shows the effect of three types of benefit plans on an employer's total cost of employment. It assumes that the employee needs health insurance (@ $2400/year), has a gross pay of $20 000, and the dental practice also has a retirement plan to which it contributes 5% of each employee's pay.

per month ($2400 per year). Their gross pay is $10 per hour ($20 000 per year) and the tax rate is 25%. Two options are available. The first option is to receive full pay, fewer taxes, and then buy health insurance with after-tax dollars. The second option is to have the amount withheld from their paycheck as part of a tax-free, flexible benefit plan and then receive the difference (less taxes) as pay. Box 26.8 shows the practical effect on the employee. The employee has an increase in net spendable income of $600 simply by having the insurance taken out as a pretax benefit instead of paying for it with posttax dollars. The employer saves approximately $282 through the second option because it pays the unwithheld expenses (11.75%) on the reduced taxable income. This sounds like the perfect "free lunch," with both sides winning. The government, through the tax deductibility of employee benefit plans, ends up subsidizing the difference in cost.

These 125 plans (named for Section 125 of the Internal Revenue Code) allow employees to choose between cash salary (taxable) and non-taxed benefits. Because the employee may take the compensation as cash, the employer can finance the entire cost of the benefit through employee salary reductions. These plans offer significant advantages (such as flexibility and cost control). Still, they have the disadvantage that the employee may lose the money allocated to the benefit plan if it is not used by the end of the plan year. (This is the "use it or lose it" rule.)

Flexible benefit plans are easy and inexpensive to operate. (The employer should use a benefits specialist to set up the plan.) The unwithheld expenses they do not pay on benefits offset the administrative costs. For example, if three employees reduce their salaries by $200 per month, the employer does not pay the unwithheld expenses on $7200 of the employees' salary per year. That translates into total savings on employee taxes for the employer of approximately $850. The more employees shelter, the more money the employer saves in employer taxes. However, the employer should not view these flexible benefit plans as a tax "gold mine." The administrative expenses will often about equal the tax savings. More importantly, a flexible benefit plan allows the employer to compete effectively for employees by offering a benefit package that meets each employee's most important benefit needs at the least cost to the employer. As a result, the employer should have better, more loyal employees.

PROCESSING STAFF PAYCHECKS

Writing staff paychecks involves several steps beyond the typical office expense check. Some offices hire a payroll company to process staff paychecks. Many others use a computer program (such as Quick Payroll) to process checks. Still others use the forms and material sent by the Internal Revenue Service (IRS). All of these work. The deciding factors are the number of checks to process and the dentist's or bookkeeper's comfort level with payroll issues. This discussion focuses on the theory of payrolls so that practice owners will understand how to use any payroll system.

When employers prepare a payroll check for an employee, the IRS requires that they estimate the income tax that the employee owes, withhold it from the employee's pay, and send it to the IRS. At the end of the year, the employee calculates their actual tax liability and compares it to the amount the employer withheld along the way. If the employer withheld too much, the employee gets a refund of that amount. If the employer withheld too little, the employee owes extra tax to make up the difference.

At the end of the month (or quarter, depending on the agency), the employer sends each taxing agency a check for all the taxes that are withheld from all employees for the payroll period. The employer can use the general office checking account and does not have to have a separate or unique account for holding this money. At the end of the month, the employer sends the US Treasury all the

BOX 26.9	PROCESSING STAFF PAYCHECKS

An employee, Susan, earns $20 per hour and works 40 hours this week. She has $100 withheld weekly for medical insurance. Her paycheck for the period would be as follows:

Gross pay ($20.00 × 40)	$800.00
Health insurance	$100.00
Taxable income	**$700.00**
Federal income tax withheld, from Tax Table (Circular E)	$52.00
Social Security (FICA) withheld ($700 × 6.2%)	$43.40
Medicare withheld ($700 × 1.45%)	$10.15
State income tax withheld ($700 × 6%, state income tax rate of 6%)	$42.00
Local income tax withheld ($700 × 1.5%, city income tax of 1.5%)	$10.50
Net pay	**$541.95**

The employer will write Susan's check for $541.95 and will keep the remainder ($158.05) in an account along with other employees' withholdings to pay to the various taxing agencies. The employer must add $53.55 (7.65% of $700) as the matching portion of FICA and pay the health insurance premium for Susan.

taxes withheld from all employees for the month (federal income, Social Security, and Medicare taxes) and their matching amounts for Social Security and Medicare (Box 26.9). The employer can make one online payment, which the IRS electronically deducts from the office checking account. State and local tax agencies have similar rules and procedures.

To know how much tax to withhold, the employer must have each employee complete a Form W-4 annually. (These forms can be downloaded from the IRS website or obtained from an accountant.) This form declares the marital status and number of exemptions claimed by the employee. The employer then looks up the gross pay in the appropriate table and deducts the given amount from the employee's gross pay for taxes. (Again, computer systems have the tables built into their software.) The IRS sends a publication (Circular E) to all employers that describe these withholdings and gives tables that dictate how much the employer must withhold from each employee's check. (The employer does not have a choice. They must follow

the tax withholding table amounts.) Many US states, counties, and cities have similar income or occupational tax requirements for employers. They will also send the employer tax tables that describe how much to withhold from employees' paychecks for their various taxes. Payroll computer programs have these tables built into them to make the calculations easier. Because tax rates and rules change frequently, the employer needs to be sure to have an updated payroll package, or they might withhold the wrong amount.

Besides income tax, employers must also withhold Social Security and Medicare taxes and send these to the federal government. These payroll taxes are covered by the Federal Insurance Contributions Act (FICA) and the money collected funds these programs. Employers withhold a certain amount from employees' pay (earned income), then match it with additional company money and send the entire amount to the government. Currently, employers withhold 6.2% for Social Security and 1.45% for Medicare from wages for a total withholding of 7.65%. The employers then match this amount (totaling 15.3%) and send both to the government. There is an upper limit on the Social Security portion (currently about $150 000 adjusted for inflation). Any earnings beyond this amount are only subject to the Medicare portion of the tax.

To begin processing the payroll, the employer needs to know the number of hours worked for the week and the hourly wage for each employee. The employer finds the hours worked for each employee from a time clock or other record. The hourly wage is decided on through annual performance appraisals and reviews. The gross wage is simply the hours worked times the per-hour wage. If there is an employee benefit plan, the employer first subtracts tax-deductible amounts for benefits, which leads to taxable income. In this way, taxes are not withheld from benefits. From this, the employer subtracts the table amount for income tax withheld and calculates the amount for FICA. This results in the employee's net pay. The employer then writes the check to the employee for net pay, leaving the withheld amounts in the checkbook.

If a dentist operates as a corporation, they are an employee of the corporation. When dentists pay themselves, they withhold taxes, just like any other employee. If a dentist operates as a proprietor, partnership, or disregarded entity, they are an owner, not an employee. Instead of withholding taxes, the dentist estimates their tax liability and pays it quarterly to the government. Instead of FICA, the IRS imposes a similar tax on the earnings of self-employed individuals called SETA from the

SelfEmployment Tax Act. It is like FICA in amount and is calculated using a specific form (Schedule SE).

THE COST OF A STAFF MEMBER LEAVING

Staff compensation is the single largest expense item for most dental practices. If a staff member leaves the practice, the practice incurs additional hidden costs. These include lost production from not having the employee, additional pay for other employees to cover the lost time, the cost of advertising the position, time away from production for interviews and selection, and lower production while the new staff person acclimates to the job. Many management experts have calculated that it costs from three to four months' pay to replace a person who leaves. For a typical chairside dental assistant, that translates to $8000–10 000. If the employer can make this a smooth transition, they can keep these costs on the lower end. It obviously costs more if an employee walks out with a full schedule of patients, rather than giving several weeks' notice so that the employer can begin the replacement process. The employer must balance the cost of turnover with the cost of paying additional wages and benefits.

Part 3: Motivating Employees to Perform Well

There are no bad regiments. Only bad colonels.

Napoleon

GOAL

This part aims to describe how to motivate staff in the dental office.

LEARNING OBJECTIVES

At the completion of this part, the student will be able to:

- Differentiate between leadership and motivation.

- Describe the three factors that affect a person's performance on the job.

- Describe the major motivation perspectives and give examples of their application in the dental office:
  o Work ethic
  o Theory X and Theory Y
  o Need theories
  o Equity theory

- Define guidelines for a proper incentive plan.

KEY TERMS

ability	legitimate power
coercive power	motivation
content perspectives	need theories
equity theory	reward power
expert power	Theory X
incentive plans	Theory Y
leadership	work ethic

Before deciding on a particular wage and benefits package, it is important to understand why some people are motivated in the office and others are not. This is such an important issue that management experts have been doing research in this area for many years. Most now believe that pay and benefits are a baseline or threshold employers must meet to develop a motivated worker. Motivation then comes from the achievement, growth, and recognition gained from the job. Employers must cover both factors to have a truly satisfied and motivated worker. According to this theory, employees will be dissatisfied if they are not paid enough. However, simply paying an adequate, or even excessive, wage will not produce a more motivated worker. It may lead to a worker who is less likely to leave because of the high pay. Still, it does not make the person a better or more motivated worker.

Researchers have developed many other theories to explain what motivates employees in the workplace. Motivation refers to all the forces that direct, energize, and maintain a person's effort on the job. Highly motivated employees work hard to achieve their performance goals. If they have adequate skills, resources, and freedom at work, they will show high job performance. To be an effective motivator, the dental practice owner must know what behaviors they want and then stimulate and challenge employees to do those behaviors.

Three factors determine a person's performance on the job (Box 26.10). The first is the ability or physical and mental preparation to do the job. This includes all forms of training and experience. Employers assess this through the application and interview process and by licensing and training credentials. The second factor is the environment. A person cannot properly do a job without the proper setting, tools, and materials. Employers control the work environment to help in the work process. The third factor determining job performance is motivation, or desire to do the job. Employers must motivate through daily interactions with the people involved.

LEADERSHIP

People often think of leadership as an innate ability that certain people possess and others lack. Research has shown, however, that leadership, rather than being a genetic or personal trait (like blue eyes or black hair), is a style or behavior that people display. Leadership is creating a vision, having the power to translate it into reality, and then sustaining it over time. Leaders inspire people to perform; managers see that the organization runs smoothly. In the dental office, the dentist will fulfill both of those roles.

Leadership means working with the office's employees (dental team members) to have a shared office goal and then getting the people to "buy into" the goal and work toward meeting that goal. It is the human factor that binds the workgroup together and makes it function at its peak. Leadership involves power but is not necessarily pure power. It is the employer's ability to influence those who work for them (Box 26.11). As the owner of the practice, the owner has *legitimate* power over the people they hire to work for them. The employer can legally fire or reprimand employees and set work conditions (such as hours of employment). The employer also has *reward* power in establishing pay scales and offering raises, as well as issuing recognition and praise for performance. Conversely, the employer may also punish non-compliance by using *coercive* power. Because dentists have unique skills, training, knowledge, and certification (licensing), they also have power as an *expert* that other employees do not have. *Personal* power comes from the influence that an employer may (or may not) have over others through the force of individual personality.

BOX 26.10	THREE FACTORS OF JOB PERFORMANCE

Ability
Environment
Motivation

BOX 26.11	TYPES OF LEADERSHIP POWER

Legitimate
Reward
Coercive
Expert
Personal

Leadership then involves getting the people in the office to perform as the employer wants them to by the employer's behavior influencing the employees' behavior. The effectiveness of the employer's leadership depends on several factors. The employer's background, experience, personality, and style will affect their leadership effectiveness. An equally important factor is the background, experience, and personality of the followers in the office. If there is not an appropriate match, then the interaction is destined to fail. Finally, leaders who understand a subordinate's task are in a much better position to select an appropriate leadership style and strategy to fit the situation. To understand these interactions, employers first must understand themselves.

WHY PEOPLE WORK

Many dentists believe that a person will work harder if they are paid more. Many also believe that pay is the only reason that people work. However, modern management proposes that people work for reasons other than just pay. (After all, many people put in many hours of volunteer work for organizations that pay nothing.) Although people must meet their financial needs, they also work because of the friendships they form on the job and the sense of personal accomplishment and value they can gain from a job. It follows, then, that if people work for these other reasons, a business owner can motivate them to work harder or do better by arranging the job so that they can accomplish these needs.

Modern management experts believe that people work for three reasons: compensation (pay and benefits),

BOX 26.12	REASONS PEOPLE WORK

Compensation
    Pay
    Benefits
Psychological reasons
Social reasons

psychological reasons (personal growth and fulfillment), and social reasons (friendships and relationships in the workplace) (Box 26.12). As the manager–dentist, the practice owner must control these motivational factors to develop and encourage excellent employees. That is a difficult task in itself. To make the problem even more difficult, different employees want varying amounts and types of fulfillment in each of these areas. Obviously, motivating employees to work at their peak level can be a complex problem.

COMPENSATION

People often use pay as a comparative indicator of success. Even those who do not need money from work may use their earnings to supplement the family income or fund special needs or savings plans. So, people will only work if the pay is adequate, but adequate pay alone is not a good job motivator. And pay is only a short-term motivator. If someone receives a raise, they will work harder for a while, but the new pay level soon becomes the norm and they return to the previous work level. If an employee views the raise as recognition for work well done, that recognition can become a longer-term motivator on the job.

PSYCHOLOGICAL REASONS

People want to believe that they have a purpose in life and that their life has meaning. An important job or a job that contributes to others' well-being helps bring meaning to people's lives. Some people define themselves by the job they hold. They have strong psychological reasons for their work. Everyone continues to grow their entire life in knowledge, skill, and abilities and in spiritual and emotional ways. Many people look to their work environment to provide some of that growth, both professional and personal.

The practice needs specific tasks to be done. The purpose of the practice, after all, is not to provide a country club atmosphere or a self-help venue for its employees. However, if a practice owner understands what excites people about their jobs, they can structure the job or work setting to encourage motivated people to work better. This leads to a more successful practice.

SOCIAL REASONS

People often form friendships and personal relationships with coworkers. Daily interaction with a group of people is a social function that many enjoy in the workplace. Because people spend such a significant portion of their adult waking lives in the work setting, many look for and appreciate close personal relationships that develop. Staff members may meet socially outside the office, and their families may become close as they share personal and family triumphs and failures. This helps lead to a cohesive workgroup in the office.

The owner–dentist is in a problematic situation regarding social interaction. They want to promote a cohesive team atmosphere in the office, but they are still the boss. The employer is responsible for staff direction, evaluations, raises, and discipline. Therefore, they tread a fine line between being friendly (pleasant, warm, concerned, and engaging) to staff and being friends with them. (It is difficult to discipline or fire an employee, much less a friend.) Employers should keep a certain distance between themselves and workers. This helps insulate them from staff members claiming that the employer shows favoritism toward a particular staff member and helps remove claims of harassment.

THE WORK ENVIRONMENT

Many dentists believe that job motivation is a trait that a person either possesses or does not possess and that they can do little to influence motivation. The experience and history of US business do not bear out this belief. Most people want to do well on the job and are willing to work hard if they are reasonably sure that their hard work will result in a meaningful pay-off (financial, social, or personal). This is the point where owner–dentists can affect the environment in their practice by setting goals and reward systems that allow and encourage motivated people to succeed in their jobs. The employer can encourage those workers who value personal development to take continuing education courses and report to the group important items learned. They also can encourage work-related social activities for those who value that aspect of their job. For those motivated more by money, the employer can establish a pay system that rewards taking on additional duties or work.

How a manager arranges job tasks and the work environment profoundly affects the motivation of employees. As the manager of a small business (i.e. the dental practice), the dentist is responsible for formulating policies and an environment that enhances the practice's productivity. Employee work habits, turnover, tardiness, and performance affect productivity. By learning which factors lead to enhanced motivation of employees, employers can understand what causes workers' behaviors (good and bad), predict the effect of policy changes, and direct workers' behaviors to meet the business's needs better.

The basic paradigm of a motivation system is to define the job's objectives as to the practice needs, identify a person's needs, and then set a system that encourages constructive behavior on the job by rewarding proper behaviors and punishing or extinguishing improper behaviors. This assumes that the dentist can clearly define challenging yet attainable goals, that there is an effective ongoing system for monitoring the attainment of those goals, and that constructive methods of thinking about performance are present.

EMPLOYEE MOTIVATION CONCEPTS

Researchers have proposed that several theories help explain what motivates people at work. If employers can learn what motivates people on the job, they can structure the job to have more motivated employees. None of these theories explains all the motivation (or lack of motivation) that occurs in the workplace. However, they are all helpful in explaining some of the motivation that occurs or certain cases of motivation or demotivation.

WORK ETHIC

Dentists are highly motivated, successful workers. The practice of dentistry is inherently interesting and rewarding work with high levels of responsibility, growth, and self-fulfillment for the dentist. Dental schools have screened dentists for success and work habits through the educational process. The work has value in itself. In this sense, it is a terminal value, like honesty. Many people think that a strong work ethic is internalized among good people. However, people value the meaning of work differently. Some people do not believe that work is a terminal value (i.e. a desirable activity by itself), but instead it is an instrumental value (i.e. it produces desired consequences). These people may be hard workers, but they see the job as a means rather than an end unto itself. They view their work as simply a job. They work to get paid; their motivation is external to them. Others view their employment as a career. They have long-term outlooks and long-term employment goals. Their work fits into a life script; their motivation is internal (Box 26.13).

BOX 26.13   THE WORK ETHIC

Terminal value	<-------->	Instrumental value
Career	<-------->	Job
Internal motivation	<-------->	External motivation

These two conflicting views are seen in the extreme examples of a "workaholic" who places exaggerated importance on work, and the teenager who works only to buy clothes and gas for their car. The rewards needed to motivate them will vary with the worker's perceived importance of work. This perceived importance or "work ethic" is not an entirely fixed internal response. It is some personal combination of moral obligation, productivity, pride in work, commitment to employers, and an achievement orientation that others can influence, to a degree, by the work environment. In other words, rewards may influence the extent to which workers perceive work to be important.

THEORY X AND THEORY Y

Douglas McGregor developed a related idea concerning a manager's perceptions of human beings at work that he detailed in his 1960 book *The Human Side of Enterprise*. He described two opposing views of how managers perceive how people approach work. One he called Theory X; the other, Theory Y. Theory X and Theory Y are not distinct types but a continuum, with a theory at each end. Theory X adherents believe that workers are lazy, dislike work, lack ambition, dislike responsibility, are easily duped, and prefer to be directed. Theory X managers, therefore, are more authoritarian, task oriented, boss centered, and use external controls. On the other hand, Theory Y adherents believe that work is a natural activity for most people, that they are internally motivated, and that they willingly seek and accept responsibility. Theory Y managers are more democratic, participative, employee oriented, and people and process oriented (Box 26.14).

McGregor believed that Theory X is a destructive, self-fulfilling prophecy. Theory X beliefs lead to policies and practices that tightly control employees. (In this system, managers believe that workers see their work as just a job.) This leads to withdrawal and resentment by the workers. The manager then observes these negative behaviors that reinforce their beliefs in the nature of people, leading to tighter controls.

A manager–dentist's view of the nature of workers will profoundly affect the techniques they use to motivate

BOX 26.14   THEORY X AND THEORY Y

Theory X	Theory Y
Workers	
Lazy, lack ambition	Self-directed, seek responsibility
Prefer external control	Prefer internal control
Managers	
Close supervision	General supervision
Directive	Supportive
Authoritarian	Participative
Boss centered	Employee centered
Task oriented	Relationship oriented

BOX 26.15   ERG THEORY

Alderfer's levels	Components
Growth (personal)	Self-esteem, self-actualization, achievement
Relatedness (social)	Social and interpersonal relations, esteem of others
Existence (pay and benefits)	Physical safety and human existence

staff members and, in turn, the workers' response. A practice owner who views workers through Theory X will have much tighter control and use more external rewards than the Theory Y-oriented dentist. This highly controlling, distrustful atmosphere may be appropriate in certain situations, but the practice owner must be willing to realize the almost inevitable results: employee resentment, turnover, and dissatisfaction. On the other hand, the Theory Y manager must also be aware of that system's limitations. Too often, ideas of efficiency, production, and results are secondary to people's growth in and enjoyment of work. Purely internal rewards may not be enough to get the best results.

NEED THEORIES

Need theories are based on the supposition that everyone has needs or internal stimuli they want to satisfy. Jobs have various attributes that may or may not correlate with a person's needs. Because actions are based on some intrinsically (within the individual) determined need, people often think that everyone will react similarly. This perspective assumes that attitudes, job characteristics, and behavior are related. People's behavior is an attempt to satisfy their needs. Incentives reward people for satisfying those needs. Needs determine the motivational value of incentives. The manager's job is to decide what those needs are and then to structure the work environment to allow people to satisfy their needs best.

Abraham Maslow developed the best-known idea of human motivation. He believed that people have five different needs or internal stimuli: physiological, safety, belongingness, esteem, and self-actualization. These form

a hierarchy, with self-actualization at the top. Clayton Alderfer proposed one well-known simplification of Maslow's hierarchy. His modification collapsed the five levels of needs into three – existence, relatedness, and growth – and is known as ERG theory (Box 26.15). Alderfer believed that all three levels influence work motivation, but not equally. Existence needs are satisfied primarily by extrinsic rewards (e.g. pay, fringe benefits). Relatedness is satisfied through friendships and interaction with coworkers. Growth needs (the highest-preference needs) are intrinsic motivators and are satisfied through the opportunity to learn and advance and through positive responses. People can respond to different levels simultaneously. For example, money (E), friendship (R), and learning new skills (G) may all be motivators for a person. Alderfer's theory forms the basis of the initial proposition of this part that people work for compensation (existence), social reasons (relatedness), and personal reasons (growth).

The implications of ERG theory for dentists are important. Practice owners cannot change employees' needs but they can react to them by manipulating incentives (means) to satisfy them. Practice owners must tie existence needs to incentives to work. Formal and informal groups, and formal titles and office organization, will help meet relatedness needs in the dental office. The practice owner can influence all these. They can meet growth needs by creating a proper climate that will encourage and enable employees to develop to their full potential.

Practice owners may see the effects of unrecognized needs in the common dental office problem of staff members (often hygienists) having basic existence and relatedness needs being met and still being unfulfilled in the job role. Often, this situation results from the staff member wanting to fulfill those higher-level needs represented by growth or actualization. If no one allows and encourages these people to expand their roles, continued unhappiness and eventual departure are the almost inevitable results.

$$\frac{I_s}{O_s} = \frac{I_s}{O_o}$$

Where: I_s = Input of self
I_o = Input of others
O_s = Output of self
O_o = Output of others

EQUITY THEORY

Equity theory is based on group influences (Box 26.16). It asks whether people feel they are being treated fairly compared with others based on the value of their contribution. Each person has expected outcomes (rewards) from the work setting. These may be external (pay, promotion, benefits) or internal (recognition, social relationships, satisfaction). To get those outcomes, people realize that they must have certain inputs. These may be time, expertise, effort, education, hours worked, certification, or loyalty. Equity theory assumes that people compare themselves with others and assess the fairness of the outcome considering the inputs required. This "other" may be a specific person or group of people, or it may be a composite of a given workforce. Based on this subjective and personal comparison, employees will decide if they are equitably rewarded, under-rewarded, or over-rewarded for the input required. If the employees feel under-rewarded, they will likely put forth less effort (lower inputs), ask for a raise (increase inputs), rationalize the difference, get others to change their inputs or outcomes, or seek new employment. If employees feel overcompensated, they may increase their effort to balance the outputs, or simply justify the higher reward.

Equity theory has clear implications for the dentist who manages a practice. This theory is based on group and social norms, which are prevalent in small businesses. It involves a person's perception of the values of inputs and outcomes. Those perceptions, although not necessarily the truth, are the reality for that person and must be viewed as such. The accuracy of a person's information becomes important. People may view the group to which they compare themselves entirely differently from the dentist. This raises the problems of job values and the comparable worth of different jobs in the office. Finally, for rewards to motivate, employees must perceive them as fair and equitable, or the difference will exacerbate the issue.

Equity theory probably has more implications for pay systems than for any aspect related to practice management.

Auxiliaries in a practice will compare earnings, and any discrepancy between what a person earns and what they believe they should earn may result in problems. Consequently, the practice owner needs to pay particular attention to designing a compensation system that is equitable and well understood by employees. Practice owners should tell the employee how they relate performance to possible pay increases and what level of performance will result in a salary increase.

Employees compare their wages to other people in the dental office. Although it is easy to make a policy that "All pay issues must be strictly confidential," it is quite another to keep that confidentiality. Eventually, everyone in the office will know what everyone else is making. They will then compare their pay to others to see if they are being treated, in their mind, fairly or equitably. If the employees do not understand how salaries are determined, resentment and hostility may arise because of a lack of knowledge about how the dentist decides salaries. The hygienist may make $15 an hour more than an expanded-duty dental assistant (EDDA). Still, an employee may see that as reasonable, given the additional training and certification required of the hygienist. However, if another assistant makes 50 cents an hour more but has no additional skills, training, or work habits, the same employee will see that as inequitable and experience job dissatisfaction. This comparison with other employees in the office is called *internal equity*.

Employees make the same types of comparisons with alternate forms of employment in the same geographic area. This comparison is called *external equity*. A staff member may know other dental assistants working for other local dentists and making different wage and benefit rates. Or a person with the general training and skill level of a dental assistant may work at a local bank or grocery store for $3 more an hour and a complete benefits package. Both external comparisons lead to equity considerations outside the practitioner's control.

Employees may feel either or both types of equity problems simultaneously. Both internal and external types are important to employees and therefore are important in wage rate determinations. The prevailing economic conditions, general wage and benefit rates, and local unemployment situation all affect the amount dental practice owners must pay to attract productive employees.

INCENTIVE PLANS: USING MONEY TO MOTIVATE

Many dentists believe that money motivates all employees. All they need to do is establish a bonus or incentive plan, and all employees will work harder to make more money. Often a bonus plan can help the office to increase productivity. Unfortunately, this idea is not a panacea for poor management. Practice owners must carefully structure incentive plans, or the plans may backfire and cause more problems than they were designed to solve.

GUIDELINES FOR INCENTIVE PLANS

The dental office owner can use the following points as guidelines for incentive plans:

- **Each incentive plan must have a specific goal**
  Most employers have the simple goal of "increasing production." However, they must accurately identify the real problem. The problem may be a lack of new patients or a poor collection policy. If an ineffective recall system, poor scheduling, or poorly performing employees cause low production, the practice owner must first address that problem. By establishing goals and rewards that address the specific issue, an incentive plan can help to achieve the goal of increased production.

- **Each plan must have appropriate rewards**
  The practice owner must ensure that their incentive plan has a proper employee reward system. Not all employees are motivated by money. (In fact, many employees are internally motivated.) Certainly, the prospect of making more money motivates some employees to work harder. Others may not feel that the rewards are worth the extra work, time, and effort required. They may be motivated by the possibility of additional time off, office trips, or continuing education courses. Establishing an effective bonus plan can be difficult when office employees are motivated by different incentives.

- **Staff members must have control over critical factors needed to meet the goal**
  If the dentist is slowing down production (because they enjoy talking with patients), the staff has no real control of the problem (the dentist's style). They can therefore do nothing to increase production (schedule effectively). Staff performance must be the critical factor causing the lack of goal attainment.

- **The practice owner must be ready to manage collateral problems**
  Every action in the dental office has collateral or unintended side effects. The employee focus becomes the attainment of the goal, not necessarily the work itself. If the dentist wants to see additional patients and the schedule is full, they should be ready to work longer hours or through lunch. This will cause employee dissatisfaction.

- **Incentive plans lose their effectiveness over time**
  The lack of money can be a demotivator, but money will only be a short-term incentive. Soon employees grow to expect the bonus as pay. A guaranteed bonus decreases the motivation to work hard to achieve the bonus. However, constantly increasing the goal leads to staff frustration as practice owners expect them to achieve ever-higher production levels.

DEVELOPING INCENTIVE PLANS

Given these problems with incentive plans, dentists need to follow certain steps if they want to develop an effective plan:

- **Make sure management systems are well constructed**
  The dentist must do everything they can, as the practice owner and manager, to increase production. They need to have an excellent scheduling system; have employee job descriptions, performance appraisals, and compensation policies in line; and make sure credit and collection policies are effective.

- **Be sure the incentive system is easy to administer and understand**
  The dentist can probably pick out one or two numbers (from the end-of-month computer report) and decide if they have met their goals. The dentist also needs an easy method of dividing the bonus. Is it equal shares, based on pay, or based on hours worked?

- **Identify goals to achieve**
  Most offices simply say they "want to increase production." Is that really the goal, or is the real goal to increase staff productivity to increase doctor take-home pay? Some goals are best for individuals, others for groups. If the goal is to increase recall effectiveness and the hygienist runs the recall system, the practice owner does not need to involve others in the incentive system. Conversely, a goal of increasing new patient visits will probably need to involve everyone in the office.

- **Identify what motivates employees**
  The challenge to receive more pay may motivate some employees. Additional vacation days, money, or office vacations may motivate others. The practice owner should talk with the employees and come to a consensus on what will get the employees to buy into the incentive plan. The office owner should set a reward system that is achievable but is also difficult to attain.

- **Follow-up**
  Employees need to know how well they are doing in meeting their goals. Employees and staff should celebrate and congratulate each other when they meet the goals. If the goals are not met, the practitioner should sit with everyone and develop a plan to meet them in the next period. The practice owner needs to be careful that incentives do not become entitlements.

Part 4: Assessing Employee Performance

Start with good people, lay out the rules, communicate with your employees, motivate them and reward them. If you do all those things effectively, you can't miss.

Lee Iacocca

GOAL

This part aims to prepare new graduates to hire, compensate, and motivate staff for the dental office.

LEARNING OBJECTIVES

At the completion of this part, the student will be able to:

- Describe how to develop a performance appraisal review.
- Describe the process for terminating employees.
- Describe the areas in which a former employee might successfully sue for wrongful termination.
- Describe the use of performance appraisals in the dental office.
- Describe a progressive discipline system.
- Describe how an employee might try to "get even" for being fired.

KEY TERMS

constructive discharge
implied contract
performance appraisal
  review (PAR)

progressive discipline
unjust dismissal (wrongful
  termination)
whistle-blower

Most employees want to do well on the job. Both intrinsic and extrinsic rewards are valid goals toward which workers strive. They need and want fair and accurate appraisals based on standards of performance that explain what the business owner expects of them. Practice owners should not compare employees with each other, but instead should evaluate them based on how well each performs on the job. Appraisals must identify individual outputs or goals. They must also be honest to be effective. If employees perceive the appraisals as dishonest (e.g. performance was not adequate but was rated as adequate), then the appraisals will be ineffective. Appraisals should evaluate skill, knowledge, responsibilities, and special certification levels but not the job's worth. Employees should not view appraisals as punitive but as suggesting ways to improve. The employer must incorporate a formal response system so that the employee can relate their personal performance to the review.

Given these requirements for fair and accurate performance appraisals, it is little wonder that both manager–dentists and workers view them suspiciously. Everyone appraises each of their associates continually and informally. (Coffee room gossip frequently concerns people who are not present.) Practitioners also continually assess (informally) workers' appearance, behavior, and motivation. Yet when practice owners begin a formal review system, there is often initial resistance from staff and the owner–dentist. Employees fear job appraisals for reasons of job security and reprisals. Practice owners are fearful because of the time needed, the responsibility for objectivity, and the loss of personal power to a "system." Once a proper system is in place and working, however, both employees and employers generally find their fears to be unfounded.

PERFORMANCE APPRAISAL AND REVIEWS

A performance appraisal and review (PAR) has two general purposes. First, it justifies personnel-related actions. By objectively appraising work done, the manager has a solid basis for actions such as a promotion, rewards for past performance, a probationary review, or a warning for unacceptable behavior. Secondly, a PAR helps in counseling employees. Managers can better use staff by improving performance, assigning work more efficiently, meeting employees' needs for growth, recognizing potential, and identifying training needs.

The result of the PAR should not be a surprise to an employee. Practitioners ought to give immediate, constructive feedback every day. If an employee performs excellently at a task, the dentist should praise them on the spot. The dentist should let the employee know (sincerely) why this was a good performance and how much that means to the practice's success. The employee likely will repeat this behavior or action. Conversely, if someone does a poor job, the dentist should tell them on the spot (in private) why the behavior was unacceptable and what they can do to improve their performance. Most employees will try to improve.

PARs have several spin-offs as well. They help in the selection/hiring process. Selection of the best person for any job is a difficult task. To find the best person, employers first identify job-related behaviors and qualifications so that they can hire someone who meets those criteria. This is the basis of a PAR system. Instead of an informal, intuitive idea of the traits needed, practice owners generate a list of specific characteristics from the review process. They can use properly conducted PARs as contracts. By using PARs for feedback, goal setting, rewards, and punishments, dentists can motivate employees to accept change. Practice owners are on much more solid legal ground when they take personnel actions if a PAR system is in use. They can objectively show reasons for promotions, raises, and dismissals. The use of a PAR system can improve employee involvement in the practice. Employees who do tasks often define acceptable behaviors better than their managers. By defining goals and objectives and gaining the active participation of employees in the process, business owners improve the performance of the whole organization.

CONSTRUCTING PERFORMANCE APPRAISAL AND REVIEW

Practice owners must properly construct performance appraisals for these to be effective. PARs may harm employee motivation and performance if they are done poorly or under unsatisfactory conditions. Employers should enact the following guidelines for effective performance reviews:

- Before conducting the review, the practice owner determines the purpose (coaching, salary appraisal, criticism) and ensures that the objectives do not conflict.

- The practice owner ensures that the staff members know what is expected of them in their jobs. Many employers use the employee's job description as the basis of the PAR. This document describes what tasks the employee does on the job. It is outcome related, not attitudinal. It looks at job behaviors (what people do on the job), not attitudes (whether they like their job).

- A PAR should reflect all the duties involved in the job, but only those duties. Components should be weighted to represent their importance.

- The employer sets standards of acceptable behaviors and presents employees with the "who, how, what, and when" of performance. The PAR specifies both acceptable and unacceptable behaviors.

- The practice owner gives an immediate, constructive response so that employees know the appraisal results. Writing down a verbal appraisal gives direction to the employee and is a strong base against future disagreements.

- The practice owner develops tangible and identifiable rewards, punishments, or assistance for outcomes or specific behaviors.

- PAR is an ongoing, long-term system for performance improvement rather than a one-time punitive system. It should be followed up with "mini-reviews" of problems identified during the formal review. If PARs are used to dismiss employees, employees will perceive them as such and the system will lose all effectiveness.

- The employer seeks the employee's input during the review about their performance and problems on the job. The practice owner asks for ways to make the job easier (and, therefore, the office more efficient). Many dental staff members doubt that their dentists genuinely listen to their job problems, so they must be listened to.

- PAR does not replace continual immediate reactions in the workplace. If a staff member does a task particularly well or poorly, the owner notices and comments on it at the time. The employer then reinforces it at PAR time. The practice owner keeps a written log throughout the year of staff members' performance to help at review time.

The owner–dentist needs to consider several other issues before starting a PAR system. They need to have well-defined, written philosophies and goals. Unless the owner clearly defines the target or performance, employees cannot aim for it. The institution of such a system may require changes in the practice's philosophy, policies, or procedures. Additionally, the practice owner needs to remember that a PAR system is an ongoing review process, not a one-time effort, and must be willing to reward those who perform well through salary increases and other methods of compensation. Finally, the practice owner must be willing to spend time and energy to develop and carry out such a system.

DISCIPLINING EMPLOYEES

Most employment experts suggest that the proper way to discipline employees involves a system called "progressive discipline." In this system, the employer provides and records feedback given to an employee about their performance, suggesting ways to improve faulty performance. If the employee does not improve their performance, each round of discipline becomes progressively more severe until the employer fires the employee.

Progressive discipline encourages employees to improve performance. It also documents their poor performance. In the progressive discipline scenario, the employer gives an employee who is not performing to expectations a verbal reprimand, with methods to improve their performance. The employer notes that reprimand in the employee's personnel file. If the employee continues to perform poorly, the owner gives written notice (again with a copy in the personnel file) and methods to improve. If the employee shows no improvement, the employer suspends them for several days, warning them of possible termination. Continued poor performance leads to firing. By using this method, employees cannot reasonably claim that they did not know their performance was below standard or that their job was in jeopardy. It is also fair in that it encourages the employee to improve performance; it does not simply threaten them.

Progressive discipline requires that the employer keeps written documentation of all warnings to employees about their performance. Fortunately, this is not as big a problem as it initially sounds. As the discipline becomes more severe, the documentation needs to be more thorough. (Initial counseling may warrant a two-line note, jotted down in the employee's personnel file.) Written documentation must include the following:

- Reason for the problem.
- Corrective action to improve performance.
- Employee comments.
- Employee's signature and date.
- Employer's signature and date.

This system provides documentation of employee performance problems if the employee files charges for a breach of employer responsibility. It also helps keep discipline consistent from employee to employee. Through the act of counseling, many employees will improve their performance so that they do not need additional disciplinary steps. Finally, the dentist may find areas of policies and procedures that they need to revise to make the office work environment more effective.

Practice owners must act in all situations of poor job performance. Failure to act tells employees that the owner has no standards for work in the office. If a dentist does not take notice of an employee's sloppy work practices, then the others see that it does not matter if they are sloppy too. The result is lower standards and bad service to patients.

Taking no action is a decision that may also prevent an employer from acting in the future in a similar situation. If the employer suddenly treats one employee differently than others for a similar act of poor performance, then they are open to charges of unfairness in the workplace.

There are several aspects to remember if the practice owner decides to use a progressive discipline system in the office:

- The goal of the system is to catch poor or marginal performance early and then help employees to improve their performance in areas where there have been problems. Early coaching becomes essential. The practice owner may require an employee to take a continuing education course or do other studies, practices, or demonstrations to improve their skills. Punishment is appropriate for employees who do not improve their performance.

- The employer may repeat a step if they believe that it will help to improve performance. For example, the employer may decide that a significant amount of time has passed since the last warning and that another warning is in order. If repeating the warning and remediation work, the employer has solved the problem without escalating to a higher level. The employee should understand, however, that repeating a step may lead to higher forms of discipline.

- The employer may skip steps for serious offenses or breaches of office policy. They will generally use all the steps for routine problems, such as attendance or general work performance problems. The employer's judgment of the severity of the offense and remediation (if any) will help to define the steps to use.

Several behaviors are often excluded from a progressive discipline system. Employees are generally immediately fired for any of the following offenses:

- Reporting to work intoxicated or impaired on alcohol or illegal drugs.
- Stealing from the practice or another employee.
- Lying on an employment application or other practice document.
- Violating the confidentiality of practice or patient information.
- Causing a fight in the workplace.
- Bringing a weapon to work.
- Intentionally harassing someone (including sexual harassment).

- Insubordination.
- Extended unexcused absences.

The employer must talk with the employee about the problem and explain acceptable behavior and the consequence of failing to act appropriately.

Counseling needs to be friendly yet firm. Tell the employee the problem and try to identify a solution for the problem jointly. The practice owner must be sure that the employee has a way they can solve the performance problem. Often counseling documentation is brief, but the practice owner needs to save it in the employee's personnel file in case the performance problem continues or escalates.

If an employee is suspended from work, the employer must tell the employee the length of the suspension and that it is without pay. Usually one to several days is enough to set the stage and impress the employee with the seriousness of the problem. (Some states require employers to suspend professional people – associate dentists or some hygienists – in week-long time blocks. Practice owners should check with an attorney familiar with the state's employment law.)

For serious problems (anything more than a verbal warning), the employer needs to require the employee to sign the disciplinary record form, acknowledging that they have discussed the problem and the corrective steps required. This does not mean that the employee agrees (they do not have to agree with the employer's assessment), but that the employer has discussed the problem with them. If the employee disagrees or wants to explain their actions (there are often two sides to a story), the employer should write those on the form. If an employee refuses to sign the form, the employer must record (on the form) that the employee refused to sign.

Some management experts suggest that the practice owner should not include the progressive discipline plan in the employee manual. If they do, they should contact an employment lawyer first to check on the language and wording of the policy. The policy probably will not be used often, so if the rules are not followed exactly each time an incident occurs, the practice owner might encounter a problem. Employers need to treat employees equally. If the employer does not warn one employee about a particular performance problem but does warn another, the progressive discipline process may not protect the practice owner from legal action.

TERMINATING EMPLOYEES

Terminating (firing) an employee is perhaps the least enjoyable task a business owner can have. The employer should view firing an employee as the last option for personnel issues. If the recruitment and selection process has worked properly, the employer has given specific direction and performance responses to employees, and the compensation system is fair and equitable, firing should seldom be an issue. However, this is not always the case.

The practice may be better off by not having a particular employee around. If a staff member is not performing adequately, if the practice owner has given them notice of this and methods of improvement, and if the employee continues to perform inadequately, then firing may be in order. If an employee is found in gross violation of established laws, rules, or policies (e.g. stealing, alcohol impairment on the job, continual insubordination), firing is necessary. Finally, if a personality conflict has developed that severely impairs the effectiveness of the office team, dismissal may be in order.

GUIDELINES FOR TERMINATING EMPLOYEES

If all attempts to salvage an employee through a progressive discipline process have failed, the practice owner may decide to fire that employee. In that case, they should follow these guidelines:

- Decide beforehand what will be said and have ready all necessary information concerning the problem.

- Carefully select the day of dismissal. Most management experts suggest not firing someone on a Friday or the day before a holiday. This gives the person the weekend to stew and possibly plot revenge; the dismissed employee should be able to look for another job quickly.

- Keep all paperwork in order. The practice owner should be sure that time records are accurate (and not forged) and see if the person is due any vacation days or other benefits. If so, the employee needs to be compensated for that. The practice owner should not provoke the employee or give them any reason to involve the Wage and Hour Cabinet.

- Be firm and businesslike but sympathetic. The owner should not berate the employee for work they did not do correctly and should not argue with the employee over the validity of the information. The decision is final.

- Keep the meeting private and brief (no more than 15 minutes). The employee's final paycheck, including compensation, any benefits owed, or severance pay, should be given to them then.

- Inform the employee what will be said in future references requested by other potential employers.

- Encourage the employee to seek employment counseling or job placement services and provide the names of several agencies that might help.

- Take care of housekeeping duties, such as the return of office keys, instruments, personal effects, or other materials.

- Manage the effect of the firing on the other employees. If the other employees are not aware of all the problems, they may be wondering if they are next to be fired. If they know the problems, this will be less of an issue. The practice owner must not discuss the shortcomings of the released employee with the other employees; this invites defamation and slander actions.

LEGAL ISSUES IN DISMISSAL OF EMPLOYEES

Three primary issues are involved in firing employees: unemployment compensation problems, wage and hour laws, and legal suits related to unjust dismissal. Of these, the unemployment issue is by far the more common. Although far less common, the unjust dismissal case is much more serious. Wage and hour law problems are in the middle on both counts.

Unemployment Insurance

Unemployment insurance premiums depend on an employer's employment history, just as automobile insurance depends on a driving record. When a former employee collects unemployment compensation, it is credited against the employer's "account." Premiums may vary as a result. Unemployment compensation is available to people who lose their jobs through no fault of their own. People cannot collect unemployment if they quit a job, if someone fired them for unwillingness to work on the job, or for other due cause. If the person tries to collect unemployment or contests the firing (saying that they were not fired for cause), the unemployment department may call the employer into a hearing on the matter. This is where excellent records help. If the employer has documented the problem through performance appraisals, written warnings, and suggested improvements, they will have no problem. Without these records, the employer may see their unemployment insurance rates increase.

Wage and Hour Laws

The federal government sets employment rules through the FLSA. Each state has a Wage and Hour Cabinet or commission (they go by slightly different names) that enforces the state's wage and hour laws. Generally, this organization only becomes involved with an office if someone files a grievance against that employer. (It occasionally makes routine "field audits.") If an employee (or usually, a former employee) files a grievance concerning employment practices, the cabinet may require an employer to produce evidence to refute the claim. This is a case in which the employer is guilty unless they can prove their innocence. Excellent employee records are essential. The cabinet may use all timesheets, pay records, office policies, and vacation schedules in the review. If the employer has kept excellent records and has followed the laws about fair employment in the state, they should have no problems. If the employer cannot refute the claim, they may have to pay back overtime, vacation, or benefits, plus penalties.

Unjust Dismissal (Wrongful Termination) Suits

According to the employment-at-will doctrine, if an employee does not have a specified term of employment (such as in a contract), then that employee works "at will." Either side can end the employment relationship at any time for any reason (at the will of either party). The corollary of this is the "fire at will" doctrine, which says that an employer can fire a (non-contracted) employee at any time for any reason. Although these general principles are still in force, the courts have eroded them over time as legislatures have limited the right of employers to fire employees. Four areas have been singled out that may result in a wrongful termination lawsuit (Box 26.17):

- **Antidiscrimination**
  An employer may not fire an employee for a "wrong" reason. Several laws contribute to this list, but they generally include race, color, national origin, gender, age, disability, pregnancy, and religion. Although written statutes protect many of these groups only for large employers (15 or more employees), courts often hold the small employer to the standards of the larger employer. Many state and local laws apply these standards to all employers in their jurisdiction. The essence is, do not discriminate in hiring or firing practices.

- **Oral contract**
  Oral contracts are just as binding as written contracts. The problem with oral contracts is that when it is time to interpret them, each side has a different memory of what was said. However, if the court finds that an employer made an oral promise of job security to an employee, it may find that this is a legally binding contract.

- **Contrary to public policy**
  An employer may not fire an employee for actions that are in the public's interest. This includes requirements

BOX 26.17	**EXAMPLES OF WRONGFUL TERMINATION**

- **Antidiscrimination**

  An assistant is pregnant. The practice owner terminates her because she does not plan to return after having the baby; the practice owner wants to go ahead and get a "steady" employee. Her wrongful termination suit will probably win.

- **Oral contract**

  A dentist has told an assistant that their employment is guaranteed as long as their performance is good. As a result of the closing of a local plant, the practice is in steep decline, and the dentist terminates the assistant. Even though the economic problems of the practice were not foreseen, the oral contract is binding as long as the assistant's performance is good.

- **Public policy**

  The dentist has instructed an assistant to scale "small bits" of calculus when necessary, even though this is contrary to the state's Dental Practice Act. The hygienist threatens to inform the state board of dentistry if the practice continues. The dentist fires the hygienist, citing a bad attitude and not being part of the team. The wrongful termination suit will probably be upheld because the hygienist was acting in the public's interest and according to the law.

- **Implied contract**

  The dental office manual states that employees will be retained if their performance appraisals are good. If the dentist terminates an employee who has good performance appraisals, they may be subject to wrongful termination suits based on this principle.

such as jury duty or military duty. It also covers employees who raise questions about work procedures that are illegal or especially dangerous. This is the basis for whistle-blower court decisions. In these, employees who have been fired for informing on their company's illegal or immoral actions have won wrongful termination suits.

- **Implied contract**

  The employees' handbook, office manuals, employment applications, or performance appraisals often contain language that implies job security. These "implied contracts" are not direct agreements, but sometimes the courts interpret them as a form of promise or contract.

Such documents must include language that advises that an employer is an at-will employer and that none of the documents is or implies a contract.

Constructive Discharge

Many employers try to get around these problems by forcing or enticing the employee to quit. The employer may offer a good letter of recommendation or a severance bonus if the employee resigns. The employer might assign the employee excessive overtime or work or give them a pay cut with the intention that the employee will become dissatisfied and quit. Often employers take this approach when they fear a wrongful termination suit or other problems resulting from the firing. The courts generally rule that this is a constructive discharge, or in fact a firing. They typically uphold a constructive discharge claim when evidence shows that the circumstances the employee was under were "unreasonable" and the employer was trying to make the employee quit. Damage awards in these cases are similar to those for wrongful termination awards.

Retribution by a (Former) Employee

A former employee may try to "get even" with an employer for being fired. Some such actions are legal, others are not. Besides the previously mentioned FLSA, a former employee may file a complaint claiming an unsafe workplace with OSHA. The former employee may call the state's board of dentistry and lodge a complaint against a practice. If the employee knows that an employer has cheated on taxes (e.g. not reporting cash income from patients), the employee can report the employer to the IRS and receive a bounty of 25% of all back taxes, penalties, and interest collected. This is in addition to the aggravation the former employee knows they caused. In these cases, prevention through best business practices and records is the best defense.

Former employees have also been guilty of mischief, from trivial to significant. The employer must collect office keys at the time of firing to avoid internal mischief or theft. If an employer has any question about a fired employee's (or spouse's) intent, they need to change the locks on the doors immediately. If a security system is in place, they must change the access codes. The employer must also have a current back-up of the computer system data to avoid mischief or data catastrophes and have the back-up off-site. The employer needs to be prepared for possible slanderous or libelous statements from the disgruntled employee.

Maintaining Daily Operations

CHAPTER 27

Part 1: Office Operations

Efficiency is doing things right; effectiveness is doing the right things.

Peter Drucker

GOAL

This part aims to describe several techniques that improve the efficiency of office operations.

LEARNING OBJECTIVES

At the completion of this part, the student will be able to:

- Compare efficiency and effectiveness.

- Describe what factors affect capacity.

- Describe how to affect capacity utilization.

KEY TERMS

capacity
capacity utilized

effectiveness
efficiency

EFFICIENCY AND EFFECTIVENESS

In operating a productive practice, the dentist needs to be both efficient and effective.

EFFICIENCY

Efficiency looks at how cheaply something is done. The focus is cost. The intention is to save money, time, or effort regardless of quality. To become more efficient, people must simply lower costs. Efficiency measures productivity at the individual process level, regardless of the collateral effects of the decision (Box 27.1). It often requires conforming to norms. In this way, the process is no worse than others in the industry. It examines internal, technical issues. The result is to improve profitability by working harder and quicker.

In a dental practice, efficiency comes from doing procedures correctly the first time, without remakes. If this does not happen, not only does the practitioner have the cost of additional materials, staff, and lab charges, they have also lost the additional production they could have had during the time spent on the remake. Clinical decision-making is the prime factor that increases clinical speed.

Business Basics for Dentists, Second Edition. James L. Harrison, David O. Willis, and Charles K. Thieman.
© 2024 John Wiley & Sons, Inc. Published 2024 by John Wiley & Sons, Inc.

BOX 27.1	EFFICIENCY VERSUS EFFECTIVENESS

Efficiency	Effectiveness
How cheaply you do something	How well you do something
Costs	Quality
Process	Outcomes
Working harder, quicker	Working smarter

EFFECTIVENESS

Effectiveness looks at how well something is done. Here, the focus is on the benefit or outcome of the process. The intention is to improve quality to a higher level than the individual process, thereby raising performance levels. It measures how well the job is done or the correctness of a product or service. Effectiveness, then, is a quality measure, not a cost measure. It examines external, strategic results. The outcome of effectiveness is improving profitability by working smarter.

As an example of the difference in a dental practice, a practitioner can be more efficient (lowering costs) if they use a foreign lab. However, they may be less effective in crown and bridge work because of more remakes and lower patient satisfaction. So here, effectiveness trumps efficiency. Using the foreign lab costs less, but the practitioner is not doing their job as well. Simply doing something less expensively does not necessarily lead to more profit. Dental practitioners must ensure that they are efficient and effective in all office decisions.

CAPACITY

Capacity is the ability of the office to see patients. It is the maximum number of patient visits (or appointments) that the office has available for a given period. How practice owners plan and organize the office ultimately decides their ability to see patients. This configuration can (and should) change over time. As the practice matures, the number and type of patient visits change. Although capacity defines a dental practice's ability to see patients, marketing brings those patients in and fills available chair time. Both sides (driving demand and then seeing those patients generated) need to be satisfied for full capacity. The practitioner's practice philosophy guides the changes made in the operational and marketing systems to achieve those goals.

WHAT DETERMINES CAPACITY

All the management decisions the practice owner makes in the office affect capacity.

NUMBER OF OPERATORIES

The number of operatories has an obvious and essential effect on a practitioner's ability to see patients. However, the practitioner must ensure that proper staffing levels support the operatories. Without staff support, seven operatories will not let a practitioner see more patients than one operatory. The additional six operatories become nothing but expensive waiting rooms. Generally, practitioners assign one chairside assistant to one operatory. The assistants are responsible for chairside assisting during patient procedures, set-up, break-down, and disinfection of the operatory between patients.

OPERATOR SPEED

A practitioner's speed when doing patient procedures determines the length of appointments and, therefore, the number of available appointment slots. Operator speed is not dependent on "hand skills" and physical speed. Speed in completing patient procedures depends on the practitioner doing the procedure correctly without remakes. This means that the practitioner and staff are knowledgeable about each step of every procedure and take their time to do procedures correctly, instead of just doing them quickly. Operator speed then increases automatically with experience. As staff members become more accustomed to the practitioner and better trained in specific procedures, the practitioner can move more quickly through procedures without "wait time" for mixing materials, repositioning patients, or other small inefficiencies. That training does not just "happen." It is the practitioner's responsibility to ensure that staff training is an ongoing office function.

OFFICE HOURS

The more hours a dental practice opens, the more appointments are available. There are some obvious limitations. Most people want time away from the office for personal and family enjoyment. Although working 80 hours a week opens many appointment slots, most practitioners are unwilling to make the sacrifices involved in the trade-off. (The typical practicing practitioner works about 35 hours per week, according to the American Dental Association [ADA].)

Many patients want to visit a dental office during non-traditional hours (evenings and weekends). If an office keeps "bankers' hours" (9–5, Monday through Friday), then they may lose some patients to other practitioners who are open during those "off" hours. Although the marketing and operational considerations encourage the use of off-hours, staff considerations do not. If staff work more than 40 hours per week (in most states), they must receive overtime pay. Staff members generally do not want to work evenings or Saturdays for the same reasons practitioners do not. (They would rather spend time on personal or family pursuits. They may have children in daycare or after-school programs.) So, although there are reasons to work extended hours, the practice owner must consider the trade-offs.

Early in a practitioner's practice lifecycle, the dentist needs to generate patients for the practice. To do this, they may keep more off-peak hours (evenings and weekends). If they cannot fill the available appointments, they may close the office for traditional business hours to decrease costs. As the practice becomes more mature, the number of patients waiting for treatment increases. The practitioner can then cut back on off-peak hours, forcing patients into the more traditional appointment slots. Patients who cannot make these appointments may go elsewhere for treatment, but the practitioner will generally have other patients waiting to fill the appointment slot.

NUMBER AND TYPES OF STAFF MEMBERS

Operational decisions only significantly affect facility costs if the practice owner expands the office to increase capacity. The dentist pays rent regardless of the number of hours worked. Utility costs may be higher with additional or evening hours, but the lights are on for all working hours regardless. The biggest cost item is staff cost. If a practitioner has existing staff members work additional hours, they may have overtime costs. They may have to offer differential pay to induce someone to work non-traditional hours. They may also have extra costs due to hiring additional part-time staff members.

Many practitioners hire part-time staff. They may hire them to work during a busy time of the day (e.g. evenings) or do a particular function in the office (e.g. collecting accounts). With either type, office owners only hire people when needed most, improving office efficiency.

Chairside Assistants

As a rule, a practitioner needs one chairside assistant for each operatory. (If a practitioner has seven operatories and one assistant, they cannot see many more patients than with one operatory and one assistant.) Having fewer assistants leads to the extra chair being unused.

Expanded Functions

If the state of practice allows expanded functions by trained (or certified) dental assistants, additional operatories can significantly increase capacity. These staff members can complete intraoral procedures while the practitioner sees additional patients.

Receptionists

Receptionists are necessary for a smooth and efficient operation. A lack of receptionists will decrease recall patient visits (because the receptionist is too harried to manage the recall system effectively). This also leads to a decrease in overall patient visits (because of inadequate scheduling procedures.) As a rule, one receptionist can handle up to 1000 patients per quarter (18–20 per day) without decreasing effectiveness. As the number of patients increases above this, office capacity decreases unless additional receptionist help is hired.

Hygienists

Hygienists increase capacity by freeing the practitioner to see other patients (if adequate chairs are available). If the office does not have enough operatories available, the hygienist trades chair time with the practitioner. The total capacity remains the same. Hygienists contribute to increased production and profit in the office. They also generate demand for the practice by seeing additional diagnostic (recall) patients who have other work to be done.

OWNER WANTS, NEEDS, AND DESIRES

The owners' wants, needs, and desires heavily influence office capacity. Some practitioners do not want a large "run and gun" practice. They prefer a more intimate, personal style of practice. Neither extreme is right nor wrong, merely personal preference. Regardless of the practitioner's desires, an efficiently run practice that fully uses available capacity will be more profitable than a less efficiently run one.

OFFICE SYSTEMS

The way in which office systems are structured also affects capacity. If a practice owner organizes patient scheduling around 10-minute time blocks, they can see more patients than if they use 15-minute blocks (assuming adequate patient demand and operator ability). If the instrument management system cannot provide enough sterile instrument sets, there will be a capacity limitation.

CAPACITY UTILIZATION

Capacity utilization measures the actual use of potential appointment time. It is calculated by dividing capacity (potential patient visits) by the number of actual patient visits for a period. The result is the percentage of available appointments (chair time) that the office fills: 90% use and above is very good; 80–90% is OK, and below 80% shows that the office needs to use its resources better. Early in the practice cycle, capacity utilization may decrease as available appointment time goes unused. As capacity utilized increases above 90%, it signals the need to expand capacity or to become more efficient to increase profit.

Capacity utilization is the primary measure of office efficiency. It does not depend on the number of operatories (chairs) or staff. (Both eight-operatory and one-operatory offices must have their capacity well used.) Because a significant part of dental office costs is fixed, it becomes important to use those fixed costs efficiently. Both large and small offices can be efficient. This measure suggests whether this is happening.

INCREASING PATIENT VISITS

Patient visits are the driving force of a profitable dental practice. The key to maintaining efficiency (high capacity utilized) is increasing capacity as the patient load dictates. There is a need to anticipate growth in patient visits. (Practice owners do not want to turn people away because they do not have the capacity to see the patients, especially early in the practice life when they are trying to build a patient pool.) So, the practitioner increases capacity in anticipation of additional patient visits.

A practice's service mix describes the types of dental procedures the office does. There are three types of patient visits: diagnostic, basic services, and complex (major) services. Diagnostic visits involve new patients and routine "recare" (recall) procedures. These visits are when the practitioner identifies additional work that a patient needs. Basic care includes restorations, endodontics, and surgical procedures. These visits prepare the way for the complex visits, which generally involve laboratory work and multiple-visit procedures. Each type of visit is necessary for a profitable practice. Expanding the service mix (by taking continuing education to increase or improve the types of procedures done) increases the number of patient visits within the office.

Internal and external marketing efforts are common ways to generate additional patients. These include making more non-traditional hours available, changing credit and collection policies, and increasing insurance plan participation. Aggressive dental practitioners may buy another practice or merge practices to increase the patient pool.

DAILY SCHEDULING

Hours

Practitioners typically work about 40 hours a week, 32 of which are in direct patient contact. Most offices do not work more than a nine-hour day; they find longer days too exhausting, although a few offices work fewer, longer days. For example, some work three 12-hour days. Most state employment laws require that a lunch break (unpaid) is provided after four hours of work. This break varies from 30 minutes to an hour.

Many offices schedule early or late hours to accommodate working patients. If a practitioner does this, they must be sure not to work late one day and open early the next. This does not give employees enough time away from work. Evening hours are lucrative. Many patients who work (and have dental benefits) enjoy the evening-hour appointments. Saturday hours can be lucrative. However, often patients schedule these visits with good intentions, but when the time comes they find that they would rather have time off. They then cancel or do not show up for a visit, leaving the practitioner and the staff in the office on a beautiful Saturday.

DAILY HUDDLE

The daily huddle is a short meeting at the beginning of each day. During the meeting, the staff discuss the schedule for the day, looking for potential conflicts or problems. For example, if the office has one nitrous oxide–oxygen analgesia unit and two patients require the service, one must be rescheduled. This is also the time to discuss if periodic maintenance patients require radiographs, to ensure that the office has contacted all patients for appointment reminders, and to affirm that the laboratory has returned cases for scheduled patients. Each check avoids a scheduling problem and improves patient flow and treatment.

WAYS TO BECOME MORE EFFICIENT

A practitioner can become more efficient without changing the capacity of the office. A practitioner can streamline processes, using new or improved procedures to replace old ones. New materials may set more quickly or allow fewer steps in a process, decreasing the time required for placement. Using a new technology (such as digital radiography) allows for less time in treatment. Over the long haul, practitioners can save more in time (and additional procedures) than the technology costs to install. Adding a staff member is a significant investment, but if they increase office collections more than they cost, the addition is a good investment.

If the office is not fully using its capacity, then the primary focus must be on increasing the percentage of capacity that it does use. A practitioner can increase patient visits or decrease capacity (and the associated costs). Increasing visits involves all the internal and external marketing efforts described elsewhere in this book. Office owners should also check scheduling to ensure that they use the available time to their best advantage. Practitioners can decrease capacity by decreasing hours, making the time that they and the staff are in the office more productive. (Practitioners do not want to decrease hours so much that it is difficult for patients to schedule appointments.)

Practice owners can also decrease capacity by decreasing the number of staff members or their work hours.

If the office fully uses its capacity, there are different solutions to the efficiency question. If there are adequate patients and a practitioner has not reached their maximum personal capacity, then they can increase office capacity by moving to new office space, adding operatories, adding staff to maximize the use of the space, or increasing the hours in which they see patients. If, on the other hand, a practice owner's capacity is as large as they want it to be, then they ought to increase efficiency and profitability. A practitioner can do this by combining an increase in fees, a stricter credit and collection policy, and changing insurance plan participation (eliminating lower-paying plans).

Part 2: Office Accounting Systems

Don't go around saying the world owes you a living; the world owes you nothing; it was here first.

Mark Twain

GOAL

This aims to outline an office accounting system for tracking income and expenses.

LEARNING OBJECTIVES

At the completion of this part, the student will be able to:

- Describe the elements of common dental office accounting systems.
- Describe the purposes of the income accounting system.
- Properly enter charges, payments, and adjustments.
- Accurately compute current balance and accounts receivable.
- Accurately "proof" the day sheet postings, accounts receivable, and month-to-date figures.

- Accurately enter and compute typical transactions including:
  - Charge and payment
  - Patient payment
  - Insurance payment
  - Medicaid payment and adjustment
  - Professional discount
  - Returned check.
- Correct a posting to the wrong account.
- Properly write checks and record them in the check register.
- Describe how to prevent embezzlement in the dental office.

KEY TERMS

account guarantor	cash control
account ledger	cash flow
account payable	cash transactions
account receivable	charges
annual report	credit card transactions
assignment of benefits	credit memo
audit trail	current balance
back-ordered supplies	day sheet
bank deposit	disbursements
bookkeeping	credit card
bulk payment	checkbook
business analysis	register
summary	embezzlement

end-of-day (EOD)
  procedures
end-of-month (EOM)
  procedures
end-of-year (EOY)
  procedures
first in, first out (FIFO)
holdback (discount)
negative
  account balance
office credit card
packing slip
payment or collection
  (credit or debit)

petty cash
positive account
  balance
posting
previous balance
production adjustments
production or charge
  (credit or debit)
shipping invoice
specific allocation
statement
third-party carriers
transaction history
walkout statement

Every business must have a system for recording all the business transactions that occur each day. A dental office is no exception. It is a business. The compilations of those financial transactions are the "books" of the practice. Most practitioners delegate part of the bookkeeping function to staff members, professional bookkeepers, or accountants. However, understanding office bookkeeping is essential for several reasons. When a practitioner starts a practice, they need to establish a bookkeeping system that provides accurate information that they can use to improve the practice. Having other people do these functions can be expensive; until the practice has grown, practitioners may decide to keep their own books to decrease expenses. Finally, a practitioner needs to understand bookkeeping systems so that they can review them regularly to ensure their accuracy. Embezzlement is a sad but all too frequent occurrence in offices where the dental office owner trusted staff members and did not adequately oversee the bookkeeping function.

A dental practice needs to keep books of practice income or charges to patients for services that its staff have done. Some patients will pay on the day of service; other payments will arrive in the mail. Besides these routine transactions, dental practices need to record other transactions from time to time (e.g. no fee, a reduced fee, write-offs). Transaction records will give a dental practitioner information about each patient's status and comprehensive information about the practice's financial condition. The dental office owner also needs a series of "books" that account for expenditures or the money that goes out of the office. This system must keep a running tally of how much money is available, to whom the dental office owner owes money, and the categories of spending for management information and

tax reporting purposes. Finally, the dental office owner must combine the income and expense information into a series of books for tax reporting and management analysis. The office owner will work with an accountant, tax expert, or management consultant to use this information to improve practice performance and reduce the tax burden.

Fortunately, computerized systems have become the norm for dental office patient accounting. These systems replace the physical books of paper systems with computerized databases. The functions in these two types of systems are similar. The practitioner still needs to know the terminology and understand how to record items so that they can use the system effectively. If the practitioner turns over the entire accounting function to a staff member without adequate oversight on their part, they are inviting the problems of errors and embezzlement. Each major computer system has a report function built into its software. The systems can print more reports than a practice owner can likely use. The problem is deciding which of these reports is useful. Chapter 20 describes the data that is needed. The computer program can deliver the data for a practice owner's use. The practice owner needs to use established computer software rather than trying to develop their own. Unless computer programming is a hobby and someone wants to spend recreational hours writing computer programs, their time is better spent working in and developing the office.

Dental offices have three primary office accounting functions (Box 27.2). The first is to record and account for the money they collect from patients, insurance companies,

---

BOX 27.2   **DENTAL PRACTICE ACCOUNTING NEEDS**

- Determining income
  - Cash and checks
  - Insurance payments
  - Credit card payments

- Who owes money
  - Patient accounts and receivables
  - Third-party accounts and receivables

- Recording expenses
  - Expenses by categories
  - Tax purposes
  - Management purposes
  - Checkbook balance

or others for the services provided. Second, they must also track patients who do not pay at the time of service and thus owe for all or part of the fee. The dental practice accomplishes both through the office management system (e.g. Eaglesoft, Dentrix, Softdent). The final function is to record the payments they make to others for materials and services used in the office (e.g. lab services, supplies, payroll). The practice owner generally does this through a readily available commercial program, such as Quick-Books. (Some management programs have primitive checkbooks built into them, but the common commercial programs are so powerful and easy to use that most practitioners use them.)

The system described here is for patient financial records, not treatment records. These are two separate functions. One program generally serves for both cross-linking patient charts (for treatment histories) and accounts (for financial histories), but these are two different functions.

Most service industry businesses (such as dental practices) use "cash basis" accounting. (The other method, "accrual basis," is used more in larger manufacturing businesses.) When using cash-based accounting, the business recognizes income when it receives it (i.e. when the check crosses the receptionist's desk) and records an expense when they pay it (i.e. when they write the check). A dental practice will use the cash basis for both income and expenses. (This does not mean that a practice only accepts cash payment, but that all transactions are considered cash transactions, whether cash, check, credit card, or another form of payment.)

ACCOUNTING FOR INCOME

Businesses with many cash transactions use a simple cash register to record daily transactions. Dental offices do not have the number of cash transactions that a fast-food outlet or retail store has, so the dental office will have a different method of recording or registering payments.

PURPOSES OF INCOME ACCOUNTING SYSTEMS

Generally, any income accounting system used in the dental office serves five primary purposes.

OFFICE COMMUNICATIONS

It is a method of communication between the front office and the production areas of the office. The receptionist needs to inform the production area assistants who will be coming in and the procedures for which to prepare. After the visit, the doctor, assistants, or hygienist informs the front-office personnel what procedures they did and the plan for the next anticipated visit (if any). Many practitioners do this in person by walking the patient to the front desk and communicating verbally with the receptionist and patient. Others prefer a more efficient written method. If a practitioner saves 1 minute per patient and sees 20 patients daily, they can either see an additional patient in the time saved (making additional income) or leave the office 20 minutes earlier. Either way, the practitioner wins.

At the beginning of the day, the receptionist posts a copy of the day's schedule in the operatory area (or each operatory) and the sterilization area. The receptionist then prints a "routing slip" for each patient and places these in the sterilization area. This routing slip specifies the procedure scheduled and often other information such as balance due and medical history alerts. Through this communication, the assistants can prepare appropriate instruments and trays for the given procedure for each patient. Staff generally place routing slips with the tray and take them to the operatory. After the visit, the office staff or doctor notes on the routing slip what procedures they did and variations from the usual fee (if any). (Offices with networked computer systems often provide this information directly in the sterilization area and operatories, saving time, paper, and possible error.)

DOCUMENTATION FOR PATIENTS

An income accounting system provides a receipt to patients, showing the procedures billed that day, evidence of any payment received, and their new balance. When dental practices enter a procedure on a patient's account, accountants say they have "posted" it to the account. The receptionist completes the receipt after posting the procedures and asking for (and hopefully gaining) payment from the patient for the new current balance (previous balance + charges − adjustments). The receptionist then prints a "walkout statement" for the patient that records this information as they prepare to leave the office.

INSURANCE BILLING

An income accounting system provides information for third-party carriers (insurance companies) for billing and payment purposes. The more quickly the practice sends accurate information to them, the more quickly the dental practice or the patient will receive reimbursement. The dental office may transmit this information to the insurer either through a mailed paper form or electronically over the internet.

TRANSACTION HISTORY

An accounting information system lists the transaction history (charges, adjustments, and payments) for each patient within the account. The account is the billing unit. The dental office sends one bill to the account guarantor of each account because they are responsible or have guaranteed to pay the account. Each account may contain one or many patients. For example, the father may be the guarantor for an account that contains the spouse and their five children. Or in a divorce situation, the father may be the guarantor for an account in which the child is the only patient. The mother may have custody of the child, but the father is responsible for paying for the child's healthcare. If the mother is also a patient of the practice, she may be her account guarantor and the only patient on that account. In such a case, the office sends the child's bill to the father but sends the mother's bill to her.

The account or account ledger is the history of all the financial transactions for the account. The current balance is the amount the guarantor presently owes the dental practice for all transactions on the account. A positive account balance says that the guarantor owes the practitioner. An account may show a negative account balance if an overpayment exists. Generally, this occurs when a third party overpays or a practitioner changes planned treatment procedures that they have already initiated. (For example, the endodontic procedure that a practitioner initiated changes to a less expensive extraction, although the patient had already paid for the endodontic procedure.) In these cases, the dental practice may write the patient a check for the overpayment, or if the patient desires, the office can retain the patient's portion of the negative balance to credit it toward future work. Insurance companies will always want the check for a negative balance.

DAILY TRANSACTION JOURNAL

Finally, the accounting information system provides a day sheet or a record of each day's transactions for the practice (and each practitioner in a multipractitioner office) that summarizes the charges made, payments received, and any adjustments made. The computer program accumulates the day's transactions to form a monthly ledger. The program then accumulates monthly ledgers into an annual report. Some practice owners rely on their computer back-up procedure to ensure that their records are complete. Others print a copy of the day sheet and keep it in a binder as an additional data back-up procedure.

COMPONENTS OF ACCOUNTING SYSTEMS

Computerized accounting systems are composed of a series of related databases. Databases are computer programs that save large amounts of information concerning a specific item, allowing the program to relate that information to other, similar cases. The common databases used by these systems include account information, patient information, third-party database, procedure database, practice history database, and specific databases.

- **Account information** defines each account and its guarantor. The account information relates to each patient associated with the account, but the program stores the information about each patient in a different location. Generally, the program stores transaction histories with each account.

- **Patient information** defines the patient elements (e.g. name, address, age, etc.) and ties them to an account.

- The **third-party database** establishes the third-party carriers, their addresses, and, generally, what each plan pays for each procedure.

- The **procedure database** defines practitioners' procedures by specifying ADA code procedure numbers. This file also includes the normal fee for each procedure and the fee allowed by each insurance plan.

- The **practice history database** holds daily and monthly activity reports (day sheets and monthly summaries).

- **Program-specific databases** store information for the individual program. Examples include dunning messages (little notes that appear on patients' bills), schedule databases, prescription databases, medical history messages, and many other types of information.

These computer programs use each database as needed, pick up the information they require from that database, and then move to the next database, adding the required information. For example, if a practitioner does a two-surface alloy on a patient with insurance, the program first identifies the patient from the patient database. It then relates that patient to the account, checking to see the account' balance. It finds the insurance information from the third-party database, which tells the main program how much the practitioner expects the third-party carrier to pay for this specific procedure. It checks the procedure code file to decide how much the practitioner typically charges for this procedure. The main program then calculates the amount the patient needs to pay, enters any payments made, and saves that information in the patient's updated transaction file and on the practice's day sheet.

ACCOUNTING TERMINOLOGY

A charge is the full fee required by a dental practice to do the service. It is the same as the production figure. Payments may come from the account guarantor or patient as cash, check, or charge card or may come in the mail from third-party payers, such as insurance companies or employers. Adjustments are the amounts for which a dental practice does not bill. This may result from the patient being a friend or family member or may be required by a managed care insurance plan. A production (or charge) adjustment is a change in the amount of a patient's account from changes in procedures done. A payment (or collection) adjustment is a change in how much money the dental practice expects to collect from the patient. Either production or collection adjustments can be credited to the account (decreases the balance due) or debited from the account (increases the balance due). In the previous example, the practitioner had initiated and charged an endodontic procedure but then changed this to an extraction. The practitioner has a charge credit (negating part of the endodontic procedure) and a new charge for the extraction. Suppose a practitioner does a procedure on a family member or a managed care patient, "writing off" 50% of the amount due. In that case, the practitioner enters a payment credit because the production remains unchanged. When the computer calculates the new "current balance," it uses the formula Previous Balance + Charges − Payment − Adjustment = Current Balance (Box 27.3).

A credit is an accounting entry that decreases the account balance. A debit is an entry that increases the account balance. Adjustments may be related either to production (or charge) or to payment (or collection) adjustments (Box 27.4). Either type may be a credit or debit to the account. The practice wants to keep the types separate to keep an accurate tally of office production and collections. The practice also wants a separate payment adjustment for each type (e.g. Delta Dental, Aetna) to track the discounts for each plan. This way, the practice can calculate the overall reimbursement rate for the different plans. The last part of this chapter on dental insurance discusses how to do this.

BOX 27.4	TYPES OF ADJUSTMENTS	
	Credit (decreases balance)	Credit (decreases balance)
Production (Charge)	Entry error	Entry error
	Redo a procedure	
Payment (Collection)	Cash courtesy	Insurance did not pay full amount
	Bad debt write-off	
	Patient refund	
	Insurance refund	

BOX 27.3	INCOME ACCOUNTING FORMULA

Previous balance
+ Charges
− Payments
− Adjustments
= Current balance

New previous balance = Old current balance

INCOME ACCOUNTING SYSTEM PROCEDURES

Patient Encounter Procedures

Specific patient encounter procedures vary by office and the amount and use of technology in the office. The essentials remain constant.

At the beginning of the day, the people working in the sterilization area and each operatory need to know who is coming in and what procedure is planned at the visit so that trays, equipment, and operatories can be set up appropriately. There are three common methods. If the office uses a paper scheduling system, the receptionist makes a photocopy of the day's schedule and posts it in the sterilization area and each operatory. These must be hidden from patient view for patient privacy and to comply with the Health Insurance Portability and Accountability Act (HIPAA). If the office uses computerized scheduling with computers in each area, the staff can pull up the day's schedule on the computer system or print out a copy of the day's schedule. Finally, as already mentioned, many offices print out a routing slip for each patient planned for the day. Sterilization areas use the routing slip to set up trays. They then place the slip with the tray that goes to the operatory.

PATIENT WALKOUT PROCEDURES

Once the practitioner does the dental procedure, they need to tell the front office what they did for charge purposes and what they plan for the next appointment for scheduling purposes. If each operatory has a computer station, many offices have the staff directly enter the procedure on the patient's ledger. When the patient arrives at the front desk to leave, the receptionist has the patient's bill ready, waiting for payment. If the office uses a routing slip, then staff enter the procedures for the day and plan for the next appointment on the slip. The patient then walks the routing slip to the front desk, where the receptionist enters information on the patient's ledger, asks for payment, enters any payment into the system, and schedules the next appointment. If a patient pays in cash, the transaction must appear in the payment section of the day sheet. The receptionist then prints a walkout statement detailing the day's procedures, charges and payments, and an account summary. Even if a patient has a "no charge" visit, the receptionist should give them a walkout statement to verify their previous balance, if any. Finally, if the office uses mailed insurance forms, the receptionist prints out an insurance form of the day's procedures to put in the mail.

END-OF-DAY PROCEDURES

The office needs to close and "proof" day sheets each day. Proofing means that the practice owner verifies or proves the correctness of the entries and the mathematics. The computer program will do the mathematics correctly, but correct results only happen if staff have made the entries correctly. Proofing is important to ensure the accuracy of the accounting and to guard against the possibility of staff embezzlement. Day-end proofing includes proof of posting, accounts receivable proof and control, cash control, and bank deposit verification. Proof of posting verifies that staff members have correctly entered the day's transactions, accounted for adjustments, and credited payments correctly. Accounts receivable proofing verifies the accuracy of the total accounts receivable and keeps a running tally of the amount. Cash control checks that staff have accounted for all cash transactions. This cash may be as patient cash payments or in "petty cash." Bank deposit verification ensures that the staff has included all payments in the bank deposit for the day. End-of-day (EOD) checking takes just a couple of minutes each day. It is sound business practice on the part of the practice owner.

The dental office must close the day sheet at the end of the day's operation and not later. If staff members have made entry errors, they need to address them quickly so that their effect will not multiply through subsequent days. Computer systems will not make mathematical errors, but data entry errors are still a problem. (The receptionist may have entered a collection credit instead of a collection debit, for instance.) The receptionist or office manager will generally make all entries. The practitioner needs to verify the entries and the proofing procedures each day. Again, this is not paranoia, but sound business practice.

By the end of the day, front office staff must have completed several procedures:

- **Complete a bank deposit ticket**
  Generally, banks prefer their own preprinted deposit tickets rather than those printed by a computer system. The front office stamps all checks as they receive them with the dental practice's stamp (available from the bank) that states: "For Deposit Only, to the Account of Dr. XXXX, Account # 111-222-333-4."

- **Check that the deposit ticket total matches the day sheet "receipts" total**
  This is to verify that the front office has reported all money taken in for the day (cash and check).

- **Check the office schedule against the day sheet**
  Verify that all patients seen in the office for the day have a corresponding entry on the day sheet. This forces a numbered receipt for each patient visit. The practitioner should check that all procedures the practice did (and charged for) were charged the "usual and customary" amount unless the dentist has specifically authorized an adjustment.

- **Verify "proof of posting"**
  The practice owner should check that the numbers add up as they should. If the staff know that the practice owner regularly looks at the numbers, they will be much less likely to take liberties with the money.

- **Take the day's deposit to the bank**
  The practitioner ought to take the day's receipts to the bank each day. (This may not be possible if they work late hours.) The practice owner wants the money in their account quickly. The owner also wants all checks, and especially significant cash, out of the office (or in the practice safe) quickly. In that way, if the office is the victim of a break-in or robbery, they will lose less.

- **Occasionally verify the mail**
  The practice owner should occasionally (unannounced) open the mail and post checks to patient ledgers themselves. This verifies the accuracy of the postings and decreases the likelihood that a front-office worker might try to embezzle personal or insurance payment checks from the practice.

- **Close the day**

  Once the practice owner has verified that all the day's numbers are correct, they need to close the day in the computer system. The computer system will have routines for doing this. Essentially, closing the day accomplishes the following procedures:

  - Total all numbers that were entered into the system for the day. These include production, collections, adjustments, and other accounting numbers.
  - Reset the accounting numbers to zero for the new, upcoming day.
  - Print out a paper copy of the day sheet for the office's financial records.

- **Back up the computer**

  Front-office employees must back up the computer (data) daily after they have completed all other functions.

END-OF-MONTH PROCEDURES

The office needs to do a couple of additional procedures at the end of each month. Again, management computer systems have built-in procedures that do these functions:

- **Close the day**

  The business office staff need to be sure they have closed the current day to include any transactions from that day in the monthly totals.

- **Calculate monthly totals**

  Add up the month's totals for all running tally numbers (production, collections, etc.) and store a printout of them electronically or in a physical file.

- **Reset monthly totals**

  Reset those numbers to zero for the upcoming new month.

- **Print out monthly reports**

  Print a paper copy of monthly totals if the practice owner keeps a paper file.

- **Age accounts**

  Most offices age their accounts when they run the end-of-month (EOM) procedure.

END-OF-YEAR PROCEDURES

End-of-year (EOY) procedures are like EOM procedures, except that they account for the entire year. The computer system will guide the user through the procedure:

- **Close the month**

  Front-office staff must have closed the current month to include transactions from that month in the yearly totals.

- **Calculate yearly totals**

  Add up the year's totals for all running tally numbers (production, collections, etc.) and store a printout of them either electronically or in a physical file.

- **Reset yearly numbers**

  Reset those numbers to zero for the upcoming new year.

- **Print out annual reports**

  Print a paper copy of annual totals if the practice owner keeps a paper file.

- **Back up the software's data**

  Many offices run an additional (safety) back-up for the entire year and store it with the tax records.

TYPES OF PATIENT PAYMENTS

Staff should encourage patients to make payments when a procedure is completed. This may be in the form of cash, check, or credit card. The receptionist informs the patients of the total amount owed. They then receive the payment, enter it into the computer system, and print a walkout statement. After the receptionist gives this to the patient for verification, they stamp the back of the check with a bank deposit stamp and place it and any cash in a secure area of the desk.

CASH

The practice owner must deposit all money taken into the office in the office's bank account. If they take any cash from patient payments for personal use, they must be sure to use the accounting system totals for income tax determination rather than the checkbook or bank statement. Practice owners may be tempted to pocket cash without entering it into the accounting system. They may know others who do it and get away with it. However, the risks are not worth the little income (income tax savings).

Note that it is not a good idea to take cash for personal use without reporting it to the Internal Revenue Service (IRS) as taxable income. The IRS takes a dim view of people who intentionally do not report income. If a practice owner does this, several negative things may happen:

- If the owner does not include cash payments as income, they will be guilty of income tax evasion or tax fraud, not just a "mistake," if the IRS catches them. Conviction is a felony and carries a jail term (not just a monetary penalty).

- Employees will see that taking cash (i.e. stealing) is OK. They may be tempted to do similarly. Because the owner may "rake the cash drawer," they may have no idea how much cash is there or even how much is supposed to be there. Consequently, the owner may have no idea how much cash may be missing.

- A disgruntled or fired employee may want to "get back" at the practice owner. If the former employee reports the owner to the IRS for tax evasion, the former employee gets a "reward" or bounty of 25% of any back taxes and penalties that the owner owes. An employee who knows that a business owner cheats the IRS can be difficult to fire or control in the office.

PATIENT PAYMENT BY PERSONAL CHECK

Many patients pay with personal checks. They should make out the check to the practitioner's name or the name of the office or practice (if it is different). The front-office staff stamp each check (on the back in the "endorsements" section) when they receive it. This stamp has "For deposit only" with the bank and account number. (Banks will generally send businesses these stamps, although there may be a small fee.) That way, if someone steals a check, they cannot cash it; they can only deposit it into the practice's account.

PATIENT PAYMENTS BY CREDIT OR DEBIT CARD

Most offices allow and encourage patients to make payments by credit or debit card. From an accounting perspective, these payments are no different from any other. They are a payment on the day sheet and the patient account.

The practice owner sets up a merchant account with a bank to oversee credit and debit card transactions. (Banks offer different rates, fees, and options, so the practice owner should shop around.) The overseeing bank may hold these payments in a separate account or deposit them directly into the office checking account. When the practice owner transfers this money to the checking account, they do not have to report it. They had already counted it as income when they entered it into the accounting system. Other banks will directly deposit the credit card transaction amount into the checking account the day it occurs. The bank will then summarize the transactions in an EOM statement.

Credit and debit cards charge a fee for each transaction and a monthly service fee. (See Chapter 22 for a detailed discussion.) The banks call this a "holdback" or "discount." The office staff do not need to enter each transaction fee into the checkbook but rather the entire monthly discount amount. They enter it as a bank expense in the checkbook.

ACCOUNTING FOR TRADITIONAL INSURANCE PAYMENTS

If a patient has dental insurance covering all or part of the fee, then the accounting becomes more complex than for a simple cash transaction. The question is whether the dental office accepts "assignment of benefits." This means the insurer will send (assign) the benefit (payment) directly to the practice instead of the patient. Chapter 22 discusses this in more detail.

If the practice does not accept the assignment of benefits, accounting is easy. The front-office staff charges the patient (actually, the account) the full fee and collects it as a fee for service (FFS). They then print a completed insurance form for the patient to submit, and the patient is responsible for getting reimbursement from the insurer.

If the practice does accept the assignment of benefits, staff collect from the patient only the portion that the insurer does not pay. There are two options here. First, the practice can submit the insurance form to the insurer. The insurer sends the reimbursement to the practice. The practice waits until the insurance "clears" and then charges the patient the difference. The second option is to estimate (through the computer system) what the insurer will pay and charge the patient their expected amount immediately (at the time of service). When the insurance company sends payment for its portion, the front-office staff reconcile their estimate with the actual payment. If there is a difference, the practice either charges or reimburses the difference, depending on whether the total payments are too large or too small. They then close the claim in the computer system so that it will not continue to track it as open (unpaid). The second option speeds cash flow through the practice but may require adjustments after the insurance clears. The practitioner also needs to be sure to keep accurate and up-to-date information on the computer system on how much every plan pays for each procedure.

With any of these systems, the practitioner should get a pretreatment estimate of benefits from the insurer, especially for large cases or insurance plans with which the practitioner is unfamiliar. The insurer will send an explanation of benefits (EOB) to the practitioner and the patient. This estimates the patient's coverage: what the insurer will pay for the procedures that the practitioner has submitted for this patient. It is not a payment or even a contract for payment. It is a good-faith estimate of what the insurance company will pay. It can (and occasionally does) change from when the practitioner receives the estimate to when they submit the claim for reimbursement. This does not allow or disallow treatment. That is between the practitioner and the patient. The insurer pays (or not) for certain procedures, according to the contract with the patient, practitioner, or employer. The pretreatment estimate defines this payment so that no one is surprised.

Insurers will often send one check to pay for services done for several patients. These "bulk payments" will have a form (explanation of payments) that details the patient payments included, what procedures the payments cover, and the amount of each payment. When the office receives these bulk payments, the front-office staff allocate them to the proper procedures on the correct patient accounts.

ACCOUNTING FOR MANAGED CARE PAYMENTS

If a dental practice participates in a managed care program, it will have signed a contract agreeing to the terms of the program, one of which is a reduced fee for procedures. Two options exist for these payments, depending on the specific program(s) in which the practice participates. In one, the practice charges and collects from the patient a contractually agreed price for each service. In this case, the front-office staff enter the full fee value as the charge and then add a collection adjustment of the difference between the full fee value and the contractually agreed fee. This is a "managed care adjustment" or discount. In the second method, the practice submits the full fee value to the managed care insurer like a traditional insurance plan. The managed care insurer then sends payment along with an explanation of the payment that details how much it reimburses and how much (if anything) the practice may charge the patient. The difference between the full fee and the total payments (from the insurer and patient, if any) is the managed care adjustment. Chapter 21 describes the financial impact of managed care participation on the dental practice.

TRACKING WHO OWES MONEY (ACCOUNTS RECEIVABLE)

Immediate payments are easy to account for on the day sheet. A bigger problem comes when patients do not pay immediately, or have a third party that pays all or part of the bill. The practice needs to track the amounts that patients and insurers owe so that the practice can be sure that they pay properly. (See Chapter 22 for a discussion of how to set financial policies for the office.)

All management computer systems have a method for tracking accounts receivable. Most systems call them *account aging reports*. These reports categorize accounts by the time since the patient made the last payment. The generally accepted categories are 30, 60, 90, and 120 days. An account that falls into the 60-day category has yet to have a payment made in at least 60 days and possibly as many as 89 days.

Simply printing the report does not solve any problem. The practice owner must use the information on the report. This means calling patients, writing letters, or denying future appointments until the patient brings the balance up to date. The older the account, the more difficult it is to collect. The real value of these reports is to prevent problems by identifying slow payers early so that the office staff can encourage them to pay what they owe.

For patients who have insurance, there are two theories for determining the aging of accounts. (Most dental office software will let a practice choose which method to use.) The practice can "start the clock" for payments when they bill the procedure, or start it when the insurance has cleared and the practice is certain what the patient's portion of the bill is. If a practice uses the first method, it needs to have good information about the patient's insurance plan to estimate the patient's portion accurately. This is less of a problem with common plans in the dental office, but is more of a problem with seldom-used plans.

The practice also needs to keep track of insurance forms and pretreatment estimates submitted to insurance companies. If the practice does not get a response from the insurance within 30 days (some offices use 14 days), then the practitioner (or staff) will follow up with a telephone call to find out what the problem is. Insurance companies are not usually in a hurry to pay out money, so claims and pretreatment estimates may sit on someone's desk if they have questions. The practice's computer program will track "open" (unpaid) claims and pretreatment estimates that insurers have not returned; front-office staff should use this feature regularly.

MULTIPRACTITIONER OFFICES

Accounting for income becomes more complex in multipractitioner offices. The problem is allocating charges and payments to a particular provider rather than the office as a whole. (If the providers are all on salary or other fixed compensation, then there is no need for allocation; simply tally the office totals no matter who provided the service.) There are two standard methods of allocating payment to providers: first in, first out (FIFO), and specific. FIFO is an accounting term that means the payments go to the first procedure completed on the transaction history. Specific allocation states that the practice will credit the payment to the specific procedure.

For example, Dr. Alpha sees Mrs. Jones and does $300 worth of dental procedures. On the next visit, Dr. Baker does a $400 procedure, which requires a $200 down payment. Mrs. Jones pays $300. Who gets credit for the $300 payment? The FIFO procedure says that Dr. Alpha gets credited. Because those procedures were the "first in" the account, they are the "first out" as well. (This says that the well is filled from the bottom up.) The specific method says to credit Dr. Baker because the requirement for the down payment takes precedence over the age of the receivable. Either way works; the practitioners must be sure to list in advance which method the office will use. (The FIFO method is more common.)

RECORDING EXPENSES: PAYMENTS TO OTHERS

The practice owner also will need a system to record and categorize expenditures for the office. They need this information for two purposes: to know how much cash is in the account and to record expenses for tax and management purposes. Most practice owners have two methods for paying office expenses: a credit card and a checkbook (or e-payment account).

CHECKBOOK SYSTEMS

The office checkbook is the system for managing cash in the practice. A checkbook system can be paper or electronic. It records and categorizes payments made by the business. A practice owner needs to have two checking accounts: one for the office that contains only office expenditures and another personal account that has only personal expenditures. This way, accounting becomes much easier because the practice owner does not need to decide, after the fact, if an item is an office expense or not. All checks written from the office account are business expenses. The categories established for the checkbook register should be the same ones used for tax reports and management information. That way, the owner will not have to recategorize entries when they run reports. (Box 27.5 gives a listing of the categories.)

The front-office staff deposit all income (cash payments, personal checks received from patients, insurance checks, and credit card payments) into the office checking account. (The total amount of the daily deposit must be the same as the daily receipts on the computer system.) Practice owners then make all office payments from the checkbook and pay the office credit card with a check from the office checking account. If the practice owner borrows money, they add the loan to the checkbook balance, but it is not income for tax purposes.

The check register is the mechanism for recording and allocating office costs. Registers may be paper products (they are available from any office supply house) or they may be part of a computerized check system. Check registers identify checks issued for the month and allow the practice owner to categorize each expenditure for tax reporting and business management purposes. The purpose of the register is not to keep a running tally or balance of the checking account. The practice owner does that in the checkbook and on the check stubs. Instead, the register allocates or categorizes expenses into categories. It then summarizes the categories for the month and "posts" them to an annual report.

The annual report summarizes all office expenses for the year, broken down by category. These categories are the same as on the checkbook register. The annual report is what the practice owner takes to the accountant for tax processing. If a practice owner has done an excellent job in these bookkeeping chores, they will save hundreds or thousands of dollars in tax preparation fees.

TYPES OF CHECKBOOKS

Binder Checkbooks

Some practitioners still have checkbooks that fit into three-ring binders, which the bank has provided. The least expensive method is to get the checkbook from the bank and then purchase a good register from an office supply company. Bank checks come in two styles. If a practice owner processes their own payroll, they need to get the type called "payroll stub checks" that have an extra section for recording tax withholdings on employees' checks. The practice owner must keep meticulous records of employee withholdings on a separate payroll record. Nevertheless, it is important that employees see the total amount of their pay (gross) and all the money that various taxing agencies require that employers withhold and pay for them. Although this will not necessarily make employees happier about their pay level, the lack of this information can cause confusion and dissatisfaction.

Computer Check Systems

Many dental office management programs have check-writing and register elements included. Most practice owners use commercially available accounting systems such as Quicken/QuickBooks. These systems can print the physical check, keep an accurate register, determine staff pay and withholdings, produce financial statements, and transfer funds electronically. They are the most effective method available today for tracking expenses in the office. They all operate using the same principles and nomenclature as traditional checkbook systems.

Electronic Checks (e-Banking)

Many banks allow and encourage patrons to use electronic bank services. These systems are handy for accounts from which someone regularly writes checks (like many dental offices). In these systems, a payee (to whom to send payment) is set, and the owner adds a payment amount online. Statements are available at the end of each month. Specific systems differ significantly. Banks have different options and requirements, and a practice owner ought to explore all options.

BOX 27.5	LISTING OF ACCOUNTS FOR OFFICE CHECKBOOK

Category	Deductible?	Category	Deductible?
Dental supplies	Yes	Staff costs	Yes
Dental laboratory	Yes	Associate expense	Yes
Office expenses	Yes	Wages (net)	Yes
Office expense	Yes	Withholdings paid	Yes
Office supplies	Yes	Employee benefits	Yes
Postage and shipping	Yes	Pension/profit sharing	Yes
Office cleaning	Yes	Uniforms	Yes
Marketing	Yes	Temporary services	Yes
Advertising	Yes	Taxes	
Professional relations	Yes	FICA (payroll) taxes paid	Yes
Legal and professional	Yes	Unemployment taxes	Yes
Accounting	Yes	Property taxes	Yes
Legal services	Yes	Licenses	Yes
Management consulting	Yes	Owner's expenses	
Insurance office (business)	Yes	Draw	No[b]
Returns and allowances	Yes	Automobile expenses	Partial[c]
Miscellaneous	Yes	Continuing education	Partial[c]
Bank charges	Yes	Dues and publications	Yes
Other interest expense	Yes	Meals	Partial[c]
Office space and equipment	Yes	Personal insurance	No
Office rent	Yes	Personal taxes	No
Loan payment	Yes/No[a]		
Equipment lease	Yes		
Utilities	Yes		
Repairs	Yes		

[a]"Loan payment" is part interest expense and part principal payment. The interest portion is deductible. The principal portion is not deductible. Depreciation is a non-cash expense and not included in the checkbook.

[b] Draw from a proprietorship or partnership is not deductible. The owner's salary from a corporation is deductible for the corporation.

[c]Current tax law allows for partial deductibility of these expenses.

PROCEDURES FOR WRITING AND ENTERING CHECKS

Regardless of the type of system used, there are standard procedures for writing checks and keeping an accurate checking account.

- **Verify the accuracy of the order**
  If a practice receives a box of supplies or other articles, a designated office employee needs to thoroughly examine all the items and compare them to the enclosed "shipping invoice" or "packing slip." If items are incorrect or missing, they will call the supplier immediately to see that they ship the correct items. Further, the employee needs to keep a list of items that are "back-ordered" (the supplier was out of stock, but will send them when they are in stock) so that they do not order them again or pay for them twice.

- **File (save) the invoice**
  An invoice is a charge for payment from the supplier. It lists the material or services provided and the charges for each. An invoice is proof of the expense. Most practitioners keep invoices in an "accordion file" (available at all office supply stores). Some arrange them by expense category (e.g. dental supplies), whereas others keep them by month, relying on the check register for the accuracy of category totals.

- **Wait for the statement**
  Some suppliers send an invoice with each order (especially suppliers that the office uses infrequently). Their invoice states "pay from this invoice" or something similar. These suppliers generally do not send a statement. Others (especially those with whom the practice has several orders through the month) will send an EOM statement and mail an invoice for each order. The practice employees must learn which supplier operates in which manner. A statement of the account summarizes all a practice's invoices and payments for the month and presents a new monthly total due. The practice employee needs to verify that all the invoices entered on the statement are correct and that they have entered any credit memos. (A credit memo is like an invoice but gives credit to an account for returned items or over-billed amounts.)

- **Write the check**
  Complete the entire check. Enter the corresponding invoice number or account number on it. If there is a question of whether an invoice was paid, the practice owner can look at the canceled check to verify the invoice number. (If this is a paycheck for an employee, the practice owner should note the dates the paycheck reflects.)

- **Enter information into the register**
  If a practice uses a paper system, staff must reenter the information from the check on the register. The payee is the person or organization to which they write the check. It may be a staff member, supplier, or self, as the practice owner's draw. Checks are numbered consecutively. If the practice owner makes a mistake on a check, they write "void" in the register for the payee and destroy (shred) the check.

The practice owner lists their personal draw in a separate category. When they transfer money from the office account to a personal account, the practice owner draws on the practice's assets. They categorize this as a "draw" in the check register. This is not a tax-deductible expense item. (If the practice owner practices as a corporation, they are an employee. In this case, their salary is deductible to the corporation like for any other employee.) If the practice owner writes personal or non-professional checks from this account (such as life insurance payments), they must post them as a draw. This is so that these non-deductible expenses are not deducted on tax returns.

If the expense does not fall into a predetermined category, it is placed in the "sundry" or "miscellaneous" column or category. Again, only professionally related expenses are entered in the body of this register.

ACCOUNTING FOR CREDIT CARD PURCHASES

Practice owners need a credit card (MasterCard, VISA, etc.) that they use only for office purchases. (They will obtain a separate credit card for personal purchases.) Generally, the higher the interest rate, the lower the annual fee; the reverse is also true. If a practice owner routinely pays off their credit card balance the month it is due, they ought to get a card with a lower annual fee. If they do not routinely pay off the balance, they ought to pay the higher annual fee in return for lower monthly interest rates. The practice owner needs to consider getting a card that pays for rebates (cash, frequent flyer miles, etc.) if they pay off the credit card regularly. If the practice owner makes many office purchases (e.g. office supplies, lab, and dental supplies) with this card, they may have several free trips each year. (If the practice owner uses the frequent flyer miles for business-related trips, such as for continuing education, the trips are not taxable income. Personal use may result in the IRS treating it as assumed income.)

The practice owner often makes many business-related purchases with an office credit card. They want to include the cost of these business expenses as deductions for tax purposes. They write one check from the office checkbook to the issuing bank for monthly credit card purchases. They will then allocate the purchases to the correct categories. For example, the practice owner may have purchased professional supplies, advertising materials, and paid for continuing education courses with a credit card. They should write one check to the bank to pay for the credit card purchases, but should categorize the separate purchases for tax and management information. If the practice uses a computerized checking system, they will generally run separate accounts. The practice owner then uses all the accounts when determining and printing EOM and EOY reports. If they use a paper system, they will need to run a separate sheet for credit card purchases, adding them to the register allocations for tax reporting purposes.

RECONCILING THE BANK STATEMENT

The practice owner will receive a bank statement each month that details the initial balance, all checks written, deposits made for the month, and an ending balance. The owner needs to check the accuracy of the statement. (Banks do make mistakes!) This is called *reconciling* the statement to the checkbook. The procedure follows:

- The owner verifies that all transactions (checks and deposits) have "cleared" or have been processed by the bank. They should be sure that the bank recorded the transaction amount correctly. The owner may have written some checks that the payee has not yet cashed, or they may have written checks since the bank issued the statement.

- The owner subtracts the amount of the checks that have not cleared from the ending balance and adds the amount of any deposits that are not recorded.

- They then subtract any bank charges and add any returned checks.

- This ought to equal the current checkbook balance. If not, the practice owner needs to check item by item to detect the source(s) of the error.

EXAMPLE PATIENT ACCOUNTING TRANSACTIONS

Box 27.6 shows sample accounting transactions for the most common transactions in the office. It shows the difference between production and collection transactions and credit and debit transactions.

PETTY CASH AND CASH CONTROL

Many business checking accounts are not interest-bearing accounts. That is to say, the bank does not pay the holder interest on money in checking accounts. (The business owner ought to see if the bank has a "sweep" or another type of account that does pay interest on checking account balances.) The practitioner needs to manage the money in their bank accounts to maximize the interest earned from these assets. They also need to keep an accurate balance of the amount in the checking account so that they do not fall below the minimum balance, which generally initiates fees. However, the owner does not want to keep too much money in an account that does not pay interest. If the account does not pay interest, they ought to have a separate account (often a money market–type account) that does. Any extra cash is "swept" (transferred) into the interest-bearing account, earning interest. They should

also delay payments to others until they are due so that they keep the money as long as possible. (The owner must not be late with a payment, initiating interest or penalty charges, but there is no reason for the payment to be there early either.)

Most offices have a petty cash drawer or box. They use petty cash for small purchases, such as postage-due or delivery charges. Front-office staff will also use it to provide change for the occasional patient that pays cash for dental services. It will contain several hundred dollars in various bill denominations and some coins as well. The practice owner needs to track the petty cash and make one person responsible for the petty cash account. They need to make the responsible party understand that this is not "free" money but that they are responsible for it. The office needs to simple book that lists all petty cash expenditures. That way, they can keep a running tally of the amount, an accurate listing of how much cash has been used and who has used it.

PROTECTING AGAINST EMBEZZLEMENT

It is a sad fact that many dental offices fall prey to embezzlers. *Embezzlement* sounds like an innocuous, white-collar crime, but it is another word for "stealing." Some statistics show that as many as one in three dental practices may be a victim. Embezzlement may be as innocuous as taking a book of postage stamps (worth $30) or may involve the purposeful and systematic theft of thousands of dollars from the practice. The best defense against embezzlers is to be constantly aware, to know their patterns, and to be involved enough in the day-to-day office finances to discourage any would-be embezzlers.

Research shows that employers often consider an embezzler a "model" employee. Embezzlers work long hours (to cover their tracks) and "relieve" the practitioner of the need to be involved in the finances (to keep them ignorant of the problem). Embezzlers maintain a high degree of control of systems, seldom taking a vacation or allowing anyone else to help with "their" functions in the office. They generally present apparently thorough and complete reports, but they seldom show any account cards, bank statements, or other details of the accounting systems. All of this is allegedly to free the practice owner from "worrying about" accounting problems. In fact, it keeps the practitioner from discovering problems with the "books" of the practice.

Intelligent, enterprising, and unscrupulous people can devise many ways to steal from a dental practice. Cash transactions are difficult to trace, especially if the office does not issue a numbered receipt for every transaction. Staff can alter or destroy cash receipts, pocketing

BOX 27.6   EXAMPLE PATIENT ACCOUNTING TRANSACTIONS

	Date	Family member	Professional service	Charge	Payment	Charge adjustment	Payment adjustment	Balance
A	9/12	Mary	Restoration	$150	$150			$0
B	9/13	Chris	Crown	$1000	$200			$800
	9/22		Ins Check # 223344		$500			$300
C	9/13	Larry	Prophy	$80	$60		$20	$0
D	9/14	Betty	Restoration	$150	$100		$30	$20
E	9/15	Joe	Ex, Rad, Pro	$135			$135	$0
			Rest	$150	$65		$85	$0
F	9/20	Sam	Surgery	$300	$300			$0
	9/21	Sam	Posted in error			($300)	$300	$0
	9/21	Samantha	Surgery	$300	$300			$0
G	9/6	Louise	Rec, Pro	$95	$19			$76
	9/20		Ins Check # 45678		$79			($3)
H	3/6	Tom	Restoration	$185	$50			$135
	8/10	Tom	Bad debt				$135	$0
I	7/12	Sarah	Rec, Pro	$95	$95			$0
	7/19	Sarah	Bad check				($95)	$95
	7/19	Sarah	Bad check charge			$20		$115
	7/26	Sarah			$95			$20
J	7/19	Bob	RCT	$600	$600			$0
	7/25	Bob	RCT			($600)		($600)
	7/25	Bob	Debride, Ext	$175			$425	$0

A. Mary has a restoration and pays for it at the time of the visit. Her new balance is zero.

B. Chris has a crown on #3 ($1000 total charge). Chris pays $200, leaving a balance of $800. Chris's indemnity insurance company pays $500. Chris new balance is $300.

C. Larry receives a dental prophylaxis. A professional courtesy discount of $20 (a payment credit) was given. He pays the rest and has a zero balance.

D. Betty has a restoration done. The regular fee is $150. Her insurance plan allowable charge is $120. The required $30 is adjusted. Betty pays $100. Her balance is $20.

E. Joe has a capitation plan for his third-party plan. The contract specifies that practitioners provide exams, radiographs, and prophylaxis (a $135 value) at no charge. The practitioner then must only charge him $65 for a restoration (full fee $150). The rest is adjusted off his account (a payment/collection credit).

F. The practitioner incorrectly entered periodontal surgery and payment on Sam Smith's ledger. It should have been entered on Samantha Smith's account (a different account). It is entered as a "negative charge" (production debit) and a payment (payment credit) and reentered, correctly, on Samantha's account.

G. Louise had an exam and prophylaxis. The total charge was $95. The practitioner expected the insurance to pay $76. She paid her portion, $19. The insurance check came two weeks later for $79. Louise now has a negative balance due of $3. The practitioner could write her a check for $3, but she would rather just leave it on her account and use it against her next visit. This would be a payment credit if the practitioner wrote the check.

H. Tom had a restoration on #30, total charge $185. He paid $50 that day. Five months later, the practitioner sent Tom's account to the collection agency. The practitioner "wrote off" his bad debt (a collection or payment credit of $135).

I. Sarah had an exam and prophylaxis, total charge $95 (production debit). She paid with a check that "bounced" (payment debit). The bank returned it a week later marked *insufficient funds*. The office policy is that there is a $20 charge for all "bounced" checks (payment debit). The practitioner called Sarah; she assured us the problem was taken care of and to redeposit the check (payment credit). This time, the check was good. She owes the practitioner $20 for the bad check.

J. The practitioner started a root canal on Bob. Bob paid in full at the initial appointment. When he returned for completion, the practitioner found a crack running through the tooth, making it unrestorable. The practitioner extracted the tooth and rebated the cost of the endodontic therapy, charging him $100 for the debridement (previous appointment) and $75 for the extraction. The practitioner wrote him a check for the difference ($425).

the money. Employees have made checks out to their own debtors, having the practice unknowingly pay off personal debt. Other staff members have made fraudulent adjustments to a patient's account when the patient pays with cash, pocketing the adjustment. Some give favors to patients in return for kickbacks. False patient accounts are another likely source of embezzlement. One employee even set up a new joint bank account with the employee's and practitioner's names on the account. The employee then deposited patient checks in the new account and withdrew money from the account. All of this was unknown to the practitioner.

To avoid embezzlement, practice owners must actively protect themselves through preventive measures. The owner should always assume they might be a victim of staff embezzlement. They do not need to be paranoid, but being involved with accounting is the responsibility of a business owner. The practice owner can take several steps to decrease the likelihood that someone will embezzle from them:

- **Lead by active example**
  The practice owner must act legally and ethically in all financial transactions. They must only take cash from the office with proper accounting. They must expect others to behave similarly.

- **Hire the right people**
  The owner must recruit and hire trustworthy and ethical people to manage the office's financial systems. They need to thoroughly check the references and backgrounds of the people they hire.

- **Arrange job duties**
  The practice owner must set up the office job duties so that two or more people share some financial duties of the practice. They should have different people making collection calls, processing the mail-in and insurance checks, or preparing bank deposit slips. This form of check and balance discourages a would-be embezzler because others are looking at the details of the accounting system.

- **Manage staff time**
  The practice owner must insist that employees take vacations and maintain regular working hours. Although an employee who never takes a vacation and is willing to stay late (while the practitioner is not there) sounds like a dream worker, they are a problem waiting to happen.

- **Institute proper accounting procedures**
  The practice owner must be sure that each patient encounter has a corresponding transaction slip (or walkout statement). At the end of each day, the owner ought to check the day sheet to verify all patient transactions, especially adjustments. They should check the deposit slip against the day sheet to be sure that all money collected goes to the bank. Periodically (and unpredictably), the owner should audit the practice's financial records and ensure that everyone in the office sees them doing the audit. Although they may not find a problem, the fact that they are looking will discourage many people from even trying to steal.

- **Periodically audit the system**
  All computer systems have some form of audit trail. An audit trail lists all computer transactions, even if someone has deleted or overwritten them. There is a history of those changes that no one can erase. If a practitioner suspects embezzlement, the first place to look is the audit trail to see if anyone has altered or deleted any transactions.

The practice owner can also do several things about accounts payable and disbursements to discourage embezzlement:

- The dentist (or their spouse) must sign all checks drawn on the practice and must not grant signatory authority to a staff member. (The practice owner can have the staff member write or print the check. However, the dentist must verify and sign it.) A rubber stamp signature is an invitation to someone to act fraudulently.

- The owner needs to maintain a copy of every invoice and mark the check number on the invoice.

Part 3: Instrument Management Procedures

One only needs two tools in life: WD-40 to make things go, and duct tape to make them stop.

G. Weilacher

GOAL

This part discusses an instrument management system for the office so that the new practitioner can effectively manage this office function.

LEARNING OBJECTIVES

At the completion of this part, the student will be able to:

- Describe the goals of an instrument management plan for the dental office.

- Differentiate between the classifications of risk potential for dental instruments.

- Describe the types of surface disinfectants.

- Describe the proper sterilization procedure for the dental office.

- Describe office design considerations for instrument sterilization procedures.

- Describe procedures to sterilize instruments in the office properly.

- Describe a sterilizer monitoring program for the office.

KEY TERMS

cleaning instruments
critical instruments
dental healthcare personnel (DHCP)
housekeeping surfaces
instrument sets
non-critical instruments
semi-critical instruments
sterilizer monitoring

The instrument management plan for the office accomplishes several goals, as outlined in Box 27.7. The first goal is to prevent the spread of disease between patients and staff members. How dental offices handle both clean and dirty instruments has an obvious relationship to these goals. A properly designed instrument management plan also keeps instruments in good repair. This allows practitioners to buy only the instruments they need to keep costs as low as possible.

CENTERS FOR DISEASE CONTROL AND PREVENTION

The Centers for Disease Control and Prevention (CDC) dictates instrument management procedures through its website: https://www.cdc.gov/oralhealth/infectioncontrol/index.html. The Occupational Safety and Health Administration (OSHA) has adopted these CDC guidelines in its recommendations for worker safety in the office. This section does not try to describe that report in detail but discusses how to apply it in the dental office.

Practice owners must closely link any instrument management plan to the OSHA plan for the office. Because of the potential for sticks by dirty, sharp instruments, practice owners must have a plan in place that protects staff from injuries and follows up in case of an injury. The section on OSHA compliance discusses these issues.

Many new practice owners assume that staff members, especially those who have been "in the business" for many years, know how to manage instruments. That

BOX 27.7	GOALS OF AN INSTRUMENT MANAGEMENT PLAN

- Prevent cross-contamination

- Assure worker safety

- Provide enough instruments for operations

- Maintain instruments properly

- Allow change in instrumentation

- Keep costs low

- Be compliant with regulations

may not be the case. They may not be trained, may have been trained improperly, or may have been trained before many current guidelines were promulgated. Regardless, it is the practitioner's responsibility as owner and manager of the practice to ensure that all staff members know and follow proper instrument cleaning and sterilization procedures.

TYPES OF PATIENT CARE ITEMS

The CDC has classified instruments according to their potential for spreading infection in the dental office. Depending on the classification of the instrument (Box 27.8), they require different types of sterilization or disinfection. If a semi-critical item tolerates the sterilization procedure, it should be sterilized. If not, a high level of disinfection is acceptable.

Patient care devices that do not require sterilization are subject to one of three levels of disinfection: high, medium,

or low. Environmental surfaces (floors, cabinets, etc.) require one of two levels of disinfection: medium or low. Box 27.9 describes these levels of disinfection.

DENTAL OFFICE REQUIREMENTS

INSTRUMENT SETS

Modern dental operatories do not include large storage areas. Practitioners store instruments in the sterilization area and take them to the appropriate operatory as needed for each patient. This allows smaller operatories with less cabinetry. It also requires fewer instrument kits because practitioners do not need to store multiple copies of each kit in each operatory. As the number of procedures increases or changes over time, the office can add or change instrument kits in response.

BOX 27.8   CLASSIFICATION OF RISK POTENTIAL FOR SPREADING INFECTION

Category	Item definition	Examples	Transmission risk	Method of processing
Critical	Penetrates soft tissue Cuts hard or soft tissue	Burs, surgical instruments	High	Sterilization
Semi-critical	Touches mucous membrane or non-intact skin	Bite blocks, x-ray blocks	High to moderate	Sterilization High-level disinfection
Non-critical	Contacts intact skin	Facebow	Low	Cleaning and disinfection

---

BOX 27.9   SURFACE DISINFECTANTS

Category	Definition	Examples	Uses
High-level disinfectants	Destroy all microorganisms except bacterial endospores	Glutaraldehydes, hydrogen peroxide, hypochlorites	Heat-sensitive items, immersion only (do not use on environmental surfaces)
Intermediate-level disinfectants	Destroy bacteria, most fungi, and viruses; tuberculocidal	Environmental Protection Agency (EPA)-registered hospital disinfectants with the claim of tuberculocidal activity, iodophors	Clinical contact surfaces; non-critical surfaces with visible blood or debris
Low-level disinfectants	Destroy bacteria, some fungi, and viruses; not tuberculocidal	Quaternary ammonium compounds; EPA-registered hospital disinfectants without claim of tuberculocidal activity	Housekeeping surfaces

There are two standard methods of distributing instrument sets to the operatories: trays and cassettes. The staff must package instruments from trays for sterilization and then reset fresh trays with sterile instruments. This involves additional staff time and increases the possibility of injury each time they handle instruments. Cassettes have the advantage that hands do not touch the instruments. Staff members can place the entire cassette in the cleaner and then the autoclave. Cassettes carry a higher initial cost than trays. Dental offices also need a larger (more expensive) autoclave to accept cassettes (particularly large cassettes) over bagged instruments. Cassettes should be color-coded or have colored tape or other markers applied to show the types of instruments contained (e.g. operative, or endodontic).

Plastic tubs (color-coded) contain all the special materials needed for a procedure. These materials and equipment are *non-critical* instruments that do not need sterilization after use. For example, an endodontic tub contains sealers, points, and other supplies used in endodontic procedures. If an instrument does need sterilization, it is placed into a separate tray or cassette for processing.

NUMBER OF INSTRUMENT SETS AND TYPES NEEDED

Several factors dictate the number and type of instrument set-ups a practitioner needs. A practitioner does not want to run out of instrument set-ups, but they also do not want to have too many set-ups, because they are expensive. First, the practitioner determines the office instrument processing cycle. Many offices process once per day. Others process twice daily (at lunchtime and again at the end of the day). Larger offices that have a dedicated sterilization clerk will process instruments continually. Next, the practitioner estimates the number of patient visits per processing cycle. If the hygienist sees a patient for an hour and the office processes instruments every four hours, they need a minimum of four hygiene set-ups. If the practitioner might do two endodontic procedures in a cycle, then they need a minimum of two endodontic set-ups. Once the practitioner decides the minimum number of instrument sets they need, they should add 50%. (For example, if the practitioner decides they need six operative sets, they should get nine.) This covers a hectic day, processing backlogs, or the possibility of a set being dropped or otherwise deemed unusable.

INSTRUMENTS WITHIN THE SETS

The practitioner needs to decide the specific instruments they want within each set of instruments. They ought to use the minimum number that gives excellent results. Dental suppliers have instrument markers (small plastic rings that fit securely on dental instruments). The practitioner should get a different color for each type of set-up (e.g. blue for operative, green for prophy). Within those set-ups, the employees place the instruments in the order in which they will use them. Place the color-coded bands on the instruments in descending order. This method allows staff to quickly put the instruments in the proper order and decide if any instruments are missing during processing.

STAFF CONSIDERATIONS

As previously mentioned, OSHA requirements dictate instrument processing procedures. Practice owners must train and monitor dental healthcare personnel (DHCP) for properly performing procedures. They must wear PPE and thick protective gloves (not patient care gloves) when they process instruments.

Larger offices often have staff members whose only job is to process instruments. In these offices, instrument processing will be a continuous procedure. Many smaller offices do not need to process instruments constantly. Instead, they process instruments at several points in the daily routine, often at lunchtime or the end of the day. Some offices make each staff member responsible for cleaning and packaging their own instruments. Others make one staff member responsible for all the processing.

OFFICE DESIGN CONSIDERATIONS

The design of an office needs to provide for easy transportation of instruments to and from the sterilization area. Therefore, it ought to be centrally placed near the operatory patient areas. Ideally, it should have a separate traffic pattern from patients so that patients cannot be in contact with dirty instruments or wander into the sterilization area.

The size of the sterilization area will vary with the available floor space, the number of operatories, and normal patient flow. It needs to have ample counter space (at least 10 linear feet) and needs to be divided into "dirty" and "sterile" sides. Dirty instruments stay only on their side, and sterile instruments on theirs. (Some offices use signs or tape on the counters to designate clean and dirty areas in the sterilization room.) Storage for dirty instruments (trays or cassettes) must never mingle with storage of clean trays or cassettes. Storage cabinets will ideally have clear plastic doors that can be quickly taken apart and cleaned. There must be a large, deep sink with a spray attachment on the dirty side of the counter.

The instrument processing area must allow instruments to flow in a single loop for optimal workflow and aseptic technique. The staff bring contaminated instruments into the area, clean, package, sterilize, and store them continuously, like on an assembly line. The more automated the process becomes, the less chance there is for operator error in processing. The sterilization area must be separate, not shared or mingled with other functions. Some small offices combine the dental lab or general storage area with the sterilization area. This invites cross-contamination. Although space limitations may dictate some compromises, the practice owner should try to keep a dedicated area for instrument processing. OSHA guidelines require an approved eyewash station in the instrument processing area. That are should also have compressed air and vacuum lines for cleaning and lubricating handpieces before sterilization.

STERILIZATION AND DISINFECTION PROCEDURES

OPERATORY BREAKDOWN

The practice owner needs to schedule enough time (10 minutes) at the end of each appointment for operatory breakdown, cleaning, and set-up. DHCP should place all sharps into an approved and labeled sharps container. They should place all soaked or saturated material and all tissue (teeth or surgically removed tissue) into appropriate biohazard bags. They may put all other waste into the waste system. Before transferring instruments to the processing area, they must place them in covered containers. DHCP then disinfect smooth surfaces and remove and discard barriers.

In the dental operatory, surfaces that do not touch the patient can still become contaminated with saliva, blood, or another infectious residue. Their likelihood of having any infectious residue dictates their cleaning method. The CDC classifies them as either clinical or housekeeping surfaces (Box 27.9).

Housekeeping surfaces, such as floors, walls, and sinks, have a limited risk of disease transmission. Dental practice employees decontaminate them with less rigorous methods than patient care or clinical surfaces. Most of these surfaces only need to be cleaned with a detergent and water, or hospital disinfectant approved by the Environmental Protection Agency (EPA). Thorough cleaning once a day is more important for these surfaces than disinfection (Box 27.10).

BOX 27.10	OPERATORY SURFACE ASEPSIS

Type

- Clinical contact
  - Between patients
  - Housekeeping

- End of day

Methods

- Barriers

- Preclean and disinfect

Clinical surfaces often are touched with contaminated gloved hands or are spattered or sprayed during procedures. Examples include light switches and handles, drawer pulls, pens, and curing light triggers. Barriers are the most effective method of preventing contamination on these surfaces, especially those that are difficult to clean (such as knobs on operating equipment). If the office does not use barriers, the surface requires thorough cleaning followed by an EPA-registered hospital disinfectant.

RECEIVING AND CLEANING

The receiving area is where the office stores instruments before they process them. Staff discard any disposables not previously removed from the trays in the operatory. Cabinets above the counter, with shelves for cassettes, trays, or instruments, provide safe storage until staff can complete the cleaning procedure (Figure 27.1).

Cleaning does not sterilize the instruments; it only prepares them for sterilization. If instruments cannot be processed immediately, they need to remain wet so that the material does not dry onto them. Many practices use puncture-resistant plastic holding tubs for this purpose. Individual instruments should be placed into wire mesh baskets to reduce the chance of an accident. Cleaning removes the obvious material (e.g. blood, cement, material) that the staff members did not remove previously. The solutions used include enzymic cleaners or detergents. In most practices, the cleaning area includes a large, deep stainless-steel sink with a spray attachment.

There are three methods of cleaning: hand scrubbing, ultrasonic, and dishwasher-style cleaning systems. Hand scrubbing has fallen out of favor because of the

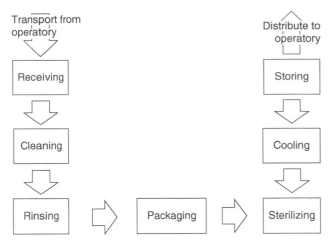

FIGURE 27.1 Instrument processing cycle.

apparent problem of potential worker injury. Ultrasonic cleaners are often plumbed directly into the existing sink drains. Many offices recess them into the countertop to improve the ergonomic transfer of cassettes at elbow height. The practice owner should be sure that the ultrasonic cleaner is large enough to hold the largest cassette. Instrument washers are devices approved by the Food and Drug Administration (FDA) for cleaning instruments and cassettes. They operate similarly to a home dishwasher.

When DHCP are ready to process instruments, they remove the instruments from the holding solution. They gather instruments from trays (in tray systems) and bind them with a rubber band. They then place them in the ultrasonic cleaner or washer-disinfector. They remove cassettes (in cassette systems) from the holding solution and place them into the cleaner. DHCP then run the ultrasonic or washer-disinfector according to the manufacturer's instructions. After the cycle is complete, DHCP remove cassettes or bundles of instruments and place them in the sink to rinse them thoroughly to remove chemical or detergent residues. They then place them on a rack or towels in the next area to dry.

PACKAGING

When the instruments have dried, DHCP inspect and clean any instruments with any remaining material. At this time, they replace any broken or damaged instruments. They also sharpen cutting instruments that have dulled. They then place the instruments in their proper place in the cassette, close the cassette, and place it in an appropriate sterilizer bag (along with a sterilizer monitor strip), and seal and label the bag. After this, no one reopens the cassette until it is next used in the operatory. In tray systems, the staff member removes the rubber band holding the instruments and verifies their cleanliness, replacing or sharpening them as required. They then package the instruments in an appropriate sterilizer bag (along with a sterilizer monitor strip) and seal the bag. DHCP must always wear heavy-duty puncture-resistant gloves whenever they are working with instruments.

STERILIZATION

DHCP sterilize the bags or bagged cassettes according to the sterilizer manufacturer's directions. They must take special care to load the sterilizer according to the manufacturer's directions. The sterilizing agent (steam or vapor) must circulate properly within the sterilizer to ensure proper function. At the end of the cycle, the instruments need to cool in the sterilizer to avoid burns. If this is not possible (because of time constraints), the practice owner needs to have the staff member use tongs to remove instrument packages and let them cool on the countertop. A "hot" sign needs to mark these packages properly.

HANDPIECE STERILIZATION

Dental handpieces are critical instruments that require sterilization. They are also expensive instruments that must be appropriately cared for and maintained. Fortunately, modern handpieces will last many sterilization cycles. Staff must follow several steps for handpiece sterilization:

- Purge the handpiece of water.

- Spray lubricant through the handpiece into the turbine area to lubricate and protect it before sterilization (following the manufacturer's directions).

- Bag the handpiece and add an indicator strip.

- Sterilize the handpieces.

- Store the handpieces properly (usually in an upright position).

Despite best efforts, the practice owner will need to have handpieces repaired periodically because of wear and tear from the sterilization process. This is a cost of doing business.

STERILIZER MONITORING

Most states require that practice owners monitor the effectiveness of their sterilization procedures. Each state's laws vary regarding frequency and type of testing, but generally follow the CDC guidelines:

- Use mechanical monitoring for every load. Staff must check the timer and indicators on the autoclave to ensure it has operated according to specifications. Many modern sterilizers have printouts for each load as a record of effectiveness.

- Place a chemical indicator inside every package. Most offices use a color-change test strip with each load (or in each bag) to ensure that heat has penetrated the load.

- Monitor each sterilizer with a spore test once per week. Subjecting live organisms and spores to the sterilization cycle accomplishes the actual monitoring. Practice owners then send these to an appropriate lab to be cultured. If nothing grows, the procedure was effective. Several businesses contract with healthcare facilities for this monitoring function.

STORAGE

Staff members then store sterile instrument packages on the clean side of the sterilization area to ensure their sterility during storage. If the office uses trays, they generally set instruments on trays and store the set trays rather than setting trays at the time they need them. (Schedules have a way of falling apart, and days become hectic.)

DISTRIBUTION

Staff use the daily schedule as a guide to setting trays and tubs for patient procedures. After they dismiss a patient and disinfect the operatory, they carry the appropriate tray (and tub) for the upcoming patient to the operatory. They wait to open sterilization packs in the operatory in front of the patient. Not only does this reduce contamination of the instruments, but opening them in the presence of patients reassures them that the instruments are sterile.

OTHER OFFICE INSTRUMENT ISSUES

DENTAL WATERLINES

Biofilms often form from oral fluids being sucked back into dental instruments (e.g. handpieces, ultrasonic scalers, three-way syringes). There are presently no federal regulations, per se, concerning dental office waterline management. There is presently no epidemiologic evidence that shows that waterlines in dental offices pose a safety risk to patients or DHCP. However, the CDC considers exposing patients or staff to water of uncertain microbiological quality a concern. It recommends that water used as a coolant/irrigant in non-surgical procedures meet the standards for drinking water as established by the CDC and the American Public Health Association. Manufacturers have engineered many modern dental units to prevent contamination. DHCP must be sure to follow the manufacturer's recommendations. The CDC further recommends that all instruments connected to public water lines must be run for 20–30 seconds at the end of a procedure to physically flush any patient-generated material that might have entered the instrument or waterlines.

MERCURY EFFLUENT

When a practitioner removes an amalgam restoration, the pieces of the old filling, dust, and slurry from the procedure are all collected through the high-speed evaluation system. This usually empties into the local sewer system and, after treatment, into the public water supply. Heavy metals, such as mercury, are well-known health hazards, even in small amounts. Consequently, many people are concerned that dental offices are adding a significant amount of mercury to the public water treatment system. Some offices have added a mercury trap that captures the mercury and other metals before they enter the public sewage system. This may be a requirement for all dental offices in the future.

Part 4: Office Supply and Lab Management

Inventories can be managed, but people must be led.

Ross Perot

GOAL

This part aims to describe several techniques to manage office supplies and laboratory cases.

LEARNING OBJECTIVES

At the completion of this part, the student will be able to:

- Describe the purpose of an inventory management system.

- Describe the ideal inventory management system.

- Describe the types of supplies used in a dental office.

- Describe how to manage supplies that arrive in the office.

- Describe the purposes of a laboratory management system.

- Describe how to choose a dental laboratory.

KEY TERMS

back-order	order lead time
bulk buying	reorder point
invoice	rotating stock
Material Safety Data Sheet (MSDS)	stock-out
	terms of payment

Most dental offices have an "inventory" of materials and medicaments they use when treating patients. These are really supplies. Common business language lists inventory as a product that will be sold to customers. Inventory and supplies are accounted for differently for tax determination, but for the purposes here they can be thought of similarly.

A well-designed and implemented inventory system satisfies several purposes. It ensures that the practitioner has supplies when they need them. If the practitioner "stocks out" and does not have impression material for a large case, they will lose the income and possibly the patient's goodwill. Practice owners must ensure that supplies are current and have not expired. Many materials have expiration dates associated with them. The material may not perform as expected if it is too old. A system helps to control supply costs and lets the practice owner change materials without excessive cost or time.

Dental practices have several types of supplies that they routinely use in the office. The ones often thought of are dental materials. These include all types of cement, restorative materials, medicaments, and operating supplies used in patient care. Dental offices also need general office supplies, such as paper hand towels, toilet tissue, cleaning supplies, and hand soap. Finally, dental practices need business office supplies, such as stationery, copy paper, pens, paper clips, and toner cartridges. They may purchase each of these categories of supply from a different vendor. A large wholesale store may provide the best price on paper products, whereas an office supply store may have the best selection and price for office supplies.

INVENTORY SYSTEMS

In the ideal inventory system, supplies are ordered with just enough lead time to fill and ship the order (Figure 27.2). The practitioner runs out of supply just as they receive the order to replenish the supply and put it on the shelf. This keeps supplies fresh and cuts storage costs to a minimum. In reality, practice owners cannot live nearly this close to the line. They need to learn precisely how much material they need or when they need it. Suppliers may run out of a product to send and back-order the supply. They may delay shipping or find that some of the current supply needs to perform more adequately. Practice owners know that they will carry some excess supply, as shown in the realistic inventory system in Figure 27.3. They want to reduce excess inventory and storage costs to a reasonable extent.

Practice owners can buy supplies in bulk; that is, a large quantity that lasts a long time. The advantages are the lower cost per unit that vendors offer for quantity purchase and the freedom from worrying about running out of supply for an extended time. However, bulky items may lead to increased space and cost of storage. Materials that have a shelf life may expire and be wasted. So there is an apparent balancing act here.

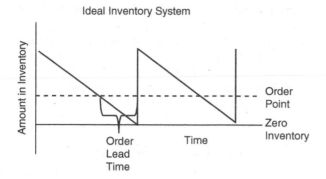

FIGURE 27.2   Ideal inventory system.

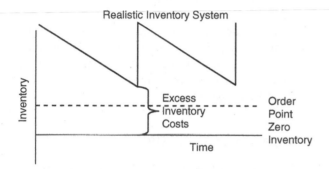

FIGURE 27.3   Realistic inventory system.

Any chemicals or materials come with a Material Safety Data Sheet (MSDS). Generally, the manufacturer packages them with the product, although sometimes the practitioner needs to go online to get the MSDS. OSHA requires that the practice owner keeps these available in case a patient or staff member has an accident with the material. These sheets list required emergency procedures and antidotes for the chemicals in the product. Emergency department personnel can then provide appropriate care based on the contents of the MSDS.

Some materials (e.g. composite restorative material) require refrigerated storage to achieve optimum shelf life and performance. In these cases, OSHA requires that dental practices have a separate refrigerator from another that staff use to store food products (e.g. lunches). In this way, practitioners avoid any potential cross-contamination.

Dental practices generally rotate their stock of supplies. This means they place the newest material at the "back of the line" of supply. This ensures that the practice uses the older supplies first, which helps prevent supplies from passing their expiration date.

ORDERING SUPPLIES

A couple of common ordering systems exist. In the first (informal) system, a designated staff member checks the inventory weekly, noting any supplies running low. They then list any needed products for order. The informality of this system leads to some apparent caveats. A different person generally looks at clinical and business office supplies. Each person needs to know how much material the office typically uses so that they can decide on an accurate order point. This may take some experience and growing pains as the person acclimates to the job. The practice owner might set rules such as "Order impression material when the second to last box of material is opened" to guide an employee who is learning to manage the inventory system.

A more formal system requires a card for each inventory item. Staff members place a small colored dot sticker on the box of supplies at the reorder point. They rotate stock, and when they pull the box with the sticker from inventory, they pull the card and place it in a "to order" box.

Once the office decides to order, the practice owner must decide from whom to order. Dental suppliers want to be a practitioner's "full service" supplier, providing dental materials, equipment, office supplies, equipment repair, computers, software, and management advice. In short, the suppliers want to provide all a practice owner's support services. When supply houses find that a practitioner has entered practice, they will generally send a sales representative (or rep or detail person) to the dental office to gain its business. These representatives take orders for supplies, bring samples of new materials, return incorrect orders, and make a practitioner aware of special offers. It is advantageous to have one (or two) suppliers as the practice's primary suppliers. If an office suddenly finds that they have run out of a supply, or a piece of critical equipment stops working, a supplier will more likely work extra to see that the practitioner is satisfied if they have a primary account with them. The office can also order materials from mail order or online suppliers. The price will probably be lower because the supplier does not have the expense of representatives driving to the office regularly to take orders. The practitioner may have a problem if a piece of equipment breaks or if the supplier back-orders a supply or, for another reason, the practice needs immediate service from a supplier.

Practice owners can buy ordinary paper and office supplies from business supply stores or warehouse clubs for less than from the dental supplier. However, there is a convenience factor for the "one-stop shopping" that supply houses offer. If the practice owner accumulates several small orders into one larger order, they often save through lower shipping costs. The owner also can negotiate with vendors. If they find something they want from a competing vendor, they should show the special price to the primary supplier and ask them to meet it. Often the supplier will. Practitioners need to watch for specials from vendors. They will often offer free material or additional products if the practitioner purchases during a convention or dental meeting from the convention floor.

RECEIVING SUPPLIES

When the order arrives from the supply house, office employees must verify that the supplier has shipped all material as ordered. Each shipment will contain a packing slip that details all items shipped in the package. Sometimes there is also an invoice, though often the supplier sends the invoice separately. An invoice, or bill, is a document the seller provides that details the goods' products, quantities, prices, and payment terms.

If something is missing or shipped incorrectly (wrong item, size, or damaged goods), the practitioner must call their sales rep and inform the rep of the problem. The practitioner does not want to pay for items they did not order, nor do they want to keep items they ordered that are faulty. Different supply houses have different procedures for returning incorrect or damaged merchandize. Many practitioners will have the representative pick up the supply on their next visit. The representative will issue a credit memo for the material that was incorrect. The practitioner needs to track these to be sure they are listed on their monthly statement. If the vendor is out of an item, they will say that it is "back-ordered," which means that they will send it when they receive it from the manufacturer.

PAYING FOR SUPPLIES

The large supply houses send the practice owner a monthly statement with each invoice noted and a total of all monthly charges. The practice owner pays for the supplies when they receive this monthly statement, not from each separate invoice. This statement has all the invoices from the month collected together. In this way, the owner only pays once, even if they have made and received several orders during that time. Often the owner can pay supply invoices by credit card. (This practice depends on the vendor's payment rules.) Doing this allows the owner to pay for the supplies later and increases the rebate tally on the office credit card. The practice owner must not miss the payment due date. Most houses charge interest if they do not have the payment in hand by the due date. The invoice gives the terms of payment. The most common is "Net/30," meaning the net payment is due 30 days from when the invoice was issued.

Some suppliers, especially those that a practitioner orders from infrequently, will post "pay from this invoice" or similar words on the invoice. This means that they will not send the practice a separate monthly statement. The owner pays the vendor as stipulated on the invoice.

LABORATORY CASE MANAGEMENT

The practitioner or staff members can do all laboratory procedures in the office. However, most dental offices find that outsourcing these procedures is convenient and cost-effective if the practitioner has additional patients to see instead of doing the laboratory procedure. These may be procedures that the practitioner does not have the materials, machines, or knowledge to do; they may be procedures that the practitioner can outsource for a lower cost, or they may be procedures the practitioner does not enjoy doing. Regardless, the practice owner needs a system to monitor work that goes out of the office to ensure timeliness, quality, and cost-effectiveness.

CHOOSING A LABORATORY

From several perspectives, deciding which laboratory to use for various procedures is an important decision. The practitioner needs to have a good working relationship with the laboratory technician who does work for them. The practitioner might need to call the lab and discuss problem areas with the case or ask questions about procedures or techniques. The lab is the expert around materials and techniques, so the lab workers can help the practitioner decide if a particular type or brand of material will work in each situation. A healthy, open discussion is often necessary to gain optimum results for a patient. The practitioner needs to visit the labs in the area and interview them as if they were a potential employee (which is really what they are doing).

The practitioner might have several different labs for different procedures. This may be based on their quality history, price, or the special materials and techniques they employ. Lab A may do excellent porcelain work, Lab B does extraordinary denture cases, and Lab C may work with the practitioner in coordinating implant cases. Use each lab for its strength to gain the best result for patients.

Laboratory personnel may change over time. The technician who had been doing the work for a practitioner may leave for another lab or retire. Often the only way the practitioner knows is if there is a noticeable change in the returned work. If the practitioner sees a problem, they should call the lab to discuss the issue. The practitioner may have to investigate a different laboratory if the lab cannot resolve the problem.

PROCESSING CASES

There is a cost trade-off for most procedures. The practitioner can send many impressions to the lab for model pouring and preparation, or they can do these procedures in house. This allows them to save money and check the work before sending it out. The practitioner needs to decide which types and what degree of cases they process internally. Digital impression systems allow the practitioner to send an electronic image to the laboratory for the preparation and construction of the restoration.

Most states require that a practitioner write a paper prescription or authorization for the work they want the lab to do. This authorization lists the exact procedures they want to be completed and any necessary materials, shades, or special instructions. Many states require the practitioner to retain a copy for a certain number of years.

When the case (all impressions, opposing casts, bite registrations, prescriptions, etc.) is ready, the practitioner sends it to the laboratory. If the lab is local, it may have a courier who will stop by the office to pick up the case and deliver it back when complete. If the lab is distant, the practitioner must be sure to box the material so it will not be damaged in transit. Further, the practitioner needs to be sure to note on the authorization when they need the case back in the office for try-in or seating. The practitioner will then note on the schedule that they require a lab case for the appointment. Staff check at the morning huddle the day before the appointment to ensure that the lab has returned the case. If not, they will call the lab to ensure they deliver the case on time.

Part 5: Dental Insurance Management

Beaver: "Gee, there's something wrong with just about everything, isn't there Dad?"
Ward: "Just about, Beav."

Leave It to Beaver

GOAL

This part introduces the various forms of third-party plans that practitioners encounter when in practice. It discusses their conceptual background and how they affect the dental practitioner.

LEARNING OBJECTIVES

At the completion of this part, the student will be able to:

- Discuss the purchaser, provider, and patient relationship regarding payment for dental services.
- Discuss the assumption of risk.
- Describe common payment mechanisms.
- Define various utilization incentives.
- Describe the historical origins of third-party payment plans.
- Recognize the role of dental practice in third-party management.
- Describe the carrier's responsibility to the practitioner and the patient.
- Discuss the patient's role in the third-party process.
- Recognize the different areas of the American Dental Association claim form and discuss the importance of each.
- Describe various techniques that can maximize benefits for the patient.
- Discuss the effects on office finances of the following payment mechanisms:
  - Medicaid
  - Medicare
  - Indemnity plan
  - Service corporation plan (Delta Dental)
  - Health maintenance organization (HMO)
  - Capitation plan (cap plan)
  - Preferred provider organization (PPO)
  - Contract dental organization (CDO)
  - Independent practice association (IPA)
  - Direct reimbursement.
- Describe contract provisions of interest to practitioners.
- Discuss how the practitioner might effectively use third-party plans to their advantage.

KEY TERMS

adverse selection
any willing provider
assignment of benefits
cafeteria (flexible)
  benefit plan
capitation plan
  (cap plan)
closed panel
contract dental organi-
  zation (CDO)
cost shifting
dental health main-
  tenance organiza-
  tion (HMOs)
dental maintenance
  organization (DMO)
diagnostic-related
  group (DRG)
direct reimbursement
  (DR)
employee benefits
fee for service (FFS)
first party
fourth party
freedom of choice
indemnity insurance

independent practice
  association (IPA)
least expensive alterna-
  tive treatment (LEAT)
managed care
managed dental care
medical loss ratio
Medicaid
Medicare
most favored
  nations clause
open panel
overall reimbursement rate
plan utilization control
preferred provider
  organization (PPO)
relative value unit
second party
third party
table of allowances
traditional den-
  tal insurance
two-tiered treatment plan
unbundling
voluntary provider
  network

A dental practice has several stakeholders, or parties, who have an interest in the care the practitioner provides in the dental office. The "first" party is the practitioner and the "second" is the patient. For many years, these were the only parties who had a vested interest in the practice of dentistry. However, when insurers began to reimburse for dental services, they became an interested "third" party. The employers who purchased the insurance contracts soon realized that they were the "fourth" party and also had a vital interest. Depending on their contract, the price they paid and the services they bought for their employees were entirely different. It is important to remember that there are four different perspectives on the issue of third-party reimbursement for dental care (Box 27.11). The practitioner has one set of desires; the patient, the insurer, and the employer each have different wants and needs in these programs. Each group lobbies in the marketplace for provisions that are beneficial for their group. The "ideal" third-party program balances all these perspectives.

BOX 27.11	STAKEHOLDERS OF A DENTAL PRACTICE
First party	Practitioner
Second party	Patient
Third party	Insurer
Fourth party	Employer

Benefits for routine dental services are unlike traditional insurance in some crucial respects. Dental needs are almost universal, unlike house fires, automobile accidents, or major surgery. So, a dental plan, especially the component that pays for routine dental services, is more of a simple prepayment plan than a true insurance policy.

Employee benefits, such as dental plans, are typically bought by employers to increase employee compensation and, hopefully, morale and productivity. Plan administrators place bids with the employer for the dental plan contract. The employer (possibly in concert with a union or worker representation) then picks a contract that best meets everyone's needs. The plan may be financed through an employer contribution, employee contributions, or a combination of the two. In traditional indemnity insurance contracts, the carrier does actuarial studies to determine how many people will probably use the services and at what level. The insurers use that information to establish utilization estimates and policy rates.

PAYMENT MECHANISMS

Dental practitioners customarily see four basic types or methods of payment for services.

FEE FOR SERVICE

Fee for service (FFS) is simply an out-of-pocket expenditure by patients for the care that they receive. This still accounts for a significant portion (approximately 45%) of the dental care payments in the United States today. The obvious advantage for the practitioner is the low interference in the practitioner–patient relationship. The downside for both patient and practitioner is that consumers will purchase less dentistry because the cost to the consumer (patient) is higher than if someone assists in paying.

TRADITIONAL (INDEMNITY) DENTAL INSURANCE

Indemnity insurance pays the patient for their financial loss from dental care. The plan estimates how much care a given population (e.g. the employees at XYZ Corp.) will need. The insurer then pays the patient for part of their financial loss (dental care). If the insurance company has estimated too low, the insurer loses money. If its estimates are correct, then the insurance company makes money. The insurer carries the risk of overutilization of services. Traditional dental insurance stimulates demand for dental services because the patient's out-of-pocket expenditures are lower than FFS.

MANAGED DENTAL CARE

Managed care is a system where the third party (insurer) contracts with practitioners to provide a certain level of dental care. Instead of insurance, managed care is a form of prepayment for services. It is the practitioner's responsibility to decide the amount and type of care that the patient requires. However, the contract may stipulate the amount the practitioner can charge the patient for the service. Because the practitioner contracts ahead of doing the services, they carry the risk that patients may overutilize by demanding more services (either in the type of services or the number of services per patient). If, on the other hand, patients underutilize services, the practitioner stands to profit.

GOVERNMENT PAYMENT PLANS

Government plans are a small part of the dental marketplace in the United States. Dental care is viewed as a consumer service (rather than a true health service) by many people, and so individuals are responsible for their own services. The government directly provides some care to special populations at the federal level (e.g. Indian Health Service, National Health Service Corp., Uniform Military Services) and state and local health departments. The government also pays for some care in private offices, primarily through Medicaid and, to a small degree, the Medicare programs. Many government plans adopt the characteristics of managed care plans. Many negotiate contracts with private managed care plans to administer the government plan.

POLICY LIMITATIONS

Each third-party plan has specific incentives (and disincentives) for patients to use dental services. The provider (practitioner) looks for maximum reimbursement, maximum coverage, minimum administrative expense, and no interference in the practitioner–patient relationship (including closed panels). The patient wants maximum reimbursement and coverage, giving the lowest out-of-pocket expense.

Patients want "freedom of choice," but are willing to forgo this if the savings are substantial enough. The purchaser (employer) wants an adequate plan at a low cost. Employers are concerned with providing a satisfactory benefit for employees with minimal administrative costs and problems. They do not care about freedom of choice unless employees complain that they cannot find adequate dental providers. The third-party carrier is looking to reduce its own risk and maximize profit for its owners and shareholders. Carriers are looking for a small payout (low medical loss ratio) and minimum administrative expenses. Balancing all these different perspectives and needs is an impossible task. To attempt it, insurance plans use many mechanisms to encourage or discourage patient treatment:

- **Exclusions** are procedures that the plan does not cover. Most insurers exclude experimental procedures. As those procedures become more commonplace, insurers begin to include them as covered procedures. Some plans may exclude orthodontics, temporomandibular disorder (TMD), or other treatments as cost-limiting measures.

- **Limitations** are limits to payment of benefits for procedures or the number of times a plan will pay for a procedure. Most plans limit prosthetic replacement to once every five years, regardless of who does the procedure. Many will limit payment for orthodontic treatment to once in a lifetime. Others limit recall exams to every six months (to the day). Patients often do not understand limitations, so it is in the practitioner's interest to have a staff member (receptionist) who understands each plan.

- **Annual maximums** are the maximum amounts in a given calendar year that an insurer will pay in total benefits for a person. Most plans set an annual maximum (or payment cap) near $1000, which has not changed (even with inflation) in many years. Practitioners frequently plan treatment to occur at the end of one year and the beginning of the next. This way, they can help the patient maximize insurance coverage for two years. Some plans also have a lifetime maximum for certain procedures (such as orthodontics).

- **Deductibles and copays** limit the third party's benefit payments. The patient is responsible for part of the costs, either the first dollar amount (deductible) or a percentage of the cost (copay).

- **Open-panel plans** allow covered patients to receive care from any practitioner and allow any practitioner to participate. These are often called "freedom-of-choice" plans.

- **Closed-panel plans** allow covered individuals to receive care only from a specific group (panel) of practitioners who have signed contracts and agree to terms of participation with the third-party carrier. Closed panels allow managed care organizations (MCOs) to limit the number of providers in the plan. In that way, they can guarantee a group of patients for each of those who do participate.

Insurance is generally regulated by state not national government. Therefore, there is not uniformity about the rules and laws concerning dental insurance benefits. For example, in some states if a specific service is not covered by a contracted (managed care) plan, the dentist may charge any fee for this "non-covered service." Other states require the dentist to follow the plan's fee schedule for the service, even though the service is not reimbursed by the plan. Or if a tooth is restored and the patient's non-compliant behavior results in a broken tooth within a time limit, some managed care contracts require the dentist to replace the restoration at their own expense. Each state's department of insurance sets the rules for these contracts.

METHOD OF REIMBURSEMENT

Third-party plans have developed many ways of determining reimbursement for services. If a dental practitioner understands these methods, it will allow them to help patients to maximize their benefits and enable the practitioner to evaluate the financial impact of third-party plans.

USUAL, CUSTOMARY, AND REASONABLE

Usual, customary, and reasonable (UCR) represents the fee a practitioner usually charges for a particular procedure. The insurance company determines the customary fee based on what practitioners in the same area are charging for similar procedures (Box 27.12). A reasonable fee justifies

---

BOX 27.12 "USUAL, CUSTOMARY, AND REASONABLE" FEE

- A patient's plan pays 80% of the UCR or practitioner's fee, whichever is less. The practitioner charges (and submits) a claim for a filling for $100. The insurance company compares that fee to its UCR for the area.

- If the UCR is more (say, $120) then the insurance company pays 80% of the charge, or $80 (80% of $100).

- If, however, the UCR for the procedure is less (say $90), then the insurance company will pay only 80% of this lower fee, or $72 (80% of $90).

---

particular circumstances that may affect the fee usually charged for the procedure. Wide differences between communities have made this system controversial. Third-party carriers generally reimburse based on a percentage of the lesser of the practitioner's usual fee or the fee that the third party has determined is customary for the area. The fee that the carriers use as their "customary" fee is a closely held corporate secret. This often causes problems between practitioners and patients who feel they are being overcharged based on insurance carrier information.

TABLE (SCHEDULE) OF ALLOWANCES

In this method, the insurer sets a maximum dollar limit for each covered procedure, regardless of the fee the practitioner charges. It pays the fee charged (or a percentage of it) up to a specified amount from a table that lists the allowable (maximum) charge. Above that, the practitioner may (or may not) charge the patient the difference, depending on the rules of the insurance contract.

LEAST EXPENSIVE ALTERNATIVE TREATMENT

The least expensive alternative treatment (LEAT) method states that the third party will reimburse for what it decides is the least expensive method of correcting the patient's problem. For example, a practitioner might replace a patient's missing tooth with an implant, a fixed bridge, or a removable partial denture. The practitioner can recommend to the patient and do any service the practitioner wants. However, the third-party payer will only reimburse for the LEAT (i.e. the removable). Others may "downcode" a posterior composite restoration to a less expensive amalgam restoration. This keeps the insurer's payout lower and places the burden of justifying treatment choices on the practitioner.

CAPITATION (PER CAPITA)

Capitated plans reimburse a practitioner a given amount for each participating patient who has signed up to be a practice patient. The practitioner is then responsible for providing a certain level of care in return for receiving the capitation payment. Patients are responsible for paying for (or a portion of) procedures not covered by the plan. The theory is that the practitioner makes enough money on capitation payments, based on the panel of patients, to cover the preventive services of those patients who come for dental care. Capitation plans have implied financial incentives for the practitioner not to see patients or do extensive dental work on them.

OTHER INSURANCE TERMS

A few additional insurance terms are essential to understand:

- **Adverse selection** occurs when only high-risk individuals sign up for a particular insurance. The insurer cannot spread the risk over a sufficient number of people. The insurer then either must increase rates dramatically or suffer a loss. This often happens with voluntary participation plans such as flexible (cafeteria-style) employee benefit plans. Only the employees who plan to use the plan sign up and pay to participate in the plan.

- Insurers speak of a **medical loss ratio**. This is the percentage of premiums that the third party pays out (to the medical provider) for covered services. It is a loss for the insurer. It is income for the provider. The ratio typically runs from 50% to 90% paid out as medical (or dental) benefits to providers. The providers prefer a higher percentage payout. The insurers prefer a lower ratio, retaining as much as possible to convert to profits.

- **Coordination of benefits** applies to people with coverage by more than one insurance plan. (For example, both husband and wife receive different dental insurance through their workplaces.) Practitioners must be careful about plan rules to help patients maximize their entitled benefits. As an industry rule (called the "birthday rule"), a person's primary carrier is through their work, and the secondary carrier is through their spouse. A child's primary insurer depends on which parent's birthday occurs first in the calendar year. Practitioners submit reimbursement for the dental procedure to the primary carrier first. Once the practitioner has received payment, they submit the remainder to the secondary carrier. Some carriers have special rules concerning dual coverage. The practitioner must not assume anything and must call the insurer or ask for a pretreatment estimate of benefits for the patient.

- **Predetermination** is a system under which a practitioner submits the proposed treatment plan to the insurer before beginning work. After review, the plan administrator will determine the patient's eligibility, covered services, copay, and maximum benefit. This is intended as an aid for the practitioner, so the patient knows how much the insurer will pay and what their portion will be. Some insurers require predetermination before treatment that exceeds a given dollar amount. Many practitioners set in-office limits at which they send claims for predetermination. Practitioners also call this pretreatment estimate, prior authorization, or preauthorization. The insurers claim that they are not authorizing treatment, only payment for the treatment.

- **Bundling** happens when the insurer combines several procedures into one procedure, generally to lower the total payout. For example, a typical recall visit may consist of a periodic oral exam, bitewing radiographs, and dental prophylaxis. If the insurer combines these procedures into a new code, lowering the cost over separate billing of the procedures, then bundling has occurred. Similarly, **unbundling** happens when the dental practitioner breaks a standard procedure into parts, increasing the total fee. For example, a composite restoration generally includes acid etching, bonding, and placing common liners. If the practitioner charges separately for these procedures, by raising the total fee, then unbundling can been said to have occurred. The profession does not like bundling because it lowers reimbursement. Third-party payers do not like unbundling because it raises reimbursement. Both sides charge fraud against the other when it occurs.

CHARACTERISTICS OF THIRD-PARTY PLANS

Each of the various plans has its own characteristics that are more or less valuable to each interested group. Box 27.13 shows the major types of plans and their characteristics.

BOX 27.13 MAJOR PLAN TYPES AND THEIR CHARACTERISTICS

Type of plan	Contract is between
Traditional fee plan	
Fee for service	Practitioner and patient
Indemnity insurance	Insurer and patient
	Practitioner and patient
Direct reimbursement	Patient and employer
	Practitioner and patient
Managed care plan	
Contract dental organization	Practitioner and insurer
Capitation plan	Practitioner and insurer
Independent practice association (IPA)	Practitioner and IPA network
Government plan	
Medicaid	Practitioner and government
	Patient and government

BOX 27.14

CHARACTERISTICS OF A FEE-FOR-SERVICE PLAN

- Not a third-party plan
- Generally, not tax advantaged
- Reimbursement based on an agreed price
- Patients carry the risk of overutilization
- Open panel
- Leads to disparities in oral health

FEE FOR SERVICE

FFS is not a third-party plan (Box 27.14). It only involves the first two parties to the transaction (practitioner and patient). It is the baseline or reference point for comparing all other reimbursement plans.

FFS is the oldest form of payment for dental services and still accounts for nearly half of all dental payments. Patients pay the practitioner directly for their dental care. Reimbursement is based on an agreed price between the practitioner and the patient. Patients are not reimbursed by any third party for their financial loss. If they have a lot of work done, they (the patient) pay individually for the above-average dental service use. In theory, those who most value dental services will pay for them. FFS is an open panel system; patients can go to any practitioner who agrees to see them.

FFS dentistry is not without its problems. Dental care is expensive. Only those who can afford dental care receive its benefits, leading to significant disparities in oral health between those who have adequate finances and those who do not. Practitioners must be especially diligent with their credit and collection policies to ensure that they collect the amounts owed from patients. The amounts that patients pay for services are generally not tax deductible. (Medical-dental expenses greater than a specified percentage of adjusted gross income are deductible for those who meet the limit and itemize deductions.) In contrast, most third-party plans offered through an employer are tax deductible. This means that the government covers some of the plan's cost, giving more "bang for the buck" than with non-tax-deductible plans.

TRADITIONAL DENTAL INSURANCE PLANS

Dental insurance plans provide reimbursement to patients for the cost of dental care they incur. This reimbursement is usually from the employer as a form of employee benefit. The money may flow directly from the employer to the employee (patient) in direct reimbursement (DR) or through a traditional insurance company.

TRADITIONAL INDEMNITY CARE PLANS

Traditional indemnity insurance is also known as "regular" or traditional dental insurance (Box 27.15). As with any insurance product, it "indemnifies" or pays for a loss. (Here, the loss is the patient's cost for the dental procedure.) The contract is between the patient and the insurer. No contractual relationship exists between the insurer and the practitioner. Practitioners often agree to process forms, accept the assignment of benefits, and send pretreatment estimates as a convenience for the patient. The patient owes the practitioner for the service, no matter their reimbursement from the insurer. These plans typically try (and succeed) to place the practitioner between the patient and the insurer by requiring documentation and mediation of disputes for services or fees.

Indemnity insurance is an open-panel product. The agreement, again, is between the insurer and the patient. The insurer does not care where the patient receives treatment because the insurance reimburses the patient. Employers purchase these insurance contracts from major insurance companies. They generally provide them as a benefit to all employees, because allowing freedom of participation would lead to adverse selection.

Indemnity insurance reimburses the patient, not the practitioner. The practitioner charges the patient for

---

BOX 27.15

CHARACTERISTICS OF A TRADITIONAL INDEMNITY CARE PLAN

- Insurer reimburses (indemnifies) patient for financial loss
- Open panel
- Reimbursement based on:
  - Table of allowances
  - Usual, customary, reasonable fee
- Insurer carries the risk of overutilization
- Plan control (deductibles, copays, maximums)
- Needs groups of subscribers
- Leads to overtreatment

the procedure. The employee (patient) sends a receipt to the insurer for reimbursement of their financial loss. The insurer pays the patient an agreed amount. The practitioner (the provider) may accept "assignment of benefits" in which the patient agrees that the reimbursement (benefit) is sent (or "assigned") directly to the practitioner instead of to the patient first. The insurer agrees (through the contract) to reimburse the entire cost of the service, part of the cost through patient copays, or a portion through a table of allowances, in which it will reimburse a certain amount for a given procedure, regardless of the fee charged. (The patient is then responsible for the remainder of the charge.) The insurance company may have internal limits for employees (either family or individual) or exclusions for certain services.

From the patient's perspective, traditional indemnity insurance is simple, there is freedom of choice of a practitioner, and it lowers out-of-pocket expenses significantly. Most researchers believe that traditional insurance leads to overtreatment compared to uninsured patients.

Practitioners like indemnity insurance because it is an open panel with freedom of choice. Therefore, practitioners see minor interference in the practitioner–patient relationship. Traditional insurance stimulates demand for services and, once systems are in place, is relatively simple because there are standard forms to complete. However, practitioners may experience cash-flow problems waiting for the carrier to reimburse and may have traditional patient collection problems for the copayments and uncovered procedures.

From the employer's perspective, indemnity insurance is an expensive benefit to provide. Employers generally do not care about freedom of choice, only about providing a cost-effective benefit for their employees. They often believe they can get more value from a capitation plan or preferred provider organization (PPO).

DIRECT REIMBURSEMENT

DR is also known as "paid dental." It is a plan that the dental associations are supporting as an alternative to managed dental care. It is promoted through the professional press, by advising employers and practitioners, and by assisting with computer software for employers to monitor and administer the DR program. It is promoted especially to smaller employers who do not have traditional insurance plans. Several third-party administrators will set up and administer a plan for a business.

DR is an open panel with complete freedom of choice (Box 27.16). It is a contract between the employer

---

BOX 27.16 CHARACTERISTICS OF DIRECT REIMBURSEMENT

- Promoted by organized dentistry
- Open panel
- Most like fee for service
- Practitioner charges and collects from the patient
- Employer reimburses patient for financial loss
- Reimbursement based on
  - Table of allowances
  - Usual, customary, reasonable fee
  - Annual maximum
- Patient carries risk of overutilization

---

and the employee (patient). The employee goes to any practitioner and has dental work done. The patient pays for the work. The patient then takes the paid receipt to their employer's benefits office. The employer reimburses the employee for the cost of care. This reimbursement may be total, involve copayments, or be based on a table of allowances. The employer may set individual maximums, or overall company maximums, use a "first come, first served" basis, exclusions, or other methods to limit its potential cost. A typical DR plan might pay for 100% of the first $100 spent on dental care, 80% of the next $500, and 50% of the next $1000 for a total annual amount of $1500.

From the patient's perspective, DR is simple. The patient can go to any practitioner. There may be increased out-of-pocket expenses or limitations compared to other types of plans. Depending on the plan's limitations, patients may view it more or less favorably than other types of plans.

Practitioners support DR because of its open-panel character and no interference in the practitioner–patient relationship. DR stimulates demand like traditional insurance. It is simple for the practitioner (no forms to complete), but the practitioner may have collection problems like with FFS patients.

From the employer's perspective, employee disenchantment about internal limits may exist. Employees then complain to the employer rather than to an insurance company. Employers often would prefer to contract out the administration of their dental plan rather than self-administer one. They can typically get more bang for their buck out of a capitation plan or PPO.

MANAGED CARE PLANS

A managed care plan is any plan in which the practitioner signs a contract to provide services for a contractually set fee. To make managed dental care plans work effectively, insurers or MCOs must exercise control over the participating practitioners in contracts and guidelines for treatment (Box 27.17). An open-panel arrangement allows a patient to go to any practitioner and receive the same level of reimbursement for a given service. (This is also called freedom of choice for the patient.) On the other hand, a closed panel denotes that patients may only go to a certain "panel" of practitioners if they wish to receive full benefit from their dental plan. (Depending on their plan, patients may receive either a reduced or no reimbursement at a non-participating practitioner's office.) Most patients have a price at which they will switch providers. Closed panels are effective at moving patients to participating providers. Some programs require the participating practitioner to be a member of the panel, but accept "any willing provider" as a member of the panel rather than limit the number of providers in an area. It is not then truly a closed panel but requires that participants agree to the terms of the contract if they participate.

Practitioners claim several problems with managed care programs. These generally revolve around the issue of the managed care plan reimbursing at a lower level than other plans and practitioners' efforts to manipulate the system to avoid the problem without compromising patient care. One common problem is the temptation for "two-tiered treatment plans." FFS and traditional insurance patients receive one plan and managed care patients receive another, less aggressive plan. Practitioners sometimes spread treatment out, "pacing" it based on the payment plan rather than patient needs. They claim a loss of control of the practitioner–patient relationship. These problems create new ethical dilemmas. (They do not create "poor dentistry.") Managed dental care offers many new opportunities to exercise poor judgment through the apparent no-win situations practitioners face.

PREFERRED PROVIDER ORGANIZATIONS

PPOs are also called contract dental organizations (CDOs). The dental profession uses CDO because the claim is that there is nothing "preferred" about these providers except that they have signed a contract. Calling them preferred providers infers a difference in quality that is not there.

Exclusive provider organizations (EPOs) are pure PPOs. They pay for patients to receive care only from their list of providers. If a patient receives treatment from a practitioner not on the EPO panel, the plan does not cover the services. (Usually, it makes some allowance for out-of-area emergencies). Point of service (POS) plans (described later) are not pure PPO plans.

CDOs work on a table of allowance payment method (Box 27.18). They are often weighted toward preventive services. The contract is between the insurer and the participating provider. The practitioner must sign a participating agreement (contract) to participate. When the practitioner signs the contract, they agree to accept their schedule of allowance as the full payment for services. The practitioner may not legally charge the patient more than

---

| BOX 27.17 | CHARACTERISTICS OF A MANAGED CARE PLAN |

- Trades groups (blocks) of patients, not individuals
- Costs and benefits are calculated in the aggregate
- Contract is between provider and insurer
- Uses provider networks (closed panels)
- Shifts financial risk (overutilization) to providers
- Emphasizes cost-efficient care
- Optimal versus adequate care
- Is secondary market
- "Brokered care"
- Dental healthcare opportunity

| BOX 27.18 | CHARACTERISTICS OF A PREFERRED PROVIDER ORGANIZATION |

- Also known as a contract dental organization
- Trades blocks of patients for contractually reduced fees
- Practitioner charges and collects from the patient for service
- Reimbursed based on a table of allowances
- Closed panel
- Practitioner carries the risk of overutilization
- Tendency to undertreat
- May have (limited) non-plan participant reimbursement

the contracted price. Non-subscribers may react negatively to reduced fees offered to plan patients.

From the practitioner's perspective, CDOs trade reduced fees for the guarantee of patients for the practice. CDOs are closed panels. They only contract for participation with a certain number of practitioners. This keeps the number of patients per practitioner at agreed levels. The advantage for the practitioner is that "warm bodies" are available, especially during the practice start-up and building phases. This contributes to paying some of the fixed costs of the office if the dentist has slack chair time. The level of the discount may not cover office overhead expenses, however. The practitioner needs to run the break-even point or other financial analyses to assess the financial impact of participation. The disadvantages of CDOs are that the practitioner receives less than their usual fee for many procedures. Practitioners may lose patients to participating providers if they are not plan participants. Contract provisions may make it difficult for practices to enter or leave the plan.

From the patient's perspective, economic incentives encourage them to receive care from a participating provider. This reduces the cost of dental care for the patient. As a trade-off, the patient loses freedom of choice if their traditional practitioner is not a plan provider.

POINT-OF-SERVICE PLANS

POS plans are a hybrid type of PPO. In the POS plan, the patient can remain in the network or go to a provider outside the network. If they stay in the network of providers, their cost is less. If they go to a practitioner not in the network, the plan reimburses them, but at a lower level than if they stay in network. The different levels of reimbursement are strong financial incentives for the patient to remain in the network. However, POS plans allow a patient the choice of a provider at a cost.

From the practitioner's perspective, they will gain more patients if they contract as a network provider. The reimbursement is usually less than the full fee. If they accept patients from the plan as a non-network provider, they receive their full fee from the patient. However, fewer patients will come to them for care since the cost to the patient is higher.

CAPITATION PLANS

Capitation plans are also known as cap plans, DMOs, and dental health maintenance organizations (DHMOs). These are managed care plans (Box 27.19). They are a contractual arrangement between the practitioner and the plan. Cap

---

BOX 27.19	CHARACTERISTICS OF A CAPITATION PLAN

- Trades blocks of patients for contractually reduced fees
- Practitioner:
  - Receives monthly "per capita" reimbursement (PMPM)
  - Charges and collects a reduced fee from patients for services
  - Reimbursed based on a table of allowances
- Closed panel
- Preventive oriented (in theory)
- Practitioner carries the risk of overutilization
- Tendency to undertreat

---

plans pay practitioners a monthly amount per person enrolled through the practitioner's office. This becomes a monthly "per capita" or per member, per month (PMPM) payment. In exchange, the practitioner agrees (generally) to provide a dental exam, radiographs, and prophylaxis twice per year at no charge to the patient or plan. The practitioner then provides other services at a reduced fee, like with a PPO. Cap plans are closed panels in which a portion is a per capita fee, and a portion is a table of allowance fee structure.

These plans have a preventive orientation. In theory, they encourage more preventive treatment, when dental care is most effective and least expensive. Once practitioners get patients to a maintenance level of care (the theory goes), the patients require less work and become more "profitable." The theory breaks down in several areas. Patients do not all stay long term with the program. People move and are transferred through the workplace. They enter and leave the plan for their own reasons. And the high degree of personal responsibility inherent in preventive dental services requires high patient compliance.

There are several advantages for practitioners. The practitioner can budget a more stable cash flow and plan resources for expenditures. These programs may provide additional patients during the practice-building phase. However, as with any managed care plan, these patients can overwhelm a practice if the practice does not control the number of patients. Because the plans end up reimbursing at reduced rates (from a full fee), they often only cover costs. There is typically inadequate profit built in to operate with traditional dental practice systems. The practice shoulders the risk of increased utilization in this plan.

The plans become most profitable to the practitioner when patients do not come in for treatment, an idea that is anathema to many practitioners. Many patients view these plans as traditional "dental insurance." They may have difficulty finding a provider who is acceptable to them.

INDEPENDENT PRACTICE ASSOCIATIONS

IPAs are also known as voluntary provider networks. In this form of reimbursement plan, providers band together to negotiate and compete for contracts (Box 27.20). These are contracts to provide services for groups of potential patients. The providers attempt to eliminate the "middle man" (in this case, the insurer) by negotiating directly with the employer or purchaser. This allows higher reimbursements for providers or more competitive prices for the purchasers. It is conceptually like a DR managed care program.

The program reimburses on any basis that the IPA negotiates. This may be indemnity, service, or capitation based. Most are service based, although capitated IPA plans are increasing in number. From the patient's perspective, these are closed panels, so providers are limited. Other than that, the reaction depends mainly on the plan's structure.

The advantage for practitioners is that they have some control over contract provisions because the provider network negotiates the contracts. However, if the contract is not competitive with others in the marketplace, it will not be bought by the plan purchasers (employers). So IPAs,

over time, end up being comparable to other third-party plans in the area. These plans generally have less than full reimbursement. There are also potential problems with the Fair Trade Commission and price-fixing from practitioners banding together to negotiate prices. There are many of the same problems as with other managed care plans, although these plans are more practitioner friendly. There is often practitioner disillusionment because practitioners think they will have more control over contract provisions than they actually have.

REFERRAL PLANS

Referral plans are not genuinely third-party reimbursement plans, but the public views them as a type of dental insurance (Box 27.21). A referral plan contracts with the practicing practitioner to do dental services at a reduced fee. In return, the patients who sign up with the plan are sent to participating providers to receive discounted cost dental care. (This is a closed-panel arrangement.) Patients who sign on with the plan pay a nominal fee (a few dollars a month), which pays for the administration and profit of the plan. No money for service flows through the plan. Practitioners still must collect from the patient for the care rendered. They gain a patient base for the reduced fee that they are contractually obligated to charge.

GOVERNMENT PAYMENT PLANS

The government pays for a limited amount of dental services in private offices, mainly through two programs, Medicare and Medicaid.

MEDICARE

Medicare is also known, erroneously, as Social Security. (They are two different programs.) Medicare is a federal program. It is health insurance for older (older than 65) and disabled Americans (Box 27.22). It is a major medical

---

BOX 27.20 | **CHARACTERISTICS OF AN INDEPENDENT PRACTICE ASSOCIATION**

- Providers band together and bid on blocks of patients
- Trades blocks of patients for a contractually reduced fee
- Eliminates "middle man"
- Must compete in the marketplace with other plans
- Practitioner's payment type depends on the plan
- Capitated
- Table of allowance
- Closed panel
- Practitioners carry the risk of overutilization
- Tendency to undertreat
- Problems of restraint of trade

BOX 27.21 | **CHARACTERISTICS OF A REFERRAL PLAN**

- Trades blocks of patients for a contractually reduced fee
- Eliminates "middle man"
- No third-party payments
- Practitioner's payment is a table of allowance charges
- Closed panel

- Government-sponsored health insurance for older (+65) Americans or disabled Americans

- Very little dental coverage or impact

- Medicare Advantage plans may include dental coverage

(hospitalization) policy. Participants can buy additional, optional coverage for physicians and other health services. Medicare reimburses based on diagnostic-related groups (DRGs), which are tables of allowances for hospitals based on the disease rather than on hospital cost.

From the patient's perspective, Medicare is medical insurance for retired people. (Often, older Americans cannot get any other health insurance when their medical needs are the highest.) It does not cover long-term (nursing home) care and does not cover many "optional" services, such as dental care. The typical dental practitioner sees little impact from Medicare. Some hospital practitioners (such as oral surgeons) may see some impact if a covered person has a disease or accident involving the jaws. This program profoundly affects the way physicians practice.

Medicare has several different types of plans to pay for doctor visits, pharmacies, and other health services. (Original Medicare does not currently cover routine dental services. As mentioned, it does cover some hospital-related services.) Private insurers offer several types of supplemental plans, which must follow strict guidelines. One type of plan is an "Advantage Plan." These plans may be medical PPOs, HMOs, or other types of medical payment. Many Medicare Advantage Plans offer extra benefits such as dental care, eyeglasses, or wellness programs. The dental benefits vary tremendously according to the providing company and the plan. Most have network providers, operating as DHMOs or EPOs; some are operated as DR plans, others as POS plans. Since they vary so much, it is impossible to tell the financial impact on the dental practitioner without getting the rules and reimbursement schedule for the specific plan under consideration.

MEDICAID

Medicaid is a combination of state and federally funded programs. It is known by many other names, including medical assistance (MA), medical assistance plan (MAP), "The Medical Card," and "The Card." It also has individual state-associated names, such as "MediCal" in California and "KMAP" (Kentucky Medical Assistance Program) in Kentucky. Coverage varies from state to state. Some states pay for more comprehensive dental services than others. Some states have no dental component at all. The federal government reimburses the state a given amount for each dollar the state spends on Medicaid.

Medicaid is a health subsidy for poor people (Box 27.23). Although each state's dental program is different, most reimburse preventive care for younger people. They may reimburse emergency and diagnostic services for adults. Each state reimburses differently. These programs often pay relatively well for kids, especially for preventive and diagnostic procedures. This encourages provider participation. The theory behind this is that if dentists treat children early in their lives, they will not need much dental work as adults. This increases the state's effectiveness in spending scarce resources (money for indigent dental care). Many states have moved to managed dental care programs for their dental Medicaid programs. This is an apparent effort to hold down costs to the state and receive the maximum amount of indigent care for a dollar.

From the patient's perspective, patients often assume that Medicaid is complete dental coverage. (Generally, it is not.) But Medicaid does provide dental care for many people who could not otherwise afford it. In some areas, it may be difficult for patients to find a practitioner who accepts patients with Medicaid.

For the practitioner, Medicaid fulfills a social responsibility. At the professional level, practitioners have a monopoly, granted through the state licensure mechanism, to practice dentistry. (No one can legally do dentistry except a licensed practitioner.) Practitioners must retain public trust or risk losing their monopoly. Public trust involves some method of responding to the dental needs of all members of the public, both the unfortunate and the fortunate. Medicaid brings

- Combines federal and state programs

- Qualification based on family income

- Provides payment for indigent care

- Coverage and requirements vary from state to state

- Many states have some coverage for dental services

- Many are managed care (closed panel) plans

- Usually preventive oriented

several disadvantages to the practitioner as well. States often set unrealistically low reimbursement rates. Practitioners may not legally charge the patient the difference between what Medicaid reimburses and the UCR fee. They may, however, charge patients for procedures that Medicaid does not cover. These patients may show a low appointment consciousness.

PROCESSING INSURANCE CLAIMS

The ADA has developed a standard numbering system for practitioners' treatments, called the Current Dental Terminology (CDT) code. This "Code on Dental Procedures and Nomenclature" is standard across the industry. The ADA periodically updates the code to ensure practitioners can code current procedures and materials for payment and reimbursement. Note that these are treatment codes (based on the treatment that practitioners do). They are not based on the diagnosis, as are most medical insurance codes. Practitioners can purchase a book from the ADA that explains the code. Office management programs incorporate the code into their programs and update it as needed through software updates. Nearly all third parties accept these standard descriptions of treatments.

INSURANCE CODE CATEGORIES

Insurers generally group procedures by type for reimbursement purposes. The specifics are not industry standard but vary somewhat from insurer to insurer and plan to plan, depending on the details negotiated with the purchasing employer. Insurers group procedures into four categories: preventive, basic, major, and other (Box 27.24). The insurers then reimburse a certain percentage of the cost of each procedure in each group. Typically, they reimburse well for preventive services, less for basic services, and even less for major and other services. Often, they do not apply deductibles to preventive services. Because of the considerable variation between insurers and among specific plans by insurers, practitioners need to have the patient bring their insurance booklet (from their employer's benefits office) to the appointment. The booklet will list the plan's specifics so that the practitioner can enter the information into the office management system for more accurate estimates of patient payments and insurance benefits. Each plan also has a contact point (telephone, fax, or internet) where staff can ask about coverage for a specific patient. Box 27.25 illustrates how different indemnity plans can result in different reimbursements and patient payments.

The tables of allowance reimbursement plans differ in that each insurer gives a list of allowable procedures and payments. Depending on the plan, the insurer reimburses

---

BOX 27.24   INSURANCE CODE CATEGORIES

Preventive services

- Diagnostic
- Radiographic
- Preventive

Basic services

- Restorative
- Endodontic
- Basic surgery

Major services

- Crowns
- Removable prosthetics
- Fixed prosthetics
- Periodontics

Other services

- Orthodontics
- Implants
- Adjunctive services

---

part or all of the charges, and the patient is responsible for the allowable charges.

THE AMERICAN DENTAL ASSOCIATION INSURANCE FORM

Almost all third-party plans accept the ADA's standard Dental Claims Form for submission of dental benefits. This paper form is the basis of claims that practitioners submit electronically. The form can be completed by hand, writing the information on a preprinted form and mailing it to the insurer. The only time practitioners do this is when they do not use an office computer management system. Most management software will print a paper form (on plain paper) based on the information the practitioner enters into the program. They can then mail this form to the insurer. Currently, the most common method is submitting claims electronically. In this method, front-office staff members use the management software at the end of the day to process claims for the day. The software checks the claims to be sure that the practitioner has entered

BOX 27.25	**EXAMPLE INDEMNITY PLAN REIMBURSEMENT SCHEDULES**

Two indemnity plans reimburse according to the following schedules:

	Plan #1	Plan #2
Preventive	100%[a]	100%[b]
Basic	80%	50%
Major	50%	50%
Other	50%	25%
Deductible	$250	$100
Annual max.	$1000	$1500

The patient has agreed to a treatment plan. The costs for the patient and insurers under each coverage are as follows:

		Plan #1		Plan #2	
Service	Fee	Patient	Insurer	Patient	Insurer
Initial exam	$75		$75	$75	
FMX rays	$85		$80	$25	$60
Prophylaxis	$90		$90		$90
Restore #2	$160	$160		$80	$80
Restore #7	$110	$110		$55	$55
FPD #3 × #5	$2000	$1035	$965	$1000	$1000
Total	$2420	$1520	$1000	$1235	$1285

[a] Deductible does not apply to preventive.
[b] Deductible applies to preventive.

the needed information. It then accumulates all claims and sends them via the internet to a claims-processing company. This clearinghouse company checks all the claims for completeness, returning any that need additional information. It takes the rest and combines them from all subscribed providers. It then sends batches of claims to each insurer. This way, the insurance carrier receives the claim the day the office submits it. The clearinghouse has checked it for completeness, so processing is quicker. There is a cost associated with electronic claims processing. However, it is generally no more than the cost of the time, paper, and postage associated with traditional processing.

A key element in speeding up reimbursement (and therefore cash flow) from the carriers is to complete the insurance form correctly. If the practice mails forms, the dentist must complete all the information on the form. If filing electronically, the submission process will check that the practitioner has entered all required information (but not

that it is correct). Regardless of how the practitioner submits, several key points keep claims from being delayed. The practice must update the CDT codes in the computer whenever the ADA updates them. Many plans limit the frequency or recency of replacement of crowns and bridges. The practitioner needs to show if this is an initial placement or the date of the prior placement. If it is not an initial placement, the practitioner needs to include an explanation in the narrative and should only use the "Notes" section for notes regarding treatment needs. Most carriers remove claims with notes from the automatic process to have an adjuster look at the claim. Notes like "Please pay promptly" or "Have a nice day" may therefore slow down the claims payment process.

When the practitioner completes an insurance form, each section has essential information. The insurer will return the claim if any fields are blank. Some common problem areas on the form are the following:

- **Header information**
  The practitioner must note whether this is a statement for work they have done or a request for predetermination of benefits. The insurer processes these differently.

- **Policyholder/subscriber information**
  The insurer needs to verify the subscriber's eligibility to be sure that the insurance plan covers them.

- **Patient information**
  The insurer must verify the patient's eligibility. If the patient is a dependent (e.g. a child), then the insurer needs to know the patient's age to verify eligibility.

- **Other coverage**
  If the patient has secondary insurance, then the insurer needs to know to check for coordination of benefits.

- **Record of services provided**
  This is the section where the practitioner enters the services completed, along with other information (e.g. date of service, procedure code). The insurer pays based on the patient's plan's requirements and the procedures that the practitioner submits.

- **Authorizations**
  This section authorizes the practitioner to file the claim (by the patient's signature) and authorizes the insurer to send payment to the practitioner instead of the patient (assignment of benefits). Both signatures may be kept on file for electronic filing. In this case, the program prints "Signature on File" in these spaces. The practitioner must have the signature on file.

- **Ancillary claim or treatment information**
  This section of the form contains information that the insurer may use to allow or deny the claim.

Orthodontics often has a lifetime maximum. Insurance usually pays for prosthetics once every five years. If this claim was for treatment resulting from an occupational injury, then the patient's workers' compensation insurance is probably responsible for the claim. If it is the result of an accident, then another insurer (health or automobile) may be responsible for paying the claim.

FILING INSURANCE CLAIMS

For many practitioners, being paid on time and appropriately is their top priority. In most practices, the majority of payments for services, in whole or in part, involve insurance carriers. Insurance carriers require a lot of information to process claims. For example, they need to verify that the plan currently covers the patient, that the plan covers the procedure, and that the practitioner is licensed and possibly contracted by the plan. Correctly submitting and verifying this information by hand is time-consuming for both the practitioner and the carrier. The technology that most professionals are adopting to simplify the claim reimbursement process is some form of electronic claim processing. The electronic transmission of insurance claims to insurance carriers, MCOs, and other healthcare payers helps practitioners enhance their cash flow and improves the efficiency of their billing processes.

Historically, an increasing number of insurers have mandated electronic claims filing to lower their costs. This movement has also been supported by governmental (Medicare, Medicaid, etc.) payment procedures, which mandate that all claims be submitted electronically by hospitals and clinics. HIPAA has also pushed the move to electronic claims. The HIPAA Transaction Rule requires the adoption of defined formats for electronic claim submission. This has simplified the sharing of healthcare payment information, especially claims information.

INSURANCE COMPANY PROCESSING

When the insurance company receives a claim, it begins its process.

The first step is for computers to check the forms and verify the patient's eligibility. The software checks the procedures and patient eligibility if the form is a predetermination of benefits. If the case has a questionable prognosis or is beyond normal procedures, the company sends the claim to a consultant who reviews the case. The dental consultant reviews any pictures, models, radiographs, or explanations that the practitioner has sent and decides on the eligibility of the procedures and appropriateness of the care. (This has been a problem with many practitioners.)

They then issue an estimate of benefits or a similar form that describes what they will reimburse. Depending on the case's complexity and the insurer's backlog, this may take several weeks.

If the form is for payment of services, then the computer calculates allowable amounts for the patient's specific plan. The insurer then writes a check for reimbursement and prints an EOB or similar form that describes how much it paid for each procedure.

METHODS OF FILING CLAIMS

Practitioners can submit claims through several methods, depending on their resources and the insurance company's requirements:

- **Paper submission**
  A dental practice can complete a paper form and mail (or fax) it to the insurance carrier. Most office software packages allow the practice to individually or batch print computer-generated forms. The software inserts information from the patient record and checks for missing information. The practitioner must ensure that the information in the system is complete and correct. There are the added costs of postage and slower return of payments. Staff time to process the claims adds to the costs. When the insurance company receives the claim, they need to enter it into their system, which requires extra time and cost.

- **Direct data entry**
  The advantages of filing claims online are available to practitioners who choose not to use their practice management software. The practitioner or a staff member enters the provider, patient, and claim information into a formatted webpage and submits the claim for processing using direct data entry. Office personnel log into a clearinghouse using a secure internet connection. To save the practitioner time if they submit similar claims in the future, the clearinghouse can save the patient, provider, and claim information in a secure system. However, office personnel must take the time required for data entry.

- **Direct file submission**
  Most practices have adopted some form of electronic file submission. This uses office management software to complete an electronic file of the information that the carrier needs to process the claim. Practitioners who only submit claims to one or two third-party payers may choose to submit their claims directly to each payer utilizing the payer's proprietary software. However, practitioners who

send claims to various third-party payers find that sending claims to a single clearinghouse (which sorts, prepares, reviews for accuracy, and sends claims to the correct payer) is the most practical option. The office's practice management software creates the claims-to-be-processed electronic file and submits it to the clearinghouse through a secure connection over the internet. Most software vendors have a preferred clearinghouse. Others allow the practitioner to choose a clearinghouse. By eliminating the need to fill out and store paper claims, electronic claim submission helps to simplify the billing processes and record-keeping. Electronically submitted claims are processed more efficiently, leading to quicker reimbursement. While errors, omissions, and other issues frequently cause paper claims to be denied, electronically submitting claims can reduce lost or incomplete claims. Office personnel can easily track claim status through a secure internet connection.

METHODS OF RECEIVING PAYMENT

There are several standard methods of receiving payment from insurance carriers. Regardless of the method, the carrier will also send an EOB form that details which patients and procedures the check covers. The front-office staff must verify the payments and credit the patient's account in the office computer system for the payment received. Payment methods include the following:

- **Paper checks**
  Most insurers will issue a paper check for payment for services if the practitioner prefers this method. The check often includes several claims aggregated into one bulk payment. The carriers also send an EOB that details the aggregated payment. Some insurance companies have announced they will no longer issue paper check payments to providers.

- **Virtual credit card**
  Some insurers make payments through a virtual credit card (VCC). In this method, the insurer establishes a VCC number for the practice. It then makes payments to this card for services the dentist has provided. The dentist redeems the card by transferring money from their point-of-sale (office) computer to their bank account. (The insurer sends an electronic EOB detailing the payment as well.) Some insurers only allow VCC payments. For others, it is an option. Using a VCC has a cost. When receiving VCC payments, providers incur considerable charges in transactions and other fees. These expenses might account for 5% of the overall transaction. Considering the possible

volume of reimbursements at an office, this can be a sizable amount.

- **Electronic funds transfer**
  Since the passage of the Affordable Care Act (ACA), the healthcare industry has worked to become more efficient, moving from predominantly paper-based transactions to electronic ones. One requirement of the ACA was the selection of a healthcare electronic funds transfer (EFT) standard, and the Department of Health and Human Services (HHS) chose EFT via the Automated Clearing House (ACH). Like direct deposit, the ACH network enables the electronic transmission of claim payments from the insurer directly and immediately to the provider's bank account. Since the HHS rule's introduction in 2014, the number of claims paid by ACH has increased, and every day more payers and providers (including dentists) switch to electronic payments. Compared to paper checks and VCC payments, EFT is a simple, secure, quick, and economical alternative to accepting claim reimbursements. On average, processing an EFT using ACH only costs a dental business roughly 34 cents.

HOW TO MANAGE INSURANCE PLANS IN THE OFFICE

The practitioner cannot change the insurance plans that are in the local marketplace. They can decide whether to participate in those plans. They can also manage, to a degree, the plans' effect on office scheduling and operations.

HOW TO MANAGE TRADITIONAL INDEMNITY INSURANCE PLANS

Traditional indemnity insurance is a contract between the insurer and the patient. The insurer has agreed to indemnify ("make whole" or reimburse) the patient for losses suffered because of dental care. For the patient, those losses are the financial cost of paying for the care. As the practitioner/provider of services, a practitioner has a contract (written or implied) that if the patient agrees to have the recommended work done, the patient will pay for the service (as an FFS patient). If the insurer reimburses the patient for financial loss, so much the better for the patient (and the practitioner because it encourages people to "purchase" care). But there is no contract between the insurer and the provider, only between the insurer and the patient. As a convenience to the patient, practitioners may agree to let the insurer send their reimbursement check (the insurance benefit) directly to them instead of to the patient.

This procedure (assignment of benefits) lowers the patient's cash outlay and apparent out-of-pocket expense. Still, it does not change the fundamental agreement between the patient and the practitioner or the patient and the insurer (Box 27.25). The patient owes the practitioner the full fee charged, regardless of the reimbursement from the insurer. Many savvy practitioners send letters to their patients in the last quarter of the year informing them of their insurance benefits remaining for the year and any needed dental treatment. Because the insurance is a "use-it-or-lose-it" proposition, many patients will schedule their treatment to maximize their benefit for the year. Many practitioners will also schedule large cases at the end of the year so that some of the work is covered by this year's insurance and some will be initiated and covered by next year's. In this way, they can help to maximize the patient's reimbursement.

HOW TO MANAGE MANAGED CARE PLANS

Participating in limited reimbursement insurance plans is like driving a car down the highway at 75 miles per hour in second gear. The person is getting where they need to go, but is working very hard to get there. At some point, they need to shift to a higher gear or risk burning out the engine. To effectively manage managed care plans in the office, practitioners need to understand the problems involved from a financial and practice philosophy perspective.

OVERALL REIMBURSEMENT RATES

The fundamental problem with managed care programs from the practitioners' perspective is not the concept of capitation, prepayment, risk shifting, or the payment method. It is simply that the overall reimbursement rates are too low to maintain profitability. To track this reimbursement rate, the accounting system must be set up to give the practitioner the needed information. It should charge the full fee value for a procedure, then adjust the managed care discount from that. (Some offices charge the reduced fee. This does not allow the office to see how much the fee was discounted for the plan.) The total reimbursement rate is the total plan charges (at the prevailing full fee rate) divided into the total plan billings (charges minus adjustments plus any capitation payments).

The overall reimbursement rate is where the cost controls hit the practitioner. It is also where the plan administrator sells the plan to various employers. If the administrator must sell a plan that reimburses 80 cents on the dollar, it will cost them more than a plan that reimburses 60 cents on the dollar. Prices to employers for the plan must reflect this difference in reimbursement rate. The employer is more concerned with the plan's cost to the employer rather than the percentage payout. The only time the employer cares about payouts is if employees complain about poor performance by the plan.

The practice needs to track the reimbursement rate over time. Plan administrators will change the payout amounts. As the fee and procedure mix change, the reimbursement level may change (Box 27.26). The practitioner cannot assume that it will remain there because the reimbursement rate was 85% of their fee. Figure 27.4 shows two plans over time. One plan has had steady reimbursement rates (with annual fluctuations). The second plan shows a steadily decreasing reimbursement rate. Practitioners need to carefully consider whether they ought to continue to participate in the second plan.

WORKING ON THE MARGIN

A detailed analysis of office costs shows that many costs (e.g. rent, staff, etc.) are fixed, regardless of the number of patients seen in a given time. The only costs that vary directly with production are those associated with a dental

---

BOX 27.26 **HOW TO CALCULATE REIMBURSEMENT RATE**

Example #1

Last month, this PPO plan resulted in $8000 of charges. The practitioner adjusted $2000 because of the plan's requirements. The overall reimbursement rate was 75%.

Charges	+ $8000
Adjustments	− $2000
+ Cap Pmt (if any)	+ 0
Amount realized	$6000

Reimbursement rate = 75% of the full fee

Example #2

Last month, this capitation plan resulted in $6000 of charges. The practitioner adjusted $3000 because of the plan. The practitioner also received a capitation payment of $1000 for the month. The overall reimbursement rate was 67%.

Charges	$6000
Adjustments	− $3000
+ Cap Pmt (if any)	+ $1000
Amount realized	$4000

Reimbursement rate = 66% of full fee

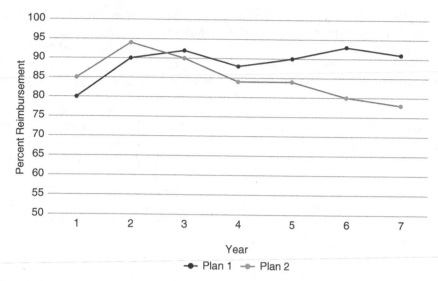

FIGURE 27.4   Tracking reimbursement rates over time.

lab, supplies, and office supplies. These are the marginal costs of seeing additional patients. The decision on participation in managed care insurance plans is as follows:

- If the question is "Do I go in the back and read a newspaper or see a managed care patient?" the financial outcome is better if the practitioner sees the patient.

- If the question is "Do I see a managed care patient or see a private, full fee-for-service patient?" then the outcome is better if the practitioner sees the private patient, not the managed care patient.

- If there is empty chair time, it is financially worthwhile to fill that chair time with the less lucrative managed care patient rather than leave it empty.

- If the question lies between "Do I add an operatory and assistant (or associate) to see managed care patients?" the answer is much more complex. The practitioner probably needs to discuss it with an accountant or management or financial advisor to investigate the answer thoroughly.

The practitioner should try to limit the amount of managed care in the practice mix. If the practice has more than 25% from a single plan or managed care is 50% of the total practice production, then the practitioner may be in the dangerous position of "needing" the managed care programs. Then, if the administrator changes the rules or reimbursement rates, the practitioner will have no choice but to stay because the practice now depends on these plans.

PLAN UTILIZATION CONTROLS

The risk that traditional indemnity insurance programs face is that more people than planned will use dental services and file claims. In other words, there will be "overutilization." Traditional indemnity insurance companies use many techniques to limit this risk and the resulting payout amount. Because the plan administrator in an alternative payment plan has shifted the risk onto the provider, the administrator has little incentive to control this risk. As a result, many of these plans are offered to the public and employers without these risk-reducing factors built in.

A common control method is to place a yearly maximum on the amount the plan will pay to any given individual for any given year. Preexisting condition clauses, copayments, deductibles, and other methods that force patients to pay out-of-pocket expenditures all accomplish the same goal. Because practitioners assume the risk in many of these managed care programs, they should likewise have controls built into the contract to protect themselves from significant losses associated with overutilization. When negotiating with a plan administrator, the practitioner should insist that patients have yearly maximums, copays, and other loss prevention measures written into the plan before the practitioner agrees to participate.

POOR PATIENT UNDERSTANDING

Insurance contracts are complex. The adage "The large print giveth, and the small print taketh away" must have been coined by a sage who was studying his own insurance coverage. When the complexities and vagaries of a host of managed care programs are brought to the public, it is little wonder that they do not understand them.

Good third-party reimbursement programs, both traditional insurance and managed care, go out of their way to explain their programs to the subscribers. It is really their obligation to fully inform their clients of the coverage, limitations, and rules associated with the various plans. However, they are not always diligent, and patients do not always listen. So, most of the population do not understand their plan but merely make assumptions about their coverage. This may be based on misinformation or incomplete information provided by the plan administrators or on the patient's historical coverage that they assume applies to the new program. When negotiating a contract, the practitioner needs to ask to see the information that the plan provides to its potential subscribers and the information that it provides once they are participants. They should then check the accuracy of the plan description. It is not the practitioner's obligation to explain insurance or managed care plans to their subscribers, but it is often in their best interest to do so. The practitioner needs to have a copy of the plan's information and coverage brochures handy so that if a question of coverage arises, they can easily show the patient the coverage rules.

COST SHIFTING

If a practitioner uses managed care patients to augment their schedule, working on the margin, then the managed care program patients are not fully contributing to the overall office overhead. Instead, the practitioner shifts that cost onto the full-pay and traditional insurance patients or takes home less income.

HOW TO REDUCE MANAGED CARE IN THE PRACTICE

Given these problems, why would anyone participate in managed care? Practitioners' needs change over time. When the practice is young, it is time to gain as many new patients as possible, even if they are not all excellent full-paying clients. As the practice grows, the practitioner may begin to "shift gears" by holding steady the number of managed care patients and then gradually eliminating the programs as full-pay clients begin to fill the practice. Other times, practitioners may need to participate from a defensive strategy. If many patients leave the practice because of changing plan types, the practitioner may need to preserve that patient base through participation. If a major employer in the area accounts for a large portion of the patient pool,

the practitioner may need to participate if that employer shifts to a managed care plan.

If a practitioner is taking on several managed care plans and wants to drop out of them, they need to do some analysis before jumping. The practitioner must maintain or improve practice volume and profitability and must be sure that they have potential patient visits to take the place of the lost managed care patients. The practitioner ought to increase marketing expenditures (both internal and external) in anticipation to drive new patient visits. They also need to look at the entire practice philosophy and operation. For example, they may be moving from a high-volume, low-fee practice to a lower-volume, higher-fee style. If so, they need to closely examine the type and scope of services that they provide, as well as their case presentation technique, patient financing options, and staff competencies, to ensure that they can cater to a higher-end clientele.

Practitioners may use POS plans to reduce the amount of managed care in the practice. A practitioner may initially be an in-network provider for a POS plan. This increases the number of patients, although the reimbursement levels may be lower than desired. As the practitioner builds a patient base, they may switch to be an out-of-network provider for a given plan. They hope that many of the patients will remain with the practice. This allows greater reimbursement among these patients, though it will decrease the number of patients. (Some will leave the practice due to the higher cost.) The practice will see probably see fewer new patients from the plan.

The practitioner will probably eliminate plans one at a time rather than all at once. They will, therefore, need to decide the order of plan elimination. The practice owner should rank all plans by their total reimbursement rate and the percentage of practice production. They then eliminate the worst-performing and smallest plan(s) first. If a plan accounts for a small proportion of the practice revenues (less than 5%), the practitioner can eliminate it easily. With larger plans, they may need to stop accepting new patients (called "going on hold") before eliminating the plan (assuming the plan allows this process). This allows them to gradually wean the practice off reliance on the plan. By continually (quarterly) reviewing and eliminating the poorest-performing plans, the practitioner may be able to completely remove their participation in managed care plans.

Box 27.27 gives an example of an analysis of managed care plans. If the practitioner has empty chair time, they should not eliminate any plans. All three contribute more than the variable production costs (about 21%). If there is not a lot of empty chair time, they should eliminate the Cap plan first. Its reimbursement is the least and

	BOX 27.27	ASSESSING MANAGED CARE PROGRAMS

A practitioner participates in three managed care programs, two preferred provider organizations (PPOs) and a capitation (Cap) plan. The numbers for the latest quarter are given. Which plan(s), if any, should the practitioner eliminate from the practice?

	PPO1	PPO2	Cap plan
Charges	$7000	$14000	$7000
Adjustments	−490	−2300	−2500
Capitation payments	$0	$0	+ $1000
Total return	$6510	$11700	$5500
Return (%)	93%	83.5%	78.5%

is a relatively small part of the practice. Next, the practitioner should eliminate the worst-paying plan (PPO2), if there are enough patients to fill most empty time slots. (It is a relatively large portion of the practice.) If not, the practitioner may need to eliminate PPO1 and build the practice until they can afford (from a patient visit perspective) to eliminate PPO2.

These options are based purely on financial considerations, without regard to personal beliefs about managed care, how hard the practitioner wants to work, or other personal concerns that may influence the decision.

The practitioner should have a strategy for handling current patients who are members of discontinued plans. They need to decide what they (and the staff) will tell patients. Some patients will remain with the practice even after the change. The practitioner should let the patients know if they will make any special arrangements for payments if they remain in the practice. Other patients will leave, even though the practitioner has treated them for years. The plan's cost-saving incentives are too strong for them to refuse. The practitioner must decide if they will refer patients to another participating practitioner or let them "fend for themselves." The practitioner must ensure that the staff know the policy (and the state law) regarding transferring patient records and radiographs.

Managing Risk in the Office

CHAPTER 28

Part 1: Office Risk Management

I'm built for comfort; I ain't built for speed. But I got ev'ything that a good girl need.

Willie Dixon

GOAL

This part aims to make students aware of common risks encountered in the dental office and to develop plans to minimize those risks.

LEARNING OBJECTIVES

At the completion of this part, the student will be able to:

- Describe the methods of managing risks in the office.

- Describe the common types of office insurance:
  - Business liability insurances
  - Business premises and personal injury insurance
  - Employment practices liability insurance
  - Professional liability insurance
  - Loss-of-use insurance
  - Property insurance
  - Building contents insurance
  - Business overhead expense (BOE) insurance
  - Employer insurances
  - Workers' compensation insurance
  - Unemployment compensation insurance.

- Describe the elements needed to prove professional liability.

- Define standards of care and their use in dental practice.

- Differentiate between poor work and poor outcomes.

- Describe the common areas of professional risk exposure for practicing dentists.

- Describe the common elements of a patient record.

- Describe the use of patient records in a possible malpractice action.

- Describe the possible avenues of resolution for poor work or poor outcomes.

- Describe the typical dental malpractice insurance policy.

- Define the National Practitioner Data Bank and its effect on dentistry.

Business Basics for Dentists, Second Edition. James L. Harrison, David O. Willis, and Charles K. Thieman.
© 2024 John Wiley & Sons, Inc. Published 2024 by John Wiley & Sons, Inc.

KEY TERMS

board of dentistry
capacity
causation
claim
claims made
covered loss
duty
equipment failure
exclusions
failure to diagnose
failure to refer
fee disputes
indemnity

informed consent
loss exposure
malpractice
managed care
negligence
occurrence
ownership of dental records
patient abandonment
patient records
peer review process
periodontal disease claims
policy
poor outcomes

poor technique
poor work
professional liability
reasonable and prudent
risk (loss) prevention
risk control (risk avoidance)
risk management
risk reduction
risk transfer
standards of care
swallowed object claims
wrong tooth claims

Risk management is the process of identification and minimization of the possible sources of negligence to which a dentist is exposed. These may develop from a dentist's role as a practitioner or as a business owner. The owner and manager of the practice must see that the practice examines the sources of risk and works to decrease them as much as possible.

THE RISK MANAGEMENT PROCESS

In the risk management area, the best remedy is prevention. The major task of a practicing dentist is not simply to buy insurance (although that ought to be part of the whole risk management package). Instead, the major task of the practitioner should be loss prevention. The risk management process is divided into several steps.

IDENTIFICATION OF POTENTIAL LOSS EXPOSURE

The initial task is to evaluate the practice to detect liability exposures. Dentists need to decide why someone might sue them. They need to examine the dental procedures they do. Removing a deep bony third molar impaction that wraps around the mandibular canal exposes a dentist to more risk than if they refer that procedure to an oral surgeon. Emergency department patients are notorious for failing to follow up on treatment, resulting in poor treatment outcomes and possible claims of professional negligence. If a practitioner collects accounts aggressively, they may encourage retribution (through a lawsuit) by dissatisfied patients. If a practitioner has inadequate or outdated patient record systems, they may have difficulty proving

that an event or conversation occurred. If a practitioner does a procedure so seldom that they are not proficient at it, or if they continually have less than optimum outcomes with a particular procedure (e.g. an endodontic technique), the dentist may be open to a claim of bad work. If a practitioner has an older facility, they must keep it in good repair. The ultimate risk avoidance technique is to quit practicing dentistry. Nobody will sue a dentist for dental malpractice or business negligence then. Most practitioners agree that they can accept a certain amount of risk if they can manage it effectively. Risk is often expressed as a combination of two variables, likelihood and impact. Graphically, this is shown in Figure 28.1. Some risks may be likely but carry a low impact. For example, the possibility that a patient may inadvertently walk out with a pen is high, but the financial cost is low. On the other hand, the

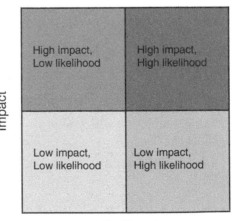

FIGURE 28.1　Risk assessment matrix.

possibility of a fire destroying the office and a dentist's livelihood is low, but the impact is extremely high. Practitioners would have a different way of managing the two risk exposures. The area of most concern is the area of high impact and high likelihood. Risks in this quadrant need immediate attention and review. Dentists should try to lower the impact, the likelihood, or both. Risks in the high-impact, low-likelihood areas often require insurance to cover the loss. Dentists typically manage the risk of low impact and high likelihood by using risk management techniques (such as staff training) to lower the likelihood of occurrence.Identification of potential loss exposure requires practitioners to honestly evaluate themselves and their staff members' skills and abilities. Occasionally, that evaluation may identify problems or deficiencies that the dentist does not want to confront. (These may be clinical, interpersonal, or management related.) However, the dentist must face them. Dentists must remember that recognizing areas of vulnerability to a liability claim is the first step to reducing the likelihood and severity of a claim against them.

EVALUATION OF RISK MANAGEMENT CONTROL TECHNIQUES

A control mechanism ensures that a dentist's process works as designed and intended. Several categories of control techniques exist:

- **Risk avoidance** negates a potential loss because a practitioner avoids or does not do the risky procedure. If a dentist refers all bony third molar impactions to an oral surgeon, they avoid the risk associated with that procedure. An oral surgeon accepts that risk because of their generally higher level of skill, training, and expertise in that specialized area. Practitioners often use this technique for risks that have a high impact.

- **Risk (loss) prevention** reduces the possibility that a loss will occur. This technique occurs before a potential loss, and is therefore preventive in nature. If a practitioner keeps excellent patient records, including notes of clinically relevant telephone conversations with patients, they may prevent a malpractice action. Removing snow from steps in the winter prevents this as a source of negligence. Using this technique moves the risk from a high likelihood to a lower likelihood category.

- **Risk reduction** is like prevention but instead decreases the severity of a loss. If dentists decrease the impact that a loss may have, the resulting patient damages will also be less. If the practitioner has a current emergency kit, they must know how to use the drugs and materials. If the practitioner and staff members are currently trained in cardiopulmonary resuscitation (CPR) and other emergency protocols, then they have reduced the risk of a claim of negligence by a patient in case of a medical emergency. Dentists taking continuing professional education courses sharpen their skills and knowledge in challenging clinical cases. In both examples, proper preparation has decreased potential loss. This technique moves the risk from a high-impact to a lower-impact category.

- **Risk transfer** implies assigning the risk to someone else. The most common form of transfer occurs when a practitioner buys insurance coverage for a possible professional negligence suit. Here, the dentist has contractually transferred the financial loss to the insurance company in exchange for annual insurance premiums. Risk transfer can also work against the dentist. If they participate in managed care contracts that require them to sign a "hold harmless" clause, then they have increased the practice's liability exposure by not allowing a transfer of risk to the managed care company. This technique is used for risks with a high impact but low likelihood.

SELECTION AND IMPLEMENTATION OF CONTROL TECHNIQUES

Once a dentist identifies the risks associated with the practice, they need to decide which techniques can prevent, reduce, or avoid the liability and resulting loss. The selection and application of such techniques depend on the practitioner's assessment of the effectiveness and cost of each when applied to a potential loss. Examples of controls include:

- Training staff in medical emergencies and CPR.

- Securely transmitting electronic data.

- Locking sensitive paper documents in a cabinet.

- Using password protection and encryption for computer files.

- Buying appropriate insurance.

REASSESSMENT AND REEVALUATION OF TECHNIQUES

Practitioners must regularly reassess and reevaluate risk exposures and techniques for managing them. As a dentist grows professionally and financially, and as the practice grows, they will need to adjust methods and techniques to manage risk exposures and potential losses.

OFFICE INSURANCES

If they are the owner of a dental practice, a dentist needs to have two major types of liability insurance: business and professional. These insurances cover them if they are negligent, leading to someone's injury. If the dentist is an employee, they will not need to carry business insurance (e.g. office liability and workers' compensation), but they still need a professional liability policy. If they are an independent contractor, they are an independent business person, and the owner's policies usually do not cover them. Here, the dentist needs to be sure to have general liability, workers' compensation (if they hire employees), and business overhead insurance. Although the two overlap, this book contains a separate chapter on personal insurance needs (Chapter 8).

BUSINESS LIABILITY INSURANCE

The grouping of business liability insurance covers the proactive owner–dentist like any other business owner. Some practitioners advocate not carrying general or professional liability insurance, hoping not to get sued, or trying to hide assets so that the injured party cannot collect significant amounts. This is a dangerous strategy. Lawyers and judges are adept at piercing through these veils of protection. The practitioner may find themselves facing large legal and damage payments. The cost of insurance is insignificant compared with the cost of losing a liability suit. Most insurers will develop packages of business liability insurance for practitioners. These packages will cover the office owner for the risks they perceive as important, with coverage in appropriate amounts.

BUSINESS PREMISES AND PERSONAL INJURY INSURANCE

A general liability policy (GLP) for the office covers the practice owner in the event they are negligent and that action leads to injury of a patient or other person in the dental office. This is often called "slip and fall" insurance, from the common occurrence of someone slipping on ice or water, falling, and getting injured. This covers the business owner as a general business, not from professional liability. As explained in Chapter 14, a business owner must first be negligent before they are liable for damages. As a rule, $2 million per occurrence and $4 million aggregate coverage is presently adequate.

Practitioners can buy many additional coverage policies or "riders" for liability insurance. A practitioner wants to be sure that their policy covers employees in their cars or in the dentist's car while doing work-related errands. If an employee runs a case to the lab and has an accident, it is the dentist's accident. Many states allow a liquor legal liability rider. Suppose a dentist entertains at a place where they serve alcohol (such as at a staff Christmas party or drinks after a continuing education course). In that case, they may be liable if someone has an accident. The dentist may also purchase a business umbrella liability policy, like personal excess liability coverage. Like all these riders, a practitioner needs to decide how much risk they are willing to take and how much they are willing to pay to sell that risk to an insurance company.

EMPLOYMENT PRACTICES LIABILITY INSURANCE

Employment practices liability insurance (EPLI) protects practice owners from legal and settlement costs that might result from an employee suing for many work-related grievances, including sexual harassment, discrimination, slander, or wrongful termination. This is especially important for small businesses, such as dental practices, that do not have an employee manual or a human relations (HR) department to manage employee hiring, pay, benefits, complaints, or other problems. Using good and fair employment practices, including hiring, disciplining, and record-keeping to help prevent problems, is the first step to gaining protection. Buying insurance coverage is the next step.

EPLI coverage is often a policy endorsement added to the business owner's general business liability policy. Like other insurance policies, the owner's employment history (such as the number of employees, established rules and handbooks, past suits, and employee turnover) will affect the rates they pay. Many of these policies are issued on a claims-made basis. Like a malpractice claims-made policy, the business owner is only covered while the policy is in effect. Since a claim or suit may happen long after the alleged incident, owners should be sure to keep the policy current and purchase a tail policy if they leave or end the practice.

PROFESSIONAL LIABILITY INSURANCE

Because professionals have a special relationship with their clients (i.e. the dentist–patient relationship), a dentist needs to carry professional liability (malpractice) insurance to cover this possibility. Professional liability (malpractice) insurance is separate from a general (slip and fall) liability. This is a specialized insurance field, so few companies write this type of insurance. A later section in this chapter discusses this insurance in more detail.

LOSS-OF-USE INSURANCE

A couple of insurances cover practitioners in case they lose the ability to practice in the location. These are beyond a personal income disability policy, which is described in Chapter 8.

PROPERTY INSURANCE

If the practitioner owns the building they practice in, they must insure the physical structure. Commercial property insurance covers the building in much the same way that homeowner's insurance covers a home. The practitioner must be sure to insure the replacement value of the building. The price of constructing a new space can appreciate quickly. If the building is in an area prone to floods, storms, wildfires, or earthquakes, they should be sure to include coverage for those events.

BUILDING CONTENTS INSURANCE

Practitioners need to insure the physical contents of the practice, whether they own or lease the space. This type of insurance covers dental equipment, supplies, leasehold improvements, patient records, furniture, and fixtures in case they are damaged or destroyed. What could damage them? Fire, water damage from fighting a fire, theft, explosions, broken water pipes, or any of a host of problems can damage property. Building contents insurance seems like an expensive luxury until a dentist gets to the office and finds that a water pipe has burst, flooding the reception room and business office. Often lenders will require that dentists purchase this insurance to cover them in case of loss.

Practitioners have the option of covering their equipment at its present (current) value or at replacement value. The present value is the value of the equipment when the loss occurs. Assume that a dentist purchases a dental chair for $10 000 and insures it for the present value. If the chair is destroyed the day after it is insured, the present value is what the dentist paid for it. However, assume that the accident causing the loss did not occur for five years. That same dental chair may now have a present value of only $3000, yet to buy a new one (replacement value) would cost $12 000. Although replacement policies are more expensive, they are generally worth the extra premium paid.

BUSINESS OVERHEAD EXPENSE INSURANCE

If dentists are unable to practice because of a disability or other reason, office costs continue regardless. Although the landlord may be pleasant, they are not going to forgo the rent because someone cannot practice. Likewise, the banker needs the loan payment, and the staff still need to be paid if they are to stay in a dentist's employ. An office, or business, overhead expense (BOE) policy helps a practitioner to pay many office costs if they are unable to work. The dentist needs to carry personal disability income insurance to be sure that they provide for the family budget in case of disability. BOE policies do much the same for the office costs. Premiums are deductible, so benefits are taxable. Because the benefits go to pay deductible expenses, the deductible expense offsets the additional taxable income.

Business interruption coverage is the core of BOE insurance. This coverage pays the practitioner either direct costs or a set amount if they must shut down the business. If a practitioner has a major loss (such as a fire), they may have many months without practice income while they repair and refurnish the office. The practitioner needs to ensure that the policy covers them for interruption causes that are outside the building, such as a citywide power loss. Many do not.

Some practitioners opt not to carry BOE insurance. Instead, they plan to use their accounts receivable to pay office costs if they are unable to work. This is a risky plan. Typical accounts receivable may equal 1–1.5 months' billings. If the disability lasts longer than this (and many do), then the practitioner would run out of money to pay the bills. At that point, the practitioner would need to tap into personal savings or income to make regular payments. If they do not keep the staff on the payroll, the staff will probably leave, looking for employment elsewhere. Even if the practitioner weathers this storm, they will then have a cash-flow problem when they reopen the office. The practitioner will have used up their accounts receivable, so no cash flows into the office. It will be just like starting up again. The practitioner will need to go to the bank and borrow working capital, and then pay off the loan.

INSURANCES PROVIDED FOR EMPLOYEES

Practitioners need several insurances to provide for employees. If a dentist does not have employees, they obviously do not have to provide these insurances. As a proprietor or a partner in a partnership, practitioners do not cover themselves for (or receive any benefits from) these insurances. If a practice is a corporation, then the dentist is an employee of the corporation. The corporation must provide these insurances for them, the same as all other employees. They may also receive the same benefits if qualified.

WORKERS' COMPENSATION INSURANCE

This is an insurance that business owners must, by law, carry on all of their employees. (It is optional in some states, but business owners are still responsible for any claims.) It covers a business owner if an employee is injured on the job. This insurance covers medical expenses that are injury related and provides some disability payment (lost wages) if the accident disables the worker. Workers' compensation is a pure no-fault system. It does not matter whose fault the injury was. Workers' compensation pays for it because the injury occurred while the person was on duty. In return for the no-fault provision, workers' compensation laws have virtually eliminated the ability of the injured worker to sue the employer for negligence.

Specific workers' compensation rules vary state by state, but they all have several common elements:

- Workers' compensation provides benefits for accidental injury while on the job. The definition of an injury usually includes repetitive trauma, such as carpal tunnel syndrome. The compensation also includes occupational diseases, such as black lung disease for a coal miner or hepatitis for a dental worker who contracted it through an accidental needlestick.

- Benefits include lost wages (about one-half to two-thirds of weekly wages), medical benefits, and death benefits.

- This is pure no-fault insurance. Whether the employee's actions caused the accident or the employer did nothing wrong (had no fault), the insurance still pays benefits.

- The employer pays the entire cost. The cost of coverage may not pass to employees. There are stiff fines if the employer does not provide this coverage.

- Employees generally give up the right to sue employers for negligence if workers' compensation insurance covers the accident. This is called the *compensation bargain*.

Workers' compensation provides four types of benefits:

- **Medical payments** pay for physician services, durable medical equipment, prescriptions, and most other conventional medical treatments, such as psychological therapy. This is without a limit and a waiting period or copay.

- **Rehabilitation services** may be physical or vocational rehabilitation and are beyond medical payments. The worker may also receive disability benefits during the rehabilitation phase of treatment.

- **Death benefits** go to survivors of someone killed in a work-related accident. These include both a lump sum and a weekly income benefit.

- **Disability payments** pay a worker who is disabled while on the job.

A business owner's payment (or premium) for workers' compensation insurance is based on the number of employees and the annual payroll. Workers' compensation is a federally mandated system operated by the state. Each state has different rules concerning eligibility for benefits, costs, and owner requirements. A business owner can find a private insurance company that writes these policies. Many office liability carriers will include a workers' compensation policy in a package of insurance. These packages may be more expensive, but they are easier for the practitioner. The question becomes a cost-versus-convenience trade-off.

Whether worker's compensation insurance covers the owner–dentist depends upon the form of the business and the state in which the dentist practices. Many states allow business owners to be covered if they want. If a practitioner is a proprietor or a partner, they are an owner, not an employee. Therefore, in most states the owner–dentist does not fall under the workers' compensation laws. (Their employees are covered.) Such dentists do not pay premiums on themselves and they are not eligible for benefits. If, on the other hand, a dentist practices as a corporation, they are an employee of the corporation (though also an officer) and must be part of the workers' compensation system unless they opt out. Worker's compensation rules for limited liability company (LLC) members, family members, and employees also vary by state. Finally, worker's compensation generally does not include independent contractors. Again, each state is different and specific applications of the rules are confusing. Practitioners need to check with their workers' compensation carrier in the state of practice to know how these specifics apply.

UNEMPLOYMENT COMPENSATION INSURANCE

Unemployment compensation is a tax, but it operates as an insurance product. This is another joint federal–state program. Practitioners pay two unemployment taxes, State Unemployment Taxing Authority (SUTA) and Federal Unemployment Taxing Authority (FUTA). Practitioners pay state "contributions" (taxes) monthly. At the end of the year (January 30 the following year), the state checks to see how much the business owner paid into the state unemployment pool the previous year. If the amount was less than the federal requirement, the owner makes an additional payment to the federal government to make up the difference. Dentists only pay FUTA once a year, and the amount depends on the amount they have paid to the state (SUTA).

The system is complex. However, the total premiums paid are small. Payments will vary depending on the practice's history regarding staff unemployment. Generally, the employer can take a credit against FUTA for contributions to state unemployment (SUTA) funds up to a certain percentage of employee earnings. An accountant or payroll manager will provide this information. If a practitioner's staff has many claims, the business owner becomes a higher risk and rates go up. If there are few or no claims, rates and payments go down. This insurance, like worker's compensation, varies somewhat between states.

OTHER INSURANCES

Practice owners may also provide other forms of insurance for employees as employee benefits. These may include medical, disability, or life insurance. Business owners can check Chapter 26 for a detailed look at those insurances.

PROFESSIONAL RISK MANAGEMENT

This book has previously discussed the ideas of risk management as it relates to the personal and business risks that dentists face. These are the same risks that all Americans or all US business people face. However, professionals face an additional risk that most other business owners do not. That is the risk that the dentist may be negligent in their performance of their professional duties. Most practitioners have adequate malpractice insurance, believing that this satisfies the problem of risk management.

PROFESSIONAL NEGLIGENCE AND LIABILITY

Professional risk management closely aligns with quality assurance in the office, although risk management takes a more realistic view of the problem. Dentists must identify potential sources of professional risk exposure, train themselves and their staff to reduce the number and impact of these exposures, and continually work to improve the quality of dental care delivered in the office.

Negligence is the failure to act as a reasonable and prudent person in a similar situation would act. As described in Chapter 14, this definition is not absolute and opens the door to interpretation and changing definitions as social customs change. If a dentist's negligence causes an injury to someone, then the dentist is liable or must restore that person's loss. This generally means that the dentist must financially reimburse the injured person for the damages that the dentist's negligence caused. This may be through personal or insurance sources.

ELEMENTS TO PROVE PROFESSIONAL LIABILITY

The same cause-and-effect relationship exists in professional liability issues. If a dentist is negligent in the delivery of healthcare, they may be liable for the damages that result. These damages may include repair of the problem, lost earnings from missing work or reduced performance or ability, and pain and suffering experienced by the injured patient. (Obviously, significant discretion is available for judges and juries in awarding damages.)

An additional level must be satisfied in professional liability to prove professional negligence. The idea is similar but with a different "twist." Someone must prove each element to establish professional liability.

- **Creation of duty**
  When professionals agree to treat a patient, they create a practitioner–patient relationship. When this relationship exists, the practitioner has a legal duty (obligation) to act according to the standards of care for the profession. These standards involve using the required skill, knowledge, and care that members of the profession display. If a practitioner does not accept a person as a patient, they have not created a practitioner–patient relationship and therefore have no duty.

- **Breach of duty**
  If a practitioner fails to possess or use the skill, care, and knowledge that a reasonably well-qualified member of the profession would display under similar circumstances (i.e. fails to live up to the standards of care), then they have breached the duty owed to the patient. This is equivalent to the idea of negligence in a civil liability case.

- **Causation**
  If the breach of duty leads to injury or harm to the patient, then causation has been proved. The connection between the breach and injury must be both "actual" and "foreseeable."

- **Damages**
  The patient must establish that an actual loss occurred from the injury. That loss may be either monetary (e.g. lost wages) or personal (e.g. disfigurement, pain, and suffering).

STANDARD OF CARE

Malpractice actions do not hinge on the absolute notion that any injury is malpractice. Instead, these actions are based on what a "reasonable and prudent" professional in a similar situation would have done. This is known as a *standard of care*. These standards cover the practitioner's knowledge, skill, care, and judgment. They involve the technical level of expertise needed to complete a procedure successfully, the knowledge of how to interpret signs and symptoms, the behavioral accomplishment of treatment, and the ability to diagnose and properly plan for a patient's treatment. So, the standard of care involves both the technical performance of an extraction and the knowledge and judgment of when an extraction is and is not appropriate therapy.

There are no written standards of care published by the American Dental Association (ADA) or other professional organizations. (Some organizations are trying, with mixed success, to compile them.) These standards evolve over time. The technology and knowledge of the profession influence them as well as the wants, needs, desires, and sophistication of the public. Posterior composites, gold foil restorations, silicate restorations, and implant prostheses all enter current standards of care in a dynamic interchange. Standards are not an absolute definition or a "prescription" for how dentists must handle every patient procedure. Instead, they are a set of expectations for how a "reasonable and prudent" dental practitioner would behave in a similar professional situation.

Although the standards of care are constantly evolving, they are determined by a consensus of "experts" in the field. Experts have background and training that gives them an actual or inferred level of professional expertise. In a malpractice case, both sides bring experts to the trial to bolster their points of view. The experts who interpret the prevailing standards are often specialists in their field. To this extent, the law holds generalists to the standards that a specialist would hold. For example, if a case involves extracting an impacted third molar, the experts are usually oral surgeons. The courts would then hold the generalist to the same standard of care as the surgeon.

Standards of care vary by state or region, although these differences are becoming smaller with time. Some practitioners in rural, inner-city, or poverty-stricken areas claim that the standard of care is different in those areas. The standard of what is proper care is the same in all areas; patient acceptance of treatment may be different. With the increased speed of communication, ease of travel, and increase in third-party payers, these arguments are becoming less viable as well.

INFORMED CONSENT

For a dentist to have true informed consent from a patient, they must prove each of the following points concerning the treatment:

- **Capacity**
  The patient must have the capacity to make healthcare decisions for themselves. From a legal perspective, this means (in most states) that the patient must be at least of legal age (18 years old) or an emancipated (married) minor. From an ethical standpoint, the patient must have the mental ability to decide. These decisions can be difficult for the patient who is in emotional turmoil or physical pain or is approaching senility and is intermittently capable but at other times incapable.

- **Information provided**
  The dentist must provide information concerning the proposed treatment. This includes the nature of the treatment, the proposed time, and the cost to complete the procedure. Treatments within the general understanding of the patient from past treatment history do not need to be explained. The patient's treatment decisions will consider the risks involved in the treatment. To that end, dentists must discuss complications that commonly occur because of the procedure. They should also inform the patient of reasonable alternatives to the proposed treatment and the associated risks. Dentists do not need to discuss every alternative and every risk of every alternative. However, they must discuss the material and foreseeable risks in which a reasonable person would be interested. There is some room for interpretation in what is "material," "foreseeable," and "reasonable." That is what juries are for.

- **Patient comprehension**
  The patient must comprehend (understand) the information provided. Dentists must use uncomplicated language to discuss the treatment and alternatives, not technical dental terminology or jargon. Suppose the patient does not understand the language. In that case, the practitioner must get an interpreter to ensure that the person understands the oral description and has a chance to ask questions about the proposed treatment. Dentists may use written communication and other visual aids as appropriate to supplement (not replace) oral discussions.

- **Voluntary agreement**
  The agreement must be voluntary, without coercion, deception, duress, or other influence. A patient cannot be tricked or coerced into agreeing. An oral agreement

is adequate. A written (signed) agreement supplements an oral agreement, but it is not an ironclad defense for the dentist. (The patient can say "I didn't really understand what I was signing.")

- **Patient authorization**
  The patient must positively authorize the treatment. In effect, the patient must positively say "Yes, do the treatment." If they are uncertain or do not affirm the desire for treatment, the practitioner has not gained informed consent. The dentist should not do anything the patient has not authorized, even if they believe it is in the patient's best interest. The law says that what to do with a patient's body is their decision, not the dentist's. If a practitioner does dental work that the patient did not authorize, they may be guilty of malpractice and assault.

A patient may not legally consent to malpractice. If a dentist advocates or does a procedure they know is not within the standard of care, then the dentist has committed malpractice. This happens whether the patient has consented to the treatment or agreed not to hold the practitioner responsible. So, suppose an 18-year-old patient with healthy teeth and periodontium requests full-mouth extractions and dentures and the practitioner performs the requested service. In that case, they are committing malpractice and are liable for the results, even if the patient signed in the record that they understand this and will not hold the dentist responsible. This extreme case is straightforward. The problem comes in interpreting the standards of care in borderline cases.

Dentists must also allow informed refusal. Informed refusal means that the patient fully understands the treatment, the alternatives, and the outcomes, but they refuse the dentist's advice about treatment. If the patient is making a truly informed decision, the dentist must accept that decision. The practitioner needs to explain the possible outcomes of the lack of treatment. If the patient still refuses the advice (even after adequate explanation), the practitioner needs to document the advice and refusal in the patient's record. Even after this initial refusal of treatment, the dentist must again recommend treatment at subsequent follow-up or recall visits for as long as the condition remains and the dentist–patient relationship exists. Some dentists dismiss patients from the practice who do not accept their full advice. They believe that this opens them to charges of "supervised neglect," in which they know of a problem and are guilty of negligence because they contributed to the problem by allowing the patient to continue to decline under their care. If practitioners adequately express and document their recommendations, they will be on a sound legal footing.

COMMON AREAS OF PROFESSIONAL RISK EXPOSURE IN PRIVATE DENTAL PRACTICE

Several areas of common professional risk exposure happen in the dental office. These may result in resolution through any avenue described later in this chapter.

POOR WORK

Poor work is a simple failure to do a procedure at the level of the standard of patient care. It can occur for a variety of reasons, even to competent practitioners:

- **Poor technique** occurs when the technical aspects of a case are not up to the standard of care. If a dentist leaves an overhanging margin on an alloy or crown that can lead to future caries or a periodontal problem, they have committed bad work.

- **Failure to diagnose** a disease or problem is a common source of poor work. A dentist must give the patient a diagnosis of any disease within their area of expertise. They may be liable for the results if they fail to diagnose periodontal disease and inform the patient of the problem and likely outcomes. Often a dentist may claim that they did a proper exam and found everything to be within normal limits but did not document that fact. An example is an oral cancer screening. If a practitioner finds no oral cancers in an intraoral exam, their record should note that fact. This will help protect them from a future claim of "failure to diagnose" if someone later finds intraoral cancer in the patient. The dentist reminding a patient of needed or suggested treatment at each recall visit supports an ongoing diagnosis.

- **Failure to refer** to a specialist is another form of bad work. Although the courts understand that some diagnoses or technical procedures are out of the scope of a typical generalist, they also understand that practitioners need to recognize these cases and refer them to a specialist for evaluation and possible treatment. Dentists must be most interested in improving patients' health, not their personal pocketbooks.

- **Equipment failure** may be outside the dentist's control, yet still their responsibility. If a practitioner is doing an endodontic procedure and the file becomes lodged in the canal and breaks, they have had an equipment failure, considered poor work. As a rule, the practitioner is responsible for any equipment or supplies they should have known might be defective.

POOR OUTCOMES

A poor outcome does not necessarily involve poor work. It may involve a patient who is not satisfied with the result. Dentists have all seen denture cases in which the technical denture is clinically acceptable. The patient is simply not satisfied with the results. (The dentist might have had a suspicion when the patient walked into the office with a bag of seven other dentures that did not "work right.") A dentist may have also seen the opposite case of a patient with an anterior crown that looks terrible to their eye, yet the patient is delighted with the outcome, although the technical work was poor. This category of risk exposure is difficult for many dentists to accept, yet the courts have ruled that it is real and valid.

Poor outcomes are widespread in cases that involve patient values, such as esthetics. A practitioner's notion of what is acceptable may differ entirely from the patient's. Patient communication is a critical issue in these cases.

PATIENT COMMUNICATION PROBLEMS

Communication is a two-way street. Dentists may believe they have adequately expressed their side of the issue, but the patient either did not truly understand or did not adequately express their side of the issue (Box 28.1).

Patient communication problems fall into the following categories:

- **Lack of treatment plans**
  Lack of a plan is the basis of most patient communication problems. Without a treatment plan, patients do not know what to expect and may be surprised by the treatment or its cost. Detailed and written treatment plans are one of the best methods of avoiding dental malpractice litigation.

- **Unrealistic patient expectations**
  Being unrealistic often leads to liability problems. These expectations may be the result of the patient not adequately expressing goals and desires concerning their dental treatment, or the practitioner may make implied or actual promises of treatment that they do not fulfill. Either way, it is in the practitioner's interest to ensure that the patient has realistic expectations of the outcomes before beginning treatment.

- **Lack of informed consent**
  Lack of consent becomes the basis of many dental malpractice lawsuits. Informed consent is the ethical and legal doctrine requiring that dentists give patients sufficient information to make a free, rational treatment choice. This also implies the right of informed refusal. Informed consent relates to the treatment planning and patient communication issues discussed previously.

- **Poor work or outcomes by another dentist**
  These issues typically arise from a fee issue or third-party problems. A dentist redoes poor work from another dentist; however, the third-party carrier will not pay to redo the recent work. The patient then seeks various methods to have the first dentist pay for the poor work. Practitioners are understandably reluctant to criticize their fellow practitioners. They really do not know the circumstances, decision process, patient compliance, or a host of other issues that can negatively affect treatment outcomes. Therefore, dentists should avoid saying or giving the patient the impression that the previous dentist did faulty or poor work.

  Three options are available if a practitioner encounters poor work by a previous dentist (either negligent treatment or undiagnosed disease). The first is to contact the other dentist directly. Often the other dentist can inform the present dentist of problems or circumstances affecting treatment that the patient could or would not discuss. The previous practitioner might also offer to respond directly to the patient to try to correct the problem. The second avenue is to discuss with the patient various professional methods, such as peer review or mediation, to resolve the problem. However, when a dentist sees grossly or continuously faulty work, they have an ethical obligation to report the issue to the appropriate body of the local dental society or regulatory boards or bodies.

- **Fee disputes**
  Fee disputes typically arise from patients who are not completely satisfied with the dental work they have received. When the practitioner pursues aggressive collection techniques, the patient responds with a malpractice complaint. The practitioner's job is to balance their right to collect the money owed with the possibility of

BOX 28.1	**COMMUNICATING WITH PATIENTS**

- Personally discuss benefits and risks
- Personally discuss alternatives and consequences
- Encourage the patient to ask questions
- Use lay or common terms
- Get a commitment from the patient to proceed
- Keep well-documented records

triggering a lawsuit. Before sending anyone to a collection agent or attorney, the practitioner should be confident that the work is clinically acceptable. A statute of limitation (SOL) specifies when someone has to bring a lawsuit. The limitation may differ by type of suit (property, personal injury, medical negligence) and varies by state. For example, some states have an SOL of one year from the date of discovery for adult malpractice actions. (The patient has one year from when they knew or should have known about a problem to sue.) Many experts recommend waiting until after the SOL expires before pursuing aggressive collection techniques. The dentist should check with an attorney in the practice state. Many nuances in these laws can affect the dentist's decision.

- **Auxiliary treatment problems**
  The practitioner is generally responsible for the actions and work of the auxiliaries employed in their office. If a staff member has committed an act of malpractice, the dentist is also liable through the doctrine of agency. So, if a hygienist accidentally injures a patient by dropping an instrument in their eye, both the dentist and the hygienist will be liable.

- **Patient abandonment**
  Once a dentist–patient relationship is established, the dentist must continue that relationship for the patient's care. The patient may end the relationship at any time. The dentist may end the relationship but only under certain conditions. They may not end the relationship in the middle of treatment. (What constitutes the "middle of treatment" is open to interpretation.) The dentist may end the relationship if the patient is in a stable condition and will not be harmed by a delay in treatment while they seek care elsewhere. If, for example, the dentist is in the middle of root canal therapy, they must complete the endodontic treatment and probably place an adequate provisional restoration. If the dentist has done a surgical procedure that usually involves follow-up appointments for dressings, suture removal, or other care, they must complete that course of treatment. If a patient owes the dentist money, the dentist still must complete the procedure and ensure that the patient is dentally stable before ending the relationship. The notion here is that dentists must not harm (or even potentially harm) a patient by ending the relationship. If a dentist refuses to continue to treat a patient, they have violated the duty to treat that they established in the initial relationship, opening the dentist to charges of abandonment if the patient's oral health declines.

BOX 28.2	ENDING A RELATIONSHIP WITH A PATIENT

- Reason for termination
- Date it becomes effective
- Treatment remaining
- Referral to or source for a new dentist
- Method of continuing emergency care
- Offer to transfer records to a new provider
- Office policy regarding record transfer

ENDING THE DOCTOR–PATIENT RELATIONSHIP

When a practitioner ends a relationship with a patient, they must inform the patient verbally and in writing (Box 28.2). (The dentist should keep a copy of the written correspondence.) The dentist's letter should state why they ended the relationship and ensure patient health through referral, emergency care, and an offer to send records to a new dentist.

Insurance problems have led to a new set of malpractice issues. Although managed care does not cause poor ethical decisions and malpractice by the practitioner, it causes new problems in the dentist–patient relationship that can lead to accusations of malpractice. The single most significant influence is the temptation to perform less than optimal care. The pressure for minimal treatment may come from the dentist, the plan administrator, the patient, or the employer. Despite the pressure, the dentist is still responsible for the treatment rendered.

The dentist needs to remember that the best treatment for a patient is the best treatment, no matter how much money they make (or do not make) when doing the procedure. A dentist is obligated to recommend and do treatment that is at least at the standard of care, regardless of the method or amount of payment. If a practitioner cannot abide by the rules established in a managed care contract, they should not participate in the managed care program.

PATIENT TREATMENT RECORDS

The patient treatment record is the official document of all treatment procedures, referrals, professional communications, recommendations, and advice the dentist renders to patients in the dental office. The written treatment record (or its computer equivalent) is the basis of knowledgeable patient treatment. It serves as the recorded history of treatment and recommendations in case of professional liability issues.

COMPONENTS

Patient records may be paper or electronic in form. They need to have the following components:

- **Identification data**
  This is the demographic information about the patient, their name, age, responsible party, Social Security number, insurance carrier, etc.

- **Health Insurance Portability and Accountability Act (HIPAA) disclosure**
  The patient needs to read and acknowledge having received the office's HIPAA disclosure.

- **Consent form**
  The doctrine of informed consent that is customary in the United States requires that healthcare providers inform patients of the nature of the proposed services, the possible outcomes (positive and negative) of the treatment, and the alternatives to the proposed treatment in language that the individual can understand. Simply having a patient sign a consent form does not adequately gain the patient's informed consent. The dentist must present the proposed treatment so that the patient can understand. The dentist should orally explain the procedure, give written explanations (especially if the procedure is difficult or complex), and gain the written understanding of the patient on a "consent form." This may be general consent for treatment or specific consent for a procedure that has additional risks not present in common procedures, such as the removal of a bony-impacted third molar.

- **Medical history**
  The written medical history should include oral follow-up (consultation when indicated) of any abnormal conditions. The history should note drug usage (prescription and over the counter), allergies, substance abuse (including alcohol and tobacco), and family history of a disease.

- **Dental history**
  This section needs to include the patient's chief complaint and their past use of dental services.

- **Clinical exam**
  Dentists frequently note this section graphically as charts (caries, periodontal, and soft tissue exam). They may also include radiographs and photographs.

A complete exam is standard for all initial patients; updates are done on routine recall examinations.

- **Diagnosis**
  The dentist must write the diagnosis of findings clearly in an understandable form. This is the basis of the treatment plan.

- **Treatment plan**
  The treatment plan is a written statement of the proposed treatment to address the defined diagnoses.

- **Progress notes**
  This section chronicles the patient's treatment visits to the office. Dentists need to note any treatment or advice rendered to the patient and any changes in the proposed treatment plan or sequence, laboratory services ordered, or medications prescribed.

- **Completion notes**
  A summary of treatment, including postoperative radiographs and photographs if indicated, concludes the record. The dentist should record recommendations concerning continued or follow-up care.

THE VALUE OF GOOD RECORDS

The individualized dental record must contain all the information concerning a patient's treatment. If many practitioners (e.g. partners, associates, hygienists) all make entries in records, the office depends on accurate entries by every member of the team. Even for an individual practitioner, the records are an indispensable source of information. Memories are notoriously faulty after months (or years) have passed. Most practitioners cannot accurately remember having an encounter with a patient, much less any specific diagnostic finding, treatment recommendations, or treatment outcome that occurred during that encounter.

Patient records also are the cornerstones of any malpractice case defense. The adage that "if it isn't in the record, it didn't happen" is, unfortunately, accurate. Because patient records are critical to preventing and resolving patient problems and disputes, a few words concerning their use are in order.

- **All entries must be accurate and thorough**
  Practitioners must make entries when the event occurs rather than later. The patient's record is a legal document. When the dentist or staff member writes in a record, it must only be in blue or black ink. (Colored chart notations are OK.) A practitioner should not use slang or common language. They should use only objective, factual, and medically

accurate information, avoiding disparaging or personal comments. ("Patient was a real pain in the butt today" is a highly inflammatory statement. "Patient appeared agitated, was demanding and uncooperative in treatment" says the same thing in a more factual way.) If a practitioner has a shorthand system for chart notations, they must post a list so that all office personnel use it consistently. If the dentist sends a record or copies to another office or expert witness, they should include a copy of the shorthand definitions so that nobody misunderstands them.

- **Records must be neat and legible**
  For paper records, all entries must be typed or written legibly in ink and signed or initialed by the person who makes the entry. The dentist should review and countersign the entry if a staff member makes it. Computer records should be as complete as handwritten records, and data should be backed up regularly. Practitioners should follow computer program recommendations for security and staff identification when anyone enters data into patient records.

- **Never attempt to alter records**
  If a dentist makes an entry in error, they should put a single line through the entry, followed by the reason for the correction and the correction itself on paper records. The practitioner must not use correction fluid or tape, must not scratch over an entry until it is solid ink, and must not attempt to erase an entry. A note explaining an incorrect entry (beside the original note) should occur in a computer record. Dentists must not delete or add to records in the event of potential legal action. Tampered records are more damaging to the professional than incomplete records. People can examine computer records forensically to learn when someone added or altered an entry. Any changes the dentist makes once a malpractice action has been initiated will look at best suspect and at worst fraudulent.

- **Keep separate financial information**
  Practitioners should keep financial information separate from the treatment record to the extent possible. If someone uses a paper treatment record, they should have a separate sheet for financial transactions and communications. The two files are linked if the practitioner uses a computerized record system. Many programs have a "Comments" section for making non-treatment entries.

- **All records must be considered confidential**
  Dentists must secure written patient consent before granting access to the records to any other party, except as required by a valid subpoena. The original copy of the patient's record must never leave the office unless by court order. Dentists may send photocopies to other healthcare providers, or other people may view the records (with the patient's permission) in the dentist's office. Remember, the dentist owns the physical record, but the patient also owns the information in that record. The dentist has an ethical and legal obligation to keep that information confidential, as dictated by HIPAA rules and the dental office's HIPAA documents.

- **Keep patient records indefinitely**
  Generally, dentists should retain patient records for as long as they are in practice. This serves two purposes. It improves patient oral health by providing a historical treatment record and serves as the basis of defense in a malpractice action against the dentist. From a practical standpoint, the practitioner may want to purge records of patients they have not seen in the office for several years. When a practitioner purges records, they should not destroy them but move them to another office area where they can retrieve them within a reasonable time. Some states have minimum times for which the practitioner must keep records, but it is a good idea to keep them as long as possible. If storage is a problem, then the dentist can microfilm or store seldom-used records off the premises. Computer records do not have the problem of quantity storage that paper records do. The practitioner must check with a lawyer and malpractice carrier before destroying patient records.

- **Use supporting records where appropriate**
  Photographs are excellent means of supportive record-keeping; however, they must not replace the standard written record procedure. The practitioner should keep casts for difficult or complex cases. They may substitute good photographs of casts in routine cases for satisfied patients. Casts and photographs are excellent means of documenting pre- and posttreatment oral conditions.

FORMAT OF DAILY ENTRIES

Several standard formats (Simple note, PARTS, SOAP) exist for daily entries in a patient's record. The most common is a "SOAP" note (Box 28.3). These formats intend to ensure that practitioners record important information about the patient visit systematically so that they do not miss anything important. They require the dentist to include the date and a paragraph for each heading. What is important is that the dentist is systematic in entering information.

BOX 28.3   EXAMPLE OF A SOAP NOTE

S: Patient reports "a bad pain in my upper right jaw. It keeps me up all night. Nothing makes it stop hurting." (Patient points to tooth #3.) Patient appeared tired and agitated.

O: BP: 125/80, P: 62, R: 12, T: 100.7. Tooth #3 with large, cavitated carious lesion. PA radiograph shows extensive caries on M and D of #3 with large (2 mm) periapical radiolucency on palatal root. Tooth #3 percussion sensitive +++ (#2, 4 neg to percussion) Pos R cervical lymph nodes. Patient displays generalized gross caries.

A: Rampant dental caries. Tooth #3 irreversible pulpitis with periapical abscess, questionable restorability. Patient is febrile.

P: Discussed treatment options, risks, and benefits (RCT/Crown vs EXT with FPD or implant replacement). After discussion, patient desires extraction #3. Administered 1.8 cc lidocaine with epi 1 : 100 000. Simple forceps extraction #3. Rx: PenVK 500 mg #28 one q6h until gone. Patient instructed to return of further pain, fever, or swelling. Patient advised of need for extensive dental care.

SOAP NOTES

SOAP is an acronym for:

- **Subjective**
  What the patient said was their reason for the visit. The dentist may also include their observations about the patient.

- **Objective**
  The objective findings related to the patient's chief complaint. This includes the results of any tests or measurements.

- **Assessment**
  The assessment and diagnosis of the problem. The dentist may develop several diagnoses.

- **Plan**
  The plan and treatment for the patient. This includes any treatment done or medication prescribed and patient recommendations, instructions, or required follow-up.

For patients undergoing routine, continuing care, the SOAP note is simpler. The *subjective* section may be "Patient for routine dental care per treatment plan" or "Patient for a periodic maintenance visit." The *objective* section consists of recording vital signs and "See patient database."

Assessment is "periodontal disease treatment," "preventive visit," "caries restoration," or other descriptions. The *plan* section is then a listing of the treatment rendered.

OWNERSHIP OF PATIENT RECORDS

The practitioner owns the physical patient record (including the radiographs), but the patient has a right to control the information in the record. HIPAA dictates how the practitioner will safeguard this information. Personal and health information is confidential. The dentist may not give that information to anyone else without the patient's written consent. (The dentist needs to be sure to keep this written consent in the record.) Most states require a practitioner to provide the patient with a copy of their record within a reasonable time. The practitioner also needs to note in the chart any time they send a copy of the record to anyone outside the office. This can avoid confusion if, in the future, multiple copies of a patient's record apparently exist. The dentist should be sure to have on file a signature from the patient authorizing them to release information to a third-party carrier for claims processing. Access to records for quality assurance reviews should be limited to patients of the involved third-party carrier.

TELEPHONE CALLS

The dental office personnel must document all telephone calls (and attempted contacts) related to patient treatment in the treatment record. This includes calls that follow up treatment, advice to patients, referrals or specialist discussions, and calls from patients requesting information or clarification of treatment or advice. (Office personnel should note financial calls to or from a patient or account guarantor in the patient's financial file, ledger card, or computer financial file. Financial issues do not have anything to do with the patient's treatment and ought to be separate.) Documenting telephone calls to and from patients that the dentist receives or makes from home during non-office hours is also important. Many practitioners keep a pad of paper or "sticky notes" near the phone to jot down notes concerning patient conversations. If a dentist prescribes medications or recommends additional care during such a call, they should make a note and transfer it to the patient record the following day.

AVENUES OF RESOLUTION OF POOR WORK OR POOR OUTCOME

A patient (or the public) has four avenues to try to gain satisfaction for what they believe is poor work done by a dental practitioner. State laws vary as to when each avenue is appropriate, so the dentist should check with a local attorney or malpractice carrier if they face a potential malpractice action. (For example, some peer review boards do not handle fee disputes.)

INDIVIDUAL COMMUNICATION

The profession handles most complaints through individual communication between the dentist and the patient. Unfortunately, many dissatisfied patients are reluctant to discuss their perceived problems with the dentist. It becomes a self-fulfilling prophecy that if a dentist has a problem that results from poor communication, the patient will not express this to them. However, communication is a two-way street. The practitioner must establish an atmosphere of trust and openness so that patients and staff are not reluctant to bring problems to their attention. If the dentist can, they should resolve a problem while it is small.

PEER REVIEW PROCESS

Peer review is a system that organized dentistry has developed to resolve conflicts between patients and practitioners. Generally, it is a voluntary process. If a dentist does not want to participate, no one requires them to do so. (Some states require a peer review process before any malpractice litigation. In such cases, peer review is mandatory.) It is in the dentist's interest (and the profession's) to resolve problems fairly before they end in a courtroom. In this process, patients bring a problem to a peer review board composed of members of the local dental society. (Many states also have a statewide "appeal" board.) Generally, each side of the dispute will give their side of the tale in writing so the board can investigate or ask for additional information. In the hearing that follows, the patient voices their problem. The dentist gives their side of the story. The board may look at records, examine the patient, or ask for "experts" in the field to give opinions.

In most states, the peer review board's decision is advisory. It has no force of law, although it has the moral force of a professional imprimatur. (If the peer review board votes overwhelmingly that the work shows a problem, the dentist ought to take heed.) If a patient is unsatisfied with the outcome, they can usually still pursue malpractice litigation. Peer review has helped to decrease the amount of professional litigation. Because organized dentistry runs peer review, in many states it is only open to members of the ADA (and its affiliate state and local societies). Not all practitioners (only about 80%) are members of the organization. Those who are not cannot participate. The only disciplinary action that boards can generally take

is expulsion from the professional society. For members, this may or may not be significant. For non-members, it is meaningless.

MALPRACTICE LITIGATION

The best-known avenue for the resolution of disputes is malpractice litigation. In these cases, the dentist (the defendant) will be taken to court by the dissatisfied patient (plaintiff), who claims that the dentist was professionally negligent and therefore owes damages. Most of the cases never reach the actual courtroom. The plaintiff drops some, the defendant settles some, or the defendant's malpractice insurance carrier may negotiate a settlement. The plaintiff's lawyer handles most cases on a "contingency" basis. This means the lawyer only earns a percentage (usually about a third) of any awards collected. If the dentist wins, the attorney gets nothing. This makes plaintiffs' lawyers careful in choosing their cases. The lawyers will only take cases they believe they can win and will likely result in considerable damage awards. This process helps screen out small nuisance-type cases, but encourages others where the plaintiff does not have enough money to hire an attorney.

If a dentist receives any information from a lawyer or patient indicating a possible lawsuit, they need to contact their malpractice carrier immediately. The carrier will help and guide the dentist through the process. The carrier is interested in paying out the least amount of money for damages, so the carrier will do what it can to help the dentist in the case. The carrier will find (and pay for) an attorney to represent the dentist's interest in the case. (Some dentists believe the attorney represents the carrier's interest in the case.) The carrier will also pay any damages from the dentist's case up to the limits of their coverage. Most carriers will vigorously defend the dentist's case so that plaintiffs' lawyers do not see dental malpractice as an easy area to get a settlement. A carrier may not spend $100 000 defending a dentist in a $20 000 suit, even if it believes the case can be won. In this case, it makes economic sense for the carrier to settle the suit before trial. The dentist then may continue the suit, but the carrier is no longer involved and will not pay any losses the dentist has as a result.

LICENSING AGENCY ACTIONS

Each state has some form of board of dentistry. This is the agency that the state charges with protecting the public from poor or fraudulent dental practitioners. The agency sets rules and regulations concerning the practice of dentistry in its state and then enforces those rules daily. The agency's job is to protect the public from substandard dentists, not to protect the dentist's ability to practice dentistry. State boards have the authority to grant dental licenses. They can also revoke or suspend licenses and reprimand, censure, or probate practitioners. Most boards have investigative powers. If they receive a complaint, they can require documentation from the dentist or conduct an inspection at the practitioner's office. Many boards, by law, must investigate every patient complaint (or certain types of complaints) they receive.

Boards enact disciplinary actions for several common reasons. They may be involved if a practitioner has done "grossly or continually faulty work." (A single act or finding of malpractice *generally* does not lead to board action unless it is "grossly" or "egregiously" faulty.) The boards are often involved in cases of interpretation of the state dental laws, such as proper auxiliary use and specialty designation. Boards frequently punish practitioners who are guilty of improper prescription writing, and they guide or punish impaired providers. Most state Dental Practice Acts require "good moral character" of dentists. Based on this rule, many boards can (and do) punish dentists if they are convicted of moral types of crime. If a dentist is involved in a board of dentistry action, the results can be disastrous for them and their practice. Because these are not malpractice actions, malpractice carriers do not represent the dentist in actions by the board of dentistry.

MALPRACTICE INSURANCE

Despite a practitioner's best efforts at managing the professional risk in the office, they may, at some time in their career, be sued for dental malpractice. Those are the times for which the dentist has professional liability (malpractice) insurance.

MALPRACTICE INSURANCE TERMINOLOGY

Like general business liability insurance, several terms are common to all malpractice insurance contracts. The dentist pays an annual premium to the insurance company (*carrier*). In return, the company writes a contract (policy) in which it agrees to indemnify or repay the dentist for any covered loss while the contract is in force. Covered losses are judgments of damages against the dentist, usually in a court of law, that arise from their professional negligence. The carrier typically puts stipulations in the contract limiting the maximum amount it will pay. For example, the insurer may write a policy with limits of "$1 million/$3 million." This says that it will pay up to $1 million for a single

claim (judgment) against the dentist and up to $3 million in total judgments per year. If the dentist is successfully sued for $2.5 million in a single case, the insurer will pay $1 million. The dentist is responsible for paying the other $1.5 million. Usually, no deductibles are associated with these policies. Policies will have a long list of exclusions or cases in which the insurer will not pay. A *claims-made* policy covers the dentist for any claim made while the policy is in force. If the dentist leaves the practice, they need to purchase a "tail policy" to cover them for their work after the claims-made policy is no longer in force. An *occurrence* policy covers the dentist for their work during a given period, even if no one discovers the problem until many years later. So, a dentist does not need a tail policy if they have this type of coverage.

Some carriers will pay for the cost of medical follow-up care (often called "first aid expenses") for a patient of the practice. For example, assume a patient swallows a crown while the dentist is adjusting it before cementation. The dentist wants to send the patient to a physician or the emergency department for a chest x-ray to ensure that the crown is in the stomach and not lodged in the patient's lung. Many malpractice carriers will pay for the cost of follow-up care. (It is obviously in their interest to ensure that a more serious problem does not develop.) The dentist ought to check their policy before a problem arises.

WHAT TO DO IN CASE OF A SUIT

If a dentist suspects a patient is so dissatisfied that they might sue, they need to contact the professional liability agent immediately. They should not wait until a summons, requiring the dentist to be present for a deposition, arrives. This is probably new territory for the dentist. The agent, however, will have handled many such cases before. They can help the dentist through the process and give advice that will reduce the likelihood of a full-blown court case or even avert a claim. Conversely, inappropriate comments or actions by the dentist may hasten or intensify a claim. If a case does become serious, the insurer will find (and pay for) an attorney to represent the dentist's side of the case. However, the dentist needs to remember that the attorney works for the insurance company. Some policies say that if the insurer decides to settle the case without going to trial, the dentist does not have much say in the matter. (They call this a *hammer* clause, for good reason.) Even if both the dentist and the attorney believe they will win the case, the insurance company may find it less expensive (from its perspective) to settle before trial rather than going through a lengthy and expensive court trial. If that is the case, the company usually will settle. Other policies give the dentist the option to decide whether to settle. The dentist must read their policy carefully before signing. Not all policies contain such clauses. Some require the dentist's consent to settle. This can be a deciding factor for some practitioners in choosing malpractice insurance carriers. Most carriers will fight a suit if they believe they will win it. They do not want to have a reputation as an insurer who will readily settle a claim.

FACTORS THAT AFFECT RATES

Several factors affect a dentist's malpractice insurance rates. The area in which they practice is one of the most important. Some areas experience many more malpractice cases than others. If a dentist practices in one of these high-suit areas, the rates will be higher than in other areas. A dentist's professional history plays a significant role. If they have had previous malpractice cases, the insurer will see them as a greater risk, and therefore they will have to pay higher premiums. Each insurance company has a point at which it will simply refuse to write the dentist any more policies. The company may believe that the dentist is too great a risk for it to carry. Specialists do more complex and risky procedures than generalists. Their premiums are also higher. Dentists who use deep sedation or general anesthesia will pay a higher premium to compensate for the additional risk that those procedures carry. (Nitrous oxide analgesia generally does not lead to higher premiums.) Many plans will give a dentist a premium reduction if they complete a risk management seminar or quality assurance office review by the staff.

COORDINATION OF POLICIES

Many malpractice insurers also carry general business ("slip and fall") liability insurance and workers' compensation policies. The dentist can coordinate the three to ensure there are no gaps in their coverage. For example, a patient falls while getting out of the dental chair, injuring themselves. Is this a general or professional liability problem? If the practitioner coordinates their insurance policies, they do not have to worry about which insurance will be responsible for coverage.

Many group practices require that all providers carry malpractice insurance through the same carrier. This decreases problems if a patient jointly sues several practitioners in the same practice over a case. It simply avoids a squabble between the insurers (claiming the other should pay) that leaves the dentist in the middle.

NATIONAL PRACTITIONER DATA BANK

The federal government has been concerned about tracking healthcare practitioners with poor malpractice or other treatment records. Often these practitioners move from hospital to hospital or state to state. Their histories and backgrounds are only sometimes adequately or easily checked. The problem is primarily with medical practitioners, although it has included dentists. The government has established the National Practitioner Data Bank (NPDB) to address this problem. Any time a healthcare practitioner receives a judgment against them in which the practitioner (or a malpractice carrier) pays an award, they must notify the data bank. The data bank then develops a historical record of payments. Any time a practitioner applies for a license, credentials, or privileges, the investigating agency can receive a report on the person's malpractice history. The practitioner can request a self-query, although there is a small fee.

The profession sees several problems with the data bank. The idea of what constitutes a payment to a patient is in question. If a patient is dissatisfied with a denture and the dentist refunds their money, that may be a payment that must be reported. Payments made from personal (not professional) sources may not be reportable. Peer review intends to avoid problems, but many in the profession see the resulting reporting to the data bank as punitive. Finally, only credible investigators have access to the information (e.g. hospitals, state licensing boards, and other credentialing bodies). Practitioners are worried that the public may have easy access to the information and make false or uninformed decisions based on the information. Meanwhile, consumer advocates are calling for a more open record. So, as with many regulatory processes, the NPDB will likely evolve over time.

INFORMATION SECURITY AND MANAGEMENT

Practicing dentists deal with sensitive data every day. Modern dental offices contain a tremendous amount of information that can be misused or abused by unscrupulous, dishonest, or incompetent people. This information consists of the personal medical information of patients, personal and financial patient information, payment card information, and personal information about the employees and owners of the practice. With the instant dispersal of information through the internet, dentists must proactively and zealously protect that information from intrusion.

It is both a moral and legal responsibility for practitioners to ensure that this information does not fall into the wrong hands and is not misused. HIPAA rules and sanctions govern protected patient information. Federal rules govern large organizations' handling of financial information. Many states have rules about disposing of data that contains sensitive information. Finally, dentists as individuals would be incensed if lax security allowed their personal information to be misused. Practitioners must take the same view on the other side to ensure that the information they have on others is well protected.

TYPES OF INFORMATION

Data exists in many forms in the dental office. It may be physical (such as paper, film, or a computer screen), electronic (on a computer, the internet, office intranet, or fax), or storage media (such as computer tapes and back-up drives). This data is at risk of being accessed by unauthorized people (both inside the office and outside) any time a practice uses, stores, transfers, or disposes of it. In the old days, the biggest concern was that someone might look through the trash (dumpster dive) and find sensitive information on discarded paper forms. This information could then be used for illegal purposes. Today, computer hackers and thieves are more inventive in ways in which they can steal sensitive information, so the management of this risk needs to evolve similarly.

ELEMENTS OF A PLAN

Any plan for information security must be reasonable yet protect patients', staff members', and dentists' interests. As in all risk management efforts, the practitioner must use a reasonable level of diligence to be sure that the data is secure and used as intended. Some forms of data are more sensitive or potentially more damaging than others and must be treated differently. Reasonableness is the key here. HIPAA sets the baseline on what dentists must do with patients' personal information. The data management plan describes how the practitioner handles this and other forms of sensitive information.

COMPUTER BACK-UPS

Practitioners need to back up their computer database daily. They should be sure that their data back-up uses secure data encryption techniques. (To read an encrypted file, a data thief must have a secret key or password that enables decryption.) Many computer consultants call for redundant back-ups, one on a physical disk, the other in a secure offsite storage area. When a practitioner makes back-ups on physical media, such as a removable disk, drive, or tape, the best procedure is to take it off site. In case of an office fire or other catastrophe, the practitioner must be able to access the information. If a practitioner places media in a fireproof safe, they should be sure that the safe is rated for enough time and temperature to withstand a complete fire. It must also be waterproof, because fire departments use water for fire suppression. If the practitioner takes the media off site, they have the additional problem of securing the media to ensure that no one steals it in transit or storage. Many people have found laptops or storage disks stolen from their cars while they took a brief stop in a grocery store on the way home. HIPAA rules say that it is the practitioner who is guilty of not securing the data, not the thief for stealing it. Secure online back-ups are becoming the norm because they successfully address these problems and have become much less expensive.

DESTROYING DATA

When the practice no longer needs the data, or when they change storage media, practitioners need to destroy the information on the old media. Shredding any paper or film that has any sensitive information must be a normal operating procedure. All cities have companies that will come to the office and shred documents and destroy computer disks. For large jobs, the cost is well spent. Most will give the dentist a certificate that guarantees complete destruction of the media.

DATA IN TRANSIT

Any time practitioners move data, physically or electronically, it is at greater risk of being lost or stolen because it may be out of their control. Dentists need to take special precautions.

- For physical (paper and film) data, dentists must use approved couriers (such as UPS, FedEx, USPS, etc.) for sensitive data. For sensitive documents, the dentist must ensure that parcel tracking is available and that someone must sign for the package.

- For electronic data, the dentist must be sure that software vendors comply with HIPAA for information processing (most do). The dentist needs to use proper encryption techniques. If they use a wireless network, they need to be sure that it is properly configured for security. If a dentist emails information, they must be sure that the email provider secures it properly.

Part 2: Regulatory Compliance

*Badges? We ain't got no badges. We don't need
no badges. I don't have to show you any
stinking badges.*

Gold Hat, *The Treasure of the Sierra Madre*

GOAL

This part aims to prepare the new practitioner to be compliant with regulations that affect dental practice.

LEARNING OBJECTIVES

At the completion of this part, the student will be able to:

- Describe the types of licenses that a dental practitioner requires to practice legally.
- Describe the process of gaining a state dental license.
- Describe the process of registering to write prescriptions for scheduled drugs.
- Describe the purpose of the Occupational Safety and Health Administration (OSHA).
- Define the owner–dentist's role in worker safety in the dental office.
- Describe the office policies required by OSHA regarding bloodborne pathogens.
- Describe the Hazard Communication Program required by OSHA for the dental office.
- Describe fines and actions that may result from a dentist's failure to comply with OSHA standards.
- Describe the purpose of HIPAA.
- Define protected health information (PHI) and give common dental office examples of PHI.
- Describe why it is important to protect a patient's PHI.
- Describe the three broad HIPAA rules.
- Describe the use of the common HIPAA forms in the dental office.
- Describe present regulations and standards regarding the disposal of medical wastes.

KEY TERMS

Bloodborne Pathogens Standard
board of dentistry
blood and other potentially infectious material (BOPIM)
business associate agreement
continuing education requirement
DEA number
Drug Enforcement Administration (DEA)
Electronic Transactions and Code Set Standards rule
engineering controls
exposure control plan
general industry standards
hazard communication standard
hazardous material
hepatitis B vaccine
Health Insurance Portability and Accountability Act (HIPAA)
infectious waste
license renewal
medical waste
minimum necessary information
narcotic registration
occupational license
Occupational Safety and Health Administration (OSHA)
personal protective equipment (PPE)
privacy notice
privacy rule
protected health information (PHI)
regional clinical examinations
security rule
state dental license
treatment, payment, and operations (TPO)
universal precautions
work practice controls
written exposure control plan

There are several regulatory needs that practitioners must take care of in their practice. These issues are not exciting, but they are important. They involve complying with government regulations.

With all these regulatory and compliance issues, in the end it does not matter whether the practitioner likes them or not, whether they believe they are an intrusion into their life, or whether they believe they are effective. They need to comply. The business owner is responsible for seeing that everyone in the office complies with the general intent and details of the regulations. Several steps will help to ensure that the practitioner does comply.

- **The practitioner needs to learn the laws**
  As the leader and manager of the practice, the practice owner must be familiar with the regulations that affect the practice. They should take continuing education courses that show how to comply with these laws.

(The practice owner should also require staff to take these courses.) They should purchase material from the ADA or other sources that guide them in developing office compliance policies. They can often delegate compliance to a trusted employee and must encourage the employee to take their role seriously and remain involved. Many consultants will help a dentist set up compliance policies and develop documentation.

- **The practice owner should train new and current employees on how to follow the law**
Each regulation describes the training that practice owners must conduct with employees. Most require extensive training for new employees, retraining, and certification for ongoing employees.

- **The practice owner needs to document office compliance**
If the practitioner does the training and other compliance requirements, they must be able to prove it if a regulator requests. They must therefore document all the training and other activities that the practice does to support compliance. Often, the documentation (not the training itself) avoids a problem. Much like patient records, if the practitioner does not document it in the records, it does not happen.

- **The practice owner must do annual updates**
Practitioners often believe that they have complied with the regulations when they have done something once. Most regulations require that practice owners update all staff members annually. People forget information if they do not use it regularly. Their perspectives change, and the laws and regulations change over time. Annual refresher courses help everyone understand what to do and why they need to do it.

These regulations are not onerous. They are well-intentioned rules to be sure that dentists protect themselves, their workers, patients, private information, and the public. Each office needs to develop a culture of compliance. This culture says that the office does not grudgingly do the minimum of what it must, but looks for ways to ensure that all the affected people are protected.

LICENSES AND REGISTRATIONS

STATE DENTAL LICENSE

Completing a state or regional clinical board exam does not get a dentist a license to practice dentistry. They still must apply for a license in every state in which they will practice.

As a rule, they must also pass an exam that covers the state's dental laws before the state will grant the dentist a license. By far the biggest problem is the clinical exam. The rest is pretty much paperwork, although the dentist must know the state dental laws in detail.

A dentist must have a current state dental license certificate (the piece of paper) in hand before seeing the first patient. They must not see a patient without it because they would be practicing dentistry without a license. This is a bad way to start a dental career. The dentist may have received notice at school, by phone, or in any of several other ways that they have "passed." But unless the state makes a specific exception, a graduate cannot see patients until they have the license in hand.

Some new dentists schedule patients based on the assumption that they will pass the licensing exams. Others assume the license will arrive by a specific date. These bad gambles can have serious adverse results if the gambles do not pay off. Other new graduates hurry to have their names placed in the phone book so that it will be there for the remainder of the year. This is another bad bet that can cause trouble for the graduate if someone complains to the board of dentistry that they are purporting to be a dentist before graduating or gaining licensure. These are also bad ways to start a dental career.

Many states require a dentist to register their license at the county courthouse where they will be practicing. This may seem like a silly contrivance to pad the wallet of the court clerk. Maybe it is. Nevertheless, if the state Dental Practice Act says that a dentist needs to register, they must register. It is the law, despite how silly someone might think a particular requirement is. They need to follow the law.

All states require either annual or biennial license renewal. If a practitioner fails to renew or pay the renewal fee, they will forfeit the license. If there is a date for renewal (e.g. December 15 of the previous year), then the practitioner needs to have the application in on time. Most states require that practitioners complete a certain number of hours of continuing education courses. Some states require specific types of certifications (e.g. cardiopulmonary resuscitation [CPR], HIV education, narcotics regulations) before renewal. The dentist needs to read the state laws carefully and follow them to the letter. A dentist's ability to practice is too important. If someone wants to make a statement about the intrusion of government into their life, they need to write a letter to the newspaper editor and not use their dental license renewal as a forum to speak.

Many people hold dental licenses from several states, although they practice only in one state. Many states may accept regional board examinations for dental licensure.

However, most states only accept those clinical exams for the first five years after completion. (Some states offer licensing by credentials or reciprocity. Others do not.) Consequently, many dentists will gain licensure in many states, using that as insurance in case they may want to move to that state in the future. The annual license renewal fees are cheap compared to the problem and expense of taking a new clinical exam at some time in the future. Besides, the cost of those licenses is a tax-deductible expense of doing business. This further decreases the out-of-pocket (after-tax) expense of maintaining those licenses. The practitioner should check with the states in which they hold licenses. Some states put time limits on how long they will license someone if that person does not practice in their state.

LOCAL OCCUPATIONAL LICENSES

Many municipalities have local occupational licenses. They are generally inexpensive but are another requirement for a practitioner to meet. These licenses are often used for ad valorem or property taxes, levied by the local municipality. Other areas may have local income taxes (occupational taxes) that they levy on people who work in their jurisdiction. They may use occupational licenses to track compliance with these taxes as well. The dentist needs to check with the local dental society, an established practitioner, or an accountant about these because they will know if the municipality has such a tax and where to sign up for it.

DRUG ENFORCEMENT ADMINISTRATION REGISTRATION

Before a dentist can dispense or write prescriptions for "scheduled" or narcotic drugs, they must register with the US Department of Justice Drug Enforcement Administration (DEA). Many people call this a "license" although, in fact, it is a registration. Dentists do not need to pass a test, they only provide information concerning their dental licenses and prescription writing needs, and then send a fee. The registration is currently for three years and must then be renewed. (Note that a dentist needs a valid dental license number before registering with the DEA, but they can request an application form before they gain licensure. This may save them several weeks in the initial practice start-up time.) Each registration number is for a particular office. If someone has more than one office location, they must have more than one DEA number (and pay more than one registration fee). The DEA has a website (http://www.deadiversion.usdoj.gov/drugreg) that allows practitioners to apply for registration.

When the Department of Justice issues a certificate, it contains a number that must appear on all narcotic prescriptions. Many practitioners have their DEA number printed on their prescription forms. (A practitioner also needs this number to phone in a prescription to the pharmacy for a scheduled drug for a patient.) Some states require the dentist to use prescription pads with special characters embedded in the paper that make them difficult (or impossible) to photocopy. This is an attempt to keep patients from misusing prescriptions for narcotic drugs. Again, the dentist should check with the local dental society or practitioners to find the laws for the area.

Most dentists occasionally prescribe narcotics, especially analgesics, in their practices. Therefore, they will need a narcotics registration. In most states, a dentist can still practice without this registration; they just cannot dispense or prescribe scheduled drugs. If a practitioner does not have this registration, they can still write prescriptions for non-scheduled drugs (such as antibiotics). All prescriptions must relate to dental treatment and must be for a patient of the practice. Many dentists have got into trouble with their dental board or other law enforcement agencies for improper prescriptions. This is usually for writing non-dental-related prescriptions or for writing prescriptions for people who are not patients (often self or family).

STAFF CERTIFICATION

Individual staff members in addition to the dentist may have license compliance issues. It is usually the practitioner's responsibility to ensure that they do not hire someone the state has not properly licensed or certified. This includes checking the hygienist's license, expanded function assistant's certification, or radiographic safety certification. The practitioner needs to keep current copies of these certifications. Some states require that they post the certificates in a public area of the office.

OCCUPATIONAL SAFETY AND HEALTH ADMINISTRATION AND THE DENTAL OFFICE

The OSHA is a federally mandated program that is intended to increase worker safety while on the job. Traditionally, unions were the source of worker safety rules. The federal government began to develop these rules as the workforce became less unionized. President Richard Nixon developed OSHA in 1973. Initially, it only covered high-risk workplaces, such as construction sites and heavy manufacturing. It has gradually increased its sphere of influence to cover almost every possible workplace in the United States. Many federal laws that govern business only control the larger corporations. OSHA pertains to all businesses that hire employees, even if they hire only one employee.

Many dentists want to rant and rail against OSHA as an unnecessary intrusion into their practices. However, these rules provide guidance on good workplace techniques and conditions. OSHA compliance is not a big problem if someone takes a positive attitude and sees that it is done. The ADA has material that is useful for complying with OSHA regulations in the office. One of the big issues is to be sure that the dentist has documented all the training and other compliance measures.

PURPOSE

OSHA's goal is to protect the worker. OSHA does not concern itself with the customer, client, or patient safety. (For example, OSHA would not cite a dentist if a patient does not wear safety glasses, but it could cite them if employees do not.) OSHA develops rules and regulations for each workplace environment. It often depends on other federal agencies to make recommendations concerning the rules and standards to follow. For example, OSHA follows the Centers for Disease Control and Prevention (CDC) guidelines concerning the transmission of bloodborne pathogens when developing OSHA guidelines for the workplace.

OSHA has an open definition of an employee. Anyone who receives pay is an employee. They may be fulltime, part-time, or probationary. Professional employees, such as dental associates, also fall under OSHA rules. An owner–dentist may or may not fall personally under these rules. If the dentist practices as a sole proprietor, or as a partner in a partnership, then they are technically an owner, not an employee. OSHA is not concerned with owners unless the owner is also an employee. This happens when the dentist practices as a corporation. Here, they are both an owner and an employee of the corporation. OSHA rules then pertain to them. However, most state dental boards will apply OSHA-type standards to any practitioner, regardless of their business form. The reason is that this is the standard of care all dentists need to follow.

REQUIREMENTS FOR DENTAL PRACTICES

OSHA presently has three standards that apply to the dental office work environment. They are the Bloodborne Pathogens Standard, concerned with the transmission of bloodborne infectious diseases; the Hazard Communication Standard, concerned with hazardous chemicals; and General Industry Standards, which are not specific to dental offices but relate to safety rules for all places of employment.

BLOODBORNE PATHOGENS STANDARD

The Bloodborne Pathogens Standard is intended to prevent employees from contracting infectious, bloodborne diseases while on the job. It is based on research conducted by the federal CDC in Atlanta. It is generally concerned with handling blood and other potentially infectious material (BOPIM). BOPIM consists of blood and blood-soaked materials, such as blood-soaked gauze. In dentistry, saliva often contains significant amounts of blood, so saliva (in dentistry) is potentially infectious. Finally, any unfixed tissues, such as biopsy specimens, extracted teeth, and gingival fragments, are potentially infectious.

The OSHA standard dictates that dental offices will:

- Develop a written exposure control plan.

- Carry out specific housekeeping, laundry, and labeling procedures.

- Provide hepatitis B virus vaccination and postexposure evaluation and follow-up.

- Develop a training program for employees and keep records of their participation.

- Provide adequate personal protective equipment (PPE) and ensure that employees use it.

WRITTEN EXPOSURE CONTROL PLAN

An exposure control plan assesses each employee's potential exposure to bloodborne pathogens. Then it lists specific things the business owner will do to prevent or decrease exposure to these pathogens for employees. The first step is deciding which employees will likely be exposed to these pathogens. In the dental office, dentists, hygienists, and assistants are all at risk (by the nature of their jobs) of exposure. The receptionist may not be at any risk (unless they also help by taking radiographs or assisting occasionally).

The next step is to decide the methods of compliance for employees. The practice owner should consider five general methods when developing this part of the plan.

- **Universal precautions** mean treating everyone as if they are infectious. In this way, the owner protects all employees from a patient or infectious staff member. This means that the office staff need to use PPE on all patients, use rubber dams, sterilize all equipment, and perform routine disinfection procedures.

- **Engineering controls** are equipment that forces compliance with safety practices. Safety-engineered equipment is much more effective than simply telling someone to act in a certain way. For example, a self-sheathing needle (engineered control) is more effective at preventing needlesticks than simply telling employees not to use a two-handed recapping technique.

- **Work practice controls** reduce the likelihood of exposure by changing the way tasks are done in the office. For example, practice owners can require that employees do not recap needles with two-handed techniques or that they restrict personal habits and eating in the work area. They must label all biohazards, sharps, and sharps containers and provide red bags for all potentially infectious material. The problem with work practice controls is that the practice owner must be diligent in checking to ensure that the employees always follow these controls.

- **Personal protective equipment** is the equipment the practice owner provides for employees' protection. PPE includes gloves, masks, eye protection, protective clothing, and resuscitation equipment. The employer must provide this equipment, repair or replace it, and ensure that employees use it appropriately. The owner must provide protective outer garments for employees and see that these garments are properly laundered.

- **Housekeeping** chores must be completed regularly. The practice owner must have a written schedule of decontamination for operatories, written decontamination procedures, procedures for containing regulated wastes, and procedures for handling contaminated laundry. (Laundry must be cleaned in house by employees or laundered off premises by a laundry company or other non-employees. The owner, if the practice is not incorporated, can take laundry home for cleaning.)

HEPATITIS B VACCINE

Practice owners must provide a series of hepatitis B virus vaccine injections for employees who are at risk of exposure to the disease. This is free (at the dentist's expense) to employees prone to exposure. It must be available within 10 days of beginning employment. If the employee refuses the vaccine, the practice owner needs to have them sign a form that acknowledges refusal, but they must then provide it free if the employee ever changes their mind.

The owner must have a plan if an employee is exposed to a bloodborne pathogen (e.g. through an inadvertent needlestick). This postexposure evaluation and follow-up plan include the following elements:

- Document the route of exposure.

- Inform and test the source individual, if voluntary consent of the source is obtained.

- Test the employee:
  - If negative, use it as a baseline for three-week, three-month, and six-month follow-ups.
  - If positive, end the series.

- The dentist must have a healthcare professional's written opinion on the results.

- This is free to the employee (i.e. the employer–dentist pays the cost) and is done under the supervision of a licensed physician.

- The practice owner must maintain confidentiality of all parties.

COMMUNICATION OF HAZARDS OF BLOODBORNE PATHOGENS

This part of the plan requires that practice owners provide training in this area for all employees. They must provide this training to all new employees and annually to all continuing employees. Furthermore, they must keep records of the training (initial and annual).

HAZARD COMMUNICATION STANDARD

The second OSHA requirement for dental practices is to protect employees from potentially hazardous materials in the workplace.

DEFINITION OF HAZARDOUS MATERIAL

Hazardous material is any substance used in the workplace that could injure an employee. It is generally a chemical that can cause rashes, burns, or other physical distress. Many common products, when used in the workplace, have the potential of becoming hazardous. Common chlorine bleach is found in virtually every house in the United States. When someone uses it in the dental office (or another workplace), it is a potentially hazardous material. The practice owner cannot assume that employees have the common sense to use these materials carefully and wisely.

STEPS TO COMPLIANCE

The four basic steps for an owner to be compliant with this standard are:

- Read and know the standard.

- Begin a written hazard communication program.

- Begin a training program.

- Maintain records.

HAZARD COMMUNICATION PROGRAM

The first step in a hazard communication program is to develop a list of hazardous chemicals used in the dental office. The list needs to specify where to find the material and how to prepare it for use. All hazardous materials now have Material Safety Data Sheets (MSDSs) provided for them. These sheets describe the product, what chemicals are in it, and what to do if it is accidentally ingested or improperly used. (The practice obtains these from the supplier.) The practice owner must maintain a file of these MSDSs that is open to all employees. Suppose an employee splashes a bonding agent into their eye. In that case, the dentist can quickly pull the MSDS on that agent to give the physician at the emergency department, so they have the information they need for treatment.

The practice owner must also have a hazardous chemical training program for all staff. This program must contain the following elements:

- Inform employees of the regulations.

- Train employees in the use of MSDSs.

- Label all hazardous chemicals according to specific labeling requirements.

- Locate all chemicals in the workplace.

- List where those chemicals are encountered.

- List physical and health problems associated with chemicals.

The practice owner must provide precautions to protect employees from chemicals or other hazardous materials. These precautions include work practices, engineering controls where appropriate, PPE, and emergency procedures.

RECORD-KEEPING

The record-keeping requirement for hazardous materials is like that for bloodborne pathogens. Practice owners must provide annual training and document that they gave the training. The specific elements of the record-keeping requirement are:

- Written description of the hazard communication program.

- List of hazardous chemicals.

- Location and use of MSDSs.

- Record of training sessions.

- Employee comments on training.

GENERAL INDUSTRY STANDARDS

General Industry Standards apply to all workplaces, not just dental offices. Many are common sense. But just because they are common sense does not mean that owner–dentists have thought about them or informed employees about them.

MEDICAL SERVICES AND FIRST AID

Practice owners must have a first-aid kit available for employees. They must also have staff trained in CPR and know how to handle medical emergencies.

MATERIALS HANDLING AND STORAGE

Most materials are handled in the hazardous materials section of the dentist's compliance plan. However, other, non-hazardous materials need to be processed and stored safely. For example, the dentist should ensure that employees know how to lift and store heavy boxes safely.

BUILDING AND EQUIPMENT

Many local fire and safety codes for buildings and equipment are incorporated into smart business practices. This is a partial list of these safety features in the office:

- The automatic sprinkler system (if the office has one) must be maintained.

- The office must be designed with sufficient exits in case of an emergency.

- Exits must be readily marked, even when it is dark or if electrical power is lost.

- Exits must not be locked from the inside during working hours.

- Compressed gas cylinders must be in a locked area and securely fastened.

- Dental offices must have an eyewash station.

- Dental offices must provide adequate sanitary waste receptacles.

- Dental offices must have a written fire safety plan.

- Portable fire extinguishers must be maintained annually.

- Employees must be trained in fire extinguisher use.

- Electrical cords must be of adequate length and in good repair. Dentists must be sure that they protect employees from ionizing radiation.

- Dental offices must have a fire evacuation plan.

- Dental offices must adequately ventilate or scavenge anesthetic gases (such as nitrous oxide).

INSPECTIONS

In the past, an OSHA inspection was one of the most feared occurrences in a dental office. OSHA seldom conducts inspections now. Instead, it tries to work with professional organizations to gain cooperation from practitioners. However, OSHA still has the right and responsibility to conduct separate office inspections. OSHA inspectors are usually busy with larger employers and accident inspections. They may react if a (usually former) employee claims that the office was badly out of compliance and a dangerous workplace. If a dental office is subject to an inquiry, it will probably be an "OSHA Letter of Inquiry." About 1 in 10 of these letters leads to in-office inspections. OSHA is seeking "probable cause." Its personnel realize that many complaints are unfounded or come from disgruntled (generally former) employees. Nevertheless, they are diligent in inquiring about complaints. If a practice receives such a letter, the dentist should explain why they comply. They should not simply "promise to do better" because that admits that they were not in compliance. The practitioner must not take a potential OSHA inspection lightly. Fines for non-compliance are substantial. As with most other office issues, prevention is the most cost-effective method.

OSHA inspectors can come unannounced to the dental office, although they seldom do. They may have (or the dentist can require) a warrant for entry to the premises and a subpoena for any records. They can inspect the premises and interview any employee(s). They will have a closing conference in which they inform the practice owner of any adverse findings. If the inspectors do have any negative findings, they will send the practice owner a written notice of citation and proposed penalty. This lists any violations, how and when to fix them, and any penalties. The owner must post this notice for employees to see. The dentist has 15 working days to contest the findings or penalties.

HIPAA IN THE DENTAL OFFICE

HIPAA affects the transmission of information among all healthcare providers. This includes not only dentists, but also physicians, hospitals, pharmacies, optometrists, insurance companies, and even corporate personnel departments. Anyone who has access to health information about an individual must take special precautions to ensure that they use the patient's health information appropriately. The ADA has material that is useful for complying with

HIPAA regulations in the office. As with OSHA, a big issue is documenting how the dental office has complied with the requirements.

HIPAA was enacted by then-President Bill Clinton and affirmed by President George W. Bush. These rules address most aspects of documentation related to healthcare. HIPAA mandates that practitioners do the following:

- Develop a privacy policy for the office.

- Give a copy of this policy to all patients.

- Obtain patient consent before releasing medical information or records.

- Allow patients to restrict the disclosure and use of their medical information.

- Reveal only the minimum amount of health information necessary for the procedure.

- Allow patients to make corrections to their health information.

- Develop a formal complaint mechanism for patients who believe practitioners have misused or disclosed patient information.

- Educate staff as to their responsibilities under this law.

- Ensure that those business entities the practitioner subcontracts with follow privacy policies.

- Periodically review policies to ensure that they are effective.

- Use a standard identifying provider number in all electronic transactions.

If a practitioner fails to comply with these regulations, there are stiff criminal and civil penalties (including monetary penalties and prison terms). These rules are national minimums. If the practice state has stronger privacy rules, the dental office must follow those stronger rules.

HIPAA RULES

HIPAA contains three separate sections, with rules that define each section.

- The **privacy rule** protects individuals from wrongful use of their protected health information (PHI).

- The **security rule** safeguards PHI through security measures in the office.

- The **Electronic Transactions and Code Set Standards rule** sets standard codes for an electronic transaction involving health information.

PRIVACY RULE

The privacy rule sets the standard for using someone's health information. It is based on the notion that information about a person and their health must be private and protected. There is huge potential for abuse of an individual's health information. For example, if a potential employer knows that someone has a medical condition, the employer might be less likely to hire that person. A health insurer might refuse to insure a person, raise rates, or claim preexisting condition clauses if the insurer knows of a condition. A person could be slandered in the community if a neighbor got to know about a particular medical condition. An insurer might deny someone life or disability insurance if it found out that they did not have a "clean" medical history. Drug companies or other medical suppliers could badger someone with solicitations about their product based on their medical history. All these abuses have occurred when people's private health information was released. Especially in the age of large computer databases, it becomes easier to share information electronically and compile information from various sources on individuals. This leads to potentially invasive and abusive acts. That is what the privacy rule intends to prevent.

PHI is any information about a person that someone can track to that individual. It includes their name and Social Security, telephone, and account numbers. An address and even zip code (along with other information) could identify an individual, so it must be protected. PHI includes any information about a person's medical condition, including disease diagnoses, treatment plans, regimens and options, tests or treatments done, and consultations with other health providers. This information can be in any form, including paper (written forms, notes, photocopies, or photographs), electronic (fax, internet transmission, computer disks, or back-up tapes), radiographic (film or electronic), or even oral communication (through the spoken word, telephone, or voicemail).

It is the practitioner's responsibility to ensure that they only give information about someone to the specific people or organizations to which the practitioner has told the person they will give it. Even then, the practitioner must only give that organization as much information as it needs to complete its job.

A dental practice may disclose PHI routinely for three primary office functions: treatment, payment, and operations (TPO):

- **Treatment** means conducting medical (or dental) procedures or tests related to the patient's medical condition. For example, suppose a dentist consults with the patient's physician regarding a medical condition that is part of the patient's treatment. In that case, the dentist may disclose it to the physician without specific consent.

- **Payment** involves information that the dentist provides to third-party payers related to a person's condition so that the third party may accurately determine benefits and make timely payments. When the dentist submits an insurance form, the form contains a large amount of PHI (both personal and medical). However, the insurance carrier needs this information to process the claim. Therefore, dentists can routinely disclose this information.

- **Operations** involve normal healthcare business operations. Examples here include quality assurance programs, regulatory compliance procedures, or other uses that are normal healthcare operational activities. If the dentist has a quality assurance office review by a third-party carrier, they may reveal information to the carrier (e.g. through chart audits) without specific consent.

Dentists may use PHI routinely for TPO without the patient's specific authorization. (The patient provides a general authorization in an acknowledgment of the dentist's privacy policies.) After the patient acknowledges the dentist's privacy procedures, the office does not have to ask for specific permission to submit insurance claims, consult with other practitioners, or respond to quality assurance reviews. The dentist may also use the information for other uses if they declare them in the "Notice of Privacy Practices" and the patient acknowledges that they know this. However, the dentist may not use or disclose a person's PHI for any other purpose without signed authorization from the patient.

Providers must make a good faith effort to give every patient a written notice (Notice of Privacy Practices) that explains the routine uses and disclosures of PHI. It must also explain the patient's rights and the dentist's responsibility in using and disclosing PHI. Dentists must give every patient (or their legal representative) a copy of the privacy notice as soon as feasible (usually at the beginning of the first visit). The patient must also sign an acknowledgment that they have received and understand the policies. This acknowledgment needs to be in the patient's chart with other records. If the patient refuses to sign, the dentist may still do their work (and use the information). However, they must document the patient's refusal and try to use the information in a way that is consistent with the patient's desires. If the dental office changes its policies, every patient must sign a new acknowledgment.

SECURITY RULE

The second HIPAA rule safeguards PHI by mandating specific procedures and personnel in the office. It requires the practice owner to name a security officer for the office who conducts employee training and sets standards for office conduct regarding health information.

Security measures include defining "reasonable safeguards" for the protection of PHI. These are rules that all employees (and providers) must follow while in the office. They are self-defined and left to the imagination of the particular entity (office). They may include using a lowered voice in public areas when discussing treatment or conditions with a patient. If a provider talks on the telephone about a patient (e.g. when receiving a medical consult), they should do it in private or not use the patient's name or other identifying information if other people in the office can overhear the conversation. The provider must shred any paper with any PHI on it (old forms, computer printouts, routing slips, etc.) rather than simply throwing it in the trash. Employees need to be sure that they turn their computer screens from the view of patients and not leave them accessible when they leave the room. Dentists must strictly maintain paper chart security by storing the charts in a secure area or by ensuring that only authorized people have access to them. (For example, it is inappropriate to leave charts on counters, where nosy patients may read them.) The staff should leave voicemail messages that do not reveal PHI unless the patient has allowed this through the privacy policy.

This rule also requires that the dental practice uses the "minimum necessary information" when disclosing someone's PHI. The minimum necessary information is only the information someone needs to complete the procedure assigned to them. Again, this is a self-defined limit. As an example, dentists do not need to inform a dental laboratory of a patient's medical history unless it somehow affects the work that the laboratory is doing. Conversely, a specialist's consultation may require complete medical information but no payment history information.

Practice owners must establish sanctions and disciplinary actions for employees who violate their privacy rules. Besides notification to law enforcement officials and regulatory bodies (such as the board of dentistry), the dental office needs to have a policy that violations may result in termination of employment or other sanctions appropriate to the breach. Practice owners should clearly state this in their employee handbooks and reinforce this at HIPAA training sessions.

If a dentist subcontracts with any people or organizations, they must ensure that those subcontractors follow the dentist's rules concerning patient privacy. It becomes the practice owner's responsibility (and problem) if a subcontractor abuses a patient's PHI. For example, a dentist hires a collection agency to collect their accounts. That agency now has a large store of PHI (personal and medical) on the patients of those accounts. If the collection agency sends those patients' names and information to a financial planner to help it manage its debt loads, it has violated the spirit and letter of the HIPAA laws. Common subcontractors include collection agencies, software vendors, lawyers, and consultants. Dental labs are providers and therefore exempt from this rule through the "treatment" option of the privacy rule.

Dentists may reveal PHI to a subcontractor without patient authorization if they obtain satisfactory assurances that the business associate will use the information according to their rules. This will be a written business associate agreement. The practice owner must have a separate business associate agreement with each of the entities that subcontract for them, although the contracts will be essentially the same.

ELECTRONIC TRANSACTIONS AND CODE SET RULE

The final HIPAA Rule is the Electronic Transaction and Code Set rule. This sets standard codes for electronic transactions, such as filing insurance forms. Most vendors use the ADA's CDT-5 code set for dental procedures. However, several third-party vendors (especially governmental organizations such as Medicaid) have unique code sets. This rule will standardize those organizations, requiring all insurance companies to use the ADA code set.

This rule has a negligible impact on dental offices. It affects software developers and vendors more, especially those that use proprietary code sets. The one big item in this standard for dentists is that they must obtain and use a National Provider Identification (NPI) number. This 10-digit number will identify the dentist in all HIPAA standard transactions. All dental plans must accept one standard number. There are two types of NPI, type 1 and type 2. Type 1 identifiers are for individual healthcare providers who act independently. Type 2 numbers are for organizations, such as a group practice or a corporation (including incorporated dental practices). If, for example, a dentist is in a group practice that bills procedures under the corporate name (e.g. "Anytown Smile Center"), they need to use the entity's NPI on the claim form as the billing dentist and enter the individual's NPI as the treating dentist. The standard claim forms have space for both numbers.

HIPAA REQUIRED FORMS

The HIPAA regulations require all offices to have many forms for use with patients. Practices will use several of them frequently. Others will be seldom used, but they must still be available if needed. Many practice owners have adopted the example forms from the ADA in its *HIPAA Compliance Manual*. This is an excellent reference and starting point for those developing their office HIPAA compliance program.

- **Privacy notice**

  Each practice must develop a notice that describes the office's policies regarding the privacy of patient information. The practice must give it once to each patient. If it changes the policies, they must reissue the notice to all patients. It must be given at the time of initial service, except in severe emergency cases. The practice owner must also post it in a clear and prominent location in the office.

- **Acknowledgment of receipt of notice**

  A separate form signed by the patient acknowledges that they have received a copy of the privacy form. Besides that, the dentist must document reasonable efforts if they cannot obtain the acknowledgment.

- **Patient authorization**

  This form differs from the acknowledgment that the patient has received the privacy notice. It authorizes the dentist to use the information for purposes other than those specified in the privacy notice. For example, assume that the dentist has interacted with a particularly effective diabetes support group. Suppose that the dentist wishes to send the name of a patient with diabetes to that group so it can send literature and solicitations. In that case, the dentist must receive specific authorization for that release.

- **Patient authorization to transfer records**

  If a patient transfers to (or from) a dentist's office, the patient will generally want their records transferred so that the new doctor knows their entire treatment history, radiographic findings, and other pertinent information. Before the transfer, the dental practice must gain written patient authorization. The office will not send (or expect to receive) the original record. Instead, the practice will send a copy of the record and radiographs. States vary in their allowance for reasonable charges for duplication of those records.

- **Patient complaint**

  If a patient has a complaint about a dentist's privacy practices or compliance, they must have a means of registering that complaint. The office's compliance officer must respond within 30 days.

- **Health information access: response/delay**

  A patient may request access to the information in their record. This form tells the patient whether the dentist grants that information or not. The dentist may deny an individual access, provided that the individual is given a right to have such a denial reviewed. Grounds for denial include that the access requested is reasonably likely to endanger the life or physical safety of the individual or another person. This does not extend to concerns about psychological or emotional harm (e.g. concerns that the individual will not be able to understand the information or may be upset by it).

- **Request for additional restrictions**

  Patients may request additional restrictions on the use or distribution of their PHI. This form allows them to request these restrictions. If they are reasonable, the dentist must abide by them. For example, a patient may request that a dental office leave no answering machine messages (or send postcards) because other household members may listen to or read them. The dental office must abide by the patient's wishes in these cases. This form is where the practitioner may allow the patient to designate with whom the practitioner may discuss treatment or billing needs or questions (e.g. spouse, parent, or child).

- **Request to amend protected health information**

  A patient may request to amend their health information. This form registers the request. The dentist may agree to change the information or not. For example, a patient was in an automobile accident and claims that her front tooth was broken. She wants to remove the information from the record showing that the tooth had previously decayed through and through because she believes she can get automobile insurance to pay for an anterior bridge. The dentist does not need to (and should not) allow this request to change information.

- **Staff review of policy and procedures**

  The practice owner must train all staff in the office on the privacy rules. This form registers verification that the staff have received the training and will follow the policies.

- **Business associate agreement**

  The business associate agreement specifies for subcontractors how the dentist uses PHI and their expectations of how the business associate will use the information.

MEDICAL WASTE DISPOSAL

Regulated medical wastes (RMW) are also called *biohazardous* or *infectious medical wastes*. These materials are exposed to blood or other bodily fluids, which can lead to a real risk of infecting someone else. In the dental office, this includes used needles, blood- or saliva-soaked gauze, discarded instruments, extracted teeth, or other materials used intraorally. In the office, the staff need to separate infectious waste from general waste, and sharps waste from infectious waste. Fortunately, most dental office waste is general waste (like household or general office waste) and requires no special handling.

RMW are defined and regulated at the state and local levels. These agencies may classify medical waste as infectious, used sharps, hazardous, radioactive, or other general waste. Because of the possible hazards to people collecting, transporting, or disposing of these wastes, the practice must dispose of such hazards properly. Depending on the regulating body, there may be specific rules or precautions for different types of medical waste. (For example, most states do not allow a used sharps container to be placed in the general trash.) Regulatory compliance is further complicated because different agencies may regulate different wastes within a state.

Practice owners should check with the state's dental association to find specific requirements and lists of acceptable vendors for medical waste disposal. Many states require disposal companies to be certified, licensed, or otherwise regulated. Vendors will provide appropriate containers and establish a schedule for hazardous material disposal. Practice owners should shop around for a vendor. Online and mail-order waste disposal companies may be appropriate for the practice situation. Practice owners also need to document how they dispose of medical wastes in case a problem ever develops.

RADIOGRAPHIC MACHINES

Many states inspect machines that produce ionizing radiation (often annually). Others inspect them when the machine is bought. This inspection ensures that the machine does not emit too much radiation. The practice owner should check with the state dental board to see if they need to have this inspection done. The inspecting agency generally charges a nominal fee for the inspection.

Part 3: Quality Assurance

The quality of a champagne is judged by the amount of noise the cork makes when it is popped.

Mencken and Nathan's Ninth Law of
the Average American

GOAL

This part presents the concepts of quality assessment and quality assurance, including the approaches currently being used in dental practices.

LEARNING OBJECTIVES

At the completion of this part, the student will be able to:

- Define the three dimensions of quality and cite examples of each in dentistry.

- Discuss the history of quality assurance activities in dentistry in the United States.

- Explain the difference between quality assessment and quality assurance.

- Define standards of care and discuss why they are important.

- Discuss commonly used standards for performing a facility review.

- Review a record using accepted standards of care.

KEY TERMS

ADA's Commission of
  Dental Accreditation
  (CODA)
board of dentistry
clinical licensing exams
facility review
malpractice
patient satisfaction
peer review

records review
quality assessment
quality assurance
quality of care
standard of care
structure
technical quality
total quality management
  (TQM)

The quality of healthcare services is a major social issue. Activities directed toward the assessment and assurance of the quality of dental care are receiving increased attention. Changes in reimbursement and payment plans, heightened competition, and a rise in consumer expectations have all contributed to the increased emphasis on the quality of patient care. Consumers, government, businesses, and insurance companies are scrutinizing the quality of dental care considering the billions of dollars that they spend annually for that care.

QUALITY ASSURANCE TERMINOLOGY

Quality is difficult for most people to define. When asked whether a given good or service is of high quality, people generally have an opinion, but might have difficulty in stating the rationale for providing that opinion. In other words, it may be difficult to answer the question "What makes Burger King higher quality than McDonald's?" It may be the way they cook the burgers. Or it might be the variety of menu items, the service, or the cleanliness of the restaurants. It might simply reflect a personal preference or taste, or other criteria might be used to judge.

Dentists often equate the quality of care with technical quality – for example, does a restoration have smooth margins, proper dental anatomy, and adequate occlusion? Quality of care encompasses a much larger domain than simply technical quality. It includes issues such as the appropriateness of care provided to patients, the ability of a patient to receive care when needed (access), and the timeliness of the care provided. To include all these aspects when defining quality, healthcare professionals refer to the three dimensions of quality: structure, process, and outcome.

- **Structure**
  Structure addresses the characteristics of the setting in which the dentist provides the care. This includes the

infection control and radiation safety procedures followed in an office, the training and certification of dental office staff, the adequacy of office hours, and office cleanliness. For example, if Dr. Smith operates a roach-infested dental practice, a person would question the quality of her office and, therefore, the care provided in that office based on a structural concern.

- **Process**
  Process describes the activities between the dentist and the patient. This dimension is the one most often thought of when discussing quality. It includes the actual technical quality of care plus issues such as the accuracy and documentation of oral examinations and medical histories, the status of the recall system to ensure continuity of care, and the frequency with which the dentist takes radiographs. For example, a practitioner who never takes radiographs for diagnostic purposes would not offer high-quality care.

- **Outcome**
  The outcome dimension reflects the effects of dental care on the health and welfare of the patient. This aspect of quality is new and is still evolving. In dentistry there are two components to the outcome dimension. The first is the effect of the care on a person's health and functioning: do they feel better, look better, or eat better because of the care received? This component is difficult to measure, and researchers are doing significant work to refine approaches to measuring it. The second component is patient satisfaction with the dental care received. This is based on the belief that patients can accurately evaluate the quality of care provided by their dentist. From the consumer's perspective, if a dentist has met the patient's needs as a consumer, then the care is of adequate quality.

Several terms are important in any discussion of the quality of care:

- **Standard of care**
  A standard of care is a precise statement outlining what constitutes an acceptable level of quality. (OSHA's definition of acceptable infection control practice is a standard.) There have been efforts to develop standards of care for other aspects of dental practice; however, presently no universally accepted standards govern quality in dentistry. The standard of care is discussed in more detail earlier in this chapter.

- **Quality assessment**
  This refers to measuring the quality of any good or service compared with a set of standards. An example of

quality assessment in dentistry is the comparison of infection control procedures in a dental office with OSHA standards. If it is common practice in an office to reuse saliva ejectors, an assessment of the office will show a deficiency.

- **Quality assurance**

  This relates to quality assessment, but includes an essential additional idea. Quality assurance activities go beyond measurement and include any necessary changes to bring the quality of care into compliance with standards governing that aspect of care. In the infection control example, any policies, procedures, or actions that bring the office practices in line with OSHA standards (e.g. using a new saliva ejector for each patient) represent a quality assurance activity.

- **Total quality management**

  Total quality management (TQM) is a system used in business that attempts to involve all producers of the goods or services in identifying and resolving quality assurance activities.

HISTORY OF QUALITY ASSESSMENT AND QUALITY ASSURANCE IN DENTISTRY

The dental profession has always been involved in evaluating and ensuring the quality of dental care rendered to the public. In the late 1700s, the profession encouraged states to develop a system for licensing dentists. By the 1860s, state dental boards became legally responsible for examining and licensing dentists. Today, clinical board examinations and licensure procedures show organized dentistry's commitment to quality dental care because they help confirm that a dental graduate is adequately prepared to provide that care.

During this time, US dental education underwent significant changes. It progressed from the apprentice system through proprietary schools to university-based programs. Accreditation activities were founded on the dental profession's commitment to quality; that is, ensuring that dental schools give students the knowledge, skills, and abilities needed to render high-quality care to the public. Today, all dental schools are subject to accreditation through the ADA's Commission of Dental Accreditation (CODA). This accreditation process requires schools to evaluate critically their curricula, facility, and educational practices. It culminates in a multiple-day site visit by CODA representatives. If a dental school loses its approval by CODA, its graduates will not be eligible for licensure in most states. This, then, is a virtual death penalty for the dental school.

Dental school accreditation and licensure are important components of a quality assurance program. However, simply graduating from an accredited school and getting a dental license do not guarantee that a dentist will continue to provide high-quality patient care. To ensure that practitioners remain current in knowledge and technique, many states require that dentists participate in continuing education courses as a prerequisite for relicensure. These states often require a certain number of hours per year of participation in scientific coursework by each dentist or hygienist. Although these courses expose practitioners to current materials, they offer no guarantee that participants will learn or use the material presented.

Each state has laws that govern the practice of dentistry in that state. Most have a board of dentistry or a similar oversight committee whose job is to protect the public from incompetent or unscrupulous practitioners. They have several methods to accomplish this end. They intend clinical licensing exams to assess the technical quality of an unknown practitioner, protecting the public from poor-quality dentists. (In fact, nearly all dentists eventually pass a licensing exam, so these are not particularly effective.) Boards may also revoke or suspend dental licenses for conduct that endangers the public. Examples of this conduct may be alcohol or drug abuse, continually faulty dentistry, or conviction for a crime that shows poor moral qualities, judgment errors, or character deficiencies. There is significant room for interpretation by the individual boards and state laws.

Another form of professionally developed quality assessment activities is peer review, a system that most dental societies operate. In these systems, a dispute between a patient and a dentist can go to a committee composed of dentists trained to evaluate the situation impartially. Disputes handled by peer review committees generally relate to the quality of treatment and the appropriateness of care. The peer review process reflects one basic tenet of a profession: the ability to "police its own" and thereby maintain high standards. It also has a couple of disadvantages that are worth mentioning. First, peer review is a reactive process initiated only after the allegations of poor-quality work exist. Thus, rather than raising the overall level of quality provided by the profession, the process aims at the few poor-quality providers. Secondly, most patients who perceive receiving less than optimal care change dental providers. They will not waste the time and effort of filing a complaint with the peer review board. Thus, peer review does not become involved in many situations where the care provided may warrant it.

Malpractice litigation is another form of quality assurance in the profession. A dentist who has several instances of successful malpractice litigation brought against them may have difficulty in finding malpractice insurance and may lose patients as the public becomes aware of their incompetence.

The most recent step in quality assessment and assurance activities stems from third-party involvement. Insurers primarily became involved with quality-of-care issues as they related to efforts to contain costs. They began to review the insured's claims to detect overutilization patterns, where particular patients or groups of patients consumed "too many" services. Traditional indemnity plans quickly became aware that "overtreatment" was common among their involved providers. Third-party plans began requiring dentists to obtain a preauthorization from the plan to ensure that the services the dentist has proposed are, in the opinion of the plan, necessary and warrant coverage. Because of this concern with controlling care costs, third-party plans began to address quality-of-care issues, such as the appropriateness of the care provided and patient overtreatment.

CURRENT FOCUS ON QUALITY ASSESSMENT AND ASSURANCE ACTIVITIES

Today's healthcare arena has an increasing focus on the quality of care provided. One needs only to scan the daily papers to find an article about healthcare reform, with quality-of-care issues being a central focus. Four trends in the healthcare system contribute to the public's concern with quality.

THIRD-PARTY PLANS

By virtue of the reimbursement structure, many managed care plans (e.g. capitation plans, preferred provider organizations, etc.) provide incentives for a dentist to undertreat patients. For example, suppose Dr. Smith receives less than the usual fee for a crown for a patient covered by the local capitation plan. In that case, she may reduce costs by using lower-quality materials, providing less than ideal treatment, or not treating the patient at all.

HEALTHCARE COSTS

The costs of healthcare have risen dramatically over the last several years. Though dentistry is only a small component of the healthcare system, the costs have followed those in the medical community on their upward spiral. As patients, insurers, and employers pay more for the care received, they increasingly demand that their purchases be of high quality.

CONSUMER INVOLVEMENT

Forty years ago, patients accepted the advice of healthcare practitioners with no questions asked. After all, the doctor knows best. Today, however, patients are taking a more active interest in their own health and in the care they receive. Most want an understanding of the problem, explanations of treatment, a discussion of the options available to them, and a perception that the care they receive will be of high quality, before ever consenting to care.

PROFESSIONAL LITIGATION

People sue others for anything (or for nothing) because we live in a litigious society. This results in malpractice suits costing the system millions of dollars. To avoid or decrease the costs of a liability suit, dentists and their liability insurers are focusing efforts on monitoring quality to reduce risk. Many insurers conduct courses for students and practicing dentists, which address the methods to monitor and document the care provided in their offices.

IMPLICATIONS FOR PRACTICING DENTISTS

The current focus on the quality of care has several implications for practicing dentists. First, if a dentist participates in a managed care plan, they will likely go through a quality assessment review of the office. To counter the allegations of undertreatment discussed previously, most managed care plans have written standards for their participating providers and conduct formal annual quality assessment reviews. The format of these reviews is discussed later in the chapter. Secondly, because of the increased focus on quality and consumers' concern with quality, even traditional indemnity plans are becoming more involved in quality assessment. That means that if a dentist participates with any third-party insurer, the chances are that the insurer will review the dentist's office at some point.

Dentists generally have one of two responses to these reviews: either they are highly insulted that anyone would question their professional capabilities and resent the intrusion of the reviewer into the practice, or they view the review as an opportunity to learn something about their practice, welcoming the reviewer's comments and opinions. A word of advice: the second response may be the one to strive for. Usually, if an insurance plan has reached the point of reviewing a dental office, that plan wants to have the dentist work with it. In other words, the plan wants the review to go well. The practice owner should remember that the reviewers are usually dentists who have reviewed hundreds if not thousands of offices and thus have a wealth of experience in what works and what does not. The practice owner might learn something from the reviewer and should be open to suggestions for change!

The benefits of quality-of-care reviews for practitioners relate to professional liability premiums and practice marketing. The quality of care provided in an office, and the documentation of that care, is of obvious concern to liability insurance carriers. Like reduced health or life insurance premiums for non-smokers, the day may come when liability insurance carriers will offer a decrease in the premium to practitioners who have participated in a quality assessment review and provide care according to professional standards. Participating in a quality assessment program and receiving the "seal of approval" from a recognized entity can also have implications for marketing a dental practice. Any patient who chooses a dentist would likely be drawn to a practitioner who has evidence from an independent reviewer that the care provided in the office meets high professional standards.

QUALITY ASSESSMENT REVIEWS IN DENTISTRY

Third-party (especially managed care) plans conduct most quality assessment reviews in dentistry. Large group practices and networks also conduct quality assessments on many aspects of their business, including the delivery of care. Most of the quality assessment programs operated by those plans are similar in design. Quality assessment reviews generally contain five components: facility reviews, records reviews, laboratory work reviews, patient examinations, and patient satisfaction surveys.

FACILITY REVIEW

A review of a physical practice facility addresses the structural aspects of quality (Box 28.4). It entails an on-site visit by the quality assessment reviewer. The reviewer will tour the office and ask a series of questions of the dentist or of the office staff. This portion of the review looks at several structural aspects of the practice to find out whether these comply with professional standards. The reviewer looks for specific facility issues. For example, third-party payers are usually interested in contracting with offices with enough operatories to efficiently see the plan's patients. They will,

---

BOX 28.4	FACILITY REVIEW ITEMS

- Office cleanliness
- Equipment In good working order
- Cleanliness
- Layout of the office
- Number of operatories
- Office staff
- Staff licensure and certification
- Personnel policies
- Access to care
- Office hours
- Emergency coverage
- Recall system
- Access to care
- Infection control
- Medical emergency preparedness
- Radiation safety

---

therefore, examine the number and condition of the operatories compared with patient volume. If the dentist delegates clinical work to auxiliaries, those staff members must be duly licensed or trained to carry out the work legally and safely. Written policy manuals, regular staff meetings, and such suggest to the reviewer that the dentist is attentive to personnel issues. Constant staff turnover hinders the continuity of care and decreases the satisfaction of patients and plan members. Are the dentist's office hours sufficient to handle the patient load, or is the waiting time for appointments prohibitive for patients? The practitioner should be accessible to patients during hours when the office is closed. If not, the dentist needs to arrange for someone to cover emergencies. Does the office have a recall system with a follow-up mechanism to ensure that patients do not get "lost"? Is there equal access to care for patients with different payment sources? This question is critical to alternative care plans to ensure that their plan members are not treated differently in their access. The reviewer may want to observe infection control procedures and question the staff about their knowledge of proper procedures. The reviewer may also check to be sure that the office follows standard emergency procedures, OSHA guidelines, worker safety, and radiation hygiene practices.

RECORDS REVIEW

The quality assessment reviewer will likely ask the dentist to select a sample of records to review or will select some themselves. The reviewer will examine records of people who have been patients for some time, so that there will be sufficient treatment recorded to warrant a review. They will conduct the review at the dentist's office. If the dentist is concerned about patient confidentiality, many plans will ask that they make copies of the record and mask any identifying names, numbers, and such before the review. The reviewer will be a dentist who will be looking for specific features in the records (Box 28.5). Usually, they want to be sure that the record is complete from a medical-legal standpoint. They check that the dentist's progress notes are thorough, recording in some detail what has occurred at each appointment. The reviewer verifies that the notes are in ink and signed by the practitioner. Technical quality is difficult to judge by simply examining patient records. However, when reviewing multiple records, some technical quality facets become readily apparent, for example if the same poor margins or calculus are visible on radiographs year after year, while the bone level decreases. Extensive crown and bridge procedures may be done on periodontally compromised teeth. Note that reviewers are looking for a pattern of work that may not meet professional standards, not for one or two patients where this may be the case.

BOX 28.5   RECORD REVIEW ITEMS

Performance and documentation of:

- Medical histories
- Complete oral exams
- Diagnoses
- Treatment plans
- Radiographs
- Quality
- Frequency
- Progress notes
- Technical quality of work

COMPUTER REVIEW

Many third-party payers conduct computer reviews of a dentist's billing procedures. They do these to find mistaken or fraudulent billing practices by practitioners. They know the service profile of typical general dental practices. They then compare the billing profile to the "average" dentist, looking for any area in which the dentist charges for more or fewer procedures than that average dentist. For example, assume that an insurance plan knows that its average general dentist does about 4% of their billing as endodontic procedures. The practitioner shows about 10% of their practice as endodontic procedures. The reviewer might question why the practitioner does so many more endodontic procedures than the average dentist. On investigation, the reviewer finds that the dentist charges for the procedure when they initiated it instead of when they completed it (when it should be charged) and that many of the patients did not return for the completion of their endodontic procedure. The reviewer would probably then ask the practitioner to return to the insurance company the amounts paid for the procedures they did not complete.

REVIEW OF LABORATORY WORK

This component of quality assessment reviews is less common, but some plans include it. Usually it is informal, because to date there have been no standards to guide reviewers. When this review is conducted, the reviewer examines cases for proper work orders, adequate mounting/articulation, and acceptable model preparation.

PATIENT EXAMINATIONS

A few plans will conduct clinical examinations of patients in a dentist's office to decide on the quality of care being provided (Box 28.6). Because of the intrusion into the practice and because of the logistics in scheduling, this component of a quality assessment review is seldom done in private practices.

PATIENT SATISFACTION SURVEYS

Patient satisfaction surveys are taking on increasing importance as a quality assessment mechanism. Recent research has shown that such surveys may even be the best predictor of quality of care. They do not measure the technical quality of a procedure directly. They do examine the behavioral application of that procedure. The patient's

BOX 28.6 PATIENT EXAMINATION REVIEW ITEMS

- Appropriateness of care
- Timeliness of care
- Cost
- Lack of pain
- Office cleanliness
- Helpfulness of staff
- Interpersonal interactions in the office

assessment of how the service was provided is the basis of their assessment of quality. If a procedure was not technically acceptable, the important issue is whether the practitioner responded appropriately to remedy the problem. In this sense, the patient's perception measures whether their healthcare needs were met. Therefore, most third-party plans will conduct surveys of their plan members to monitor satisfaction levels and help detect concerns with individual providers. Patient surveys are also the one quality control mechanism that the dentist can conduct independently of any third-party plan in their own office. If the dentist wants to maintain their patient base and serve them optimally, knowledge of patients' perceptions is important.

Index

Business Basics for Dentists, Second Edition. James L. Harrison, David O. Willis, and Charles K. Thieman.
© 2024 John Wiley & Sons, Inc. Published 2024 by John Wiley & Sons, Inc.